AF182169

Skin Neoplasms: Advanced Research

Skin Neoplasms: Advanced Research

Edited by Spencer Wells

hayle
medical

New York

Hayle Medical,
750 Third Avenue, 9th Floor,
New York, NY 10017, USA

Visit us on the World Wide Web at:
www.haylemedical.com

ISBN: 978-1-63241-578-3

The publisher's policy is to use permanent paper from mills that operate a sustainable forestry policy. Furthermore, the publisher ensures that the text paper and cover boards used have met acceptable environmental accreditation standards.

Printed in China.

Cataloging-in-Publication Data

Skin neoplasms : advanced research / edited by Spencer Wells.
p. cm.
Includes bibliographical references and index.
ISBN 978-1-63241-578-3
1. Skin--Tumors. 2. Skin--Cancer. 3. Skin--Diseases. 4. Dermatology--Treatment.
I. Wells, Spencer.
RC280.S5 S55 2019
616.994 77--dc23

Table of Contents

Preface IX

Chapter 1 **Topical Rapamycin as a Treatment for Fibrofolliculomas in Birt-Hogg-Dubè Syndrome: A Double-Blind Placebo-Controlled Randomized Split-Face Trial** 1
Lieke M. C. Gijezen, Marigje Vernooij, Herm Martens, Charlene E. U. Oduber, Charles J. M. Henquet, Theo M. Starink, Martin H. Prins, Fred H. Menko, Patty J. Nelemans and Maurice A. M. van Steensel

Chapter 2 **Congenic Mapping and Allele-Specific Alteration Analysis of *Stmm1* Locus Conferring Resistance to Early-Stage Chemically Induced Skin Papillomas** 9
Kazuhiro Okumura, Megumi Saito, Eriko Isogai, Ikuo Miura, Shigeharu Wakana, Ryo Kominami and Yuichi Wakabayashi

Chapter 3 **Resveratrol and Black Tea Polyphenol Combination Synergistically Suppress Mouse Skin Tumors Growth by Inhibition of Activated MAPKs and p53** 18
Jasmine George, Madhulika Singh, Amit Kumar Srivastava, Kulpreet Bhui, Preeti Roy, Pranav Kumar Chaturvedi and Yogeshwer Shukla

Chapter 4 **IL-17 Mediated Inflammation Promotes Tumor Growth and Progression in the Skin** 30
Donggou He, Hui Li, Nabiha Yusuf, Craig A. Elmets, Mohammad Athar, Santosh K. Katiyar and Hui Xu

Chapter 5 **JWA Deficiency Suppresses Dimethylbenz[a]Anthracene-Phorbol Ester Induced Skin Papillomas via Inactivation of MAPK Pathway in Mice** 39
Zhenghua Gong, Yaowei Shi, Ze Zhu, Xuan Li, Yang Ye, Jianbing Zhang, Aiping Li, Gang Li and Jianwei Zhou

Chapter 6 **Up-Regulated Dicer Expression in Patients with Cutaneous Melanoma** 49
Zhihai Ma, Helen Swede, David Cassarino, Elizabeth Fleming, Andrew Fire and Soheil S. Dadras

Chapter 7 **Ethnicity and Cutaneous Melanoma in the City of Sao Paulo, Brazil** 61
Olinda C. Luiz, Reinaldo Josè Gianini, Fernanda T. Gonçalves, Guilherme Francisco, Cyro Festa-Neto, Josè Antonio Sanches, Gilka J. F. Gattas, Roger Chammas and Josè Eluf-Neto

Chapter 8 **Time Course and Pattern of Metastasis of Cutaneous Melanoma Differ between Men and Women** 68
Liljana Mervic

Chapter 9 **Loss of *Hairless* Confers Susceptibility to UVB-Induced Tumorigenesis via Disruption of NF-kappaB Signaling** 78
Hyunmi Kim, Alexandre Casta, Xiuwei Tang, Courtney T. Luke, Arianna L. Kim, David R. Bickers, Mohammad Athar and Angela M. Christiano

Chapter 10 **Primary Cilium Depletion Typifies Cutaneous Melanoma in Situ and Malignant Melanoma** ... 89
Jinah Kim, Salma Dabiri and E. Scott Seeley

Chapter 11 **Tumour Microenvironments Induce Expression of Urokinase Plasminogen Activator Receptor (uPAR) and Concomitant Activation of Gelatinolytic Enzymes** ... 96
Synnøve Magnussen, Elin Hadler-Olsen, Nadezhda Latysheva, Emma Pirila, Sonja E. Steigen, Robert Hanes, Tuula Salo, Jan-Olof Winberg, Lars Uhlin-Hansen and Gunbjørg Svineng

Chapter 12 **Distinct Innate Immune Gene Expression Profiles in Non-Melanoma Skin Cancer of Immunocompetent and Immunosuppressed Patients** ... 112
Beda Muehleisen, Shang Brian Jiang, Julie A. Gladsjo, Monika Gerber, Tissa Hata and Richard L. Gallo

Chapter 13 **Prognosis of Sentinel Node Staged Patients with Primary Cutaneous Melanoma** ... 124
Otmar Elsaeßer, Ulrike Leiter, Petra G. Buettner, Thomas K. Eigentler, Friedegund Meier, Benjamin Weide, Gisela Metzler, Helmut Breuninger and Claus Garbe

Chapter 14 **Dysregulated ΔNp63α Inhibits Expression of Ink4a/arf, Blocks Senescence and Promotes Malignant Conversion of Keratinocytes** ... 132
Linan Ha, Roshini M. Ponnamperuma, Steven Jay, M. Stacey Ricci and Wendy C. Weinberg

Chapter 15 **Miz1 is a Critical Repressor of *cdkn1a* during Skin Tumorigenesis** ... 145
Jan Hönnemann, Adrián Sanz-Moreno, Elmar Wolf, Martin Eilers and Hans-Peter Elsässer

Chapter 16 **Increased IKKα Expression in the Basal Layer of the Epidermis of Transgenic Mice Enhances the Malignant Potential of Skin Tumors** ... 156
Josefa P. Alameda, Rodolfo Moreno-Maldonado, M. Jesús Fernández-Aceñero, Manuel Navarro, Angustias Page, JosèL. Jorcano, Ana Bravo, Ángel Ramírez and M. Llanos Casanova

Chapter 17 **Occludin Is Involved in Adhesion, Apoptosis, Differentiation and Ca^{2+}-Homeostasis of Human Keratinocytes: Implications for Tumorigenesis** ... 167
Susanne Rachow, Michaela Zorn-Kruppa, Ulrich Ohnemus, Nina Kirschner, Sabine Vidal-y-Sy, Peter von den Driesch, Christian Börnchen, Jürgen Eberle, Michael Mildner, Eik Vettorazzi, Rita Rosenthal, Ingrid Moll and Johanna M. Brandner

Chapter 18 **Loss of Grainy Head-Like 1 is Associated with Disruption of the Epidermal Barrier and Squamous Cell Carcinoma of the Skin** ... 180
Michal Mlacki, Charbel Darido, Stephen M. Jane and Tomasz Wilanowski

Chapter 19 **Multiphoton Multispectral Fluorescence Lifetime Tomography for the Evaluation of Basal Cell Carcinomas** ... 189
Rakesh Patalay, Clifford Talbot, Yuriy Alexandrov, Martin O. Lenz, Sunil Kumar, Sean Warren, Ian Munro, Mark A. A. Neil, Karsten König, Paul M. W. French, Anthony Chu, Gordon W. H. Stamp and Chris Dunsby

Chapter 20 **Depletion of Cutaneous Macrophages and Dendritic Cells Promotes Growth of Basal Cell Carcinoma in Mice** **198**
Simone König, Frauke Nitzki, Anja Uhmann, Kai Dittmann, Jennifer Theiss-Suennemann, Markus Herrmann, Holger M. Reichardt, Reto Schwendener, Tobias Pukrop, Walter Schulz- Schaeffer and Heidi Hahn

Chapter 21 **Altered Prostanoid Signaling Contributes to Increased Skin Tumorigenesis in Tpl2 Knockout Mice** **206**
Kathleen L. DeCicco-Skinner, Sabrina J. Nolan, Monika M. Deshpande, Erika L. Trovato, Taylor A. Dempsey and Jonathan S. Wiest

Permissions

List of Contributors

Index

Preface

A skin neoplasm is an unusual growth of tissue on the skin. It can be cancerous, noncancerous or precancerous. A benign neoplasm does not spread to nearby tissues or other parts of the body and stays localized. However, it can still cause damage to organs and tissues around it. Some of the common forms of benign skin neoplasms are lipoma, cherry angioma, epidermoid cyst, etc. A malignant neoplasm is cancerous and grows uncontrollably and invades other organs. It travels through the body producing new tumors. Some of its types are squamous cell carcinoma, melanoma, basal cell carcinoma, lymphoma of the skin, etc. Some neoplasms are termed as precancerous because they can potentially turn into a cancer if untreated. Some types are actinic keratosis and Bowen's disease. This book is a compilation of chapters that discuss the most vital concepts and emerging trends in the diagnosis and treatment of skin neoplasms. The various advancements in this domain are glanced at and their implications as well as ramifications are looked at in detail. For someone with an interest and eye for detail, this book covers the most significant topics in dermatology and oncology.

The information shared in this book is based on empirical researches made by veterans in this field of study. The elaborative information provided in this book will help the readers further their scope of knowledge leading to advancements in this field.

Finally, I would like to thank my fellow researchers who gave constructive feedback and my family members who supported me at every step of my research.

Editor

1

Topical Rapamycin as a Treatment for Fibrofolliculomas in Birt-Hogg-Dubé Syndrome: A Double-Blind Placebo-Controlled Randomized Split-Face Trial

Lieke M. C. Gijezen[1,9], Marigje Vernooij[1,9], Herm Martens[1], Charlene E. U. Oduber[1], Charles J. M. Henquet[1], Theo M. Starink[2], Martin H. Prins[3], Fred H. Menko[4], Patty J. Nelemans[3], Maurice A. M. van Steensel[1,5,6*]

1 Department of Dermatology, GROW School for Oncology and Developmental Biology, Maastricht University Medical Centre+, Maastricht, The Netherlands, **2** Department of Dermatology, VU University Medical Centre, Amsterdam, The Netherlands, **3** Department of Epidemiology, CAPHRI Research School for Public Health Primary Care, Maastricht University Medical Centre+, Maastricht, The Netherlands, **4** Department of Clinical Genetics, VU University Medical Centre, Amsterdam, The Netherlands, **5** Department of Clinical Genetics, GROW School for Oncology and Developmental Biology, Maastricht University Medical Centre+, Maastricht, The Netherlands, **6** Institute of Medical Biology, Singapore, Singapore

Abstract

Background: Birt-Hogg-Dubé syndrome (BHD) is a rare autosomal dominant disorder characterised by the occurrence of benign, mostly facial, skin tumours called fibrofolliculomas, multiple lung cysts, spontaneous pneumothorax and an increased renal cancer risk. Current treatments for fibrofolliculomas have high rates of recurrence and carry a risk of complications. It would be desirable to have a treatment that could prevent fibrofolliculomas from growing. Animal models of BHD have previously shown deregulation of mammalian target of rapamycin (mTOR). Topical use of the mTOR inhibitor rapamycin is an effective treatment for the skin tumours (angiofibromas) in tuberous sclerosis complex, which is also characterised by mTOR deregulation. In this study we aimed to determine if topical rapamycin is also an effective treatment for fibrofolliculomas in BHD.

Methods: We performed a double blinded, randomised, facial left-right controlled trial of topical rapamycin 0.1% versus placebo in 19 BHD patients. Trial duration was 6 months. The primary outcome was cosmetic improvement as measured by doctors and patients. Changes in fibrofolliculoma number and size were also measured, as was occurrence of side effects.

Results: No change in cosmetic status of fibrofolliculomas was reported in the majority of cases for the rapamycin treated (79% by doctors, 53% by patients) as well as the placebo treated facial sides (both 74%). No significant differences between rapamycin and placebo treated facial halves were observed ($p = 1.000$ for doctors opinion, $p = 0.344$ for patients opinion). No significant difference in fibrofolliculoma number or change in size of the fibrofolliculomas was seen after 6 months. Side effects occurred more often after rapamycin treatment (68% of patients) than after placebo (58% of patients; $p = 0.625$). A burning sensation, erythema, itching and dryness were most frequently reported.

Conclusions: This study provides no evidence that treatment of fibrofolliculomas with topical rapamycin in BHD results in cosmetic improvement.

Trial Registration: ClinicalTrials.gov NCT00928798

Editor: Maria Fiammetta Romano, Federico II University, Naples, Italy

Funding: This study was financed by the Myrovlytis Trust (UK Charity Commission number 1122073, http://www.myrovlytistrust.org/). MAMvS and MV are additionally supported by the Dutch Cancer Society, grant UM2009-4352 (http://www.kwfkankerbestrijding.nl). The funders had no role in study design, data collection and analysis, decision to publish, or preparation of the manuscript.

Competing Interests: The authors have declared that no competing interests exist.

* E-mail: maurice.vansteensel@imb.a-star.sg.edu

9 These authors contributed equally to this work.

Introduction

Birt-Hogg-Dubé syndrome (BHD, MIM #135150) was first described in 1975 by Hornstein and Knickenberg and again in 1977 by Birt, Hogg and Dubé [1,2]. It is a rare autosomal dominant disorder characterized by the occurrence of benign, mostly facial, hair follicle tumours called fibrofolliculomas (FF)s [2], multiple lung cysts, spontaneous pneumothorax [3], and an increased renal cancer risk [4–6]. The FFs can be quite disfiguring and are often the reason why patients come to medical attention. FFs occur in around 80% of patients and usually appear after the age of 20 years as dome-shaped, whitish or skin-coloured papules. Typically presenting around the nose, they can also occur on the ears, neck and trunk [2]. Although they do not grow beyond 3–4 mm in size, their numbers increase with age. Consequently, patients can eventually have hundreds of papules that may cause emotional distress and have a strong impact on their quality of life.

Current treatment options for FFs include destructive approaches such as ablative laser, electrocoagulation, excision and other invasive interventions [7–10]. These treatments have high recurrence rates (for laser therapy it is known that FFs recur after 2–3 years or even after months [9]) and are not effective in preventing early lesions. Moreover, they have a significant risk of complications such as scarring, inflammation, hypo- and hyperpigmentation. Therefore, there is a medical need for a more targeted therapy that is suitable for chronic use, reduces the number of tumours and/or prevents the growth of new ones. Insights from genetic and cell biological studies have suggested such an approach.

BHD syndrome is caused by germline mutations in the *FLCN* gene on chromosome 17p11.2 coding for the protein folliculin (FLCN) [11,12]. FLCN's functions are mostly unknown, although recent data suggest that it might be involved in cellular energy sensing through the mammalian target of rapamycin (mTOR) signalling pathway [13]. A considerable body of data suggests that in BHD, the mTOR pathway is activated [14–18]. Thus, we theorized that BHD syndrome belongs to a larger family of disorders characterized by mTOR deregulation, such as tuberous sclerosis complex (TSC) [14,19]. In yeast, the homologue of *FLCN* is found to have opposing roles to the genes involved in TSC (*TSC1* and *TSC2*), but all are suggested to regulate common downstream targets [20]. In TSC, as in BHD, patients develop facial hair follicle tumours, called angiofibromas. These tumours strongly resemble FFs and have also been reported in BHD syndrome (Figure 1) [21,22]. Angiofibromas in TSC were coincidentally found to respond favourably to the mTOR inhibitor rapamycin. They disappeared after only a few months of oral rapamycin, which was administered after renal transplantation [23]. Oral administration of rapamycin has potential side effects that are not acceptable in the context of BHD. However, there are several studies showing that topical application is safe [24–26]. Additionally, multiple reports show successful treatment of angiofibromas in TSC with topical rapamycin [24,26–30]. Thus, we hypothesized that rapamycin oral solution might be used for the topical treatment of FFs.

We here show the results of the first double-blind placebo-controlled randomized split-face trial of topical rapamycin for the treatment of FFs in BHD. The objective of this study was to determine whether topical application of rapamycin 1 mg/ml oral solution could lead to overall cosmetic improvement and reduction in size and number of facial FFs in BHD patients. Secondly, we evaluated safety and formula acceptance.

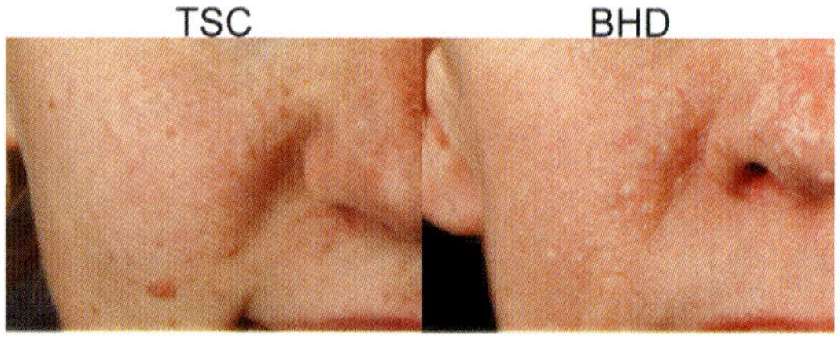

Figure 1. Skin features in TSC and BHD. Photographs taken from a TSC and a BHD patient show angiofibromas and fibrofolliculomas, respectively. Notice the resemblance between the two types of lesion.

Materials and Methods

The protocol for this trial and supporting CONSORT checklist are available as supporting information (Protocol S1 & Checklist S1). Before patient recruitment started the study was deposited at ClinicalTrials.gov (NCT00928798; http://www.clinicaltrials.gov/ct2/show/NCT00928798?term = rapamycin+BHD&rank = 1).

Ethics Statement

This study was approved by the Medical Ethical Committees of the Maastricht University Medical Centre+ and the VU Medical Centre Amsterdam, Licence number NL28245.068.09 and was conducted in accordance with the Helsinki Declaration of 1975. The individuals shown in this manuscript have given written informed consent (as outlined in PLOS consent form) to publish their pictures.

Patients

Patient recruitment, inclusion and follow-up occurred at the Department of Dermatology in the Maastricht University Medical Centre+ and at the Department of Clinical Genetics in the VU Medical Centre Amsterdam, both reference centres for patients with BHD. Patients with genetically proven BHD, a minimum age of 18 years, at least 10 facial FFs (of which at least one histologically confirmed) and a general good health were eligible for inclusion. Pregnant or lactating women, patients with proven or suspected skin or other malignancy in the past 5 years and patients who planned facial surgery in the treatment period were excluded. Because of the increased risk of renal cell carcinoma in BHD patients, screening by an abdominal ultrasound or MRI was scheduled for patients who had their last screening more than 1 year ago. Patients with concomitant disease requiring systemic immunosuppressive treatment and patients using any facial topical immunosuppressive treatment or facial topical drugs interfering with rapamycin during the trial period or within 30 days before starting therapy were excluded, as were patients with facial skin lesions other than FFs that might worsen under rapamycin, such as active infections. Next to these protocolled criteria, patients were excluded when they could not attend any of the follow-up visits, because this made monitoring of (side) effects and adverse events impossible. A biopsy of a facial FF was taken if this had not been performed earlier. Written informed consent was obtained from all patients eligible for participation.

Treatment procedures

Computer generated randomisation was performed using random permuted blocks of 2. Randomisation was stratified by participating centres. For each participant, topical treatment with a commercially available rapamycin (sirolimus) oral solution 1 mg/ml was randomized to one facial half and application of a placebo solution to the other facial half. Patients were instructed to topically apply the two formulations twice daily, for 6 months. The rapamycin solution was decanted at 2–8°C in a nitrogen atmosphere and packaged in amber glass bottles to preserve solution quality. The solvent was used as a placebo and was packaged in identical bottles. Bottles were numbered and marked 'left' or 'right' by the pharmacist, in order to conceal randomisation. Patients and investigator were both blinded for the treatment of each facial side throughout the study.

Efficacy assessment

Patients were clinically assessed at baseline, 3 months and 6 months by a single investigator (LMCG). Evaluation consisted of careful examination of the face, including assessment of facial FF number and size, as well as the change in general cosmetic FF status compared to baseline. At each visit, facial medical photographs were obtained under standardized conditions concerning: studio lighting, subject positions, predetermined camera settings (distance to subject, resolution, aperture settings, exposure time) and background. For each patient full front, left and right oblique views (45°) and left and right profile views (90°) were obtained. Photographs were evaluated twice by 3 physicians; the investigator and 2 dermatologists. All were blinded for the treatment. They assessed the size of the largest FF in a predefined area. Right and left facial halves were scored separately and 3-month and 6-month photographs were compared to baseline. The change in general cosmetic FF status was evaluated using a 7-point Likert scale (−3 = strong worsening; −2 = moderate worsening; −1 = minimal worsening; 0 = no change; 1 = minimal improvement; 2 = moderate improvement; 3 = strong improvement) [31,32]. The FF number was registered in categories, (0; 1–10;11–20;21–30; 31–40; 41–50; >50). Each of the three observers scored the photographs twice for cosmetic status, FF size and FF number. From the six Likert scores or categories obtained per patient the most frequently assigned score was used for analysis. When multiple scores were obtained in equal amounts, the score indicating the least improvement was used. The change in FF number was obtained by comparing the 6-month results to baseline results. Reduction of FF number was defined as a decrease of at least one category. Patients' impressions concerning cosmetic FF status were assessed as well, also using the 7-point Likert scale. At follow-up visits we assessed and registered side effects.

Statistical analysis

A minimum of 17 patients was needed to detect an increase in preference for rapamycin over placebo by at least 35% (from 50% to 85%), with a power of 90% and a type 1 error (2 sided) of 0.05. A minimum of 35% difference in response was considered to be clinically relevant, as a smaller difference does not justify the routine treatment of BHD patients with rapamycin. The McNemar's chi-square test was used to test for discrepancies in response to rapamycin and placebo treatment concerning cosmetic improvement and reduction in FF number. This test was also used to compare the proportion of side effects occurring between the two facial sides. Differences in FF size were tested for significance using the T-test for paired samples. A p-value smaller than 0.05 was considered to indicate statistical significance in all analyses. The inter-observer variation of scores on cosmetic status, FF size and number was measured using the intraclass correlation coefficient. For data analysis we used SPSS Statistics version 20.0.0.1 (IBM, Armonk, NY, USA) and for calculation of 95% confidence intervals (95%CI) for difference in paired proportions we used R package ExactCIdiff version 2.15.1 (http://cran.r-project.org/web/packages/ExactCIdiff/index.html).

Results

Study population

Between January 2010 and August 2010, 24 patients with BHD were recruited and assessed for eligibility to participate (Figure 2). One patient was excluded due to excessive use of alcohol and three because of frequent travelling abroad, which made follow-up impossible. After screening, but before randomisation, one person had to be excluded due to the diagnosis of a malignancy not related to BHD. A total of 19 individuals were randomised. The distribution of baseline characteristics of the study population is shown in table 1. One individual was not able to attend the 3-month follow-up visit due to immobility after back surgery, but could be evaluated at six months. This person was excluded from the data analysis of the 3-month results (n = 18). After two months of treatment, one patient had to discontinue the treatment because of a tearing eye. This patient was seen at the 3-month follow-up visit, but was considered lost to follow-up at six months. A second patient was lost to follow-up at six months due to travelling. For both, the 3-month data were carried forward in the 6-month efficacy analysis (n = 19). An additional analysis of the 6-month results was performed in which all persons that were lost to follow-up at six months were excluded from the analysis (n = 17).

Effects of rapamycin treatment

The effect of rapamycin was assessed by measuring changes in cosmetic status, number and size of the FFs.

Cosmetic improvement of the FFs as judged by doctors and patients is presented in figures 3 and 4. There were no significant

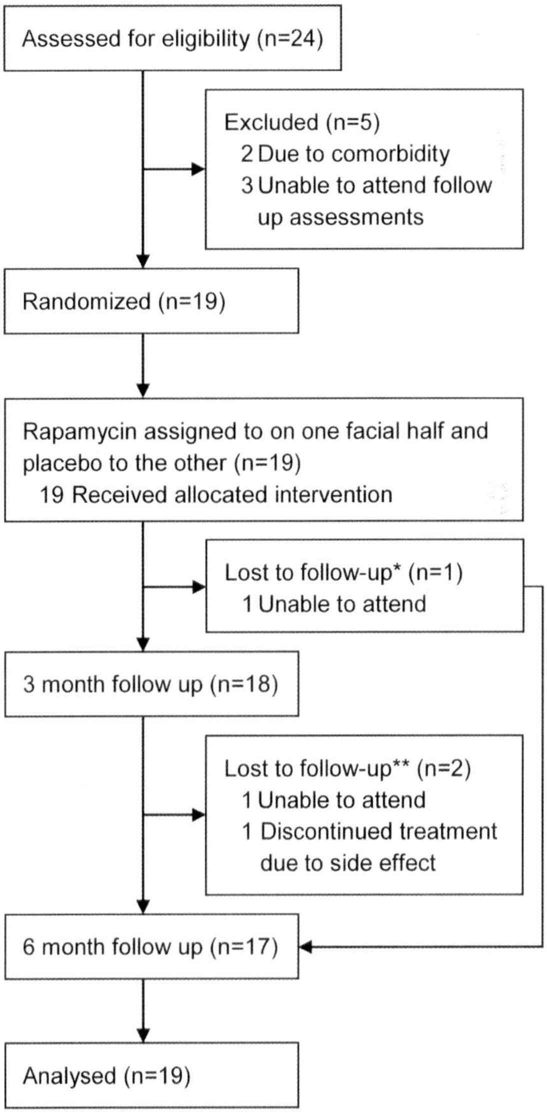

Figure 2. Trial outline. * The patient who was lost to follow-up at 3 months was excluded from the analysis of the 3 month results. ** For the patients who were lost to follow-up at 6 months, the 3-month data were carried forward in the analysis of the 6-month results.

Table 1. Baseline characteristics of included patients.

Characteristic		Number of patients (n = 19)
Gender	Male	13
	Female	6
Mean age, years (range)		52 (34–70)
Number of facial fibrofolliculomas	20–50	4
	50–100	4
	>100	11
FLCN mutation	c.319_320delGTinsCAC	1
	c.610_611delGCinsTA	9
	c.655dupC	1
	c.1177-2A>G	1
	c.1285dupC	3
	c.1408_1418del	1
	c.871+3_c.871+4delGAinsTCCAGAT	1
	c.880G>T	1
	c.250-?_1740+?del	1
Previous treatment	None	15
	Laser	4
	Surgical	1

differences between rapamycin and placebo treated facial sides. According to doctors' opinion, improvement of cosmetic status was seen in 10.5% of rapamycin treated facial halves and in 10.5% of the placebo treated sides. The difference is 0% with a 95%CI of -19% to +19%; p = 1.000 (Appendix S1). Patients reported cosmetic improvement upon rapamycin treatment more often than upon placebo treatment (47.3% versus 26.3%). The difference is 21% with a 95%CI of −14% to +51%; p = 0.344 (Appendix S1).

Both doctors and patients reported no changes in the majority of cases for the rapamycin treated (79% and 53% respectively) as well as the placebo treated facial sides (both 74%). The doctors reported minimal worsening in 16% of the placebo treated versus 11% of the rapamycin treated facial halves, whereas minimal

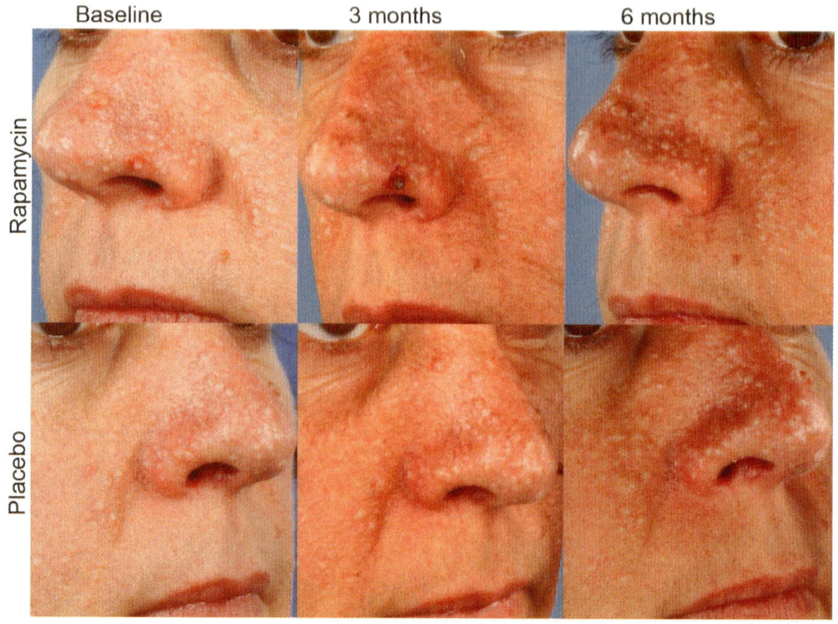

Figure 3. Photographic recording of cosmetic status during rapamycin treatment. Close up of standardised facial photographs taken at baseline, 3 months and 6 months after starting treatment with topical rapamycin or placebo per facial half. Photos of a representative patient are shown, revealing no visible improvement or worsening of the facial fibrofolliculomas.

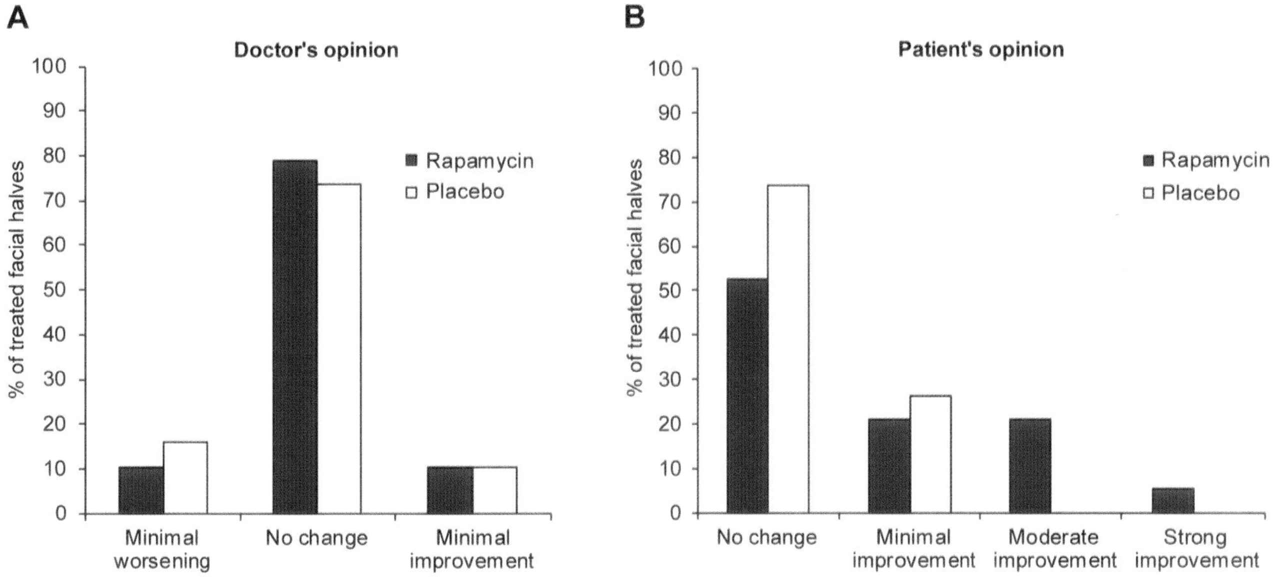

Figure 4. Changes in cosmetic status of fibrofolliculomas after treatment with rapamycin scored by doctors and patients. BHD patients with facial fibrofolliculomas were treated with topical rapamycin and placebo for six months. The degree of improvement compared to baseline was scored on a 7-point Likert scale by both doctors (A) and patients (B). Doctors and patients reported no change in the majority of cases. Patients reported improvement more frequently for the rapamycin compared to the placebo treated facial side.

improvement was observed in 11% of both rapamycin and placebo treated facial sides (Figure 4). Patients reported improvement more frequently for the rapamycin treated compared to the placebo treated facial side. Nine patients (47%) reported minimal to strong improvement of the rapamycin treated facial half, versus five (26%) reporting improvement of the placebo treated half (Figure 4). Additional analysis of the 17 patients that were seen at the 6-month follow-up showed similar results for the doctors' opinion on cosmetic improvement of FFs after treatment. Reduction in FF number was observed in 32% of rapamycin treated sides versus 37% of placebo treated sides, with a difference of 5% with a 95%CI of −20% to +31%; p = 1.000 (Figure 5 and Appendix S1)

After three months of treatment the mean change in FF size was 0.054 mm on the rapamycin treated sides and 0.027 mm on the placebo treated sides, with a mean difference of 0.027 mm with a 95%CI of −210 to +0.264 mm; p = 0.184 (Table 2).

The inter-observer variations, expressed as intraclass correlation coefficients (ICC) for cosmetic status, FF number and FF size are shown in Table 3.

Side effects of topical rapamycin

The majority of patients reported one or more side effects during the six months of treatment for rapamycin (68%) as well as for placebo (58%) (difference 10% with 95%CI −14.3 to 35.0; p = 0.625). A burning sensation, erythema, dryness and itching were most frequently reported (Figure 6). Other side effects were tearing and prickling eyes, scaling, moderate pain and a prickling sensation of the skin. Most side effects occurred in the first three weeks of treatment and resolved over time, with 71% reported at the 3-month follow-up visit and only 42% at the 6-month visit. No serious adverse events have occurred during treatment.

Discussion

This is the first randomised controlled trial in which the effectiveness of rapamycin on persistence and growth of FFs in patients with BHD was studied. We provide evidence that topical rapamycin does not improve the cosmetic status of FFs in these patients and does not reduce the amount or size of the FFs.

Previous studies in rodent and *Drosophila* models have suggested a role for increased mTOR activity in the pathogenesis of BHD, prompting this study [15–17,33]. However, other mouse models subsequently showed conflicting data concerning the nature of the link between FLCN and mTOR. In contrast to other studies, Hudon et al. and Hartman et al. found decreased mTOR activity in mice [15–17,34,35]. In human BHD tumours, the role of

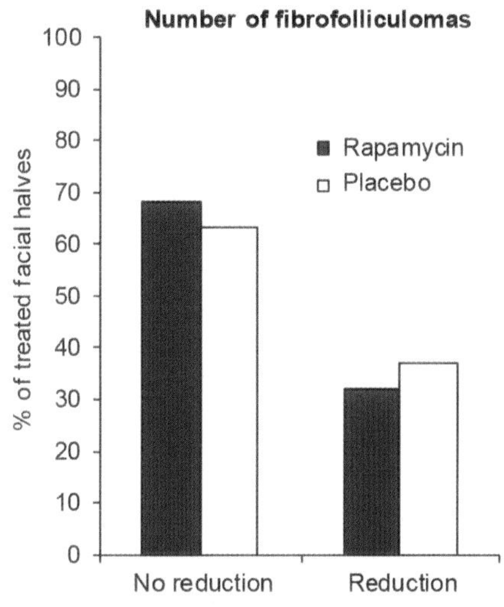

Figure 5. Changes in the number of fibrofolliculomas after treatment with rapamycin. BHD patients with facial fibrofolliculomas were treated with topical rapamycin and placebo for six months. The number of fibrofolliculomas in a predefined area of the face was determined and compared to baseline. The reduction in the number of fibrofolliculomas was stronger upon placebo treatment.

Table 2. Between-treatment comparison of mean change in fibrofolliculoma size compared to baseline (in mm) using the T-test for paired samples.

	Rapamycin	Placebo	Difference	95% CI	p-value
At 3 months	0.054 (SD 0.34)	0.027 (SD 0.27)	0,027	−0,21–+0,26	0.814
At 6 months	0.100 (SD 0.29)	0.096 (SD 0.32)	0.004	−0,16–+0,17	0.961

SD = standard deviation; CI = confidence interval.

Table 3. The inter-observer variation of scores used to measure the effect of rapamycin using the intraclass correlation coefficient (ICC).

Outcome measure	Lowest ICC (95%CI)	Highest ICC (95%CI)
Cosmetic status of fibrofolliculomas	0.517 (0.244–0.758)	0.633 (0.390–0.821)
Number of fibrofolliculomas	0.643 (0.324–0.840)	0.878 (0.757–0.947)
Size of fibrofolliculomas	0.374 (0.075–0.660)	0.653 (0.401–0.834)

95%IC = 95% confidence interval.

mTOR had also been questioned by Claessens et al. based on immunohistochemical assessment of BHD patient skin and kidney tumour tissue [36]. More recent *in vitro* studies using *FLCN* knockdown cells have not been able to confirm a direct link between FLCN and mTOR [37] (and unpublished data). The deregulation of mTOR activity found in the tumours of BHD animal models could be due to mTOR's general involvement in cancerous growth rather than a direct effect of FLCN's absence. Of note, most animal models involve knockout of *FLCN*. FFs do not have loss of *FLCN* and we have recently provided evidence that BHD-associated kidney tumours do not have complete loss of *FLCN* either [38–40]. Thus, the present state of the art suggests that there is no clear-cut relation between FLCN and mTOR. Our trial data support this assertion and we suggest that mTOR does not play an active role in the maintenance or growth of fibrofolliculomas, in contrast to angiofibromas in TSC.

We have considered alternative explanations for the observed lack of efficacy. Firstly, the concentration of rapamycin in the lotion might have been too low. However, the oral rapamycin solution that we used in this study has been shown to be an effective topical treatment for angiofibromas in TSC, without detectable levels of rapamycin in the serum [26]. A 1:1 mixture of rapamycin solution 1 mg/ml in an emollient has also shown to be effective in TSC [27]. This indicates that rapamycin in this oral solution penetrates into the skin and that the concentration of rapamycin we used is sufficient to cause a clinical effect. Propylene glycol is part of the solvent of the oral rapamycin and is known to enhance topical drug delivery [41–44]. Secondly, patient compli-

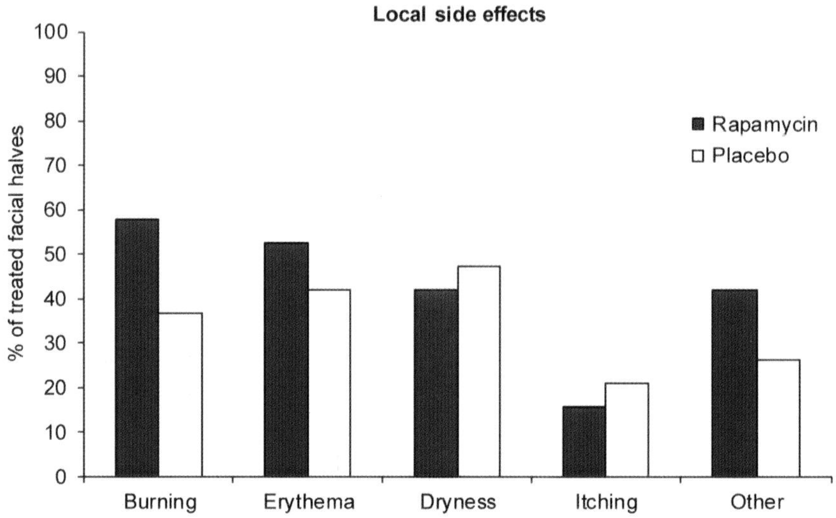

Figure 6. Local side effects of topical rapamycin treatment. Side effects of both topical rapamycin and placebo treatment were registered at each clinical assessment. Burning, erythema, dryness and itching were the most commonly reported local side effects. All side effects other than dryness and itching were reported more frequently for the rapamycin treated facial half.

ance might have been too low. To measure compliance we planned to weigh the used bottles with rapamycin and placebo solution at every follow-up visit. Because the treated surface varied widely between patients and not all bottles were retrieved, compliance could not be determined in this way. No patient reported to have deviated from the treatment protocol, but we cannot rule out non-compliance. However, as most patients experienced one or more side effects, we are confident that they did indeed adhere to protocol. Thirdly, there was moderate variation between the doctors in scoring the change in cosmetic status and the size of FFs. Small random errors in classification of cosmetic status theoretically may result in obscuring an effect of rapamycin. However, it seems improbable that large, clinically relevant differences would be missed by lack of perfect agreement. Moreover, ICCs up to 0.878 were obtained for observer agreement on FF number. For this outcome measure the results clearly show no advantage of rapamycin treatment compared to placebo treatment.

In this randomised controlled trial both doctors' and patients' opinion on the efficacy of the topical rapamycin treatment of FFs in BHD was measured, giving disparate results. Patients reported improvement in some cases, whereas doctors observed no efficacy of rapamycin treatment. All three doctors were blinded and they evaluated the treatment twice at separate time points. Patients were also blinded at the start of the treatment, but because side effects occurred more often on the rapamycin treated side blinding could have been compromised. Therefore patients might have been biased towards experiencing improvement on the facial half with most side effects. This can explain the difference in doctors' and patients' opinion on improvement of the FFs after treatment.

Most reported side effects were a sign of skin irritation. Although these irritation signs occurred more often on the rapamycin treated side, they were also reported on the placebo treated side of the face. This suggests that the excipient, which contains ethanol, may have been responsible for some of the side effects.

In conclusion, we show that topical rapamycin as used by us is not an effective treatment for FFs in BHD. It is still possible that a higher concentration or oral administration could be effective. However, very recent work provides evidence that reduced expression of FLCN does not necessarily cause increased mTOR activity. Thus, our present findings do not support further study of rapamycin or similar compounds for the treatment of FF in BHD. Development of an effective topical treatment will have to await full elucidation of FLCN's functions in cellular signalling.

Acknowledgments

We are grateful to all of the patients who were willing to participate in this trial. We thank Dr. M.B.A van Doorn for his assistance during the inclusion.

Author Contributions

Conceived and designed the experiments: MAMvS MHP LMCG. Performed the experiments: LMCG HM CEUO CJMH TMS FHM. Analyzed the data: MV LMCG PJN. Contributed reagents/materials/analysis tools: PJN. Wrote the paper: LMCG MV MAMVS.

References

1. Hornstein OP, Knickenberg M (1975) Perifollicular fibromatosis cutis with polyps of the colon—a cutaneo-intestinal syndrome sui generis. Arch Dermatol Res 253: 161–175.
2. Birt AR, Hogg GR, Dubé WJ (1977) Hereditary multiple fibrofolliculomas with trichodiscomas and acrochordons. Arch Dermatol 113: 1674–1677.
3. Toro JR, Pautler SE, Stewart L, Glenn GM, Weinreich M, et al. (2007) Lung cysts, spontaneous pneumothorax, and genetic associations in 89 families with Birt-Hogg-Dubé syndrome. Am J Respir Crit Care Med 175: 1044–1053.
4. Roth JS, Rabinowitz AD, Benson M, Grossman ME (1993) Bilateral renal cell carcinoma in the Birt-Hogg-Dubé syndrome. J Am Acad Dermatol 29: 1055–1056.
5. Toro JR, Glenn G, Duray P, Darling T, Weirich G, et al. (1999) Birt-Hogg-Dubé syndrome: a novel marker of kidney neoplasia. Arch Dermatol 135: 1195–1202.
6. Pavlovich CP, Walther MM, Eyler RA, Hewitt SM, Zbar B, et al. (2002) Renal tumors in the Birt-Hogg-Dubé syndrome. Am J Surg Pathol 26: 1542–1552.
7. Al-Daraji WI, Al-Razag ZA, Craven N, Twaij Z (2005) Multiple hereditary facial papules. Clin Exp Dermatol 30: 309–310.
8. Farrant PB, Emerson R (2007) Letter: hyfrecation and curettage as a treatment for fibrofolliculomas in Birt-Hogg-Dubé syndrome. Dermatol Surg 33: 1287–1288.
9. Gambichler T, Wolter M, Altmeyer P, Hoffman K (2000) Treatment of Birt-Hogg-Dubé syndrome with erbium:YAG laser. J Am Acad Dermatol 43: 856–858.
10. Jacob CI, Dover JS (2001) Birt-Hogg-Dubé syndrome: treatment of cutaneous manifestations with laser skin resurfacing. Arch Dermatol 137: 98–99.
11. Schmidt LS, Warren MB, Nickerson ML, Weirich G, Matrosova V, et al. (2001) Birt-Hogg-Dubé syndrome, a genodermatosis associated with spontaneous pneumothorax and kidney neoplasia, maps to chromosome 17p11.2. Am J Hum Genet 69: 876–882.
12. Nickerson ML, Warren MB, Toro JR, Matrosova V, Glenn G, et al. (2002) Mutations in a novel gene lead to kidney tumors, lung wall defects, and benign tumors of the hair follicle in patients with the Birt-Hogg-Dubé syndrome. Cancer Cell 2: 157–164.
13. Tsun ZY, Bar-Peled L, Chantranupong L, Zoncu R, Wang T, et al. (2013) The Folliculin Tumor Suppressor Is a GAP for the RagC/D GTPases That Signal Amino Acid Levels to mTORC1. Mol Cell. [Online] 2013 Oct 3. Available from: doi.org/10.1016/j.molcel.2013.09.016. [Accessed 13th November 2013]
14. Baba M, Hong SB, Sharma N, Warren MB, Nickerson ML, et al. (2006) Folliculin encoded by the BHD gene interacts with a binding protein, FNIP1, and AMPK, and is involved in AMPK and mTOR signaling. Proc Natl Acad Sci U S A 103: 15552–15557.
15. Baba M, Furihata M, Hong SB, Tessarollo L, Haines DC, et al. (2008) Kidney-targeted Birt-Hogg-Dubé gene inactivation in a mouse model: Erk1/2 and Akt-mTOR activation, cell hyperproliferation, and polycystic kidneys. J Natl Cancer Inst 100: 140–154.
16. Chen J, Futami K, Petillo D, Peng J, Wang P, et al. (2008) Deficiency of FLCN in mouse kidney led to development of polycystic kidneys and renal neoplasia. PLoS One 3: e3581.
17. Hasumi Y, Baba M, Ajima R, Hasumi H, Valera VA, et al. (2009) Homozygous loss of BHD causes early embryonic lethality and kidney tumor development with activation of mTORC1 and mTORC2. Proc Natl Acad Sci U S A 106: 18722–18727.
18. Furuya M, Tanaka R, Koga S, Yatabe Y, Gotoda H, et al. (2012) Pulmonary cysts of Birt-Hogg-Dubé syndrome: a clinicopathologic and immunohistochemical study of 9 families. Am J Surg Pathol 36: 589–600.
19. Inoki K, Corradetti MN, Guan KL (2005) Dysregulation of the TSC-mTOR pathway in human disease. Nat Genet 37: 19–24.
20. van Slegtenhorst M, Khabibullin D, Hartman TR, Nicolas E, Kruger WD, et al. (2007) The Birt-Hogg-Dubé and tuberous sclerosis complex homologs have opposing roles in amino acid homeostasis in Schizosaccharomyces pombe. J Biol Chem 282: 24583–24590.
21. Toro JR (2008) Birt-Hogg-Dubé Syndrome. In: Pagon RA, Adam MP, Bird TD, Dolan CR, Fong CT et al., editors. GeneReviews. Seattle (WA) [Online] 2008 Sept 9. Available from: http:/www.ncbi.nlm.nih.gov/books/NBK1522. [Accessed 10th June 2013]
22. Schaffer JV, Gohara MA, McNiff JM, Aasi SZ, Dvoretzky I (2005) Multiple facial angiofibromas: a cutaneous manifestation of Birt-Hogg-Dubé syndrome. J Am Acad Dermatol 53: S108–111.
23. Hofbauer GF, Marcollo-Pini A, Corsenca A, Kistler AD, French LE, et al. (2008) The mTOR inhibitor rapamycin significantly improves facial angiofibroma lesions in a patient with tuberous sclerosis. Br J Dermatol 159: 473–475.

24. Haemel AK, O'Brian AL, Teng JM (2010) Topical rapamycin: a novel approach to facial angiofibromas in tuberous sclerosis. Arch Dermatol 146: 715–718.
25. Wataya-Kaneda M, Tanaka M, Nakamura A, Matsumoto S, Katayama I (2011) A topical combination of rapamycin and tacrolimus for the treatment of angiofibroma due to tuberous sclerosis complex (TSC): a pilot study of nine Japanese patients with TSC of different disease severity. Br J Dermatol 165: 912–916.
26. Mutizwa MM, Berk DR, Anadkat MJ (2011) Treatment of facial angiofibromas with topical application of oral rapamycin solution (1mgmL(-1)) in two patients with tuberous sclerosis. Br J Dermatol 165: 922–923.
27. Kaufman McNamara E, Curtis AR, Fleischer Jr AB (2012) Successful treatment of angiofibromata of tuberous sclerosis complex with rapamycin. J Dermatolog Treat 23: 46–48.
28. Foster RS, Bint LJ, Halbert AR (2012) Topical 0.1% rapamycin for angiofibromas in paediatric patients with tuberous sclerosis: a pilot study of four patients. Australas J Dermatol 53: 52–56.
29. Truchuelo T, Diaz-Ley B, Rios L, Alcantara J, Jaen P (2012) Facial angiofibromas treated with topical rapamycin: an excellent choice with fast response. Dermatol Online J 18: 15.
30. DeKlotz CM, Ogram AE, Singh S, Dronavalli S, MacGregor JL (2011) Dramatic improvement of facial angiofibromas in tuberous sclerosis with topical rapamycin: optimizing a treatment protocol. Arch Dermatol 147: 1116–1117.
31. Leyden JJ, Shalita A, Thiboutot D, Washenik K, Webster G (2005) Topical retinoids in inflammatory acne: a retrospective, investigator-blinded, vehicle-controlled, photographic assessment. Clin Ther 27: 216–224.
32. Ozolins M, Eady EA, Avery A, Cunliffe WJ, O'Neill C, et al. (2005) Randomised controlled multiple treatment comparison to provide a cost-effectiveness rationale for the selection of antimicrobial therapy in acne. Health Technol Assess 9: iii-212.
33. Liu W, Chen Z, Ma Y, Wu X, Jin Y, et al. (2013) Genetic Characterization of the Birt-Hogg-Dubé Syndrome Gene. PLoS One 8: e65869.
34. Hudon V, Sabourin S, Dydensborg AB, Kottis V, Ghazi A, et al. (2010) Renal tumour suppressor function of the Birt-Hogg-Dubé syndrome gene product folliculin. J Med Genet 47: 182–189.
35. Hartman TR, Nicolas E, Klein-Szanto A, Al-Saleem T, Cash TP, et al. (2009) The role of the Birt-Hogg-Dubé protein in mTOR activation and renal tumorigenesis. Oncogene 28: 1594–1604.
36. Claessens T, Weppler SA, van Geel M, Creytens D, Vreeburg M, et al. (2010) Neuroendocrine carcinoma in a patient with Birt-Hogg-Dubé syndrome. Nat Rev Urol 7: 583–587.
37. Betschinger J, Nichols J, Dietmann S, Corrin PD, Paddison PJ, et al. (2013) Exit from pluripotency is gated by intracellular redistribution of the bHLH transcription factor Tfe3. Cell 153: 335–347.
38. van Steensel MA, Verstraeten VL, Frank J, Kelleners-Smeets NW, Poblete-Gutierrez P, et al. (2007) Novel mutations in the BHD gene and absence of loss of heterozygosity in fibrofolliculomas of Birt-Hogg-Dubé patients. J Invest Dermatol 127: 588–593.
39. Vernooij M, Claessens T, Luijten M, van Steensel MA, Coull BJ (2013) Birt-Hogg-Dubé syndrome and the skin. Fam Cancer 12: 381–385
40. Luijten MN, Basten SG, Claessens T, Vernooij M, Scott CL, et al. (2013) Birt-Hogg-Dubé syndrome is a novel ciliopathy. Hum Mol Genet. [Online] 2013 Juli 6. Available from doi: 10.1093/hmg/ddt288 [Accessed 31st July 2013]
41. Barrett CW, Hadgraft JW, Caron GA, Sarkany I (1965) The effect of particle size and vehicle on the percutaneous absorption of fluocinolone acetonide. Br J Dermatol 77: 576–578.
42. Poulsen BJ, Young E, Coquilla V, Katz M (1968) Effect of topical vehicle composition on the in vitro release of fluocinolone acetonide and its acetate ester. J Pharm Sci 57: 928–933.
43. Arellano A, Santoyo S, Martin C, Ygartua P (1999) Influence of propylene glycol and isopropyl myristate on the in vitro percutaneous penetration of diclofenac sodium from carbopol gels. Eur J Pharm Sci 7: 129–135.
44. Nicolazzo JA, Morgan TM, Reed BL, Finnin BC (2005) Synergistic enhancement of testosterone transdermal delivery. J Control Release 103: 577–585.

2

Congenic Mapping and Allele-Specific Alteration Analysis of *Stmm1* Locus Conferring Resistance to Early-Stage Chemically Induced Skin Papillomas

Kazuhiro Okumura[1], Megumi Saito[1], Eriko Isogai[1], Ikuo Miura[2], Shigeharu Wakana[2], Ryo Kominami[3], Yuichi Wakabayashi[1]*

1 Department of Carcinogenesis Research, Division of Experimental Animal Research, Chiba Cancer Center Research Institute, Chiba, Chiba, Japan, **2** Technology and Development Team for Mouse Phenotype Analysis, Japan Mouse Clinic, Riken Bioresource Center, Tsukuba, Ibaraki, Japan, **3** Department of Molecular Genetics, Graduate School of Medical and Dental Sciences, Niigata University, Niigata, Niigata, Japan

Abstract

Genome-wide association studies have revealed that many low-penetrance cancer susceptibility loci are located throughout the genome; however, a very limited number of genes have been identified so far. Using a forward genetics approach to map such loci in a mouse skin cancer model, we previously identified strong genetic loci conferring resistance to early-stage chemically induced skin papillomas on chromosome 7 with a large number of [(FVB/N×MSM/Ms)×FVB/N] F1 backcross mice. In this report, we describe a combination of congenic mapping and allele-specific alteration analysis of the loci on chromosome 7. We used linkage analysis and congenic mouse strains to refine the location of *Stmm1* (*Skin tumor modifier of MSM 1*) locus within a genetic interval of about 3 cM on proximal chromosome 7. In addition, we used patterns of allele-specific imbalances in tumors from F1 backcross and N10 congenic mice to narrow down further the region of *Stmm1* locus to a physical distance of about 5.4 Mb. To gain the insight into the function of *Stmm1* locus, we carried out a long term BrdU labelling experiments with congenic mice containing *Stmm1* locus. Interestingly, we observed a decrease of BrdU-LRCs (Label Retaining Cells) in a congenic strain heterozygous or homozygous for MSM allele of *Stmm1*. These results suggest that *Stmm1* responsible genes may have an influence on papillomagenesis in the two-stage skin carcinogenesis by regulating epidermal quiescent stem cells.

Editor: Amanda E. Toland, Ohio State University Medical Center, United States of America

Funding: This work was supported by MEXT's program "Promotion of Environmental Improvement for Independence of Young Researchers" under the Special Coordination Funds for Promoting Science and Technology at Niigata University, and Grants-in-Aid for Scientific Research from the Ministry of Education, Culture, Sports, Science, and Technology of Japan. The funders had no role in study design, data collection and analysis, decision to publish, or preparation of the manuscript.

Competing Interests: The authors have declared that no competing interests exist.

* E-mail: yuichi_wakabayashi@chiba-cc.jp

Introduction

Identification of the specific genetic variants responsible for increased susceptibility to familial or sporadic cancers remains an important but challenging goal with major implications for the prediction of individual cancer risk, as well as for improved strategies for prevention or targeted therapy [1–4]. Present approaches to detect low-penetrance tumor-susceptibility alleles in humans involve association studies using DNA samples from hundreds or thousands of cancer patients, and an equal number of well-matched controls. Such studies are plagued by confounding factors such as population heterogeneity, weak effects, and genetic interactions, and require a very large number of cases and controls to reach statistical significance [5–7]. For many complex-trait diseases, including cancer, low-penetrance susceptibility alleles account for a very small proportion of the total cancer risk [8], leading to considerable discussion of the best approaches to discover the majority of disease-causing alleles in human populations.

For these reasons, complementary gene mapping and validation approaches including cross-species comparisons using animal models are required to identify genes that modify disease phenotypes, including the risk of developing cancer [9–11]. Exploiting the resistance of *M. spretus* to the two-stage skin carcinogenesis model involving 7,12-dimethylbenz(a)anthracene (DMBA) initiation and subsequent promotion with 12-*O*-tetra-decanoylphorbol-13-acetate (TPA), 15 skin tumor susceptibility loci, *Skts1-15*, were identified in an interspecific F1 backcross [(*NIH/Ola*×*M. spretus*)×*NIH/Ola*] using QTL analysis [12], [13]. In addition to the *Skts* series, several other skin tumor modifier loci were identified using commonly used inbred strains or wild-derived strains. *Skts-fp1-3* were identified in a cross between the wild-derived inbred strain PWK and FVB/N [14]. *Skts-fp1* was also identified in a study involving a cross between a wild-derived outbred stock of *Mus musculus castaneus* and FVB/N [15]. We previously reported mapping of *Stmm1* and *2* (*Skin tumor modifier of MSM*), which confer resistance to skin tumor development on mouse chromosome 7 in a cross between the resistant Japanese wild-derived inbred strain MSM/Ms and the susceptible strain FVB/N [16]. In the present study, we used interval-specific congenic mouse strains to refine the location of *Stmm1* within a genetic interval spanning approximately 3 cM on proximal chromosome 7. In addition, we used patterns of allele-specific imbalances in tumors from F1 backcross and N10 congenic mice to further refine the location of *Stmm1*. High frequency of either MSM allele loss or FVB allele gain was detected in the region corresponding to physical distance of about 5.4 Mb. To gain the further insight into the function of *Stmm1* locus, we carried out BrdU chase experiments with congenic lines containing *Stmm1*. As a result, we observed a decrease of BrdU-LRCs in congenic strains heterozygous or homozygous for the MSM allele of *Stmm1* on proximal chromosome 7. These results suggest that gene(s) located within the *Stmm1* locus may have an influence on papillomagenesis in the two-stage skin carcinogenesis by regulating epidermal quiescent stem cells.

Results

A Strong Papilloma Resistance Locus, *Stmm1* (Skin Tumor Modifier of MSM), on Proximal Chromosome 7

Previous QTL analysis identified at least two independent skin tumor susceptibility loci (*Skts1* and *Skts2*) on mouse chromosome 7 [12]. We have recently identified a series of skin papilloma resistance loci, *Stmm* (*Skin tumor modifier of MSM*) loci, using F1 backcross mice between a wild derived inbred mouse strain (MSM) and a susceptible inbred mouse strain (FVB/N). Two of these loci are located in the vicinity of *Skts1* and *2* on chromosome 7: *Stmm1* was mapped near the markers D7SNP507 and D7SNP513, and *Stmm2* near the markers D7SNP6 and D7Mit10 [16], (**Figure 1A**). To confirm the presence of low-penetrance susceptibility genes in these regions, we selected resistant F1 backcross mice for further backcrossing to FVB/N mice to generate two N10 congenic mouse lines that span either the *Stmm1* (congenic line a) or the *Stmm2* (congenic line b) region (**Figure 1A**). First, these congenic lines were subjected to the DMBA-TPA skin carcinogenesis experiment, according to the standard protocol. As previously shown, FVB/N mice are highly susceptible to the two-stage skin chemical carcinogenesis. Similarly, homozygous FVB/FVB (FF) mice of congenic lines (a) (n = 13) and (b) (n = 14) were highly susceptible to skin carcinogenesis, developing on average 18 papillomas at 10 weeks after initiation, and about 40 papillomas at 20 weeks after initiation (**Figure 1B, 1C and Table 1**). In contrast, heterozygous MSM/FVB (MF) mice of a congenic line (a) developed an average of 3.6±3.8 papillomas/mouse at 10 weeks after initiation (n = 15; compared with control: $P = 3.2^{-10}$) (**Figure 1B, 1C and Table 1**), consistent with this region conferring resistance to skin papillomas. On the other hand, MF heterozygous mice of a congenic line (b) had little effect on papilloma development. The number was an average of 12.5±5 papillomas/mouse at 10 weeks (compared with control: $P = 0.13$) and 38.3±8.7 papillomas/mouse at 20 weeks after initiation (n = 14; compared with control: $P = 0.07$) (**Figure 1B, 1C and Table 1**). In summary, MF heterozygous mice of a line (a), corresponding to *Stmm1*, developed significantly fewer papillomas than FVB/N mice. On the other hand, MF heterozygous mice of a line (b), corresponding to *Stmm2*, developed about the same number of papillomas as control wild type FVB/N mice. These results clearly suggest *Stmm1* has a strong suppressive effect on papilloma development.

Table 1. Papilloma incidence in the congenic lines.

Congenic line	Chromosomal region (cM)	10 weeks			20 weeks		
		MF	FF	P-value	MF	FF	P-value
a	1.91–60.49	3.6 (0–14; n = 15)	19.8 (11–26; n = 13)	3.2E-10	17.8 (3–29; n = 15)	46.2 (36–66; n = 13)	1.50E-08
b	68.16–88.85	12.5 (4–21; n = 14)	15.8 (9–29; n = 14)	0.13	36.8 (19–50; n = 14)	44.1 (28–67; n = 14)	0.07
c	20.65–60.49	2.7 (0–13; n = 7)	19.8 (11–26; n = 13)	5.8E-07	10.5 (4–32; n = 7)	46.2 (36–66; n = 13)	2.50E-07
d	43.4–60.49	5.9 (1–11; n = 13)	24.2 (14–44; n = 10)	4.20E-07	26.5 (2–42; n = 12)	45.5 (30–61; n = 8)	0.003
e	49.01–60.49	3.7 (0–11; n = 12)	20.1 (5–44; n = 11)	1.40E-09	16.5 (0–37; n = 12)	36.7 (28–50; n = 10)	0.0003
f	52.92–54.45	2.7 (0–10; n = 9)	18.2 (12–25; n = 6)	4.88E-06	15.125 (2–39; n = 9)	47.25 (36–54; n = 6)	0.0007
g	1.91–20.65	20.2 (11–29; n = 5)	19.8 (11–26; n = 13)	0.87	39.4 (26–45; n = 5)	46.2 (36–66; n = 13)	0.17
h	1.91–51.6	20.5 (16–25; n = 3)	19.8 (11–26; n = 13)	0.31	41.5 (29–54; n = 3)	46.2 (36–66; n = 13)	0.55
i	20.65–54.45	20.8 (7–27; n = 5)	24.6 (21–29; n = 6)	0.31	30.2 (24–37; n = 5)	40.4 (32–49; n = 6)	0.04

Abbreviations: cM, centi-morgan from MGI; N.D., not determined; MF, MSM/FVB; FF, FVB/FVB. *P*-value is from standard *t*-test.

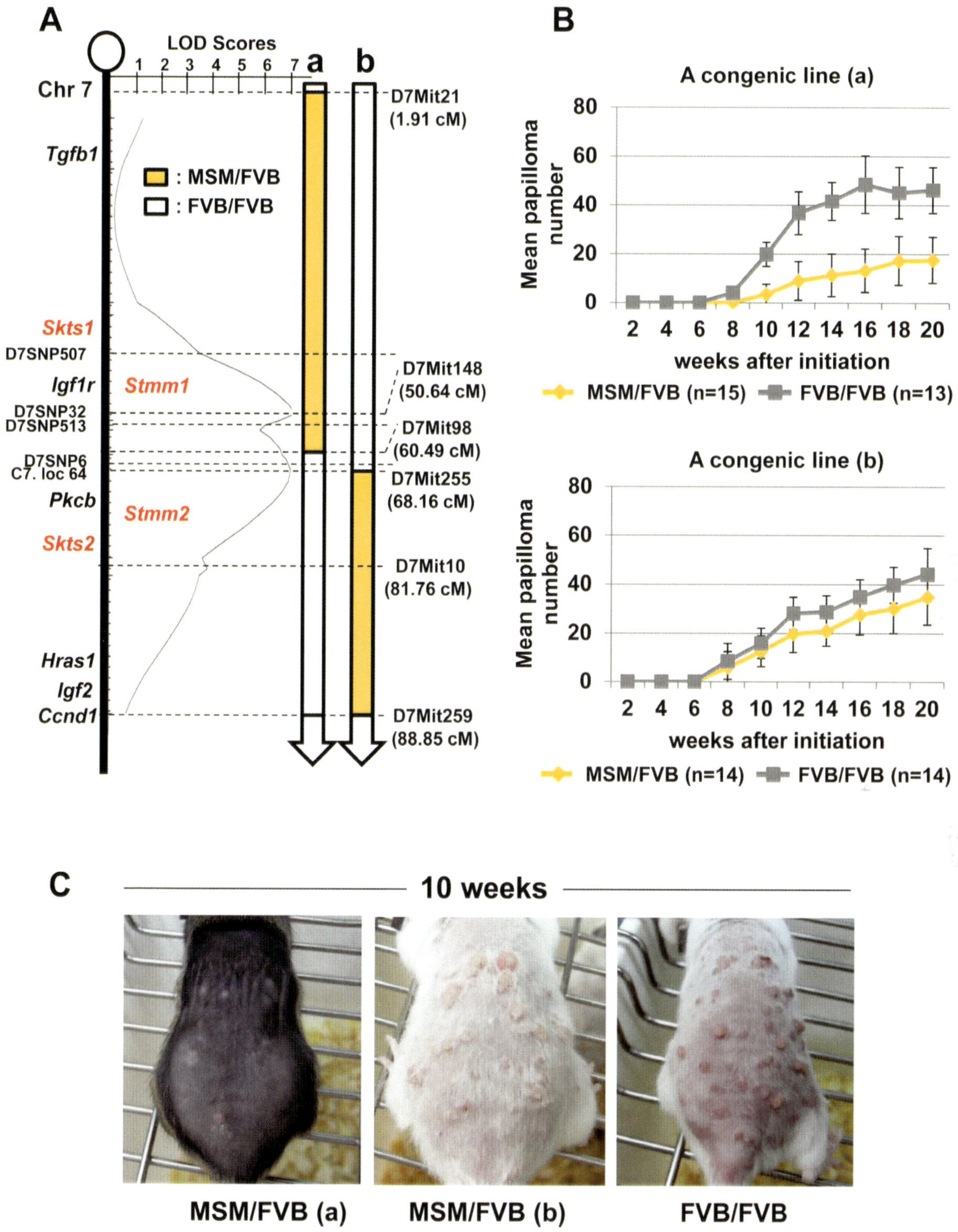

Figure 1. Genetic linkage map and papilloma incidence in congenic lines (a) and (b) on mouse chromosome 7. (A) Two significant linkage peaks, *Stmm1* and *2* were mapped in the previous report [16]. Two orange and white bars represents two congenic lines (a) and (b). The orange bars indicate the heterozygous MF region, while the white bars indicate the homozygous FF region. Several well-known genes located on chromosome 7 are indicated with other papilloma resistance loci, *Skts1, 2*, and genetic markers. Genetic positions shown are according to the Ensembl database (http://uswest.ensembl.org/index.html), the Mouse Genome Informatics Database (http://www.informatics.jax.org/). (B) Comparison of average papilloma numbers/mouse between a congenic line (a) and (b). The top panel shows papilloma incidence in a congenic line (a). The bottom panel shows papilloma incidence in a congenic line (b). The orange bars represent papilloma numbers of MF heterozygous congenic mice. The grey bars represent those of FF heterozygous congenic mice. (C) Photos of representative mice on TPA treatment. Dorsal back skin of MF heterozygous mice of congenic lines (a), (b) and a homozygous FF mouse of a congenic line (a) as a control at 10 weeks after initiation.

Narrowing down the Genetic Distance of *Stmm1* on Chromosome 7

On the basis of skin carcinogenesis experiments of lines (a) and (b), we focused on a line (a), which contains the *Stmm1* locus and showed a much stronger suppressive effect on papilloma development. A series of congenic lines (c–i) containing different overlapping regions were generated from mice of a line (a) (**Figure 2A and Table 1**). These sub-congenic lines were subjected to the DMBA/TPA chemical carcinogenesis protocol and their papilloma development was monitored for a period of 20 weeks (**Table 1**). For each congenic line, we documented the number of papillomas at 20 weeks after initiation.

Figure 2A and 2B show a genetic map and papilloma incidence of each congenic line. Of the seven sub-congenic lines (c-i) tested, four lines (c, d, e, and f) showed significant linkage with papilloma incidence (**Figure 2B and Table1**). By determining the minimum-overlapping region within the four positive congenic lines (c, d, e, and f) and by excluding the regions of the three congenic lines (g, h, and i) that did not show an effect (**Figure 2B and Table 1**), we were able to narrow down the location of the *Stmm1* region to an interval of about 3 cM (indicated by a blue arrowed line) from 54.54 to 57.52 cM (**Figure 2A and 2B**). This region does not overlap with the previously reported *Skts1* locus. These data suggest that *Stmm1* is a novel skin tumor susceptibility locus on chromosome 7, conferring resistance to papilloma development.

Allelic Imbalances in Favor of the FVB/N Allele of the *Stmm1* Locus in Skin Tumors from F1 Backcross and Congenic Mice

We carried out a detailed investigation of allelic imbalance on chromosome 7 to determine whether somatic changes would provide a more specific localization of *Stmm1*. This allelic imbalance analysis was performed using twelve informative microsatellite markers (**for detailed information, see Table 2**). **Figure 3A** shows the frequency of allelic imbalances near the *Stmm1* locus in papillomas from F1 backcross ($n = 30$) and N10 congenic mice ($n = 26$). 5/30 and 5/26 papillomas from F1 backcross and N10 congenic mice showed losses of MSM alleles across the whole region, but others exhibited regional losses involving smaller chromosome fragments (**Figure 3B**). Papillomas from N10 congenic mice showed the higher frequency of allelic imbalances than those from F1 backcross mice (17/26 vs 12/30, $P = 0.0005$), probably because other MSM alleles retained in genomic DNA of F1 backcross mice had an influence on the frequency of allelic imbalances in *Stmm1*. Two allelic imbalance peaks were detected within the minimum-overlapping region of 3 cM identified with the multiple congenic lines of *Stmm1* (**Figure 3A and 3B**), one was localized within 3.4 Mb region between D7Mit96 (100.5 Mb) and D7Mit131 (103.87 Mb), the other was within 2 Mb region between D7Mit95 (105.75 Mb) and D7Mit124 (107.68 Mb). When these two regions are combined, the total physical size of the candidate region can be cut down to about 5.4 Mb. This interval still contains a large number of genes. Further congenic and somatic mapping will refine the candidate region to facilitate gene identification.

BrdU Chase Experiments using *Stmm1* Congenic Mice

In the original report, we classified papillomas into three categories based on their diameter, and carried out linkage analysis for each category. This analysis revealed strong linkage at *Stmm1* and *Stmm2* on chromosome 7 to the total papilloma number, the number of papillomas <2 mm, and the number of papillomas of 2–6 mm in diameter. However, these linkage peaks at *Stmm1* and *Stmm2* completely disappeared when the analysis was confined to papillomas >6 mm. These results suggested that *Stmm1* and *2* genes function only at an early papilloma stage, but are not involved at the later stage of papilloma progression [16]. To gain the insight into the function of *Stmm1* locus, we carried out BrdU-LRC analysis with congenic lines (**Figure 4**). Using a thymidine derivative, such as BrdU, DNA strands of adult stem cells can be labeled at the moment they are synthesized during development. Adult stem cells are quiescent and their DNA strands segregate non-randomly. As such, epidermal stem cells can retain the BrdU label indefinitely during adulthood and are accordingly referred to as label retaining cells (LRCs). The timetable of this BrdU chase experiment is shown in **Figure 4A** (for detailed information, see Material and Methods).

As a result, heterozygous MF mice of a congenic line (a) showed significantly reduced BrdU-LRCs in the bulge of hair follicles, compared with those of homozygous FF mice of a line (a), as a positive control ($P = 9.98^{-9}$) (**Figure 4A, 4B, and 4F**). In addition, the same BrdU chase experiment was carried out using heterozygous MF mice of a congenic line having the region of D4Mit17-D4Mit15 on chromosome 4, previously found to confer strong resistance to late stage papillomas (>6 mm in diameter) [16]. Heterozygous MF mice of a chromosome 4 congenic line did not exhibit a change in the number of BrdU-LRCs compared with that of their homozygous FF littermates (**Figure 4C, 4D, and 4F**). These results suggest that gene(s) located within the *Stmm1* locus may have an influence on papillomagenesis step in the two-stage skin carcinogenesis by regulating epidermal quiescent stem cells.

Discussion

In this study, the location of *Stmm1* was refined to a genetic interval of about 3 cM on proximal chromosome 7 by using multiple congenic lines. By taking advantage of allelic alterations in papillomas from F1 backcross and N10 congenic mice, we further narrowed down the physical interval to about 5.4 Mb. We carried out BrdU chase experiments with congenic lines containing *Stmm1*, and observed a decrease of BrdU-LRCs in a congenic strain that is M/F heterozygous or M/M homozygous for *Stmm1* on chromosome 7. These results suggest that *Stmm1* modifies papilloma development by regulating epidermal quiescent stem cells.

As previously shown, we screened stage-specific papilloma modifier loci on the basis of the size. *Stmm1* and *Stmm2* were identified on chromosome 7 as modifier loci conferring resistance to papillomas of smaller size [16]. They were mapped in the vicinity of *Skts1* and *2* loci, previously identified using a wild-derived inbred mouse strain, *M. spretus* [12]. *Skts1* was narrowed down to around 15 Mb region between D7Mit193 (31.4 cM) and D7Mit248 (35.2 cM), which is proximal to *Igf1r* by congenic analysis [17]. Carcinogenesis experiments using congenic mice presented in this report show that *Stmm1* locus is distal to *Skts1* (**Figure 2A and 2B**). In addition, mice of congenic lines (d, e, and f) having only *Stmm1* region produced almost the same number of papillomas as mice of a congenic line (c) having both *Skts1* and *Stmm1* region did. Congenic lines (h and i) having only *Skts1* region didn't show any effect (**Figure 2A and 2B**). However, the number of mice in congenic lines (g, h and i) is relatively low (**Table 1**). We cannot completely exclude the possibility that the region of congenic lines (g, h, and i) has additional other *Stmm1* genes. Nevertheless, it seems likely that MSM mice do not have a modifier gene in *Skts1* region and *Stmm1* is independently capable

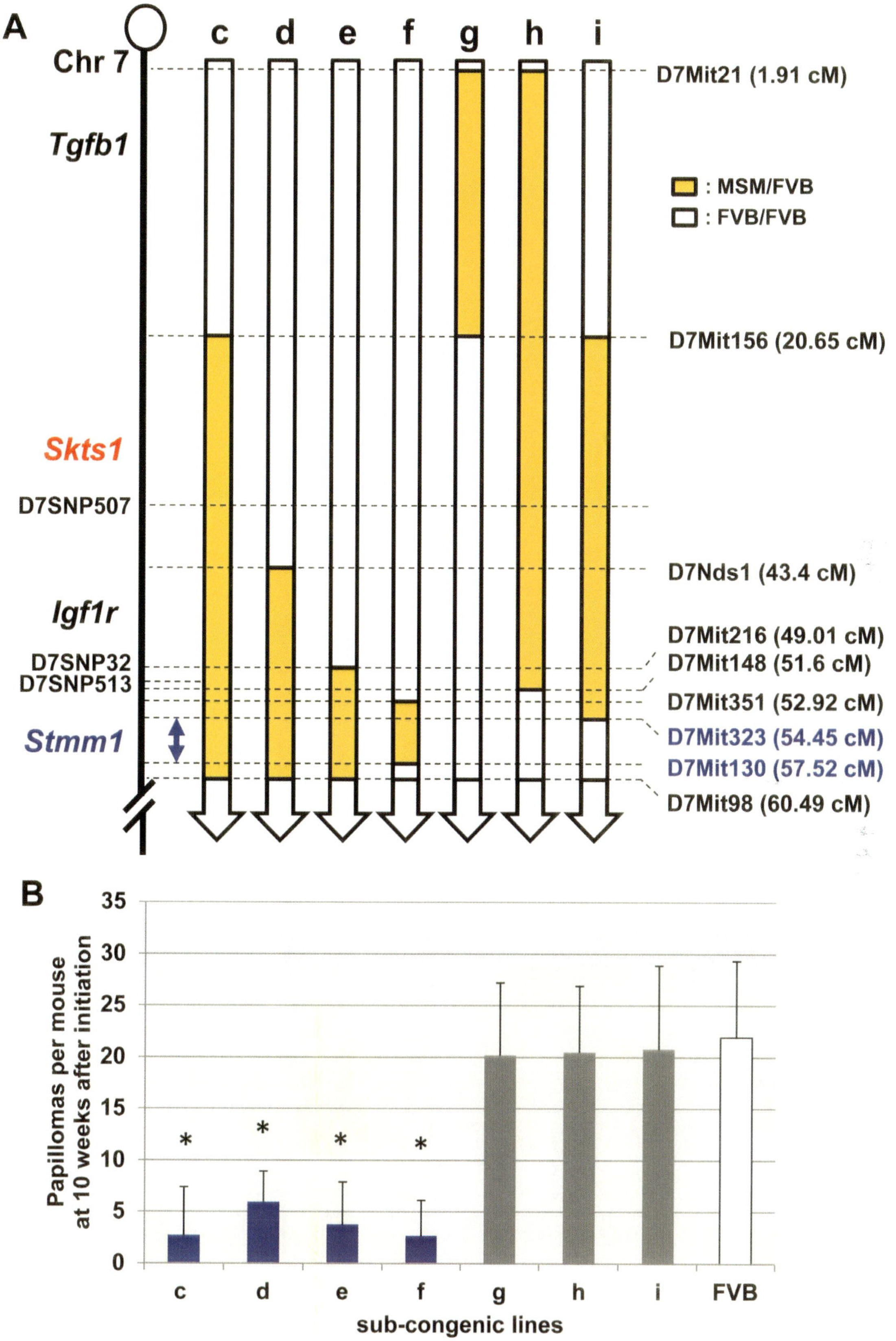

Figure 2. Summary of linkage analysis of sub-congenic lines for *Stmm1* locus on proximal chromosome 7. (A) Each bar represents a different sub-congenic line. The location of the orange and white bars indicates the region on chromosome 7. The orange bars indicate the heterozygous MF region, while the white bars indicate the homozygous FF region. The blue arrowed line indicates the *Stmm1* region narrowed down by congenic mapping. (B) Papilloma incidence of sub-congenic lines c (n = 7), d (n = 13), e (n = 12), f (n = 9), g (n = 5), h (n = 3), i (n = 5), and FVB (n = 36)

in 10 weeks after initiation. The blue bars represent congenic lines that retained papilloma resistance, whereas the grey bars represent congenic lines that didn't show resistance. Error bar represents the standard deviation (S.D.). The *P* value was calculated for papilloma number at 10 weeks by *t*-test (*$P<0.01$).

of reducing the risk of developing DMBA-TPA-induced papillomas. In contrast, mice of a congenic line (b) having *Stmm2* showed much weaker effect on papilloma suppression (**Figure 1**). *Stmm2* identified in the vicinity of *Skts2* and *Hras* on chromosome 7 showed the same effect on allele specificity of *Hras* mutation as *Skts2* did, suggesting that the same gene might be responsible for *Skts2* and *Stmm2* [16]. Although carcinogenesis experiments using congenic mice having *Skts2* have not been reported yet, data presented in this report suggests that *Stmm2* and *Skts2* genes may have a small effect on papilloma multiplicity compared with *Stmm1* (**Figure 1A**). However, a congenic line (b) does not fully cover *Stmm2* region. The interval between D7Mit98 (60.49 cM) and

Table 2. Microsatellite markers used for genetic mapping and allelic imbalance analysis.

Chromosome	Name	cM	bp
Chr7	D7Mit21	1.91	3266568–3266693
Chr7	D7Mit156	20.65	34801081–34801224
Chr7	D7Mit18	-	-
Chr7	D7Mit276	34.35	62277634–62277744
Chr7	D7Nds1	43.46	74676373–74676604
Chr7	D7Mit30	45.71	81485676–81485905
Chr7	D7Mit319	46.43	82038932–82039044
Chr7	D7Mit350	47.43	83586089–83586207
Chr7	D7Mit62	48.36	84640886–84641032
Chr7	D7Mit216	49.01	87447195–87447372
Chr7	D7Mit320	49.64	89436896–89436978
Chr7	D7Mit352	50.64	90599957–90600077
Chr7	D7Mit148	51.6	92745007–92745138
Chr7	D7Mit184	52.81	96843943–96844092
Chr7	D7Mit351	52.92	96901062–96901168
Chr7	D7Mit354	53.93	98911768–98911890
Chr7	D7Mit96	54.36	100505707–100505782
Chr7	D7Mit323	54.45	100875936–100876050
Chr7	D7Mit37	54.85	103860643–103860803
Chr7	D7Mit131	54.85	103870606–103870726
Chr7	D7Mit95	55.98	105751411–105751503
Chr7	D7Mit302	55.98	105794470–105794615
Chr7	D7Mit124	57.21	107683097–107683208
Chr7	D7Mit219	57.21	109096065–109096188
Chr7	D7Mit130	57.52	109788134–109788282
Chr7	D7Mit53	57.86	110792641–110792834
Chr7	D7Mit356	58.21	111514329–111514441
Chr7	D7Mit281	58.74	112212330–112212440
Chr7	D7Mit222	59.13	112934466–112934612
Chr7	D7Mit98	60.49	114917267–114917439
Chr7	D7Mit40	62.01	116817442–116817642
Chr7	D7Mit330	64.07	119656690–119656814
Chr7	D7Mit255	68.16	124914439–124914573
Chr7	D7Mit104	71.29	129101439–129101574
Chr7	D7Mit165	72.74	129762283–129762408
Chr7	D7Mit43	73.19	130321003–130321213
Chr7	D7Mit10	81.76	136391134–136391318
Chr7	D7Mit259	88.85	144757504–144757647

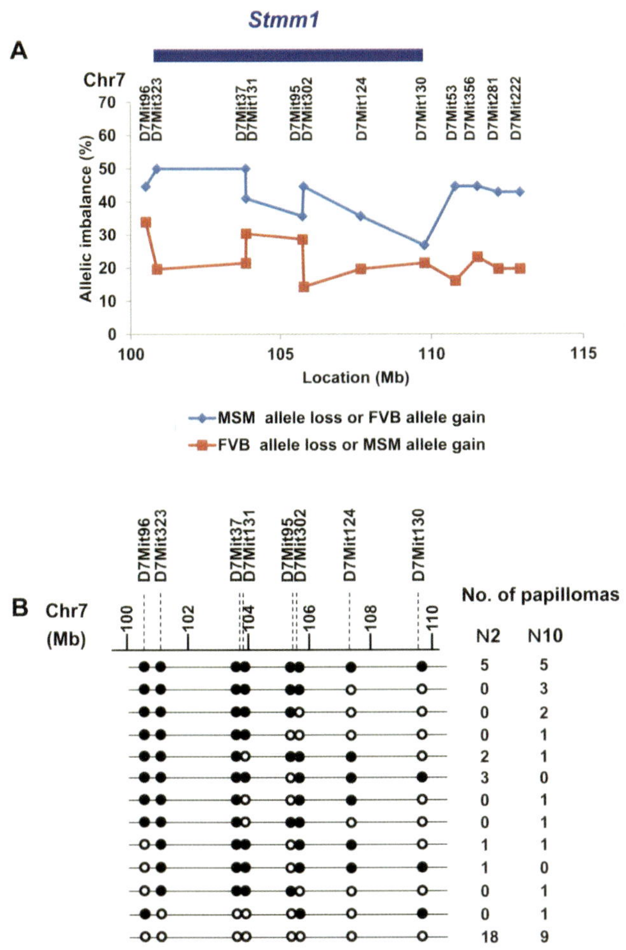

Figure 3. Allelic imbalance analysis of *Stmm1* region on chromosome 7. (A) Frequency of allelic imbalance detected by SSLP analysis on proximal chromosome 7. Data are derived from papillomas of F1 backcross (N2) and N10 congenic mice (N2, n = 30; N10, n = 26). The percentages of chromosome imbalances are plotted for different microsatellite markers (for detailed information, see **Table 2**). The blue bar represents MSM allele loss or FVB/N allele gain. The red bar represents FVB/N allele loss or MSM allele gain. (B) Detailed analysis of imbalance patterns around *Stmm1* region in papillomas. Open circles represent no imbalance; closed circles represent imbalance in favor of the FVB/N allele.

D7Mit255 (68.16 cM) is missing in any congenic line tested (**Figure 1A**). Further congenic study will give us the answer for whether *Stmm2* gene is present in this interval in the near future.

Koning *et al.* (2007) showed that low-penetrance susceptibility genes, even when present in a heterozygous state in congenic mice, can influence somatic genetic changes in tumors and that these alterations can be exploited for the rapid fine mapping of putative susceptibility loci [17]. To narrow down *Stmm1* candidate region, we carried out allelic imbalance analysis of papillomas from [(FVB/N×MSM)×FVB/N] F1 backcross and MF heterozygous mice of N10 congenic line (a) (**Figure 3**). As a result, we detected allelic imbalance showing the highest frequency in *Stmm1* region, in spite of the fact that both parental chromosomes carried the same FVB Hras gene as well as other alleles on distal chromosome 7 (**Figure 3**). This clearly shows that one or more low-penetrance susceptibility genes near *Stmm1* locus can affect somatic genetic change in tumors, independently of the effects of *Hras*. Allelic alterations with the highest rate in favor of FVB alleles were detected within the minimum-overlapping region of *Stmm1* congenic lines using the marker D7Mit323 and D7Mit37, which are located at approximately 100.88 Mb and 103.8 Mb, respectively. The physical size of this region showing allelic alterations is about 5.4 Mb. However this region still contains a large number of genes, some of which are already reported to be related to cancer. *Rrm1 (Ribonuclease reductase M1)* gene encodes the regulatory subunit of ribonucleotide reductase, the molecular target of gemcitabine. A SNP in the promoter region of *Rrm1* gene was reported to be associated with progression free survival in non-small-cell lung cancer patients treated with gemcitabine-based chemotherapy [18]. The NUP98 protein has several distinct roles within the nucleus of the normal cell. Fusion of *NUP98* to a large number of partner genes leads to the generation of leukemogenic *NUP98* fusion proteins. *NUP98* fusions are associated with a wide spectrum of hematopoietic malignancies, such as AML [19]. *RhoG* is another important caindidate gene in this region. Rho proteins belong to the Ras superfamily. They are small (21–25 kDa) molecules that share structural homology and become activated when bound to GTP. Rho GTPases have been reported to contribute to most steps of cancer initiation and progression including the acquisition of unlimited proliferation potential, survival and evasion from apoptosis, angiogenesis, and tissue invasion [20]. RhoG was recently reported to be highly expressed in human glioblastoma and mediate glioblastoma cell invasion [21]. The precise functions of these candidate genes in DMBA-TPA induced skin papilloma model remain to be elucidated yet. Further congenic and functional study will be required for gene identification in the near future.

Several lines of evidence come from studies on mouse skin tumor development where the concept that slowly dividing LRCs rather than rapidly proliferating TA (Transit Amplifying) cells are capable to expand during skin tumor promotion is long established [22]. Already in the 1980th it was shown that in mice with [3H] thymidine labeled epidermal LRCs these LRCs scarcely underwent mitosis and remained in the basal layer upon TPA treatment, whereas the proliferating cells dislocated rapidly from the basal layer undergoing terminal differentiation [23]. Furthermore, LRCs of hair follicles retained carcinogen-DNA adducts [24], and even after ablation of cycling cells in the epidermis with a chemotherapeutic drug prior to DMBA treatment, the rate of carcinoma formation was unchanged, indicating that tumor initiation occurred in quiescent (stem cells) rather than rapidly proliferating (TA) cells [25]. On the basis of these concepts, we carried out BrdU-LRC analysis using congenic mice containing *Stmm1* region. Interestingly, mice of a congenic line (a) containing *Stmm1* locus exhibited a significant reduction of BrdU-LRCs in the bulge of hair follicles (**Figure 4**). These results strongly suggest *Stmm1* gene could suppress papilloma formation by altering the behavior of adult epidermal quiescent stem cells in hair follicles. Combination of BrdU labelling, DMBA-TPA carcinogenesis and allelic imbalance analysis using congenic mice may facilitate gene identification step and functional characterization of the gene responsible for *Stmm1*.

Materials and Methods

Mice and Tumor Induction

This study was carried out in strict accordance with the recommendations in the Guide for the Care and Use of Laboratory Animals of the Ministry of Education, Culture, Sports, Science, and Technology of Japan. The protocol was approved by the Committee on the Ethics of Animal Experiments of Chiba

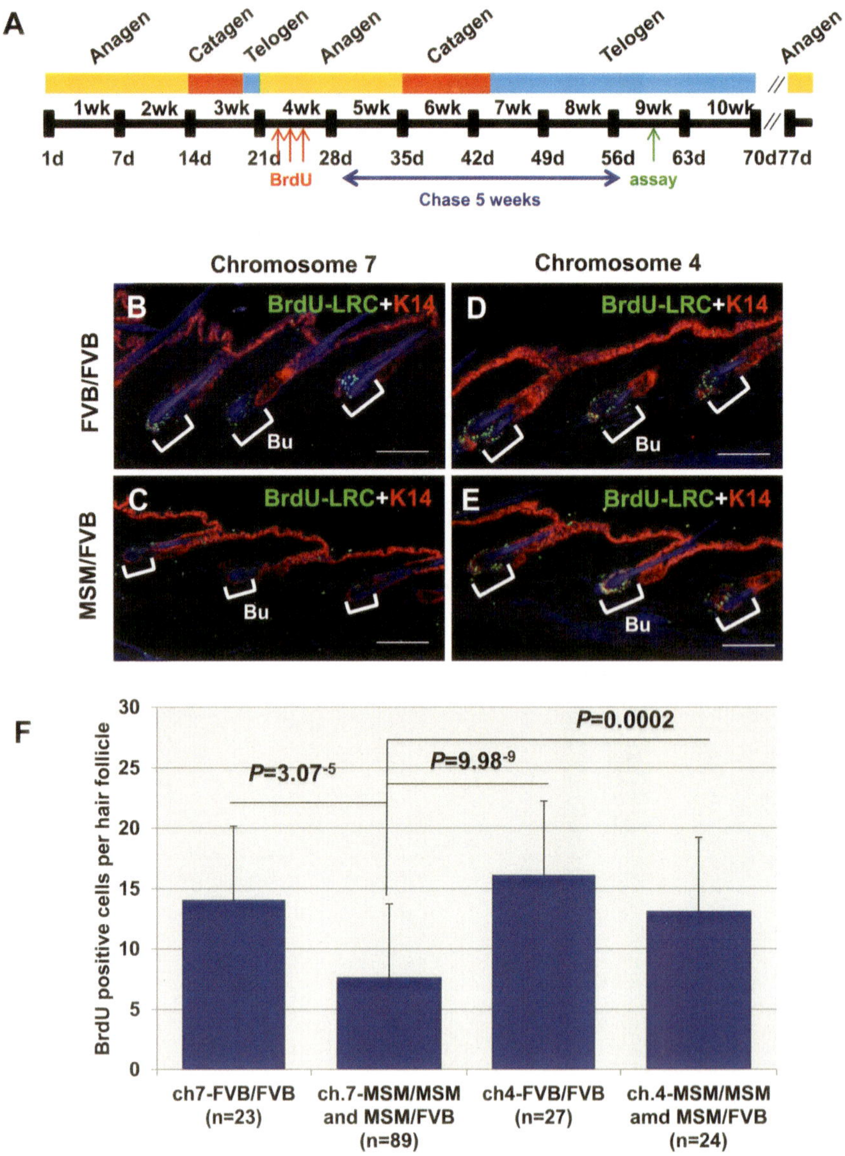

Figure 4. *Stmm1* congenic mice show a decrease of BrdU-LRCs. (A) The timetable of BrdU chase experiment. Multiple color bars indicate the mouse hair cycles (orange, anagen; red, catagen; and blue, telogen) and the bold black line below indicates the postnatal days of mice. (B) Representative double-immunostaining patterns of BrdU-LRCs (green) and Keratin 14 (K14) (red) in the skin from a FF homozygous of a congenic line (a) on chromosome 7, (C) a MF heterozygous mouse of a congenic line (a), (D) a FF homozygous mouse of a congenic line having the linkage region on chromosome 4, and (E) a MF heterozygous mice of a congenic line having the same linkage region on chromosome 4. (F) The numbers of BrdU-LRCs per hair follicle in dorsal back skin sections are plotted. The blue bars represent the number of BrdU-LRCs in each congenic line, FF homozygous mice of a congenic line (a) on chromosome 7 (n = 23), MF heterozygous and MM homozygous mice of a congenic line (a) (n = 89), FF homozygous mice of a congenic line having the linkage region on chromosome 4 (n = 27), and MF heterozygous and MM homozygous mice of a congenic line having the same linkage region on chromosome 4 (n = 24). The *P*-value was calculated for BrdU-LRC number by *t*-test. Error bar represents standard deviation (S.D.). Abbreviation: Bu, Bulge. Scale bars, 100 μm.

Cancer Center (Permit Number: 13–18). All efforts were made to minimize suffering. FVB/N mice were purchased from Japan Clea. MSM/Ms mice have been maintained in the Experimental Animal Facility at Niigata University and Chiba Cancer Centre for more than 20 years. In a large F1 backcross study using [(FVB/N×MSM/Ms)×FVB/N], papilloma resistance loci were identified by QTL analysis [16]. Resistant F1 backcross mice were selected for further backcrossing to FVB/N mice over at least 10 generations, ultimately leading to congenic lines (a) and (b) containing MSM/Ms allele of *Stmm1* and *2* on the FVB/N background (**Figure 1A**). Multiple congenic lines containing different overlapping regions were generated from line (a) mice (**Figure 2A**). These congenic mice were treated following the same skin tumor induction protocol, as reported previously [16]. In short, the mice (8–12 weeks) received a single dose of DMBA (25 μg per mouse with 200 μl of acetone) and, starting 1 week after initiation, the animals were subjected to TPA (200 μl of 0.1 mM solution in acetone) twice weekly for 20 weeks. Papilloma numbers were counted every week until 20 weeks after initiation.

DNA Preparation, Genotyping, and Allelotyping using Microsatellite Markers

DNA was prepared from papillomas, corresponding normal tail tips and kidneys. Microsatellite markers were amplified by standard methods. Each marker's order and distance were estimated from the Ensembl database (http://uswest.ensembl.org/index.html), the Mouse Genome Informatics Database (http://www.informatics.jax.org/), the NIG Mouse Genome Database (http://molossinus.lab.nig.ac.jp/msmdb/index.jsp), and the Mouse Microsatellite Database of Japan (http://www.shigen.nig.ac.jp/mouse/mmdbj/top.jsp). D7SNP markers and C7. loc64 are described in [16]. To determine susceptibility in congenic lines, unpaired two-tailed Student's t-test was used. Differences of 50% or more in the intensity ratios of the two alleles in papilloma DNA relative to the corresponding level in kidney as a normal control were defined as allelic imbalance by SSLP (Simple Sequence Length Polymorphisms) analysis, as previously described [16], [17]. Percentages of allelic imbalances in different crosses were compared using 2×2 Chi square test (Fisher's test).

BrdU Chase Experiment and Immunohistochemistry

For chase experiments, BrdU (Sigma-Aldrich) was administered by peritoneal injection to postnatal day 24 (P24) mice (40 µg per gram of bodyweight) on 3 consecutive days. Mice were then chased from day 24 to day 59. Chased skin tissues were fixed with 4% paraformaldehyde at 4°C overnight. The endogenous peroxidase activity in the specimens was blocked by treatment with 0.3% H_2O_2 and samples were then rinsed with PBS. Sections were incubated with primary antibodies diluted in blocking buffer overnight at 4°C and stained with rat anti-BrdU (1:100 Abcam) antibody and rabbit anti-keratin 14 (1:500, Covance Research). Secondary antibodies were Alexa Fluor 488-conjugated anti-rat antibody (1:100, Molecular Probes, Invitrogen) and Alexa Fluor 568-conjugated anti-rabbit antibody (1:100, Molecular Probes, Invitrogen). Nuclei were counterstained with Hard Set Mounting Medium with DAPI (Vector). All fluorescence images were obtained with a Leica TCS SPE confocal microscope equipped with a DMI4000B (10X/0.40, 20X/0.70, and 40x/1.25 oil immersion objective).

Acknowledgments

We'd like to thank Dr. Minh To for critical reading of the manuscript.

Author Contributions

Conceived and designed the experiments: KO YW. Performed the experiments: KO MS EI. Analyzed the data: IM SW. Contributed reagents/materials/analysis tools: RK. Contributed to the writing of the manuscript: KO YW.

References

1. Peto J (2001) Cancer epidemiology in the last century and the next decade. Nature. 411: 390–395.
2. Ponder BA (2001) Cancer genetics. Nature. 411: 336–341.
3. Balmain A (2002) Cancer as a complex genetic trait: tumor susceptibility in humans and mouse models. Cell. 108: 145–152.
4. Balmain A, Gtay J, Ponder BA (2003) The genetics and genomics of cancer. Nat. Genet. 33: 238–244.
5. Galvan A, Ioannidis JP, Dragani TA (2010) Beyond genome-wide association studies: genetic heterogeneity and individual predisposition to cancer. Trends Genet. 26: 132–41.
6. Stadler ZK, Thom P, Robson ME, Weitzel JN, Kauff ND, et al. (2010) Genome Wide Association Studies of Cancer. J. Clin. Oncol. 28: 4255–67.
7. Perez-Losada J, Castellanos-Martín A, Mao JH (2011) Cancer Evolution and Individual Susceptibility. Integrative Biology. 3: 316–328.
8. Manolio TA, Collins FS, Cox NJ, Goldstein DB, Hindorff LA, et al. (2009) Finding the missing heritability of complex diseases. Nature. 461: 747–753.
9. Hunter KW, Crawford NP (2008) The future of mouse QTL mapping to diagnose disease in mice in the age of whole-genome association studies. Annu. Rev. Genet. 42: 131–141.
10. Nagase H, Mao JH, de Koning JP, Minami T, Balmain A (2001) Epistatic interactions between skin tumor modifier loci in interspecific (spretus/musculus) backcross mice. Cancer Res. 61: 1305–1308.
11. DiGiovanni J, Imamoto A, Naito M, Walker SE, Beltrán L, et al. (1992) Further genetic analyses of skin tumor promoter susceptibility using inbred and recombinant inbred mice. Carcinogenesis. 13: 525–531.
12. Nagase H, Bryson S, Cordell H, Kemp CJ, Fee F, et al. (1995) Distinct genetic loci control development of benign and malignant skin tumors in mice. Nat. Genet. 10: 424–429.
13. Ewart-Toland A, Briassouli P, de Koning JP, Mao JH, Yuan J, et al. (2003) Identification of Stk6/STK15 as a candidate low-penetrance tumor-susceptibility gene in mouse and human. Nat. Genet. 34: 403–412.
14. Fujiwara K, Igarashi J, Irahara N, Kimura M, Nagase H (2007) New chemically induced skin tumour susceptibility loci identified in a mouse backcross between FVB and dominant resistant PWK. BMC Genet. 8: 39.
15. Fujiwara K, Wie B, Elliott R, Nagase H (2010) New outbred colony derived from Mus musculus castaneus to identify skin tumor susceptibility loci. Mol. Carcinog. 49: 653–661.
16. Okumura K, Sato M, Saito M, Miura I, Wakana S, et al. (2012) Independent genetic control of early and late stages of chemically induced skin tumors in a cross of a Japanese wild-derived inbred mouse strain, MSM/Ms. Carcinogenesis. 33: 2260–2268.
17. de Koning JP, Wakabayashi Y, Nagase H, Mao JH, Balmain A (2007) Convergence of congenic mapping and allele-specific alterations in tumors for the resolution of the Skts1 skin tumor susceptibility locus. Oncogene. 26: 4171–4178.
18. Dong S, Guo AL, Chen ZH, Wang Z, Zhang XC, et al. (2010) RRM1 single nucleotide polymorphism −37C -> A correlates with progression-free survival in NSCLC patients after gemcitabine-based chemotherapy. J. Hematol. Oncol. 3: 10.
19. Gough SM, Slape CI, Aplan PD (2011) NUP98 gene fusions and hematopoietic malignancies: common themes and new biologic insights. Blood. 118: 6247–6257.
20. Parri M, Chiarugi P (2010) Rac and Rho GTPases in cancer cell motility control. Cell Commun. Signal. 8: 23.
21. Kwiatkowska A, Didier S, Fortin S, Chuang Y, White T, et al. (2012) The small GTPase RhoG mediates glioblastoma cell invasion. Mol. Cancer. 11: 65.
22. Kangsamaksin T, Park HJ, Trempus CS, Morris RJ (2007) A perspective on murine keratinocyte stem cells as targets of chemically induced skin cancer. Mol Carcinog. 46: 579–584.
23. Morris RJ, Fischer SM, Slaga TJ (1985) Evidence that the centrally and peripherally located cells in the murine epidermal proliferative unit are two distinct cell populations. J. Invest. Dermatol. 84, 277–281.
24. Morris RJ, Fischer SM, Slaga TJ (1986) Evidence that a slowly cycling subpopulation of adult murine epidermal cells retains carcinogen. Cancer Res. 46, 3061–3066.
25. Morris RJ, Coulter K, Tryson K, Steinberg SR (1997) Evidence that cutaneous carcinogen-initiated epithelial cells from mice are quiescent rather than actively cycling. Cancer Res. 57: 3436–3443.

3

Resveratrol and Black Tea Polyphenol Combination Synergistically Suppress Mouse Skin Tumors Growth by Inhibition of Activated MAPKs and p53

Jasmine George, Madhulika Singh, Amit Kumar Srivastava, Kulpreet Bhui, Preeti Roy, Pranav Kumar Chaturvedi, Yogeshwer Shukla*

Proteomics Laboratory, Indian Institute of Toxicology Research, Council of Scientific and Industrial Research (CSIR), Uttar Pradesh, India

Abstract

Cancer chemoprevention by natural dietary agents has received considerable importance because of their cost-effectiveness and wide safety margin. However, single agent intervention has failed to bring the expected outcome in clinical trials; therefore, combinations of chemopreventive agents are gaining increasing popularity. The present study aims to evaluate the combinatorial chemopreventive effects of resveratrol and black tea polyphenol (BTP) in suppressing two-stage mouse skin carcinogenesis induced by DMBA and TPA. Resveratrol/BTP alone treatment decreased tumor incidence by ~67% and ~75%, while combination of both at low doses synergistically decreased tumor incidence even more significantly by ~89% ($p<0.01$). This combination also significantly regressed tumor volume and number ($p<0.01$). Mechanistic studies revealed that this combinatorial inhibition was associated with decreased expression of phosphorylated mitogen-activated protein kinase family proteins: extracellular signal-regulated kinase 1/2, c-Jun N-terminal kinase 1/2, p38 and increased in total p53 and phospho p53 (Ser 15) in skin tissue/tumor. Treatment with combinations of resveratrol and BTP also decreased expression of proliferating cell nuclear antigen in mouse skin tissues/tumors than their solitary treatments as determined by immunohistochemistry. In addition, histological and cell death analysis also confirmed that resveratrol and BTP treatment together inhibits cellular proliferation and markedly induces apoptosis. Taken together, our results for the first time lucidly illustrate that resveratrol and BTP in combination impart better suppressive activity than either of these agents alone and accentuate that development of novel combination therapies/chemoprevention using dietary agents will be more beneficial against cancer. This promising combination should be examined in therapeutic trials of skin and possibly other cancers.

Editor: Fatah Kashanchi, George Mason University, United States of America

Funding: This work was supported by a research grant from Network Project (NWP-017), Council of Scientific & Industrial Research (CSIR), New Delhi, India. The funders had no role in study design, data collection and analysis, decision to publish, or preparation of the manuscript.

Competing Interests: The authors have declared that no competing interests exist.

* E-mail: yogeshwer_shukla@hotmail.com

Introduction

Since early in the history of medicine, an association between diet and cancer has persisted. The most consistent findings on diet as a determinant of several types of cancers risk prevention is the association with consumption of fruits and vegetables [1]. To date, hundreds of natural or synthetic compounds have been found to possess promising cancer chemopreventive actions. When reviewing the literature on the effects of several dietary agents in animal and in vitro studies, there is ample evidence that specific antioxidants and other phytochemicals present in foods of plant origin protect against genotoxicity and other cancer-initiating or -promoting processes [2,3].

The concept of using a combination of agents for cancer chemoprevention has recently received much attention. Considerable evidence from laboratories studies suggests that combinations of chemopreventive agents can be more effective for the prevention of cancer than any single constituent. Recently, Xu et al. [4] showed that combination treatment of curcumin and green tea catechins prevent dimethylhydrazine-induced colon carcinogenesis rat model more potently than each of the compounds alone. In another recent study, genistein-selenium combination significantly inhibited growth of LNCaP and PC3 cells in a dose- and time-dependent manner by decreasing matrix metalloproteins-2 levels [5]. Zhou et al. [6] identified the possible chemopreventive effects of soy and tea components on prostate tumor progression in in vivo. The combination of both synergistically inhibited final tumor weight and metastasis and significantly reduced serum concentrations of testosterone and dihydrotestosterone. Our laboratory is actively investigating the hypothesis that combinations of food-based cancer prevention strategies will be a highly effective strategy for the reduction of carcinogenesis. During this course we have investigated that combination of pomegranate fruit extract and diallyl sulfide synergistically inhibited mouse skin tumor growth through reduce proliferation, inhibition of mitogen-activated protein kinase (MAPKs) and nuclear factor- kappa B (NF-κB) signaling and induction of apoptotic cell death [7]. Now, we have chosen to focus our experimental efforts on resveratrol and black tea polyphenol (BTP), two foods frequently cited to protect humans from skin carcinogenesis [8,9].

Resveratrol (3,4,5-trihydroxy-trans-stilbene), a natural plant polyphenol is widely present in foods such as grapes, wine and peanuts. One of the most striking biological activities of resveratrol intensely investigated during the last years has been its anti-cancer and anti-inflammation properties. These properties were first appreciated when Jang et al. [10] demonstrated that resveratrol possesses cancer-chemopreventive and cytostatic properties via the three major stages of carcinogenesis, i.e. initiation, promotion and progression. Since then, there has been a flurry of papers reporting the implication of resveratrol in cancer chemoprevention through a wide range of actions [11]. Most of the cancer chemopreventive evidence for resveratrol is well documented in various cancers such as those of hepatocellular, lung, skin and prostate by multiple regulatory mechanisms [12,13,14,15]. Kundu et al. [16] showed that resveratrol exert anti-tumor promoting in the 12-O-tetradecanoylphorbol 13-acetate (TPA)- induced mouse skin carcinogenesis model suppression of cyclooxygenase-2 expression by blocking the activation of MAPKs and activator protein. Previously study from our laboratory have reported that resveratrol-induces apoptosis in 7, 12-dimethylbenz[a]anthracene (DMBA)-initiated and TPA promoted, mouse skin tumors through cell cycle arrest, activation of p53 activity and alteration of apoptosis-related proteins [17].

Tea, the most widely consumed beverage has received a great deal of attention because of its polyphenolic constituents known to have strong antioxidants and inhibitory activity against tumorigenesis [18]. Many studies have demonstrated the anti-inflammatory and anti-tumor effects of BTP; it can inhibit proliferation and metastasis and induce apoptosis in various malignant tumors, including skin cancer, by modulating several different signal pathways [19,20,21]. Epidemiological studies on black tea and cancer are limited, but several investigators have demonstrated positive correlations between black tea consumption and a lower incidence of breast [22] and ovarian [23] cancer. BTP treatment has been shown to induce apoptosis in prostate cancer cells by induction of p53, down-regulation of NF-κB activity, causing a change in the ratio of pro-and anti-apoptotic proteins and inhibiting expression of activated MAPKs [24].

It is clear that resveratrol and BTP independently have biological activities for cancer prevention purposes, however, productive application of these two compounds in combination to exert synergistic effects against cancer inflammation and growth of tumor warrants further studies. Therefore, multiple properties of resveratrol and BTP in cancer prevention lead us to assume a more benefit in combining these two agents rather than the single agents for cancer prevention and therapy. Thus the present study was designed to investigate whether resveratrol in combination with BTP at low doses synergistically suppress the DMBA-initiated, TPA- promoted two-stage mouse skin tumors. Our results clearly demonstrate that a combination of resveratrol and BTP can synergistically inhibit the development and progression of mouse skin tumors then their solitary treatment.

Materials and Methods

Materials

DMBA, TPA, resveratrol, β-actin (clone AC-74) and propidium iodide (PI) were purchased from Sigma Chemical Co. (St. Louis, USA). Annexin-V and PI fluorescein isothiocyanate (FITC) detection Kit was purchased from BD (San Jose, CA, USA). Purified BTP (>98% pure) was kindly gifted by M/S Indfrag company, Bangalore, India. Hydroxylapatite and N, N-dimethylformamide was purchased from Sisco Research Laboratory (Mumbai, India). The mouse monoclonal total and phospho specific antibodies for p38, p53, c-Jun N-terminal kinase (JNK1/2) (Thr183/Tyr185), p44/42 MAPK (Thr202/Tyr204) i.e extracellular signal-regulated kinase (ERK1/2) were purchased from Cell Signaling Technology (Beverly, USA). Proliferating cell nuclear antigen (PCNA) antibody was obtained from Santa Cruz Biotechnology (Santa Cruz, CA, USA). The rabbit anti-mouse or goat anti-rabbit horse radish peroxidase (HRP) conjugate secondary antibodies were obtained from Bangalore Genei (Bangalore, India). The poly(vinylidene) fluoride (PVDF) membranes were obtained from Millipore (Billerica, MA, USA). Other used chemicals were of analytical grade and procured locally.

Animals and treatments

Male, Balb/c mice (15–18 g body weight [b. wt.]) were obtained from the Indian Institute of Toxicology Research (Lucknow, India) animal breeding colony. Prior ethical approval for the experiments was obtained from institutional ethical committee. All animals were quarantined in polypropylene cages under standard laboratory conditions (temperature 23±2°C, relative humidity 55±5%, 12/12 h light/dark cycle) and were fed solid pellet diet (Ashirwad, Chandigarh, India) and water ad libitum. After a week of acclimatization animals were used for further experiments.

Long term animal bioassay: For treatment, animals were randomly divided into 6 groups consisting 25 animals in each. Animals of all groups were carefully shaved on dorsal skin in the interscapular region of 2 cm^2. DMBA (tumor initiator), TPA (tumor promoter) and resveratrol were dissolved in acetone. In brief, treatment was given as described below for 18 weeks of duration to attain the entire period of skin tumorigenicity:

Group I- No treatment was given to the animals and served as untreated controls.

Group II- DMBA+TPA (animals were treated with single topical application of DMBA (52 μg/animal), one week later followed by topical application of TPA (5 μg/animal) thrice in a week throughout the experimental period and served as positive controls).

Group III- Acetone+Resveratrol+BTP (200 μL acetone was applied topically followed by topical treatment of 50 μM/animal resveratrol to each animal and 0.2% BTP was given as sole source of drinking fluid thrice a week).

Group IV- DMBA+TPA+resveratrol (50 μM/animal resveratrol was given topically to the animals as mentioned in group III, rest of the treatments was same as in group II).

Group V- DMBA+TPA+BTP (treatment of DMBA was similar as in group II after a week followed by TPA application and 0.2% BTP supplementation as in group II and III, respectively).

Group VI- DMBA+TPA+resveratrol+BTP (DMBA and TPA application was same as in group II, resveratrol (25 μM/animal) application and BTP (0.1%) supplementation as in group III).

During treatment period animals were carefully observed for any change in b. wt., fluid/food intake and development of skin tumor. Tumors >1 mm in diameter were considered in the cumulative number if they persist for 2 weeks or more. After completion of 18 weeks of treatments duration, the regression of pattern of tumors in terms of both number and volume were recorded up to 26 weeks in the animals of groups IV, V and VI (bearing tumor or not). These were divided into 3 subgroups and treatment schedule was as follow:

Group IV A - VI A: comprises animals' without tumor and no further treatment was given to these groups.

Group IV B and C- comprises tumor bearing animals' and treatment of TPA+resveratrol and only TPA was withdrawn, respectively.

Group V B and C- comprises tumor bearing animals' and treatment of TPA+BTP and only TPA was withdrawn, respectively.

Group VI B and C- comprises tumor bearing animals' and treatment of TPA+resveratrol+BTP and only TPA was withdrawn, respectively.

After completion of the study period (26 weeks), all the animals of groups IV–VI (A–C) were first examined for tumor volume/number regression and thereafter sacrificed. Tumor volume was calculated per mouse in each group using formula $V = D \times d2 \times \pi / 6$, where D = bigger dimension and d = smaller dimension. Skin from the painted area (with or without tumors) was excised out, cleaned, snap frozen in liquid nitrogen, and stored at −80°C until further use.

Synergy between resveratrol and BTP combination

The nature of the combined effects of resveratrol and BTP was determined using the method described by Zhou et al. [6], based on the principles described by Chou and Talalay [25]. In brief, the expected value of combination effect between agent 1 and agent 2 is calculated as [(observed agent 1 value)/(control value)] × [(observed agent 2 value)/(control value)] × (control value); and the ratio is calculated as (expected value)/(observed value). A ratio of >1 indicates a synergistic effect, and a ratio of <1 indicates a less than additive effect.

Short term animal bioassay: Animals were divided into 6 groups of 5 in each and doses for selected treatments was same as detailed in long term study section for 2 weeks period. Briefly, groups and treatments are as below:

Group I: Untreated control (No treatment).

Group II: DMBA+TPA (single dose of DMBA was applied topically one week later followed by TPA application 4 times in a week).

Group III: Acetone+resveratrol+BTP (animals were treated with acetone and 50 μM resveratrol topically, and 0.2% BTP as sole source of drinking fluid for 4 times in a week).

Group IV: DMBA+TPA+resveratrol (DMBA and TPA application as in Gr. II and resveratrol treatment as in group III).

Group V: DMBA+TPA+BTP (DMBA and TPA application as in Gr. II and BTP supplementation as in group III).

Group VI: DMBA+TPA+resveratrol+BTP (DMBA and TPA application as in Gr. II and, resveratrol (25 μM/animal) and BTP (0.1%) treatment as in group III).

At the end of the experimental period all the animals were sacrificed and skin from the painted area was excised out, cleaned, snap frozen in liquid nitrogen, and stored at −80°C until further use.

Preparation of lysates

Whole skin tissue/tumor homogenates (10%) were made as described by Kataoka et al. [26], in both, the long term as well as the short term study. The supernatants were collected and stored at −80°C till use.

Western blotting

Western blotting was carried out as described earlier [27]. Protein concentration was measured following standard protocols [28]. Proteins (60 μg) were resolved on 10–12% SDS PAGE and electroblotted on PVDF membrane. The blots were blocked overnight with 5% non-fat dry milk and probed with antibodies at dilutions recommended by the suppliers. Immunoblots were detected through chemiluminescence using kit of Millipore (Billerica, MA, USA).

Histopathological analysis

Paraffin sections (5 μm) of the skin tissues/tumors were stained with haematoxylin and eosin for histopathological analysis. Histopathological observations were made according to Bogovaski [29].

Immunohistochemical (IHC) staining

Buffered formalin fixed and paraffin embedded skin/tumor tissues were cut into sections (5 μm thick), which were subsequently de-waxed and hydrated. Then endogenous peroxidase activity was quenched and epitope retrieval was performed. This was followed by blocking of non-specific binding of primary antibody to epitopes by a preincubation step with normal serum. Sections were then incubated overnight with the primary monoclonal anti-PCNA (1:100) antibody. After incubation, the sections were again incubated with normal serum and then with HRP-conjugated secondary antibody. The colour was developed using substrate chromogen system diaminobenzidine (Dako, CA, USA). For the negative control, phosphate-buffered saline was used in place of the primary antibody. The immunostained slides were analyzed under microscope (Leica, Wetzler, Germany) attached with charge coupled device camera (JVC).

Annexin-V and PI dual staining

Annexin-V and PI FITC detection Kit (BD, San Jose, CA, USA) was used for the differentiation between apoptotic and necrotic cell population. The single cell suspensions of treated and untreated skin tissues (from short term study) were prepared using Medimachine (Beckton Dickinson, San Jose, USA). For each sample, Annexin-V/PI fluorescence was analyzed, wherein fluorescence of cells was gated and counted using 'Cell Quest 3.1 software'.

DNA alkaline unwinding assay

Strand breaks in cellular DNA were quantitated by alkaline unwinding assay using hydroxyapatite batch procedure as described previously [30]. In brief, 100 μg of DNA from treated and untreated skin tissue samples (from short term study) was subjected to alkaline unwinding and the relative amount of duplex and single stranded DNA present at the end of the alkaline unwinding was quantified.

Statistical analysis

For the statistical analysis of skin tumor appearance dynamics, the Kaplan-Meier method of tumor-free survival estimation was applied. Statistically significant differences were determined between control and treatment groups using one-way ANOVA (GraphPad Prism software) followed by Dunnett post hoc test. Values with $p<0.05$ were considered significant.

Results

Effects of resveratrol and/or BTP on tumorigenicity rate

The b. wt. of each animal was recorded every week during the entire period of the experiment. Compared with the untreated control (group I), mice on DMBA and TPA treatment (group II) showed a significant reduction in b. wt. However, there was an increasing percentage of change in the b. wt. gain of the animal of the experimental treatments (groups III–VI) (data not shown). The first day of tumor incidence in the positive control (DMBA and TPA) group II was 48th day; however, it was 63th day in resveratrol treated group IV, 58th day in BTP treated group V and 84th day in the resveratrol and BTP treated group VI. There was no tumor induction in group III. The chemopreventive potential of resveratrol and BTP was also evident by significant ($p<0.01$) increase in tumor free survival of animals. 36%, 48% and 72% of animals of group IV, V and VI, respectively, remained tumor-free till the termination of the experiment. However, in positive control group (II) 100% animals were observed with tumors by the end of 18th week (Figure 1A). The expected effect of the resveratrol/BTP combination on tumorigenicity rate (33%) was greater than the observed combination effect (28%) with a ratio of 1.17, suggesting that the resveratrol/BTP combination had a synergistic inhibitory effect on tumorigenicity (Table 1).

Protection was also seen in terms of reduction in tumor volume. The tumor volume was 130.0 mm3/mouse in DMBA and TPA group, which reduced to 52.6, 63.2 and 24.6 mm3/mouse in group IV, V and VI, respectively. The expected effect of the combined resveratrol and BTP on average tumor volume (19.7%) was higher than the observed combined effect (18.9%) with a ratio of 1.05, suggesting that resveratrol and BTP combination also had synergistic effect in reducing the tumor volume (Table 1).

Protection afforded by resveratrol and BTP was also evident in terms of reduction in the cumulative number of tumors (CNT). While the positive control group showed 230 CNT, group IV, V and VI showed 71, 89, and 25 CNT, respectively, at 18th week (Figure 1B). The observed effect (10.9%) in combination group VI was less than the expected value (11.9%), with ratio of 1.09, suggesting that resveratrol and BTP combination synergistically reduces CNT (Table 1).

When these tumor data were considered in terms of number of tumors per mice, at the termination of the experiment at 18 weeks on test, compared with 9.2 tumors per mouse in DMBA and TPA treated group, 4.4, 5.7 and only 2.5 tumors per mouse in group was recorded in group IV, V and VI, respectively (Figure 1C). Compared with the solitary resveratrol (75%) and BTP (67%) treated groups, decrease in the number of tumor per mouse in combination-treated group corresponded to 89% inhibition. The observed effect (27.2%) in combination group VI was less than the expected value (29.6%), with ratio of 1.08, suggesting that resveratrol and BTP combination also synergistically reduces CNT (Table 1).

Effects of resveratrol and/or BTP on tumor growth and regression

We further extended the work to observe regression offered by combined doses of resveratrol and BTP in tumor volume and number if any. At 19th week, TPA treatment was ceased and

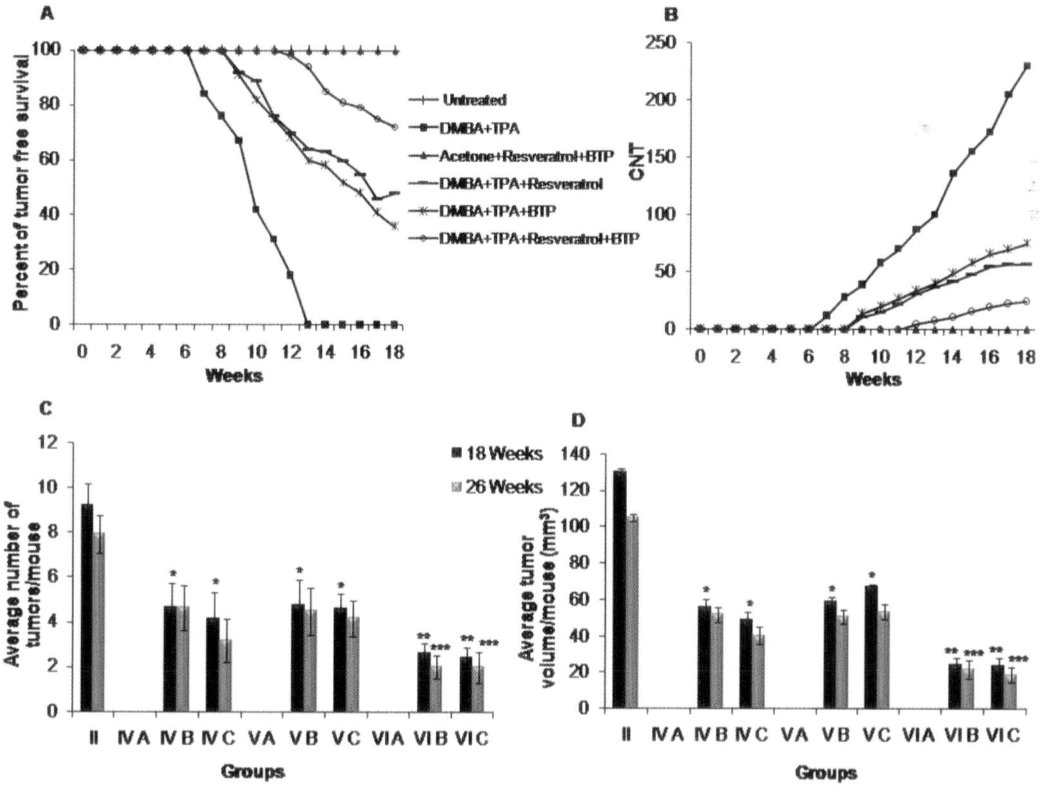

Figure 1. Effect of resveratrol and/or BTP on DMBA and TPA-induced mouse skin tumors. (A) Percentage of tumor-free survival, (B) cumulative number of tumors (CNT) per group, (C) reduction in average no. of tumors/mouse and (c) reduction in tumor volume/mouse (mm^3). The data showed are of surviving animals upto 18th weeks in (A), (B) and (C) however, mean±SD of surviving animals from 18th to 26th weeks in (D). * indicates significant reduction over DMBA and TPA treated group II at 18th week ($p<0.01$). ** indicates significant reduction over resveratrol and BTP alone treated groups at 18th week ($p<0.01$). *** indicates significant reduction after 26th weeks ($p<0.01$).

Table 1. Possible synergistic chemopreventive effect of the interaction between Res and BTP against DMBA and TPA-induced mouse skin tumorigenesis.

Treatment (Groups)	Tumorigenicity (%)			CNT (%)			ANT (%)			ATV (%)		
	O	E[a]	R[b]	O	E[a]	R[b]	O	E[a]	R[b]	O	E[a]	R[b]
Untreated control (I)												
DMBA+TPA (II)	100.0			100.0			100.0			100.0		
Acetone+Res+BTP (III)												
DMBA+TPA+Res (IV)	64.0			30.9			47.8			40.5		
DMBA+TPA+BTP (V)	52.0			38.7			62.0			48.6		
DMBA+TPA+Res+BTP (VI)	28.0	33.0	1.17	10.9	11.9	1.09	27.1	30.0	1.08	18.9	19.7	1.03

All the data are statistically significant, $p<0.01$.
[a]Expected value of Res and BTP combination = [(observed value of Res)/(control value)] × [(observed value of BTP)/(control value)] × (control value).
[b]Ratio = (expected value/observed value). A ratio of >1 indicates a synergistic effect, and a ratio of <1 indicates a less than additive effect.
O, observed; E, expected; R, ratio; Res, resveratrol; CNT, cumulative number of tumors; ANT, average number of tumors/mouse; ATV, average tumor volume/tumor bearing mouse.

morphological changes of the tumors were recorded in group IV B, IV C, V B, V C, VI B and VI C. Among these groups, in Gr. VI C, major commencement of regression was recorded from 22nd week onwards ($p<0.01$). Apparently, group VI B from which resveratrol and BTP were withdrawn showed regression in terms of both tumor volume and number (Table 2). The tumor volume at 26th week reduced to 105.4 mm^3/mouse in DMBA and TPA group II, 21.8 mm^3/mouse in group VI B and 18.9 mm^3/mouse in group VI C (Table 2, Figure 1D). CNT reduced to 198, 10 and 6 in group II, VI B and VI C, respectively (Table 2). Changes in both tumor number and volume were also observed in solitary resveratrol and BTP treated groups (IV B, IV C, V B and V C) but the extent was lesser than combination (Table 2, Figure 1D). Moreover, animals of group VI A did not show any morphological changes as well as development of tumors till the termination of the experiment (Table 2). Thus, combined supplementation of resveratrol and BTP resulted in regression in both tumor volume and number and imparts better efficacy in terms of tumor regression then either of these agents alone.

Effect of resveratrol and/or BTP on phosphorylated MAPKs

It has been reported that topical application of TPA in mouse skin results in a marked increase in the phosphorylated form of MAPKs [31], affecting fundamental cellular processes like proliferation, differentiation, and survival, thus we further evaluated the expression levels of MAPK family proteins [32]. In the present study, western blot analysis showed that the activation of MAPKs (ERK1/2 , JNK1/2 and p38) was gradually increased during progression of TPA-induced papillomagenesis in DMBA-initiated mouse skin over untreated control group ($p<0.05$), in both long and short term studies (Figure 2A and B). However, supplementation of

Table 2. Combinatorial chemopreventive effect of Res and/or BTP on tumor regression.

Groups	Treatment	Number of animals with tumors		CNT		ANT (Mean ± SD)		ATV (Mean ± SD)	
		18th	26th	18th	26th	18th	26th	18th	26th
II	DMBA+TPA	25/25	25/25	230	198	9.2±2.6	7.92±2.1	130.0±10.2	105.4±10.4
IV A	(−)Res-Non-tumor bearing	0/12	0/12	-	-	-	-	-	-
IV B	(−)Res-tumor bearing	6/6	6/6	34[a]	28[a]	5.66±1.9[a]	5.66±2.0[a]	56.1±7.2[a]	51.8±6.0[a]
IV C	(+)Res-tumor bearing	7/7	7/7	35[a]	26[a]	5.00±1.1[a]	3.71±2.5[a]	49.1±6.1[a]	40.3±5.5[a]
V A	(−)BTP-Non-tumor bearing	0/9	0/9	-	-	-	-	-	-
V B	(−)BTP-tumor bearing	8/8	8/8	42[a]	36[a]	5.25±2.1[a]	4.5±2.2[a]	59.3±6.2[a]	50.8±6.6[a]
V C	(+)BTP-tumor bearing	8/8	8/8	46[a]	34[a]	5.75±2.1[a]	4.2±2.6[a]	67.1±5.4[a]	53.6±7.5[a]
VI A	(−)Res+BTP-Non-tumor bearing	0/13	0/13	-	-	-	-	-	-
VI B	(−)Res+BTP-tumor bearing	5/5	5/5	13[b]	10[b]	2.6±2.0[b]	2.0±2.0[c]	24.2±5.4[b]	21.8±5.6[c]
VI C	(+)Res+BTP-tumor bearing	5/5	3/5	12[b]	6[b]	2.4±1.6[b]	2.0±1.6[c]	23.9±7.4[b]	18.9±8.6[c]

[a]significant reduction over DMBA and TPA treated group II at 18th week ($p<0.01$).
[b]significant reduction over BTP and Res alone treated groups IV B–C and V B–C at 18th week ($p<0.01$).
[c]significant reduction at 26th week ($p<0.01$).
(−) indicates without treatment, (+) indicates with treatment.
Res, resveratrol; CNT, cumulative number of tumors; ANT, average number of tumors/mouse; ATV, average tumor volume/tumor bearing mouse.

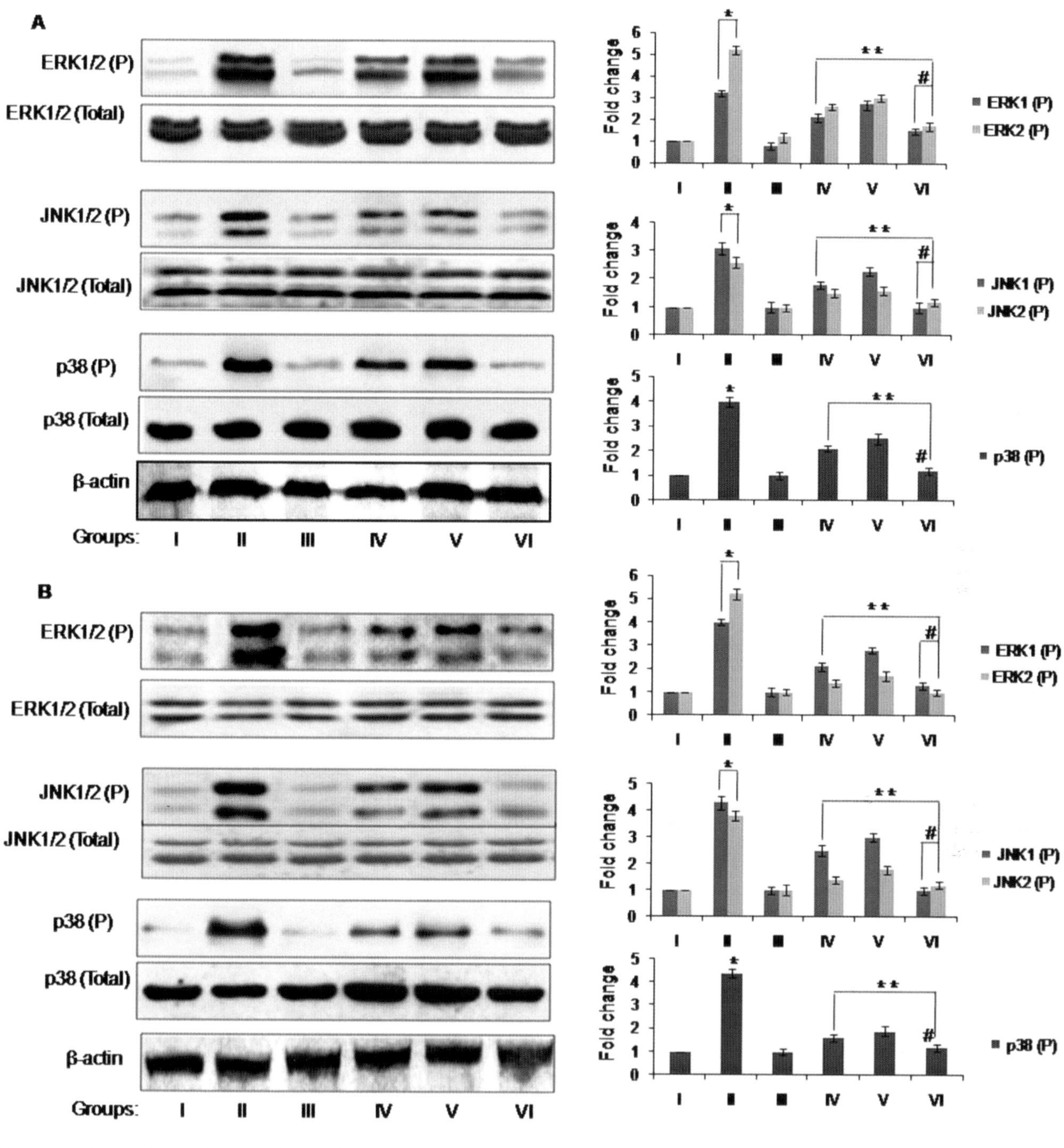

Figure 2. Western blots showing the inhibitory effect of resveratrol and/or BTP on the expression levels of total and phospho-ERK1/2, JNK1/2 and p38 in mouse skin tumors. (A) Long and (B) short term studies. Details for groups and treatments are described in Materials and methods section. The bands shown here are from a representative experiment repeated three times with similar results. Equal loading was confirmed by stripping the immunoblot and reprobing it for β-actin. The pixel density of the specific immunoreactive bands was quantified by densitometry and expressed as a fold difference against β-actin. * more than corresponding value of untreated control group I ($p<0.05$). **less than corresponding value of DMBA and TPA group II ($p<0.05$). # less than corresponding value of BTP and Res alone treated groups IV and V ($p<0.05$).

combined and solitary doses of resveratrol and BTP in DMBA and TPA treated animals, significantly ($p<0.05$) down-regulated the expression levels of ERK1/2, JNK1/2 and p38 through inhibition of their phosphorylation as compared to animals of group II, in both experimental sets (Figure 2A and B). There was no effect on the total amount of ERK1/2, JNK1/2 and p38 proteins after DMBA and TPA treatment (Figure 2A and B).

Effect of resveratrol and/or BTP on histopathology of skin/tumor

Histologically skin tumor sections from DMBA and TPA applied group II exhibited varying degrees of structural and cytological changes as compared to untreated control group I (Figure 3A). Tumors section of group II animals exhibit focal proliferation of squamous cells, presence of some necrotic cells and keratinization (Figure 3A). This clearly indicates the benign nature of tumors initiated and promoted by DMBA and TPA, respectively. However, skin sections from animals treated with resveratrol/BTP (group III), did not reveal any histopathological abnormalities (Figure 3A). The administration of both resveratrol and BTP led to suppression of DMBA and TPA induced skin tumorigenesis which was evident by skin/tumor sections (Figure 3A). Skin tumor sections of group VI showed chances towards normalization of skin as compared to group II (Figure 3A).

Similarly, in short term experimental groups' haematoxylin and eosin stained sections were showing pronounced preventive effects of resveratrol and BTP treatment when given in combination than alone over DMBA and TPA -induced changes in animals skin (Figure 3B). In group II, disorganization of epithelium, presence of necrotic cells and focal proliferative area were noticed as compared to group I (Figure 3B).

Effect of resveratrol and/or BTP on proliferation marker

IHC analysis of PCNA was used to assess the proliferation activity during tumor promotion (Figure 3A). PCNA reactivity is associated with S phase of DNA replication [33]. It was observed that PCNA labelling indices were higher in animals treated with DMBA and TPA as compared to other groups. A characteristic intense staining and higher number of PCNA positive cells were observed as shown in Figure 4A. The representative untreated control group did not show significant positive staining (Figure 4A). Further, treatment of resveratrol and BTP resulted in low expression levels of PCNA positive cells ($p<0.01$) as compared to group II revealing that effects of combinational treatment of resveratrol and BTP were superior to single treatment (Figure 4A).

Similarly, PCNA staining were analyzed to determine the proliferative status of skin after treatment with DMBA and TPA and the respective preventive treatments in short term groups (Figure 4B). It was observed that the number of PCNA positive cells were higher in animals of group II as compared to untreated animals (Figure 4B). The skin sections from untreated animals did not show significant positive staining for PCNA ($p<0.01$). Treatment with either resveratrol or BTP or both in combination in DMBA and TPA applied animals resulted in significantly low level of PCNA positive cells ($p<0.01$) (Figure 4B).

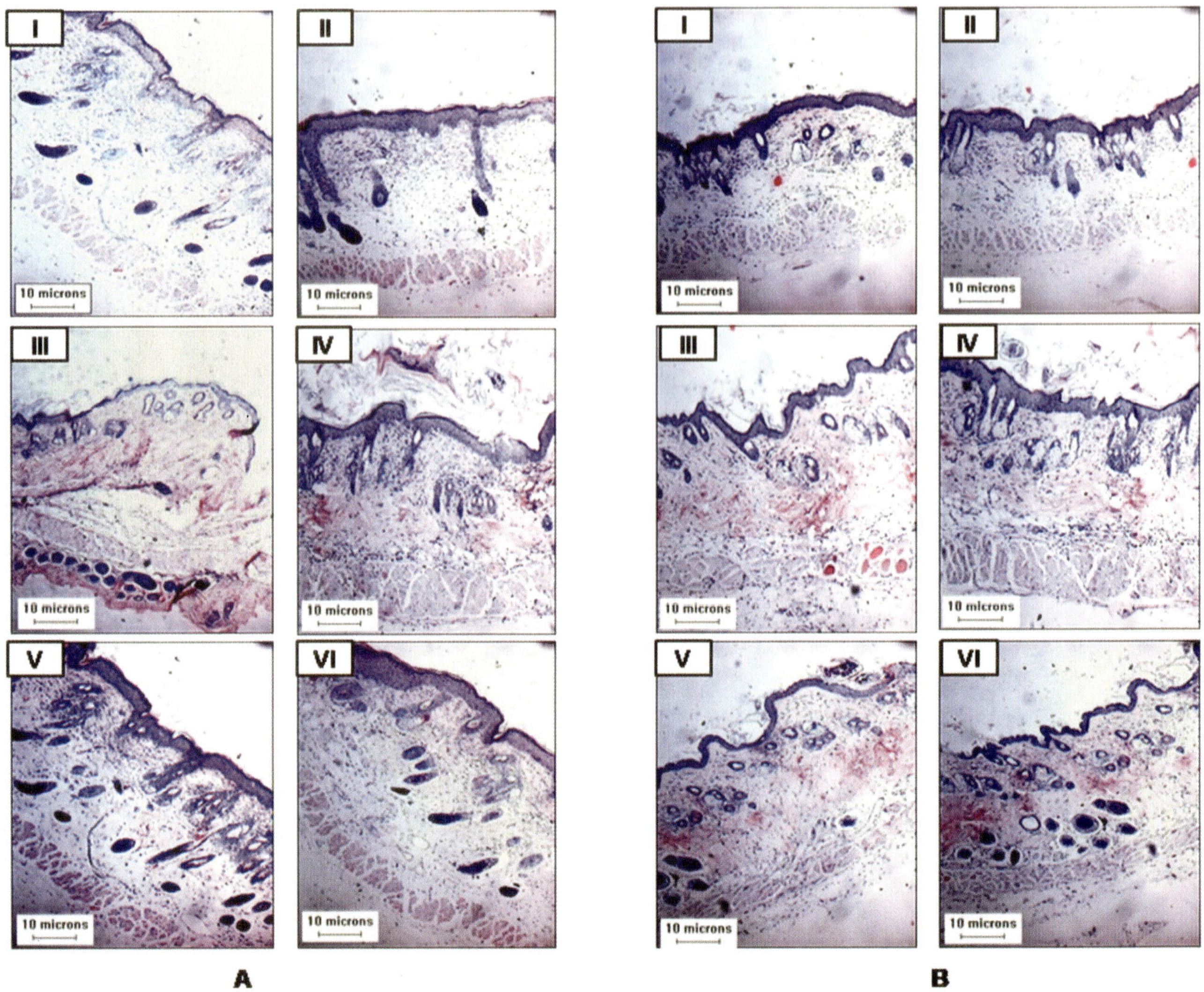

Figure 3. Histological study of mouse skin/tumors. (A) Long and (B) short term experimental groups. Details for groups and treatments are described in Materials and methods section.

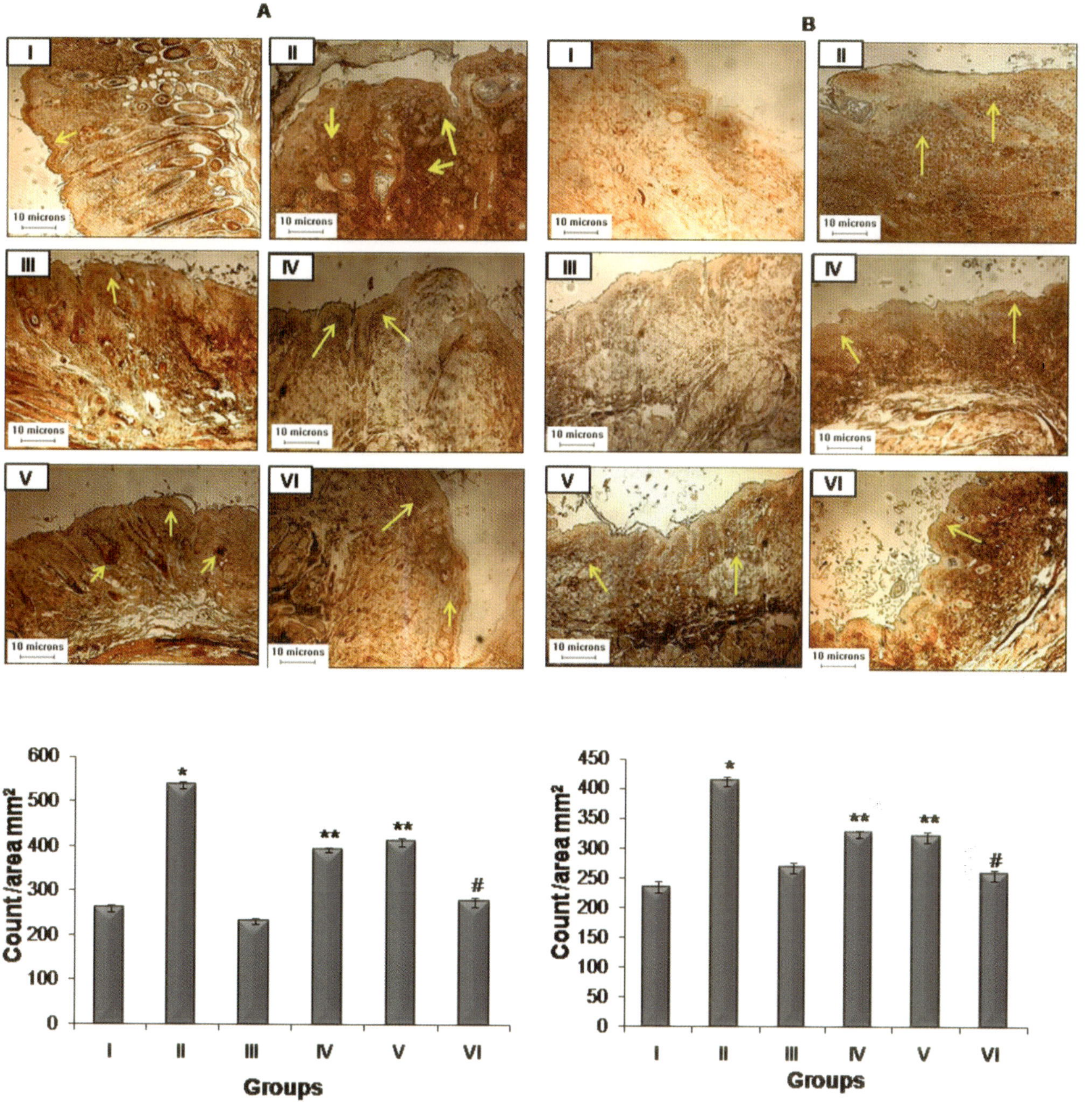

Figure 4. Effects of resveratrol and BTP treatment on modulation of PCNA expression. (A) Long and (B) short term experiments. Details are described in Materials and methods section. The brown colour nuclei mark the reactivity with PCNA indicated by arrows. Bar diagram shows mean ± SD of three independent sets analysis. *significantly increased in comparison of group I ($p<0.01$), **significantly decreased when compared with group II ($p<0.01$). #significantly decreased when compared with groups IV and V ($p<0.01$).

Effect of resveratrol and/or BTP on phosphorylation and stabilization of tumor suppressor protein, p53

p53 in response to toxic insults to DNA, triggers a chain of cell cycle regulatory events to check the proliferation of altered cells to repair or minimize the damage [34,35] and Ser 15 phosphorylation is essential for stabilization and activation of p53 [36]. To determine whether p53 is phosphorylated at Ser15 in mouse skin tumors (long term study) treated with resveratrol, BTP or their combination, we used a phospho-specific antibody against p53 at Ser15 to do Western blot analysis. Our data showed that the level of p53 phosphorylation at Ser15 was increased in group IV and V upon treatment with resveratrol and BTP as compared with DMBA and TPA group II, however, significant increase in their expression was observed in combination group VI (Figure 5). Immunoblotting showed that the increased level of wild-type p53 protein corresponded well with the increased level of p53

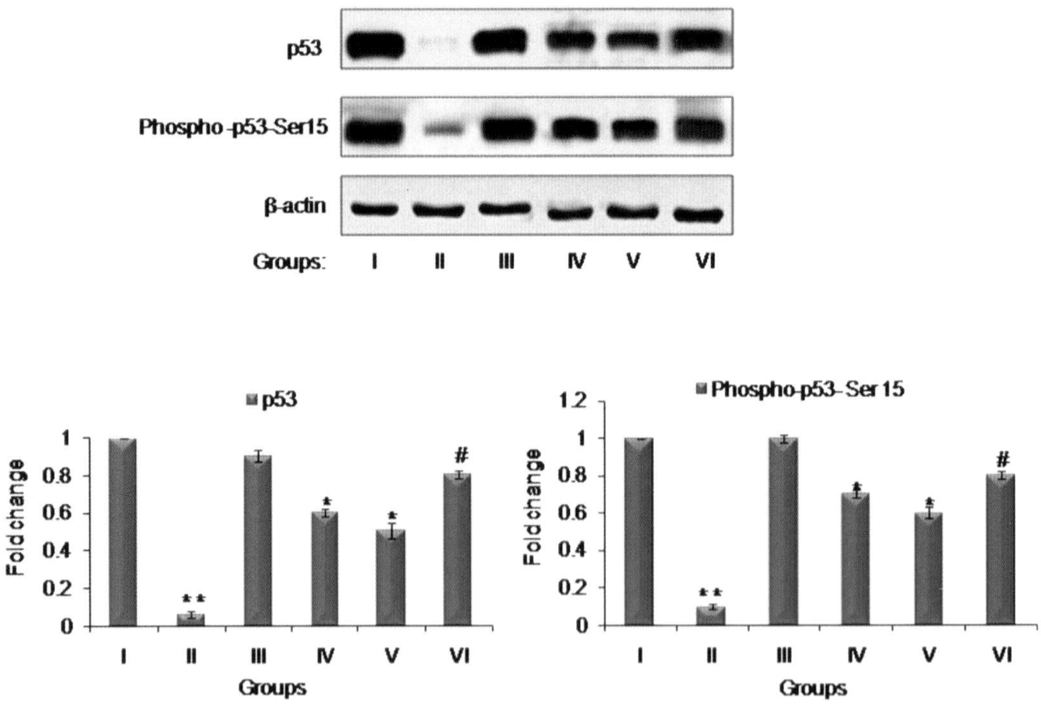

Figure 5. Effects of resveratrol and BTP treatment on modulation of p53 expression and p53 phosphorylation and stabilization. Details for groups and treatments are described in Materials and methods section. The bands shown here are from a representative experiment repeated three times with similar results. Equal loading was confirmed by stripping the immunoblot and reprobing it for β-actin. The pixel density of the specific immunoreactive bands was quantified by densitometry and expressed as a fold difference against β-actin. ** less than corresponding value of untreated control group I ($p<0.05$). * more than corresponding value of DMBA and TPA group III ($p<0.05$). # more than corresponding value of BTP and Res alone treated groups IV and V ($p<0.05$).

phosphorylation at Ser15. These results are in agreement with earlier reports from our laboratory showing inhibitory effects of resveratrol and BTP individually in DMBA induced mouse skin tumors via enhancement of wild-type p53 [17,21]. These results suggest that the combination of resveratrol and BTP more efficiently stabilized p53 and induced its phosphorylation at ser15 than either single agent.

Effect of resveratrol and/or BTP on apoptosis

Apoptosis is the most potent defence mechanism against cancer [37]. We next quantified the extent of apoptosis by flow cytometric analysis of the skin cells labelled with Annexin V/PI. Results showed significant ($p<0.05$) percent increase in apoptotic population by either resveratrol/BTP or the two in combination (6.12 ± 0.34, 5.23 ± 0.52 and 14.00 ± 0.20, respectively) over untreated (2.10 ± 0.36) and DMBA and TPA group II which recorded 1.40 ± 0.15 apoptotic populations (Figure 6).

Effect of resveratrol and/or BTP on DMBA and TPA-induced nick formation

Based on the amount of duplex DNA remaining after alkali treatment, the number of strand breaks generated per unit DNA was determined in mouse skin tissues obtained from short term study. DMBA and TPA caused a significant DNA damage ($n=1.50\pm0.17$) over untreated ($n=0.007\pm0.001$) in terms of strand breaks ($p<0.01$). Inhibition of DMBA and TPA-induced DNA alkylation damage was recorded by either resveratrol or BTP or the two in combination and prevention percentage was found to be 45.79%, 40.52% and 60.53%, respectively (Table 3).

Discussion

Chemoprevention by using dietary agents in combination is gaining the attention of researchers and consumers as a plausible approach for the management of various neoplasia. In this study, employing two-stage mouse skin carcinogenesis protocol, we are able to show that combined treatment of resveratrol (25 μM/animal) and BTP (0.1%) synergistically suppressed the skin tumors more efficiently than either of these solitary agents (Figure 1). Administration of resveratrol and BTP in combination was found to be highly effective in decreasing the CNT and tumor volume (Table 2). Earlier studies from our laboratory have demonstrated the chemopreventive potential of both the agents against mouse skin carcinogenesis, respectively [17,21]. The central finding of the study is that combined doses of resveratrol and BTP also resulted in significant regression of tumors in regard to both tumor volume and number. Also, no increase in tumor volume or occurrence of tumors was observed in groups (tumor bearing and non tumor-bearing) after withdrawal of the combined treatment. Hence, we observed that resveratrol and BTP (in combination) had superior chemopreventive effects as compared to either resveratrol or BTP.

MAPKs, comprising a family of serine and threonine kinases of ERK, JNK, and p38, are important signaling components which convert external stimuli into a wide range of cellular responses, such as proliferation, survival, differentiation and migration [32]. MAPK signalling cascades are highly relevant in the process of tumor promotion and progression induced by chemical carcinogens in mouse skin carcinogenesis, affecting not only cell proliferation, but also apoptosis by promoting the survival of the tumor cell [38,39]. Activation of the MAPKs pathway occurs in

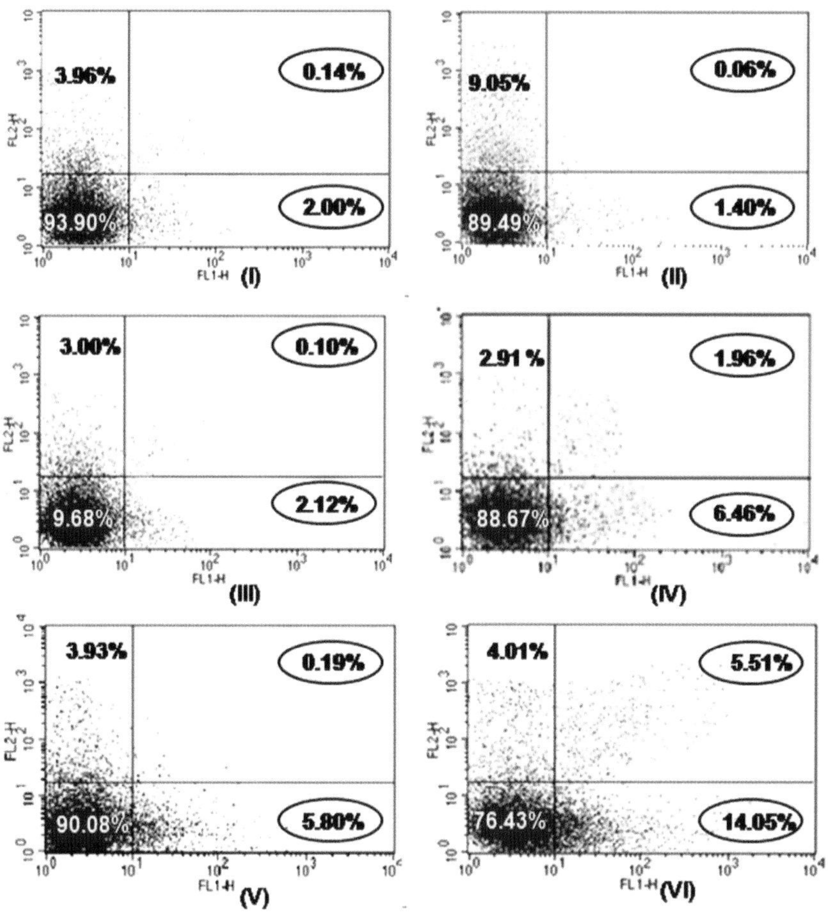

Figure 6. Representative figure of flow cytometric analysis of apoptosis in mouse skin on treatment with resveratrol and BTP. The data is representative of three independent experiments ($p<0.05$). Details are described in Materials and methods section. Figure showing cells in the upper right (UR), upper left (UL) and lower right (LR) portions portion of the picture indicates late apoptotic cells, necrotic and pre-apoptotic cells, respectively whereas cells present in lower left (LL) portion of the picture indicate percentage of live cells.

response to integrin-mediated cellular adhesion to the extracellular matrix, which plays a critical role in both tumor metastasis and angiogenesis [40,41]. In the present study, we found that topical application of DMBA and TPA (Gr. II) resulted in a marked increase in the phosphorylated form of ERK1/2, JNK1/2 and p38 protein expression; however, resveratrol and/or BTP treatment inhibited this phosphorylation. Importantly, the combined administration of both resveratrol and BTP was found to be more potent in inhibiting phosphorylation of MAPKs (Figure 2). These findings suggest a possibility that as an initial response resveratrol and BTP (in combination) modulate MAPKs activation further leads to inhibition of tumor growth and regression by apoptotic cell death.

Table 3. Number of DNA strand breaks inhibited by resveratrol or/and BTP against DMBA and TPA- induced DNA alkylation damage.

Groups	Treatment	Number of DNA strand breaks (n)
II	DMBA+TPA	1.50±0.17
IV	DMBA+TPA+resveratrol	0.81±0.18^a (45.79%)
V	DMBA+TPA+BTP	0.90±0.19^a (40.52%)
VI	DMBA+TPA+resveratrol+BTP	0.60±0.14^b (60.53%)

Data are expressed as mean ± SD of five animals. 'n' represents number of strand breaks of duplex DNA over untreated control group.
^{a}significant prevention over DMBA and TPA- induced DNA strand breaks ($p<0.01$).
^{b}significant prevention over BTP and Res alone treated groups IV and V($p<0.01$).
Values in parenthesis represents the percentage prevention offered by resveratrol or/and BTP against DMBA and TPA- induced DNA strand breaks.

In the present study, we further investigated the solitary and combined effect of resveratrol and BTP on expression of proliferation marker PCNA. Enhanced expression of PCNA, a 36 kDa co-factor of DNA polymerase δ, is one of the downstream effects of the activation of MAPK/ERK1/2 signalling and well correlated to the status of cellular proliferation [42]. Although single administration of resveratrol and BTP resulted in growth inhibition of DMBA and TPA-induced skin tumors, their combined treatment markedly inhibited the growth accompanying significant decrease in PCNA immunoexpression in tumor sections. Besides this, histologic analysis of the skin tissues of untreated animals displays major epithelial proliferation. In contrast the skin/tumor sections of mice given resveratrol and/or BTP display no indication of neoplasia. Therefore, inhibition of ERK1/2, JNK1/2 and p38 activation, suppression of PCNA upon resveratrol and BTP supplementation in combination, rather than alone treatments, suggest the superiority in synergistic effects of the two. This finding is quite intriguing, and it is tempting to speculate that a combination of resveratrol and BTP might have efficiently more influenced the cell death–related signaling pathways, ultimately leading to the suppression of well-established DMBA and TPA induced tumor in vivo, which might not possibly be achieved by a single administration of resveratrol or BTP.

To dissect the possible mechanisms in which the apoptotic and/ or anti-proliferation signaling were triggered, we also examined the expression levels of the tumor suppressor p53 protein. p53 plays a crucial role in controlling the cell cycle, apoptosis, genomic integrity and DNA repair in response to various forms of stress [35]. As aforementioned, post-translational modifications such as phosphorylation and acetylation are critical for stabilization and activation of p53 [36] our data showed that phosphorylation of p53 (Ser15) increased in mouse skin tumors treated with resveratrol and BTP, but the combination induced more efficient stabilization and phosphorylation of p53 protein at (Figure 5). Consistent with the findings of our previous reports [17,21], wild-type p53 activity also increased more in these groups (Figure 5).Thus, indicate that in mouse skin tumors, growth inhibition induced by resveratrol and/or BTP is p53-dependent and induced p53 phosphorylation at Ser15 may be attributed to stabilization of p53.

Apoptosis is a selective process of physiological cell deletion that plays an important role in the balance between cellular replication and death. Furthermore, it has been suggested that some cancer chemotherapeutics and chemopreventives exert their effects by triggering either apoptotic cell death or cell cycle transition, and accordingly, the induction of tumor cell apoptosis is used to predict tumor treatment response [43,44]. Therefore, we quantified the extent of apoptosis by flow-cytometric analysis of skin cells labelled with Annexin-V-PI. The results showed that combinatorial effect of resveratrol and BTP, leads to enhanced cell death than either of them alone. In addition, it is further noted that the administration of resveratrol and/or BTP inhibited the DMBA and TPA-induced DNA damage as revealed by the reduction in strand breaks. But combination doses exerted better effects than either of these two agents alone. This might be occurring because both of them are known to have ability to repair DNA damage [45,46].

In recent years, emerging evidence suggests that cancer-preventive agents might be combined for more effective treatment of cancer [47]. They can react together to give synergistic action to intervene cancer stages by different signaling pathways or to compensate for the opposite properties in cancer cell proliferation or apoptosis. Thus, we conclude that both resveratrol and BTP at low doses in combination synergistically inhibit established skin tumor growth than either of these agents alone accompanied by decrease in tumor volume and number. This is attributable to reduction in nick formation associated with a decrease in proliferation marker and tumor suppressor protein p53 together with an inhibition of MAPKs signaling and induction of apoptotic cell death in skin cells. Further pre-clinical and clinical trials are warranted to characterize the efficacy of dietary agents in combination with existing therapeutics for chemoprevention and chemotherapy of cancer.

Acknowledgements

The authors thank all their colleagues who were involved in the study for their excellent assistance. The authors are grateful to Director, Indian Institute of Toxicology Research (CSIR) Lucknow, India for his keen interest in the study. They are thankful to Neeraj Mathur, Scientist for statistical analysis of all the data. Authors are thankful to B. P. Chaudhari for all support of histopathological and IHC analysis. Authors also acknowledge Mr. SHN Naqvi for helping in animal experimentation.

Author Contributions

Conceived and designed the experiments: JG YS. Performed the experiments: JG MS AKS KB PR PKC. Analyzed the data: JG MS KB. Contributed reagents/materials/analysis tools: YS. Wrote the paper: JG MS YS.

References

1. de Kok TM, de Waard P, Wilms LC, van Breda SG (2010) Antioxidative and antigenotoxic properties of vegetables and dietary phytochemicals: the value of genomics biomarkers in molecular epidemiology. Mol Nutr Food Res 54: 208–217.
2. Gromadzinska J, Reszka E, Wasowicz W (2007) Anticarcinogenic activity of selenium – molecular mechanisms and epidemiological data. In: Akesson B, Mercke P, eds. Dietary vitamins, polyphenols, selenium and probiotics: biomarkers of exposure and mechanisms of anticarcinogenic action. Lodz: Nofer Institute of Occupational Medicine. pp 91–113.
3. Akesson B, Kyrtopoulos SA (2008) Compounds in food. Eur J Nutr 47: 1–2.
4. Xu G, Ren G, Xu X, Yuan H, Wang Z, et al. (2010) Combination of curcumin and green tea catechins prevents dimethylhydrazine-induced colon carcinogenesis. Food Chem Toxicol 48: 390–395.
5. Kumi-Diaka J, Merchant K, Haces A, Hormann V, Johnson M (2010) Genistein-selenium combination induces growth arrest in prostate cancer cells. J Med Food 13: 842–850.
6. Zhou JR, Yu L, Zhong Y, Blackburn GL (2003) Soy phytochemicals and tea bioactive components synergistically inhibit androgen-sensitive human prostate tumors in mice. J Nutr 3: 516–521.
7. George J, Singh M, Srivastava AK, Bhui K, Shukla Y (2011) Synergistic growth inhibition of mouse skin tumors by pomegranate fruit extract and diallyl sulfide: Evidence for inhibition of activated MAPKs/NF-κB and reduced cell proliferation. Food Chem Toxicol 49(7): 1511–1520.
8. Ndiaye M, Philippe C, Mukhtar H, Ahmad N (2011) The grape antioxidant Resveratrol for skin disorders: promise, prospects, and challenges. Arch Biochem Biophys 508: 164–170.
9. Sil H, Sen T, Moulik S, Chatterjee A (2010) Black tea polyphenol (theaflavin) downregulates MMP-2 in human melanoma cell line A375 by involving multiple regulatory molecules. J Environ Pathol Toxicol Oncol 29: 55–68.
10. Jang M, Cai L, Udeani GO, Slowing KV, Thomas CF, et al. (1997) Cancer chemopreventive activity of resveratrol, a natural product derived from grapes. Science 275: 218–220.
11. Hsieh TC, Wu JM (2010) Resveratrol: Biological and pharmaceutical properties as anticancer molecule. Biofactors 36: 360–369.
12. Bishayee A, Politis T, Darvesh AS (2010) Resveratrol in the chemoprevention and treatment of hepatocellular carcinoma. Cancer Treat Rev 36: 43–53.
13. Liu PL, Tsai JR, Charles AL, Hwang JJ, Chou SH (2010) Resveratrol inhibits human lung adenocarcinoma cell metastasis by suppressing heme oxygenase 1-mediated nuclear factor-kappaB pathway and subsequently downregulating expression of matrix metalloproteinases. Mol Nutr Food Res 54 Suppl. 2: S196–S204.
14. Roy P, Kalra N, Prasad S, George J, Shukla Y (2009) Chemopreventive potential of resveratrol in mouse skin tumors through regulation of mitochondrial and PI3K/AKT signaling pathways. Pharm Res 26: 211–217.
15. Seeni A, Takahashi S, Takeshita K, Tang M, Sugiura S, et al. (2008) Suppression of prostate cancer growth by resveratrol in the transgenic rat for adenocarcinoma of prostate (TRAP) model. Asian Pac J Cancer Prev 9: 7–14.
16. Kundu JK, Shin YK, Surh YJ (2006) Resveratrol modulates phorbol ester-induced pro-inflammatory signal transduction pathways in mouse skin in vivo: NF-kappaB and AP-1 as prime targets. Biochem Pharmacol 72: 1506–1515.
17. Kalra N, Roy P, Prasad S, Shukla Y (2008) Resveratrol induces apoptosis involving mitochondrial pathways in mouse skin tumorigenesis. Life Sci 82: 348–358.
18. Weisburger JH (1999) Mechanisms of action of antioxidants as exemplified in vegetables, tomatoes and tea. Food Chem Toxicol 37: 943–948.
19. Lu J, Ho CT, Ghai G, Chen KY (2000) Differential effects of theaflavin monogallates on cell growth, apoptosis, and Cox-2 gene expression in cancerous versus normal cells. Cancer Res 60: 6465–6471.
20. Weisberger JH, Rivenson A, Reinhardt J, Aliaga C, Braley J, et al. (1998) Effect of black tea on azoxymethane-induced colon cancer. Carcinogenesis 19: 229–232.
21. Roy P, Nigam N, George J, Srivastava S, Shukla Y (2009) Induction of apoptosis by tea polyphenols mediated through mitochondrial cell death pathway in mouse skin tumors. Cancer Biol Ther 13: 1281–1287.
22. Sun CL, Yuan JM, Koh WP, Yu MC (2006) Green tea, black tea and breast cancer risk: a meta-analysis of epidemiological studies. Carcinogenesis 27: 1310–1315.

23. Baker JA, Boakye K, McCann SE, Beehler GP, Rodabaugh KJ, et al. (2007) Consumption of black tea or coffee and risk of ovarian cancer. Int J Gynecol Cancer 17: 50–54.
24. Kalra N, Seth K, Prasad S, Singh M, Pant AB, et al. (2007) Theaflavins induced apoptosis of LNCaP cells is mediated through induction of p53, down-regulation of NF-kappa B and mitogen-activated protein kinases pathways. Life Sci 80: 2137–2146.
25. Chou TC, Talalay P (1984) Quantitative analysis of dose-effect relationships: the combined effects of multiple drugs or enzyme inhibitors. Adv Enzyme Regul 22: 27–55.
26. Kataoka K, Kim DJ, Carbajal S, Clifford JL, DiGiovanni J, et al. (2008) Stage-specific disruption of Stat3 demonstrates a direct requirement during both the initiation and promotion stages of mouse skin tumorigenesis. Carcinogenesis 6: 1108–1114.
27. Arora A, Siddiqui IA, Shukla Y (2004) Modulation of p53 in 7,12-dimethylbenz[a] benzanthracene-induced skin tumors by diallyl sulphide in Swiss albino mice. Mol Cancer Ther 11: 1459–1466.
28. Lowry OH, Rosenbrough NK, Farr AL (1951) Protein measurement with folin phenol reagent. J Biol Chem 193: 265–275.
29. Bogovaski P (1979) Tumours of skin. In: Turusov VS, ed. Pathology of tumours in laboratory animals. Lyon: IARC scientific publication no. 23. pp 1–14.
30. Nigam N, Shukla Y (2007) Preventive effects of diallyl sulfide on 7, 12-dimethylbenz[a]anthracene induced DNA alkylation damage in mouse skin. Mol Nutr Food Res 51: 1324–1328.
31. Kundu K, Chun KS, Kim SO, Surh YJ (2004) Resveratrol inhibits phorbol ester-induced cyclooxygenase-2 expression in mouse skin: MAPKs and AP-1 as potential molecular targets. Biofactors 21: 33–39.
32. Kennedy NJ, Cellurale C, Davis RJ (2007) A radical role for p38 MAPK in tumor initiation. Cancer Cell 2: 101–103.
33. Mancini R, Marucci L, Benedetti A, Jezequel AM, Orlandi F (1994) Immunohistochemical analysis of S-phase cells in normal human and rat liver by PC10 monoclonal antibody. Liver 2: 57–64.
34. Mowat MR (1998) p53 in tumor progression: life, death and everything. Adv Cancer Res 74: 25–48.
35. Meek DW (2004) The p53 response to DNA damage. DNA Repair (Amst) 3: 1049–1056.
36. She QB, Chen N, Dong Z (2000) ERKs and p38 kinase phosphorylate p53 protein at serine 15 in response to UV radiation. J Biol Chem 275: 20444–20449.
37. Lowe SW, Lin AW (1990) Apoptosis in cancer. Carcinogenesis 21: 485–495.
38. Afaq F, Ahmad N, Mukhtar H (2003) Suppression of UVB-induced phosphorylation of mitogen-activated protein kinases and nuclear factor kappa B by green tea polyphenol in SKH-1 hairless mice. Oncogene 22: 9254–9264.
39. Singh RP, Tyagi AK, Zhao J, Agarwal R (2002) Silymarin inhibits growth and causes regression of established skin tumors in SENCAR mice via modulation of mitogen-activated protein kinases and induction of apoptosis. Carcinogenesis 23: 499–510.
40. Chen W, Borchers AH, Dong Z, Powell MB, Bowden GT (1998) UVB irradiation-induced activator protein-1 activation correlates with increased c-fos gene expression in a human keratinocyte cell line. J Biol Chem 273: 32176–32181.
41. Zhu WH, MacIntyre A, Nicosia RF (2002) Regulation of angiogenesis by vascular endothelial growth factor and angiopoietin-1 in the rat aorta model: distinct temporal patterns of intracellular signaling correlate with induction of angiogenic sprouting. Am J Pathol 161: 823–830.
42. Singh RP, Tyagi AK, Zhao J, Agarwal R (2002) Silymarin inhibits growth and causes regression of established skin tumors in SENCAR mice via modulation of mitogen-activated protein kinases and induction of apoptosis. Carcinogenesis 3: 499–510.
43. Kim YS, Jin SH, Lee YH, Kim SI, Park JD (1999) Ginsenoside Rh2 induces apoptosis independently of Bcl-2, Bcl-xL, or Bax in C6Bu-1 cells. Arch Pharm Res 22: 448–453.
44. Ahmad N, Feyes DK, Nieminen AL, Agarwal R, Mukhtar H (1997) Green tea constituent epigallocatechin-3-gallate and induction of apoptosis and cell cycle arrest in human carcinoma cells. J Natl Cancer Inst 89: 1881–1886.
45. Parshad R, Sanford KK, Price FM, Steele VE, Tarone RE, et al. (1998) Protective action of plant polyphenols on radiation-induced chromatid breaks in cultured human cells. Anticancer Res 18: 3263–3266.
46. Sengottuvelan M, Deeptha K, Nalini N (2009) Res ameliorates DNA damage, prooxidant and antioxidant imbalance in 1,2-dimethylhydrazine induced rat colon carcinogenesis. Chem Biol Interact 181: 193–201.
47. de Kok TM, van Breda SG, Manson MM (2008) Mechanisms of combined action of different chemopreventive dietary compounds: a review. Eur J Nutr 2: 51–59.

IL-17 Mediated Inflammation Promotes Tumor Growth and Progression in the Skin

Donggou He[1], Hui Li[1], Nabiha Yusuf[1,2,3], Craig A. Elmets[1,2,3], Mohammad Athar[1,2], Santosh K. Katiyar[1,2,3], Hui Xu[1,2,3]*

1 Department of Dermatology, University of Alabama at Birmingham, Birmingham, Alabama, United States of America, **2** Skin Disease Research Center, University of Alabama at Birmingham, Birmingham, Alabama, United States of America, **3** Birmingham VA Medical Center, Birmingham, Alabama, United States of America

Abstract

The mechanism for inflammation associated tumor development is a central issue for tumor biology and immunology and remains to be fully elucidated. Although IL-17 is implicated in association with inflammation mediated carcinogenesis, mechanisms are largely elusive. In the current studies, we showed that IL-17 receptor-A gene deficient (IL-17R-/-) mice were resistant to chemical carcinogen-induced cutaneous carcinogenesis, a well-established inflammation associated tumor model in the skin. The deficiency in IL-17R increased the infiltration of CD8+ T cells whereas it inhibited the infiltration of CD11b+ myeloid cells and development of myeloid derived suppressor cells. Inflammation induced skin hyperplasia and production of pro-tumor inflammatory molecules were inhibited in IL-17R-/- mice. We found that pre-existing inflammation in the skin increased the susceptibility to tumor growth, which was associated with increased development of tumor specific IL-17 producing T cells. This inflammation induced susceptibility to tumor growth was abrogated in IL-17R-/- mice. Finally, neutralizing IL-17 in mice that had already developed chemical carcinogen induced skin tumors could inhibit inflammation mediated tumor progression at late stages. These results demonstrate that IL-17 mediated inflammation is an important mechanism for inflammation mediated promotion of tumor development. The study has major implications for targeting IL-17 in prevention and treatment of tumors.

Editor: Joseph Najbauer, City of Hope National Medical Center and Beckman Research Institute, United States of America

Funding: This publication was made possible by grants (AI071041 and AR46256 [HX] and ES017494 and CA138998 [MA]) from the United States National Institutes of Health. The funders had no role in study design, data collection and analysis, decision to publish, or preparation of the manuscript.

Competing Interests: The authors have declared that no competing interests exist.

* E-mail: xuhui@uab.edu

Introduction

Immune surveillance mechanisms exist to recognize and eliminate tumor cells. Defects in immune surveillance are associated with tumor progression [1,2,3]. In anti-tumor immune responses, activated T cells infiltrate into tumors and destroy tumor cells either by cytotoxic effects or elicitation of inflammatory reactions that will involve other leukocytes in the eradication of tumors [4,5]. However, chronic inflammation, an unsolved immune response, promotes tumor development [6,7]. The infiltration of immune T cells within tumors, no matter at what stages of tumor development, is associated with beneficial prognosis [8]. In contrast, infiltration of granulocytes and macrophages has been considered as a promotion factor in tumor development [9,10]. Intense inflammatory infiltrates comprised of large numbers of macrophages and granulocytes and high concentrations of inflammatory cytokines are characteristics of tumor promoting inflammation. They are considered to be the primary tumor promoting factors responsible for enhanced angiogenesis and cell growth [11].

IL-17 is an important cytokine responsible for inflammatory and autoimmune diseases [12,13]. Although IL-17 producing cells are detected in cancer patients and tumor bearing animals [14,15], studies which mostly use implanted tumor models show a controversial role of IL-17 in tumor development [14,16]. Accumulating evidence indicates that IL-17 has tumor promoting effects, especially in the context of inflammation [17,18,19]. However, mechanisms for IL-17 mediated tumor promoting inflammation remains to be fully elucidated.

Dimethylbenz[*a*]anthracene (DMBA)-initiated and 12-O-tetradecanoylphorbol-13-acetate (TPA)-promoted cutaneous carcinogenesis is a well-established animal model for inflammation associated tumor development. The two-stage chemical carcinogenesis protocol includes single exposure to the mutagen DMBA followed by repeated application of the inflammation-inducing TPA. Skin lesions can be followed from premalignant papilloma formation to progression to carcinoma [20,21,22]. Although the effects of TPA are pleiotropic, its pro-inflammatory effects are crucial to tumor promotion. In mice that are deficient either in inflammatory cytokines IL-1β or TNF-α, DMBA/TPA induced carcinogenesis is inhibited [23,24]. The arachidonic acid/cyclooxygenase (Cox) pathway of inflammation induction has a critical role in TPA induced tumor promotion [25,26]. Additionally, S100A8/9, a group of calcium binding proteins, are critical for the development of chemical carcinogenesis [27,28]. Mice deficient in the Receptor for Advanced Glycation End-products, a receptor for S100A8/A9, are resistant to DMBA/TPA induced carcinogenesis [27]. A defect in S100A9 results in increased infiltration of CD8+ T cells in tumors [29].

Our previous study showed that CD4+ T cells were primary IL-17 producing cells in DMBA/TPA induced cutaneous carcinogenesis

[15]. Moreover, DMBA/TPA induced cutaneous carcinogenesis was enhanced in TLR4 deficient mice, which is associated with an increased level of IL-17 [30]. It has been reported that IL-23, a stimulatory cytokine for IL-17 production, promotes DMAB/TPA induced carcinogenesis [31] whereas it is inhibited in IL-17-/- mice [18]. However, mechanisms for IL-17 mediated effects on chemical carcinogenesis are largely unknown.

In the current studies, we examined DMBA/TPA induced cutaneous carcinogenesis in mice that were deficient in IL-17R, IL-12p35, or both IL-17R and IL-12p35. The effect of inflammation on tumor specific T cells and tumor growth and the role of IL-17 in tumor progression at the late stage were determined. Our findings indicate that IL-17 is required for DMBA/TPA induced carcinogenesis in the skin and that blockade of IL-17 suppresses inflammation mediated tumor development and progression.

Results

IL-17R deficient mice are resistant to chemical induced cutaneous carcinogenesis

DMBA/TPA induced skin carcinogenesis was delayed and the incidence of tumors was greatly decreased in IL-17R-/- mice compared to wild type controls (Fig. 1a). Moreover, the tumor multiplicity was significantly reduced in IL-17R-/- mice (Fig. 1b and 1c). In p35-/- mice, which had a deficiency in IL-12 but not in IL-23, tumor multiplicity was significantly increased compared to wild type controls, although the incidence and kinetic of tumor development was not affected. However, mice that were deficient in both IL-17R and p35 genes (IL-17R/p35-/-), were resistant to tumor development in a similar manner to IL-17R-/- mice. These results indicate that IL-17 responses are required for DMBA/TPA induced carcinogenesis in the skin and that the effect of IL-17 on the chemical induced carcinogenesis is independent of IL-12 signals.

The development of skin tumors in DMBA/TPA treated mice is dependent on TAP induced tumor promoting inflammation [15,23]. To examine the effect of IL-17R deficiency on DMBA/TPA treated skin, mouse skin samples were harvested at the end of experiments (around 26 weeks) and subjected to immunohistochemical analysis. We found that the immigration of CD11b+ cells into the DMBA/TPA treated skin tissues was decreased (Fig. 2a). In contrast, the infiltration of CD8+ T cells was significantly increased in IL-17R-/- compared to wild type mice. The deficiency in p35 had little effect on the infiltration of CD11b+ cells and CD8+ T cells. However, similar to IL-17R-/- mice, IL-17R/p35-/- mice had an increased infiltration of CD8+ T cells and decreased infiltration of macrophages in the skin compared to p35-/- mice. The effect appeared to be selective on CD8+ T cells since the infiltration of CD4+ T cells was not significantly affected in IL-17R-/- and wild type mice (data not shown). The results implicate important effects of IL-17 on the inflammatory environment and CD8+ T cell responses in the skin during chemical induced carcinogenesis.

To determine whether the deficiency in IL-17 receptor has an effect on leukocytes in peripheral lymphoid organ, spleen cells from DMBA/TAP treated mice (26 weeks) were analyzed. Results showed that the percent and total number of CD4+ and CD8+ T cells and CD19/B200 double positive B cells were not significantly affected. However, CD1b/Gr-1 double positive myeloid cells are significantly decreased in the spleen of IL-17R-/- or p35/IL-17R-/- mice compared to p35-/- and wild type control animals (Fig. 2b and 2c).

IL-17R deficiency inhibits TPA induced tumor promoting inflammation in the skin

In the chemical carcinogenesis model, repeated treatments with TPA cause chronic inflammation which promotes tumor growth although no evidence shows that the treatment with TPA alone will induce carcinogenesis [15,23]. Inflammation induced hyperplasia is an important mechanism for the development and progression of tumors [32,33]. To test whether IL-17 regulates the development of TPA induced tumor promoting inflammation, mice were treated with TPA every other day for a total of three applications and skin samples were harvested 24 hours after the last treatment. We found that TPA induced epidermal hyperplasia was inhibited in IL-17R-/- mice compared to wild type controls (Fig. 3a). Additionally, we found that there were fewer CD11b+ macrophages and Gr-1+ granulocytes in the TPA treated skin of IL-17R-/- mice (Fig. 3b). Moreover, the levels of pro-tumor inflammatory cytokines IL-1β and TNF-α were reduced in the TPA treated skin of IL-17R-/- mice compared to wild type mice (Fig. 3c).

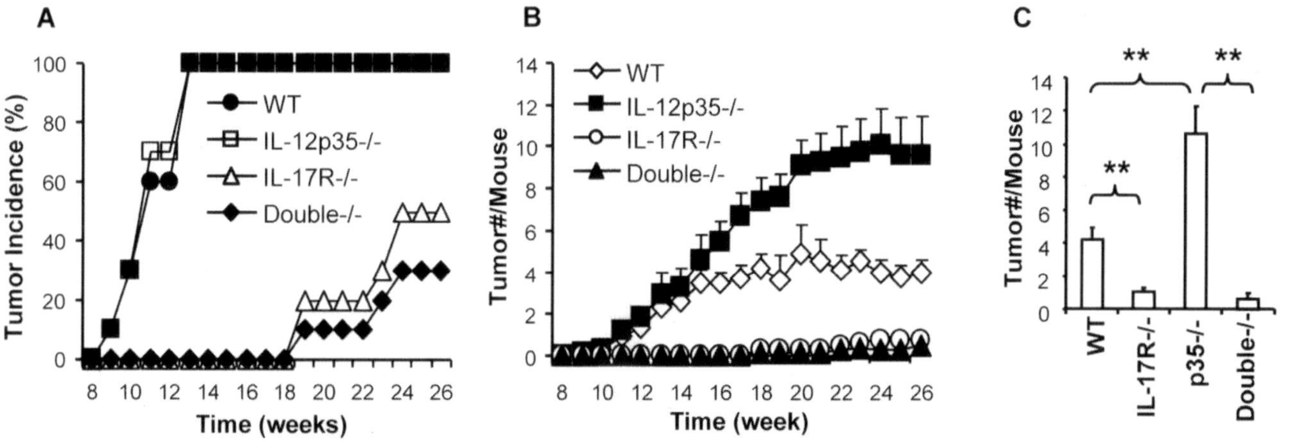

Figure 1. IL-17 receptor deficient mice are resistant to DMBA/TPA induced carcinogenesis. Mice were treated once with DMBA and then with TPA twice a week, as described in the Materials and Methods. Tumor growth was observed every week. A). Tumor incidence. B). Tumor multiplicity. C). The number of tumors was analyzed statistically at the end of experiments (26 weeks). The bar graph shows the mean number of tumors per mouse +/−SEM, *n* = 10, ** p<0.01. Data are representative of two independent experiments.

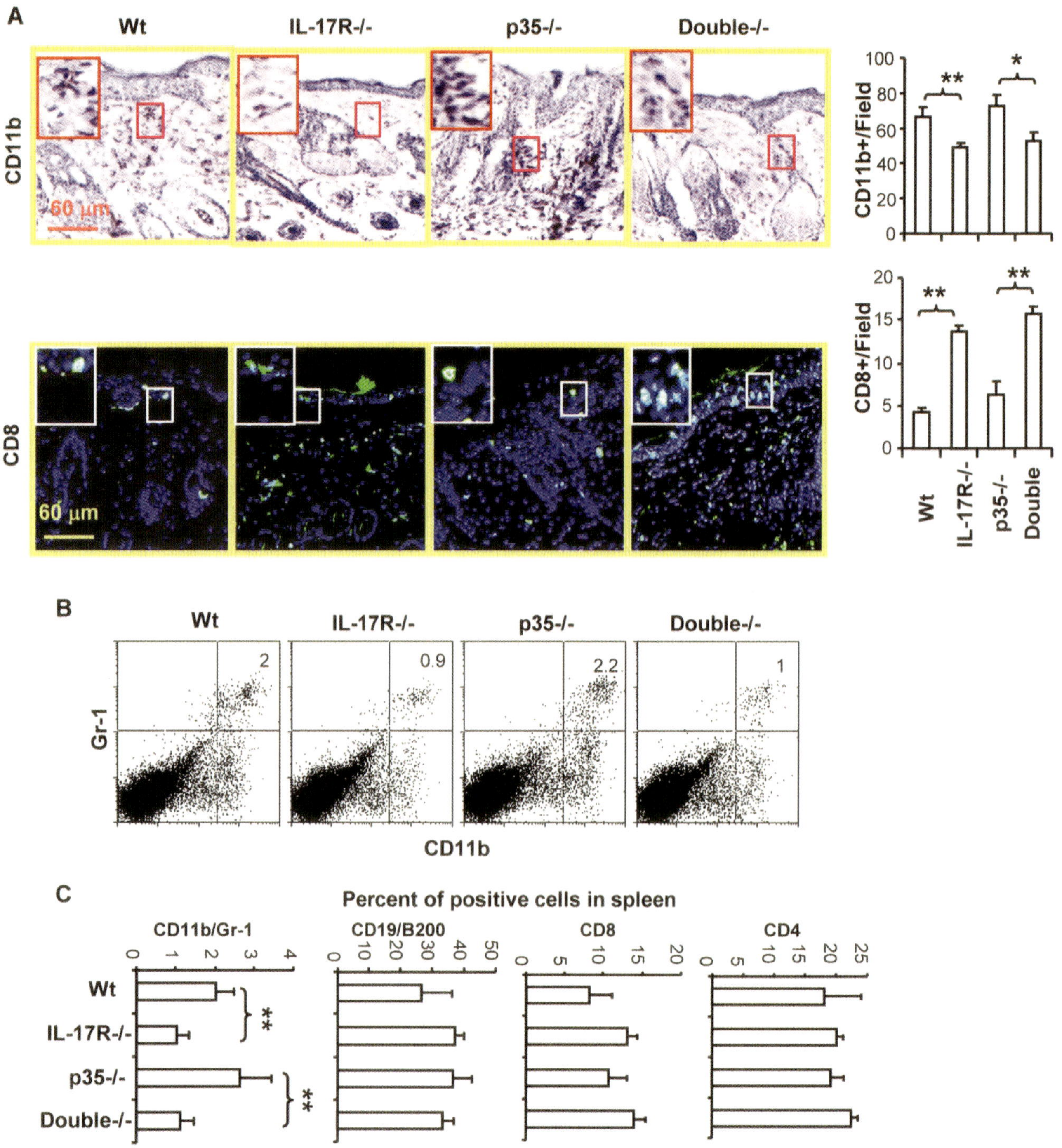

Figure 2. IL-17 has opposing effects on the infiltration of CD11b+ macrophages and CD8+ T cells in DMBA/TPA treated skin. Mice were treated with DMBA and TPA as described in figure 1 and skin tissues were harvested at the end of the experiment (26 weeks). A). Frozen tissue sections were stained with CD11b antibodies (brown) and counterstained with hematoxylin (blue, upper panels) or with anti-CD8 antibodies (green) and counterstained with a fluorescence dye DAPI (blue, lower panel). Photos were taken microscopically (20× objective). Numbers of positive cells were counted microscopically. Islets show the enlarged areas of circled squares with positive cells. Graphs show the mean number of positive cells per field +/− SEM, $n=10$, * $p<0.05$, ** $P<0.01$. B). Gr-1 and CD11b double positive cells in spleens were stained with fluorescence labeled antibodies and positive cells were analyzed in a flow cytometer. The numbers in the right upper quadrant indicate the percent of positive cells in whole spleen cells. C). Statistical analysis of GR-1/CD11b+ (myeloid derived suppressor cells), CD19/B220+ (B cells), CD8+ and CD4+ T cells in spleens (mean +/− SEM, $n=8$, ** $P<0.01$). Data are representative of two independent experiments.

Western blot analysis showed that the TPA treatment induced the expression of S100A8/A9 in the skin of wild type mice whereas it was undetectable in IL-17R-/- mice (Fig. 3d). S100A8 and S100A9, two members of the S100 family of calcium binding proteins, are abundantly produced during acute and chronic inflammation and play an important role in inflammation associated tumor development [27,28]. Similar findings were observed with Cox-2 and prostaglandin E_2 (PGE2), a main

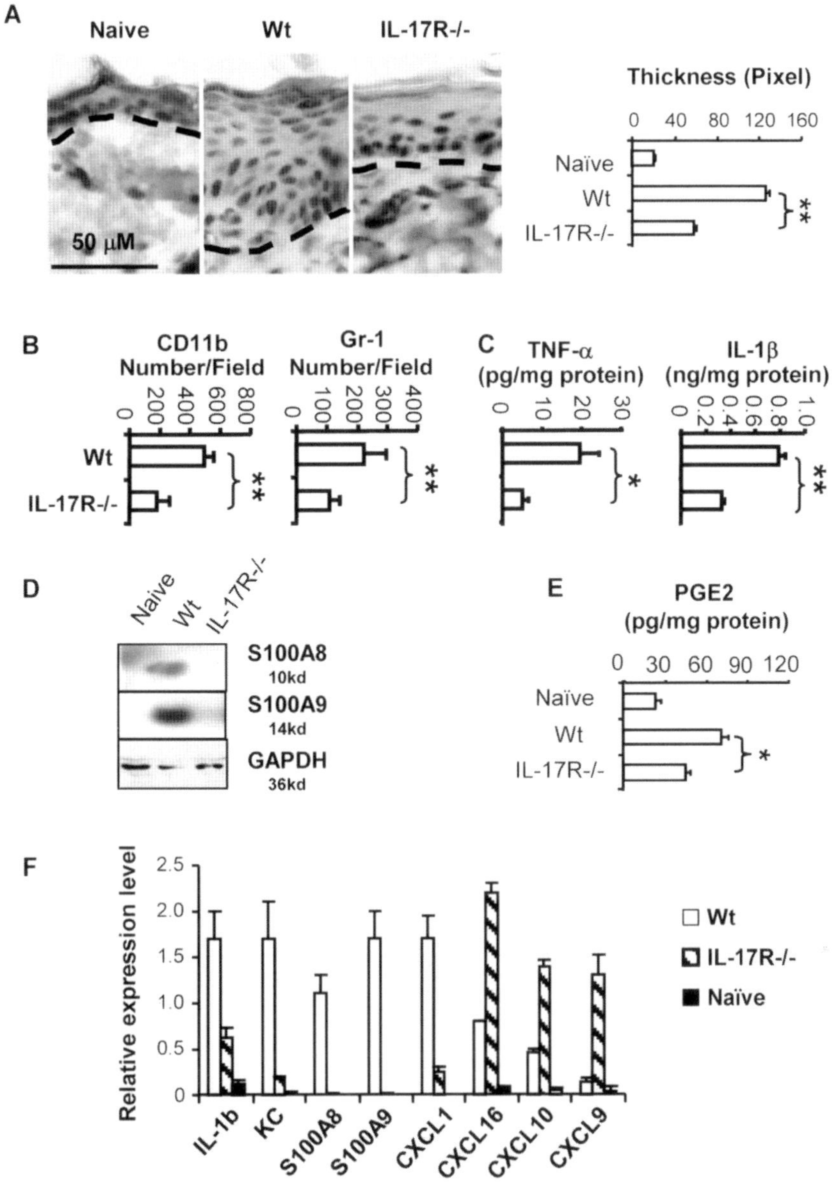

Figure 3. The deficiency in IL-17 receptor inhibits TPA induced tumor promoting inflammation in the skin. Mice were treated topically with TPA every other day for a total of three applications. Skin tissues were harvested 24 hours after the last treatment. A). Paraffin embedded tissue sections were stained with hematoxylin. Skin samples from naïve untreated mice served as controls. Dashed lines indicate the border between the epidermis and dermis. The thickness of epidermis was measured microscopically (n = 10). B). Frozen tissue sections were stained immunohistochemcially with antibodies. CD11b+ (monocytes/macrophages) and Gr-1+ (granulocytes) cells were counted microscopically (n = 6). C) Concentrations of cytokines in the skin lysates were measured by ELISA (n = 4). D). S100A8 and S100A9 proteins in the skin lysates were detected by Western blots using specific antibodies. E). Concentrations of PGE2 in the skin lysates were measured by a PGE2 EIA kit (n = 3). F). Expression levels of mRNA for chemokines and cytokines in the skin lysates were quantified by real time RT-PCR (n = 3). Data are representative of 2–3 independent experiments (mean +/− SEM, * P<0.05: ** P<0.01).

substance converted by Cox-2, which plays important roles in TPA induced inflammation and tumor promotion in chemical induced carcinogenesis [25,26]. The concentration of PGE2 was significantly higher in the TPA treated skin of wild type mice than in that of IL-17R-/- mice (Fig. 3e). Interestingly, the deficiency in IL-17R had different effects on chemokine expression in TPA treated skin tissues. Chemokines KC, CXCL1, and S100A8/A9, which regulate myeloid cell migration was reduced in IL-17R-/- mice. In contrast, chemokines CXCL16, CXCL10 and CXCL9, which are known for regulation of lymphocytes, were increased (Fig. 3f). Collectively, tumor promoting inflammation which is induced by the repeated treatment with TPA is suppressed in IL-17R-/- mice.

Pre-treatment of skin with TPA enhances the development of tumor specific IL-17 producing T cells and increases the susceptibility of mice to tumor growth in an IL-17 dependent way

Many cancers arise from the site of inflammation, which forms a microenvironment for tumor growth and progression [7]. In order to further examine roles of IL-17 in inflammation mediated tumor promoting microenvironment, mice were treated epicutaneously with TPA every other day for a total of 5 applications and then inoculated subcutaneously in the TPA treated skin area with an immunogenic mouse tumor cell line EG7 which is a mouse lymphoma cell line (EL4) transfected with ovalbumin (OVA). Results showed that the pre-treatment with TPA enhanced the growth of implanted EG7 tumors in wild type mice (Fig. 4a). It implicates that the pre-existing inflammation makes mice susceptible to tumor development. To examine whether inflammation regulated the development of tumor specific T cells, the draining lymph node lymphocytes were harvested from the mice which were pre-treated with TPA and then inoculated with EG7 tumors. The cells were then stimulated with OVA pulsed bone marrow derived dendritic cells (BM-DC) in cultures. Results showed that the pre-treatment with TPA induced a significantly higher level of tumor specific IL-17 producing T cells than those from control mice that were pre-treated with vehicle acetone (Fig. 4b). The production of IFN-γ was slightly but not significantly affected. To determine whether the increase in IL-17 producing lymphocytes was associated with the increased tumor growth in TPA treated mice, wild type and IL-17R-/- mice were treated with TPA or control acetone and then inoculated with EG7 tumor cells. We found that the treatment with TPA significantly enhanced tumor growth in wild type mice whereas it did not have a significant effect on tumor growth in IL-17R-/- mice (Fig. 4c). It is to note that the tumor growth in control IL-17R-/- mice was inhibited compared to that in control wild type mice as previously reported [34].

Neutralization of IL-17 inhibits the progression of DMBA/TPA induced cutaneous carcinogenesis in mice that have already developed tumors

Based on our results described above, which showed the suppression of TAP induced tumor promoting inflammation in IL-17R-/- mice, further experiments were to examine whether neutralization of IL-17 could inhibit inflammation associated tumor progression in mice which had already developed DMBA/TPA induced skin tumors. Mice with skin tumors (12 weeks after the DMBA/TPA treatment) were treated intravenously twice (week 12 and 16) with non-replicating adenovirus encoding neutralizing soluble IL-17R (Ad-IL-17R:Fc) or GFP as a control (Ad-GFP). The mice were kept with TPA treatment twice a week as described. Results showed that in the control mice which were left untreated, the number of skin tumors increased (Fig. 5). Neutralization of IL-17 with the administration of Ad-IL-17R:Fc significantly inhibited the progression of tumors compared to controls mice that were treated with Ad-GFP. The treatment with control Ad-GFP did not have a significant effect on tumor progression compared to mice that were left untreated (Fig. 5). The result implicates that neutralizing IL-17 can inhibit the progression of DMBA/TPA induced skin tumors.

Discussion

The role of IL-17 in tumor development is controversial in implanted tumor models [14,16,35]. It appears that in induced tumor models which are associated with inflammation, IL-17 mediated inflammation has tumor promoting effects [18,36]. However, mechanisms remain to be fully elucidated. We have showed here that mice deficient in IL-17R are resistant to DMBA/TPA induced carcinogenesis in the skin. The deficiency in IL-17R enhances CD8+ T cell mediated immune surveillance and inhibits tumor promoting inflammation in the skin. Furthermore, TPA induced inflammation promotes the susceptibility to the growth of implanted tumors in the skin and increases the development of tumor specific IL-17 producing T cells. However, this TPA induced tumor promoting effect is abrogated in IL-17R deficient mice. Finally, we show that neutralization of IL-17 inhibits the progression of DMBA/TPA induced skin carcinogenesis in mice which have already developed tumors. Our data demonstrates that IL-17 mediated inflammation promotes carcinogenesis in the skin and targeting IL-17 may be exploited to a new therapeutic strategy for tumors.

In DMBA/TPA induced skin carcinogenesis, IL-23 has been shown to enhance carcinogenesis. It is postulated that IL-23 mediated up-regulation of IL-17 production is a mechanism [31]. Similar to studies in IL-17-/- mice [18], we show that the deficiency in IL-17R render mice resistant to chemical induced

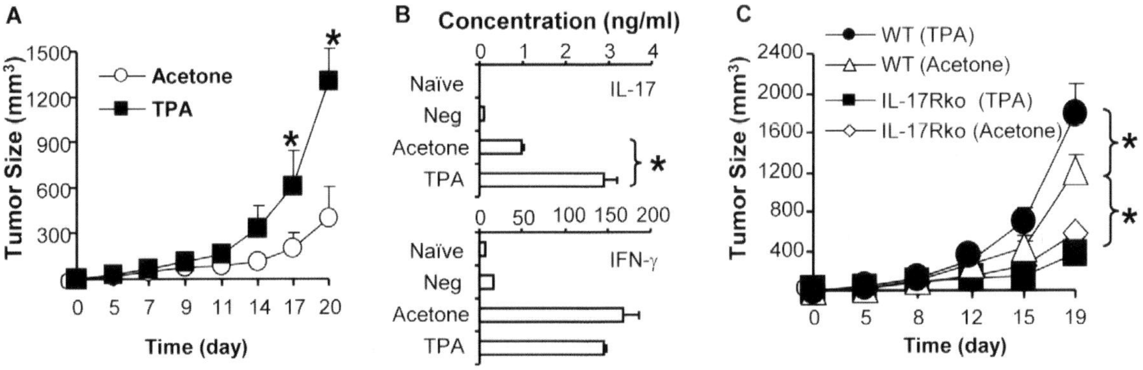

Figure 4. TPA induced promotion of tumor growth is abrogated in IL-17R-/- mice. A). TPA induced inflammation enhances tumor growth. Wild type C57Bl/6 mice were treated epicutaneously with TPA or acetone (vehicle controls) every other day for a total of 5 applications. The mice were then inoculated subcutaneously with EG7 tumor cells. Tumor growth was monitored (n = 5). B). TPA induced inflammation increases tumor specific IL-17 producing cells. At the end of experiments, the draining lymph node lymphocytes were collected from EG7 tumor bearing mice that were treated with TPA or acetone. The cells stimulated with OVA pulsed BM-DC for 4 days. Concentrations of cytokines in supernatants were measured by ELISA (n = 4). Naïve T cells with OVA pulsed BM-DC (Naïve) and immune T cells with BM-DC without OVA (Neg) served as controls in the cultures. C). TPA induced tumor promotion is abrogated in IL-17R-/- mice. Wild type or IL-17R-/- were epicutaneously treated with TPA or acetone every other day for a total of 5 applications. The mice were then inoculated with EG7 tumor cells and tumor growth was monitored (n = 5). Data are representative of 2–3 independent experiments (mean +/− SEM, * $P<0.05$).

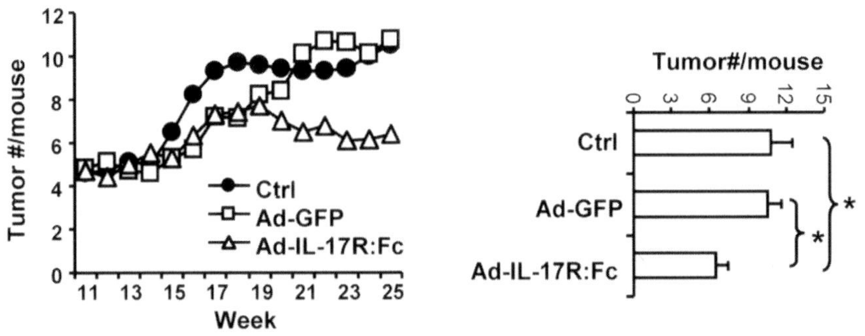

Figure 5. Neutralization of IL-17 inhibits the progression of tumors in DMBA/TPA induced cutaneous carcinogenesis. Wild type C57Bl/6 mice were topically treated once with DMBA and then twice weekly with TPA. All mice developed cutaneous tumors at 12 weeks. The mice were divided (10 mice/group) and treated intravenously with adenovirus encoding GFP (Ad-GFP), IL-17R:Fc (Ad-IL-17R:Fc) or left untreated (Ctrl) at week 12 and 16. All mice were continuously treated with TPA twice a week throughout the experiments. The tumor growth was monitored weekly. Bar graph shows the mean tumor number per mouse +/− SEM at the end of experiments (* $P<0.05$). Data are representative of 2 independent experiments.

skin carcinogenesis. Moreover, the IL-17R deficiency reverses the susceptibility of IL-12p35-/- mice to chemical carcinogenesis. It implicates that IL-17R mediated responses at least in part are attribute to increased tumor growth which is caused by IL-12 deficiency. However, mechanisms for the effect require further investigations. It is to note that in different tumor models, especially in implanted tumor models, IL-17 can have a protective effect against tumor development [37,38,39]. It suggests context dependent effects of IL-17 on tumors. Our data indicate that IL-17 has tumor promoting effects in inflammation associated tumor development in the DMBA/TPA model, which is inconsistent with reports showing that IL-17 promotes inflammation associated colon tumorigenesis [17,36].

In DMBA/TPA induced chemical carcinogenesis, CD8+ T cells are primary effector cells and required for prevention of tumor development [15]. The opposite effect of IL-17 on the infiltration of CD11b+ myeloid cells and CD8+ T cells in the inflamed skin implicates a novel role of IL-17 in the regulation of immune surveillance during inflammation associated carcinogenesis in the skin. Interestingly, similar findings have been reported in implanted tumor models by our laboratory and others [34,40]. Numerous clinical and laboratory studies show that the presence of macrophages is a hallmark of tumor promoting inflammation and is associated with a poor prognosis [9,32] whereas the presence of CD8+ T cells is associated with a good prognosis [8,41]. The effect of IL-17 on the production of chemokines has been well studied, which is considered to be responsible for its effects on the regulation of myeloid cell migration [42]. We have found that the deficiency in IL-17R reduces the expression of chemokines KC (human IL-8 analogue) and CXCL1 in TPA treated skin tissues, which are known to regulate the infiltration of myeloid cells in inflammation. In contrast, chemokines CXCL9, CXCL10 and CXCL16 which are known to regulate T cell migration are increased [43]. The differential effects of IL-17 on the expression of chemokines for myeloid cells and lymphocytes provide important clues for its effects on the regulation of myeloid cells and lymphocytes and may be important mechanisms for IL-17 mediated tumor promoting inflammation in DMBA/TPA induced skin tumors. Certainly, further studies are required to determine chemokine sources and to validate whether the effect of IL-17 on the chemokine production is associated with its effects on the regulation of leukocyte migration and development of skin tumors.

Depending on the functional status, myeloid cells including neutrophils and macrophages can have pro- or anti-tumor activities [4,44,45,46]. However, it is a common feature that the number of myeloid derived suppressor cells (MDSC), which are defined as CD1b/Gr-1 double positive cells in mice, is increased in cancer patients and tumor bearing mice [47,48,49,50]. MDSC are able to suppress anti-tumor immune responses and promote tumor growth [47,50]. The decrease of MDSC provides a good explanation for the suppression of DMBA/TPA induced carcinogenesis in IL-17R-/- mice and may be an important mechanism for the role of IL-17 in the development of tumor promoting inflammation and immunosuppression. This is in accordance with our recent studies showing that IL-17 stimulates the function of MDSC in tumor bearing mice [34]. Additionally, MDSC are able to inhibit T cell infiltration of anti-tumor T cells in tumor sites [51]. The down regulation of MDSC in IL-17R-/- mice may contribute to the increase of CD8+ T cells in the inflamed skin.

The effect of inflammation on tumor promotion is mediated by complexes of mechanisms. We have found that the deficiency in IL-17R inhibits characteristics of tumor promoting inflammation which is mediated by the repeated treatment with TPA in the skin. Inflammation associated hyperplasia is a pro-tumor change which is observed in many inflammation associated tumorigenesis [32,33]. Inflammatory infiltrates comprised of large numbers of macrophages and granulocytes and high concentrations of inflammatory cytokines are considered to be the primary factors responsible for enhanced angiogenesis and cell growth [9,32]. TPA induced epidermal hyperplasia is inhibited in IL-17R-/- mice, which is associated with significantly reduced leukocyte infiltrations and levels of IL-1β and TNF-α. Literature shows that a deficiency in either IL-1β or TNF-α suppresses the development of chemical induced skin carcinogenesis [23,24]. The reduction of IL-1β and TNF-α in IL-17R-/- mice may be part of mechanisms for the suppression of DMBA/TPA induced skin carcinogenesis.

Cox-2/PGE2 activities are significantly reduced in TPA treated skin of IL-17R-/- mice. Cox-2/PGE2 pathways have multiple effects on tumor development [50,52,53,54]. Importantly, PGE2 not only promotes cell proliferation and tumor associated angiogenesis but also induces the development of MDSC [55,56,57]. Over expression of Cox-2 enhances whereas a defect in Cox-2 suppresses TPA induced inflammation and DMBA/TPA induced chemical carcinogenesis [25,26]. Additionally, our results show that IL-17 is required for the expression of S100/A8/A9 in the TPA induced inflammation in the skin. S100A8/A9 proteins can induce the recruitment and differentiation of MDSC [58,59]. A defect in *S100a9* inhibits the infiltration of MDSC whereas it results in increased infiltration of CD8+ T cells in tumors [29]. Collectively, the inhibition of TPA induced Cox-2/PGE2 activity and S100A8/A9 expression may be a critical mechanism for the reduction of MDSC, increases of CD8+ T cells in the skin, and the suppression of DMBA/TPA induced carcinogenesis in IL-17R-/- mice.

Many cancers arise from the site of inflammation, which forms a microenvironment for tumor growth and progression [7]. Increased levels of IL-17 and IL-17 producing T cells have observed in human and animal tumors [14,16,36]. A direct proof for an association of inflammation with induction of tumor specific IL-17 producing T cells and tumor development is not known. Our data show that pre-existing inflammation in the skin, which is induced by repeated treatment with TPA, increases the susceptibility of wild type mice to implanted tumors (Fig. 4). This effect is associated with a significantly increased level of tumor specific IL-17 producing T cells in the draining lymph nodes. In contrast, a significant effect on IFN-γ producing cells is not observed. Importantly, the promotion of tumor growth in TPA treated mice is abrogated in IL-17R-/- mice. Our study provides a strong support that inflammation induced increase of IL-17 producing T cells is a mechanism for the increased tumor growth and that blockade of IL-17 can inhibit inflammation mediated tumor promoting effects.

Although tumor promoting effects of inflammation have been well documented, it remains to be explored whether targeting inflammation can have therapeutic effects on existing tumors at late stages. Our data show that neutralization of IL-17 in mice that have already developed skin carcinogenesis induced by DMBA/TPA can inhibit tumor progression (Fig. 5). It indicates a role of IL-17 in inflammation mediated tumor progression at late phases and suggests that blocking IL-17 could have therapeutic effects. However, it is to note that neutralization of IL-17 can not eliminate tumors. Mechanisms for tumor development and tumor promoting inflammation are complicated. It is known that the immune system in tumor bearing host is suppressed. It is possible that IL-17 is just part of tumor promoting inflammation factors or that blockade of IL-17 diminishes the promoting effects of inflammation but can not restore the activity of tumor specific T cells to eliminate tumors. Interestingly, a recent report shows that IL-17 producing $\gamma\delta$T cells contribute to the efficacy of anticancer chemotherapy. A deficiency in IL-17 responses inhibits the infiltration of cytotoxic T cells in the implanted colon tumors [60]. Similarly, in implanted melanoma model, Th17 cells promote the activity of cytotoxic T cells in tumors [61]. DMBA/TPA induced skin tumors are associated with persistent inflammation which may constitute a different microenvironment from that in implant tumors. It implicates that tumor treatment requires multifaceted strategies which will be dependent on tumor type, stage and microenvironment.

In summary, our studies have demonstrated that IL-17 is required for inflammation associated tumor development in DMBA/TPA induced skin carcinogenesis and IL-17 induces tumor promoting inflammation through multiple interactive mechanisms. TPA induced inflammation enhances the susceptibility to tumor growth, which is associated with an increased level of tumor specific IL-17 producing T cells. Blockade of IL-17 can abrogate the inflammation induced susceptibility to tumor growth and inhibit the progression of existing tumors in DMBA/TPA induced skin carcinogenesis. Given the important role of inflammation in tumor development, our studies implicate that targeting IL-17 may provide novel strategies for prevention and treatment of inflammation associated tumors.

Materials and Methods

Mice

IL-12p35-/- (C57BL/6 background) and wild type C57BL/6 mice were purchased from The Jackson Laboratory (Bar Harbor, Maine). IL-17R-/- mice on C57BL/6 background were provided by Amgen. IL-17R-/- mice were cross-bred to p35-/- mice to generate double knockout mice in our laboratory. The gene phenotype was routinely confirmed. All animal procedures were performed according to NIH guidelines and the protocols were approved by the Institute Animal Care and Use Committee of the University of Alabama at Birmingham (APN: 081008302).

Cutaneous chemical carcinogenesis

Detailed protocols for DMBA/TPA induced carcinogenesis were reported previously [15]. In the current studies, mice were treated once with 100 µg DMBA (Sigma, St Louis, MO) in 100 µl acetone on the shaved back skin. One week later, the DMBA treated skin site was treated topically with 10 µg TPA in 100 µl acetone twice weekly. The development of cutaneous tumors was monitored every week. Tumors which were larger than 2 mm in diameter and were present for two consecutive weeks were counted. In compliance with IACUC requests, which were based on tumor multiplicity and size, mice were euthanized around 26 weeks.

To examine whether neutralization of IL-17 affected the progression of tumors in DMBA/TPA treated mice which had already developed skin tumors, mice were treated once with DMBA and then treated repeatedly with TPA as described above. At 12-14 weeks after the treatment with DMBA/TPA, all mice developed skin tumors. The mice were then divided in three groups with similar average tumor numbers per group (10 mice/group) and treated intravenously with non-replicating adenovirus encoding neutralizing soluble IL-17R (Ad-IL-17R:Fc) or GFP as a control (Ad-GFP)(10^9 pfu/mouse) or left untreated. The treatment was repeated once 4 weeks later. This protocol has been reported in our previous studies to neutralize IL-17 and prevent autoimmune diseases in mice [62]. The mice remained to be treated with TPA twice a week and tumor progression was monitored once a week as described above.

Examination of TAP induced tumor promoting inflammation in the skin

To examine TPA induced inflammation, back skin of mice was shaved and treated with TPA (10 µg in 100 µl acetone) every other day for a total of three applications. Skin samples were harvested 24 hours after the last treatment and subjected to analysis for inflammation.

To examine whether pre-existing chronic inflammation increased the susceptibility of mice to tumor growth, mice were topically treated on the shaved back with TPA (10 µg in 100 µl acetone) or vehicle control (acetone) every other day for a total of five applications. The mice were then implanted subcutaneously in the TAP treated area with a mouse lymphoma cells line EG7 (EL4 transfected with OVA, E.G7-OVA, CRL-2113, ATCC) at 4×10^6/mouse one day after the last treatment with TPA. The growth of tumors was measured every three days by using an engineer's micrometer [34].

Analysis of T cell cytokine production

The draining lymph nodes of EG7 tumor bearing mice were collected at the end of experiments and cell suspensions were prepared as described [34]. Bone marrow derived dendritic cells (BM-DC) were generated and pulsed with OVA for 24 hours as described in our previous report [34]. The lymph node cells (2×10^6/ml) were stimulated with OVA-pulsed BM-DC (2×10^5/ml) for 4 days. Culture supernatants were harvested and measured for concentrations of cytokines by ELISA as described [34]. Naïve T cells with OVA pulsed BM-DC (Naïve) and immune T cells with BM-DC without OVA (Neg) served as controls in the cultures.

Immunohistochemical staining of skin tissues

Immunohistochemical staining of tissue sections was described in our previous studies [63]. Frozen tissue sections (5 μm) were applied for staining of CD8 and CD11b positive cells. Paraffin embedded sections (6 μm) were applied for staining of PCNA and Cox-2. The antibodies were purchased from Santa Cruz Biotechnology (Santa Cruz, CA), Cayman Chemical (Ann Arbor, MI) and BD-Biosciences (San Diego, CA). Pictures were taken microscopically (20× objective) with a digital camera (Olympus). Positive cells were counted in 10 fields of each group. Average numbers of positive cells per field were calculated and the difference between groups was analyzed statistically. The thickness of epidermis of skin sections was measured with the ImagePro Plus software.

Analysis of PGE_2 by enzyme immunoassay

The concentration of PGE2 in the TPA treated skin tissues was measured by using a prostaglandin E_2 EIA kit according to the manufacturer's instructions (Cayman Chemical, Ann Arbor, MI). Briefly, skin samples were homogenized in the buffer provided by the kit and centrifuged at 11,000 rpm for 15 min. The concentration of PGE_2 in supernatants was determined and normalized to the protein concentration in supernatants.

Western blot

Western blots were conducted as reported in our previous studies [64]. To detect S100A8 and A9 proteins, skin tissues were harvested and lysed in the RIPA buffer. Equal amounts of proteins samples were loaded onto 7.5% SDS-PAGE and then transferred to nitrocellulose membranes. The membranes were probed with anti-S100A8, A9 or GAPDH antibodies. After wash, the blots were incubated with appropriate horseradish peroxidase-linked secondary antibodies. Protein bands were revealed by enhanced chemiluminescence (ECL) system (Pierce biotechnology, Rockford, IL). Blots were photographed with Bio-Rad gel documentation system and analyzed using Quantity one 1-D Analysis Software (Bio-Rad Laboratories, Hercules, CA).

Detection of cytokines in skin tissues

Skin tissues were homogenized in the RIPA buffer. Concentrations of IL-1β and TNF-α in the lysates were measured by cytokine specific ELISA using commercial assay kits according to the manufacturer's instructions (Invitrogen). Concentrations of cytokines were normalized to protein concentrations in each sample.

Real Time RT-PCR

The expression of mRNA for chemokines and inflammatory mediators was quantified by real time RT-PCR as described in our previous report [23]. Briefly, Skin tissues were homogenized in TRIzol and total RNA was isolated according to the manufacture's instructions (GibcoBRL). Real time TR-PCR was performed with iQ SYBRO Green Supermix Kit in a MyiQ real time qPCR system according to the manufacture's instructions (Bio-Rad). The expression level of cytokines was normalized to the house-keeping gene GAPDH in each sample. The sequences for primers were The sequences for primers were The sequences for primers were : CXCL9: forward, 5′-CCGCTGTTCTTTTC-CTTTTG-3′, reverse, 5′-TCCCCCTCTTTTGCTTTTTC-3; S100A9: forward, 5′-TCATCGACACCTTCCATCAA-3′, reverse, 5′-GATCAACTTTGCCATCAGCA-3′; S100A8: forward, 5′-ACAATGCCGTCTGAACTGG-3′, reverse, 5′-CTCTGCT-ACTCCTTGTGGCTGTCT-3′; CXCL1: forward, 5′-GCTG-GGATTCACCTCAAGAAC-3′, reverse, 5′-TGGGGACACCT-TTTAGCATC-3′; CXC16: forward, 5′-ATGAGAAACAGCAA-GATGACAG-3′, reverse, 5′-CAGTGAGGAAGAAGACAAT-GG -3′; CXCL10: forward, 5′-CGTCATTTTCTGCCT-CATCC-3′, reverse, 5′-CAGACATCTCTGCTCATCATTC-3′; KC: forward, 5′-GATTCACCTCAAGAACATCCAG-3′, reverse, 5′-TGGGGACACCTTTTAGCATC-3′; IL-1β: forward, 5′-ACAGCAGCACATCAACAAGAG-3′, reverse, 5′-ATGG-GAACGTCACACACCAG-3′; GApDH: forward, 5′-AATGGT-GAAG GTCGGTGTGAAC-3′, reverse, 5′-GAAGATGGT-GATGGGCTTCC-3′.

Statistical analysis

All data are presented as means +/− SEM. Two-tailed Student's *t*-test was applied for statistical analysis with $P<0.05$ being considered statistically significant.

Acknowledgments

DH. We thank Dr. Dr. Jay K. Kolls for providing adenovirus encoding mouse IL-17R:Fc and Dr. John Mountz, Dr. Hui-Chen Hsu and Dr. Jun Li for helps in generation of adenovirus encoding IL-17R:Fc.

Author Contributions

Conceived and designed the experiments: HX CAE SK MA. Performed the experiments: DH HL HX SK. Analyzed the data: MA SK NY HX. Contributed reagents/materials/analysis tools: MA HX NY. Wrote the paper: HX DH.

Reference

1. Dunn GP, Old LJ, Schreiber RD (2004) The Three Es of Cancer Immunoediting. Annual Review of Immunology 22: 329–360.
2. Swann JB, Smyth MJ (2007) Immune surveillance of tumors. J Clin Invest 117: 1137–1146.
3. Zitvogel L, Tesniere A, Kroemer G (2006) Cancer despite immunosurveillance: immunoselection and immunosubversion. Nat Rev Immunol 6: 715.
4. Carlos TM (2001) Leukocyte recruitment at sites of tumor: dissonant orchestration. J Leukoc Biol 70: 171–184.
5. Vesely MD, Kershaw MH, Schreiber RD, Smyth MJ (2011) Natural Innate and Adaptive Immunity to Cancer. Annual Review of Immunology 29: 235–271.
6. Balkwill F, Charles KA, Mantovani A (2005) Smoldering and polarized inflammation in the initiation and promotion of malignant disease. Cancer Cell 7: 211–217.
7. Coussens LM, Werb Z (2002) Inflammation and cancer. Nature 420: 860.
8. Galon J, Costes A, Sanchez-Cabo F, Kirilovsky A, Mlecnik B, et al. (2006) Type, Density, and Location of Immune Cells Within Human Colorectal Tumors Predict Clinical Outcome. Science 313: 1960–1964.
9. Pollard JW (2004) Tumour-educated macrophages promote tumour progression and metastasis. Nature Reviews Cancer 4: 71.
10. Whiteside TL (2008) The tumor microenvironment and its role in promoting tumor growth. Oncogene 27: 5904–5912.
11. Mantovani A, Allavena P, Sica A, Balkwill F (2008) Cancer-related inflammation. Nature 454: 436–444.
12. Iwakura Y, Ishigame H, Saijo S, Nakae S (2011) Functional Specialization of Interleukin-17 Family Members. Immunity 34: 149–162.
13. Cua DJ, Tato CM (2010) Innate IL-17-producing cells: the sentinels of the immune system. Nat Rev Immunol 10: 479–489.
14. Zou W, Restifo NP (2010) TH17 cells in tumour immunity and immunotherapy. Nat Rev Immunol 10: 248–256.
15. Yusuf N, Nasti TH, Katiyar SK, Jacobs MK, Seibert MD, et al. (2008) Antagonistic Roles of CD4+ and CD8+ T-Cells in 7,12-Dimethylbenz(a)anthracene Cutaneous Carcinogenesis. Cancer Res 68: 3924–3930.
16. Maniati E, Soper R, Hagemann T (2010) Up for Mischief? IL-17/Th17 in the tumour microenvironment. Oncogene 29: 5653–5662.

17. Chae W-J, Gibson TF, Zelterman D, Hao L, Henegariu O, et al. (2010) Ablation of IL-17A abrogates progression of spontaneous intestinal tumorigenesis. Proceedings of the National Academy of Sciences 107: 5540–5544.
18. Wang L, Yi T, Zhang W, Pardoll DM, Yu H (2010) IL-17 Enhances Tumor Development in Carcinogen-Induced Skin Cancer. Cancer Research 70: 10112–10120.
19. Charles KA, Kulbe H, Soper R, Escorcio-Correia M, Lawrence T, et al. (2009) The tumor-promoting actions of TNF-a involve TNFR1 and IL-17 in ovarian cancer in mice and humans. J Clin Inv 119: 3011–3023.
20. DiGiovanni J (1992) Multistage carcinogenesis in mouse skin. Pharmacol Ther 54: 63–128.
21. Yusuf N, Timares L, Seibert MD, Xu H, Elmets CA (2007) Acquired and innate immunity to polyaromatic hydrocarbons. Toxicology and Applied Pharmacology 224: 308.
22. Owens DM, Wei SJC, Smart RC (1999) A multihit, multistage model of chemical carcinogenesis. Carcinogenesis 20: 1837–1844.
23. Moore RJ, Owens DM, Stamp G, Arnott C, Burke F, et al. (1999) Mice deficient in tumor necrosis factor-[alpha] are resistant to skin carcinogenesis. Nat Med 5: 828.
24. Krelin Y, Voronov E, Dotan S, Elkabets M, Reich E, et al. (2007) Interleukin-1{beta}-Driven Inflammation Promotes the Development and Invasiveness of Chemical Carcinogen-Induced Tumors. Cancer Res 67: 1062–1071.
25. Muller-Decker K, Neufang G, Berger I, Neumann M, Marks F, et al. (2002) Transgenic cyclooxygenase-2 overexpression sensitizes mouse skin for carcinogenesis. Proceedings of the National Academy of Sciences of the United States of America 99: 12483–12488.
26. Tiano HF, Loftin CD, Akunda J, Lee CA, Spalding J, et al. (2002) Deficiency of Either Cyclooxygenase (COX)-1 or COX-2 Alters Epidermal Differentiation and Reduces Mouse Skin Tumorigenesis. Cancer Res 62: 3395–3401.
27. Gebhardt C, Riehl A, Durchdewald M, Nemeth J, Furstenberger G, et al. (2008) RAGE signaling sustains inflammation and promotes tumor development. J Exp Med 205: 275–285.
28. Gebhardt C, Németh J, Angel P, Hess J (2006) S100A8 and S100A9 in inflammation and cancer. Biochemical Pharmacology 72: 1622–1631.
29. Cheng P, Corzo CA, Luetteke N, Yu B, Nagaraj S, et al. (2008) Inhibition of dendritic cell differentiation and accumulation of myeloid-derived suppressor cells in cancer is regulated by S100A9 protein. J Exp Med 205: 2235–2249.
30. Yusuf N, Nasti TH, Long JA, Naseemuddin M, Lucas AP, et al. (2008) Protective Role of Toll-like Receptor 4 during the Initiation Stage of Cutaneous Chemical Carcinogenesis. Cancer Res 68: 615–622.
31. Langowski JL, Zhang X, Wu L, Mattson JD, Chen T, et al. (2006) IL-23 promotes tumour incidence and growth. Nature 442: 461.
32. Mantovani A, Allavena P, Sica A, Balkwill F (2008) Cancer-related inflammation. Nature 454: 436.
33. Vakkila J, Lotze MT (2004) Inflammation and necrosis promote tumour growth. Nat Rev Immunol 4: 641–648.
34. He D, Li H, Yusuf N, Elmets CA, Li J, et al. (2010) IL-17 Promotes Tumor Development through the Induction of Tumor Promoting Microenvironments at Tumor Sites and Myeloid-Derived Suppressor Cells. J Immunol 184: 2281–2288.
35. Murugaiyan G, Saha B (2009) Protumor vs Antitumor Functions of IL-17. J Immunol 183: 4169–4175.
36. Wu S, Rhee K-J, Albesiano E, Rabizadeh S, Wu X, et al. (2009) A human colonic commensal promotes colon tumorigenesis via activation of T helper type 17 T cell responses. Nat Med 15: 1016.
37. Kryczek I, Wei S, Szeliga W, Vatan L, Zou W (2009) Endogenous IL-17 contributes to reduced tumor growth and metastasis. Blood 114: 357–359.
38. Muranski P, Boni A, Antony PA, Cassard L, Irvine KR, et al. (2008) Tumor-specific Th17-polarized cells eradicate large established melanoma. Blood 112: 362–373.
39. Hinrichs CS, Kaiser A, Paulos CM, Cassard L, Sanchez-Perez L, et al. (2009) Type 17 CD8+ T cells display enhanced antitumor immunity. Blood 114: 596–599.
40. Wang L, Yi T, Kortylewski M, Pardoll DM, Zeng D, et al. (2009) IL-17 can promote tumor growth through an IL-6-Stat3 signaling pathway. J Exp Med 206: 1457–1464.
41. Dunn GP, Old LJ, Schreiber RD (2004) The Immunobiology of Cancer Immunosurveillance and Immunoediting. Immunity 21: 137–148.
42. Kolls JK, Linden A (2004) Interleukin-17 Family Members and Inflammation. Immunity 21: 467–476.
43. Zlotnik A, Burkhardt AM, Homey B (2011) Homeostatic chemokine receptors and organ-specific metastasis. Nat Rev Immunol 11: 597–606.
44. Balkwill F, Mantovani A (2001) Inflammation and cancer: back to Virchow? The Lancet 357: 539.
45. Whiteside TL (2006) The role of immune cells in the tumor microenvironment. Cancer Treat Res 130: 103–124.
46. Clevers H (2004) At the Crossroads of Inflammation and Cancer. Cell 118: 671–674.
47. Gabrilovich DI, Nagaraj S (2009) Myeloid-derived suppressor cells as regulators of the immune system. Nat Rev Immunol 9: 162–174.
48. Marigo I, Dolcetti L, Serafini P, Zanovello P, Bronte V (2008) Tumor-induced tolerance and immune suppression by myeloid derived suppressor cells. Immunological Reviews 222: 162–179.
49. Serafini P, Borrello I, Bronte V (2006) Myeloid suppressor cells in cancer: Recruitment, phenotype, properties, and mechanisms of immune suppression. Seminars in Cancer Biology 16: 53–65.
50. Ostrand-Rosenberg S, Sinha P (2009) Myeloid-Derived Suppressor Cells: Linking Inflammation and Cancer. J Immunol 182: 4499–4506.
51. Hanson EM, Clements VK, Sinha P, Ilkovitch D, Ostrand-Rosenberg S (2009) Myeloid-Derived Suppressor Cells Down-Regulate L-Selectin Expression on CD4+ and CD8+ T Cells. J Immunol 183: 937–944.
52. Williams CS, Mann M, DuBois RN (1999) The role of cyclooxygenases in inflammation, cancer, and development. Oncogene 18: 7908–7916.
53. Warner TD, Mitchell JA (2004) Cyclooxygenases: new forms, new inhibitors, and lessons from the clinic. FASEB J 18: 790–804.
54. Gupta RA, DuBois RN (2001) Colorectal cancer prevention and treatment by inhibition of cyclooxygenase-2. Nat Rev Cancer 1: 11.
55. Backlund MG, Mann JR, DuBois RN (2005) Mechanisms for the Prevention of Gastrointestinal Cancer: The Role of Prostaglandin E 2. Oncology 69: 28–32.
56. Rodriguez PC, Hernandez CP, Quiceno D, Dubinett SM, Zabaleta J, et al. (2005) Arginase I in myeloid suppressor cells is induced by COX-2 in lung carcinoma. J Exp Med 202: 931–939.
57. Sinha P, Clements VK, Fulton AM, Ostrand-Rosenberg S (2007) Prostaglandin E2 Promotes Tumor Progression by Inducing Myeloid-Derived Suppressor Cells. Cancer Res 67: 4507–4513.
58. Sinha P, Okoro C, Foell D, Freeze HH, Ostrand-Rosenberg S, et al. (2008) Proinflammatory S100 Proteins Regulate the Accumulation of Myeloid-Derived Suppressor Cells. J Immunol 181: 4666–4675.
59. Hiratsuka S, Watanabe A, Aburatani H, Maru Y (2006) Tumour-mediated upregulation of chemoattractants and recruitment of myeloid cells predetermines lung metastasis. Nat Cell Biol 8: 1369.
60. Ma Y, Aymeric L, Locher C, Mattarollo SR, Delahaye NF, et al. (2011) Contribution of IL-17-producing $\gamma\delta$T cells to the efficacy of anticancer chemotherapy. J Exp Med 208: 491–503.
61. Martin-Orozco N, Muranski P, Chung Y, Yang XO, Yamazaki T, et al. (2009) T Helper 17 Cells Promote Cytotoxic T Cell Activation in Tumor Immunity. Immunity 31: 787.
62. Hsu H-C, Yang P, Wang J, Wu Q, Myers R, et al. (2008) Interleukin 17-producing T, helper cells and interleukin 17 orchestrate autoreactive germinal center development in autoimmune BXD2 mice. Nat Immunol 9: 166–175.
63. He D, Wu L, Kim HK, Li H, Elmets CA, et al. (2006) CD8+ IL-17-Producing T Cells Are Important in Effector Functions for the Elicitation of Contact Hypersensitivity Responses. J Immunol 177: 6852–6858.
64. Kim HK, Zhang H, Li H, Wu ZT, Swisher S, et al. (2008) Slit2 Inhibits Growth and Metastasis of Fibrosarcoma and Squamous Cell Carcinoma. Neoplasia 10: 1411–1420.

5

JWA Deficiency Suppresses Dimethylbenz[a]Anthracene-Phorbol Ester Induced Skin Papillomas via Inactivation of MAPK Pathway in Mice

Zhenghua Gong[1,2], Yaowei Shi[1,2], Ze Zhu[1,2], Xuan Li[1,2], Yang Ye[1,2], Jianbing Zhang[1,2], Aiping Li[1,2], Gang Li[3], Jianwei Zhou[1,2]*

1 Department of Molecular Cell Biology & Toxicology, the Key Laboratory of Modern Toxicology, Ministry of Education and Department of Occupational Medicine and Environmental Health, School of Public Health; Nanjing Medical University, Nanjing, People's Republic of China, **2** Jiangsu Key Lab of Cancer Biomarkers, Prevention and Treatment, Cancer Center; Nanjing Medical University, Nanjing, People's Republic of China, **3** Department of Dermatology and Skin Science, Jack Bell Research Centre, Vancouver Coastal Health Research Institute, University of British Columbia, Vancouver, British Columbia, Canada

Abstract

Our previous studies indicated that JWA plays an important role in DNA damage repair, cell migration, and regulation of MAPKs. In this study, we investigated the role of JWA in chemical carcinogenesis using conditional JWA knockout (*JWA*$^{\Delta2/\Delta2}$) mice and two-stage model of skin carcinogenesis. Our results indicated that *JWA*$^{\Delta2/\Delta2}$ mice were resistant to the development of skin papillomas initiated by 7, 12-dimethylbenz(a)anthracene (DMBA) followed by promotion with 12-O-tetradecanoylphorbol-13-acetate (TPA). In *JWA*$^{\Delta2/\Delta2}$ mice, the induction of papilloma was delayed, and the tumor number and size were reduced. In primary keratinocytes from *JWA*$^{\Delta2/\Delta2}$ mice, DMBA exposure induced more intensive DNA damage, while TPA-promoted cell proliferation was reduced. The further mechanistic studies showed that JWA deficiency blocked TPA-induced activation of MAPKs and its downstream transcription factor Elk1 both *in vitro* and *in vivo*. *JWA*$^{\Delta2/\Delta2}$ mice are resistance to tumorigenesis induced by DMBA/TPA probably through inhibition of transcription factor Elk1 via MAPKs. These results highlight the importance of JWA in skin homeostasis and in the process of skin tumor development.

Editor: Jeffrey K. Harrison, University of Florida, United States of America

Funding: This study was supported in part by the National Natural Science Foundation of China (No.30930080), the Foundation of Cancer Center of Nanjing Medical University (No. 08ZLKF08),the Jiangsu Provincial Graduates Innovative Project (Z. Gong) and the Priority Academic Program Development (PAPD) of Jiangsu Higher Education Institutions. No additional external funding received for this study. The funders had no role in study design, data collection and analysis, decision to publish, or preparation of the manuscript.

Competing Interests: The authors have declared that no competing interests exist.

* E-mail: jwzhou@njmu.edu.cn

Introduction

Viable cells suffer spontaneous DNA damage or genotoxic agent-induced DNA damages. Therefore, a network of DNA surveillance systems has developed in the cells that monitor and coordinate cell cycle progression with repair of damaged DNA to maintain genome integrity. Unrepaired DNA lesions may result in genetic instability, higher frequency of chromosomal aberrations [1,2] and eventually leading to subsequent tumorigenesis [3,4].

MAPK (Mitogen-activated protein kinase) pathways are involved in the signal transduction of a wide variety of extracellular stimuli [5,6,7]. There are three such classical pathways that activate different MAPK classes, known as ERK (extracellular signal regulated kinase), JNK (Jun N-terminal kinase) and p38, each pathway evokes distinct biological responses. The MEK/ERK pathway is activated by mitogenic stimuli and plays an important role in cell proliferation and differentiation. Activated ERK phosphorylates and activates its targets such as the transcription factor Elk1 (Ets-like transcription factor-1), member of ETS oncogene family. Activated Elk1 organizes ternary complex factor with serum response factor and binds to the serum response element of the promoter of the target genes (e.g. c-fos) and enhances their transcription [8,9,10].

The *JWA* gene, also known as *ARL6ip5* (ADP-ribosylation-like factor 6 interacting protein 5), was initially cloned from human tracheal bronchial epithelial cells after treatment with all-trans retinoic acid [11]. Several JWA homologues (e.g. GTRAP3-18, addicsin and JM4) were since identified [12,13]. Subsequent studies indicated that JWA is involved in the cellular responses to heat shock and chemical-mediated oxidative stresses [14]. JWA plays a key role in protecting cells from DNA damage induced by oxidative stress [15,16]. On the other hand, there is an increasing amount of data to indicate that JWA is a structurally novel microtubule-associated protein, which regulates cancer cell migration via MAPK cascades [17]. Our recent data have shown that JWA plays an important role in melanoma metastasis via integrin signaling pathway [18]. However, the potential role of JWA in chemically induced skin carcinogenesis has not been elucidated. The purpose of this study was to characterize the role and the related molecular mechanisms of JWA in DMBA-TPA induced two-stage skin papilloma development in conditional JWA knockout mice. Our results demonstrate that JWA deletion enhanced cellular DNA damage induced by DMBA at first stage, nevertheless attenuated tumor incidence induced by TPA at second stage and probably via inactivation of MAPK pathway.

Materials and Methods

Generation and genotype identification of JWA mice and cells

The conditional $\mathit{JWA}^{\Delta 2/\Delta 2}$ mice were created by contract service at the Model Animal Research Center of Nanjing University, Nanjing, China. Bacterial artificial chromosome-retrieval methods were used for constructing the targeting vector. In brief, an 11 kb genomic DNA fragment containing 5′ element to exon2 of the *JWA* was retrieved from a 129/sv BAC clone bMO 366n04 by a retrieval vector containing 2 homologous arms. Exon2, which encodes the majority of conserved PRA-1 (prenylated rab acceptor) domain, was flanked by 2 *loxP* sites and an *frt-Neo-frt* cassette as a positive selection marker. In theory, this deletion will cause an out-of-frame reading shift and thereby generate a premature stop codon and a loss-of-function allele (Fig. 1). Embryonic stem W4 cells were electroporated with the linearized targeting vector, selected, then expanded for Southern blot analysis. Chimeric mice were generated by injecting ES cells into C57BL/6 blastocysts followed by transferring to pseudopregnant mice. These chimeric mice ($\mathit{JWA}^{loxP/+}$) were viable and finally interbred to generate $\mathit{JWA}^{loxP/loxP}$ mice, which are healthy, fertile and have reached maturity. To generate $\mathit{JWA}^{\Delta 2/+}$ mice, $\mathit{JWA}^{loxP/loxP}$ mice were crossed with mice transgenic for *EIIa-Cre* (adenovirus early transcription region IIa promoter-Cre), which express Cre in germ cells. JWA null mutant mice ($\mathit{JWA}^{\Delta 2/\Delta 2}$) were produced by intercrossing the $\mathit{JWA}^{\Delta 2/+}$ mice. Subsequent breeding yielded genotypes for experiments. All experiments were conducted in accordance with Animal Care and Use Committee of Model Animal Research Centre.

For mice and cells genotyping, genomic DNA from the tip of tail of 4-week-old pups or cells was extracted by means of standard protocols. The following primers were used for simultaneous detection of wild-type and null JWA alleles: 5′-CCACTGT-TTCCTCTGTTG (P1, forward primer for wild-type and null JWA); 5′-GTGAAAACCACTGAGAACC (P2, reverse primer for wild-type JWA); 5′-CAGATGTTCCTCGTGTATC (P3, reverse primer for null JWA). 5′-ATCAACGTTTTCTTTTCGG (forward primer for *cre*) and 5′-ATTTGCCTGCATTACCGGTC (reverse primer for *cre*).

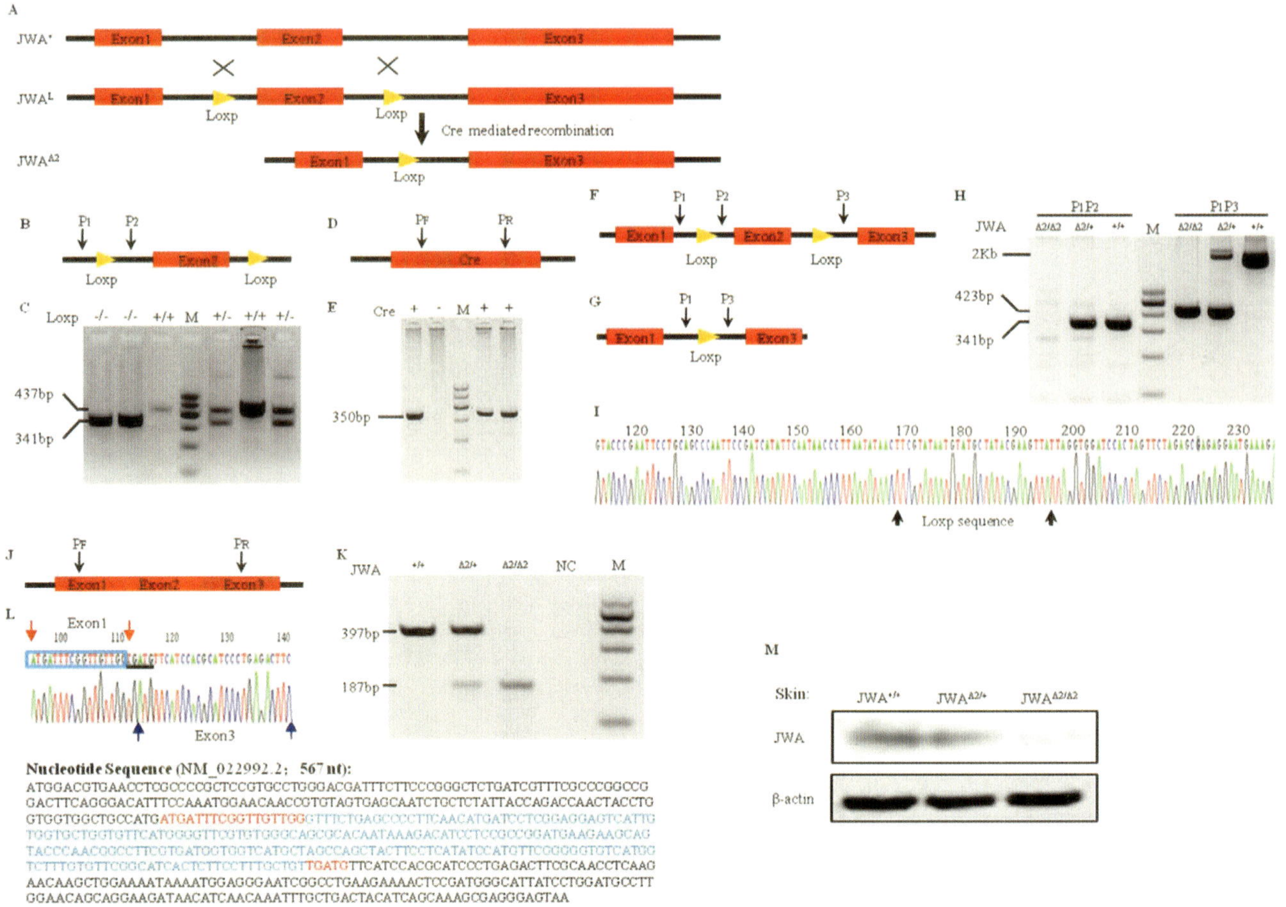

Figure 1. The construction and genotype verification of JWA knockout mice. (A) Schematic representation of JWA gene-targeting strategy. Exon2 of JWA was floxed with Loxp site (*JWA*^{L}), after Cre mediated recombination, the exon2 was deleted (*JWA*$^{\Delta 2}$). (B, C) Genotyping of Loxp mice by PCR. Forward (P1) and reverse (P2) primers used in PCR analysis were shown in (B), the products of PCR acquired were about 437 bp after Loxp inserted. (D, E) Genotyping of *EIIa* Cre mice. (F–I) Genotyping of JWA knockout mice at DNA level. The primers used were shown in (F) and (G). (H) Genotyping of *JWA*$^{\Delta 2/\Delta 2}$ and *JWA*$^{\Delta 2/+}$ mice by PCR with paired primers. (I) Sequencing result of 341 bp product after exon2 deleted. (J–L) Genotyping of JWA knockout mice at mRNA level. Primers used in RT-PCR analysis were shown in (J). PCR results were shown in (K). The sequencing result of 187 bp product was shown in (L), which is comparable with the Entrze JWA sequence (NM_022992.2). NC, negative control; M, marker. For all the experiments, markers were 600 bp, 500 bp, 400 bp, 300 bp, 200 bp, 100 bp in order. (M) The skin protein from *JWA*$^{+/+}$, *JWA*$^{\Delta 2/+}$ and *JWA*$^{\Delta 2/\Delta 2}$ mice were analyzed by Western-blot. β-actin was used as the loading control.

For mouse and cells genotype confirmation at RNA level, the RNA from mice or cells was transcribed and subjected to RT-PCR analysis by standard protocol. The following primers were used for detection of $JWA^{+/+}$ and $JWA^{\Delta2/\Delta2}$ mice: 5′-AACC-GTGTAGTGAGCAATCTTG (forward primer) and 5′-GGA-TAATGCCCATCGGAGT (reverse primer). The PCR products from genomic DNA and cDNA were subject to further sequencing analysis for final verification.

Skin papilloma induction by DMBA/TPA

All the mice used for experiments were maintained in the C57BL/6 background with at least six backcrosses from the original 129Sv/C57BL/6 founder mice. Both wild type and $JWA^{\Delta2/\Delta2}$ mice were used in this DMBA/TPA two-stage papilloma induction assay. All the genotypes of mice and cells were verified at genomic DNA and cDNA level, respectively. A total of 48 mice (8–9 weeks old) were divided into 2 groups, each with either the $JWA^{+/+}$ (n = 24) or $JWA^{\Delta2/\Delta2}$ (n = 24) genotype and identical number of male (n = 10) and female (n = 14) mice.

To induce skin papillomas, mice were shaved on their dorsal skin, and 2 days later treated topically with 25 μg of DMBA (Sigma, St. Louis, MO) in 100 μl acetone once. One week later, each animal received subsequent topical treatments of 2.5 μg of TPA (Sigma, St. Louis, MO) in 100 μl acetone twice a week for 19 weeks. Treated mice were examined twice a week for detecting the presence of skin papillomas, which were not scored as positive until they reached at least 1 mm in diameter. At the end of the two-stage model, all mice were sacrificed, and skin papillomas were counted and isolated for further histological analysis. All experiments were conducted in accordance with Animal Care Committee of Nanjing Medical University.

Histological and immunohistochemical analyses

Dorsal skin and papilloma samples were isolated and fixed in 4% paraformaldehyde at 4°C overnight, embedded in paraffin, and sectioned as 4 μm slides. The sectioned tissues on slides were stained with hematoxylin and eosin. Immunohistochemical staining was further carried out using indicated first antibodies and the Immuno Cruz Staining Systems (Zhongshan Golden Bridge Biotechnology, Beijing, China). The endogenous peroxidase activity in the specimens was blocked by treatment of 0.3% H_2O_2 and the samples were then rinsed with PBS. The specimens were probed consecutively with primary antibody against PCNA (1:100, Epitomics, California, USA), Ki67 (1:200, Abcam, Cambridge, UK) for 2 h, biotin-conjugated goat anti-rabbit IgG for 30 min, horseradish peroxidase-streptavidin complex, and then developed with diaminobenzidine.

Preparation of mouse embryonic fibroblast (MEF) and keratinocytes

On day 13.5 of gestation, embryos from $JWA^{+/\Delta2} \times JWA^{+/\Delta2}$ crossed females were harvested. Embryo head and all visible organs (heart, spleen, etc.) were removed. Remaining embryo was put in 50 ml tube and minced with scissors. 5 ml 0.25% trypsin was added and incubated in 37°C water bath for 20 min. Trypsin was inactivated using 5 ml of Dulbecco's Modified Eagle Medium (DMEM) containing 10% fetal bovine serum. The harvested cells were centrifuged to pellet at 1500×g for 5 min and then resuspended with 15 ml of fresh medium. Cell suspension was allowed to stand for 5–10 min to let the debris settle to the bottom. Top 10 ml of medium containing cells was removed and plated in a 100-mm dish.

For isolating keratinocytes, full-layer skin removed from newborn (1–2 days old) mice was treated with 0.25% trypsin (Invitrogen) overnight at 4°C. The epidermis was then peeled off from the dermis and minced into pieces smaller than 1 mm, and placed into a sterile flask, dispersed by stirring into single cells for 30–60 min, suspended in keratinocyte-SFM with supplements (Invitrogen). Cells were first incubated in dishes coated with type I collagen at 34°C in 5% CO_2 for 12 h to allow cells to attach. Unattached cells were removed by washing with PBS. Attached cells were further cultured in fresh medium, which was refreshed every 2 days.

Neutral comet assay

The keratinocytes were cultured in standard medium for 4 days, and then treated with or without 0.15 μg/ml DMBA for another 24 h. The comet assay was carried out according to the manufacturer's instructions. Briefly, cells at a concentration of 5×10^5/ml in PBS were mixed gently with pre-melted low-temperature-melting agarose at a volume ratio of 1 to 9 (v/v) and spread on glass slides which were coated with normal-temperature agarose. The slides were then submerged in pre-cooled neutral lysis buffer at 4°C for 90 min. After rinsing, the slides were electrophoresed at constant 25 V, 300 mA for 20 min, then equilibrated in Tris-borate EDTA solution, and stained with ethidium bromide. Fluorescent images for at least 50 nuclei were captured using an Olympus microscope and analyzed by CASP-1.2.2 software for tail moment.

Immunofluorescence

Cells grown on coverslips for 24 h were treated with or without 0.15 μg/ml DMBA for 24 h. After washing with PBS three times, cells were fixed with methanol for 10 min followed with PBS wash twice, and then incubated in PBS containing 5% BSA for 1 h. After washing with PBS twice, the cells were incubated with anti-phosphorate γ-H2AX primary antibody (1:300, Upstate, NY) in PBS containing 5% BSA at 4°C overnight. Afterwards, coverslips were washed twice for 5 min in PBS and incubated with Texas Red-conjugated anti-mouse antibody (1:300 in PBS containing 5% BSA) for 1 h. Finally, coverslips were counterstained with DAPI (10 ng/ml) for 10 min. The images were captured using a fluorescent microscope.

Quantitative real-time PCR

Total RNA was extracted from cells or tissues with TRIzol (Invitrogen). Total RNA (2 μg) was reverse transcribed with oligo (d18T) primer using the M-MLV reverse transcriptase for RT-PCR. The cDNA was used as template for quantitative real-time PCR analysis, preformed using SYBR Premix Ex Taq Mix (TaKaRa) with ABI Prism 7900 sequence detection system. Reactions were in triplicate for each sample and data were normalized by GAPDH levels. The following primer pairs were used for the PCR reactions: Elk1, forward primer(F): 5′-T-TTGTGTCCTACCCAGAGGTT-3′ and reverse primer (R): 5′-CTGCACCCTTTGGTGTTCC-3′; c-fos, F: 5′-CCCATCCT-TACGGACTCCC- 3′ and R: 5′-GAGATAGCTGCTCTACT-TTGCC-3′; c-myc, F: 5′-TCTCCATCCTATGTTGCGGTC-3′ and R: 5′- TCCAAGTAACTCGGTCATCATCT-3′; PCNA, F: 5′-TGCTCTGAGGTACCTGAACT-3′ and R: 5′- TGCTTC-CTCATCTTCAATCT-3′; GAPDH, F: 5′-ACAGCCGCATC-TTCTTGTGC-3′ and R: 5′-CACTTTGCCACTGCAAATGG-3′. We used the following PCR procedure: 94°C for 10 min, then 40 cycles of 95°C for 15 s, 60°C for 1 min, 72°C for 45 s.

Western blot analysis

Papillomas and dorsal skin of the mice were isolated and homogenized with a grinder for 10 min in RIPA lysis buffer as previously described [19]. Cellular protein was extracted by whole cell extract protocols from cell pellets in protein lysis buffer containing protease and phosphatase inhibitors. Western blot analysis was performed by standard procedures [18]. Membranes were incubated with antibodies detecting phosphorylated B-Raf (Ser 445), MEK (Ser 217/221), ERK1/2 (Thr202/Tyr204), JNK (Thr183/Tyr185), p38 (Thr180/Tyr182), total B-Raf, MEK, ERK1/2 , JNK, p38 and α-tubulin (1:1000, all from Cell Signaling Technology, Inc. Danvers, MA); JWA (1:1000, Imgenex, San Diego, CA, USA), Elk1, c-fos, c-myc (1:1000, Bioworld, Atlanta, Georgia); PCNA (1:2000, Epitomics, California, USA), β-actin (1/1000, Boster Technology, Wuhan, China)

Statistical analysis

Data were analyzed by Prism software 5.0 (GraphPad Software Inc., La Jolla, CA). The Kaplan-Meier method was used for comparison of the tumor development induced by DMBA/TPA. The Student's *t*-test was performed to determine statistical significance for neutral comet assay and relative expression levels. Wilcoxon rank-sum test was used to compare the difference in tumor numbers. In all the above analyses, a P value of <0.05 was considered statistically significant.

Results

Targeted disruption of the mouse JWA gene

To investigate the role of JWA in the development of mammalian skin tumors, we constructed the conditional JWA knockout mice. Exon2 of JWA was floxed with Loxp site (JWA^{L}), after Cre mediated recombination, the exon2 was deleted ($JWA^{\Delta 2}$) (Fig. 1A). The conditional JWA knockout mice ($JWA^{\Delta 2/\Delta 2}$) were produced by intercrossing the $JWA^{\Delta 2/+}$ mice. Genotyping of Loxp was shown in Fig. 1B (PCR primers location) and Fig. 1C (LoxP marker was shown in lanes contain 437 bp) and genotyping of *EIIa* Cre was indicated in Fig. 1D–E. Genotyping of JWA knockout mice were identified at genome DNA level (Fig. 1F–G for primers location; Fig. 1H for PCR products: non product for P1–P2 amplification in $JWA^{\Delta 2/\Delta 2}$, 341 bp for $JWA^{\Delta 2/+}$and $JWA^{+/+}$, 423 bp for $JWA^{\Delta 2/+}$and $JWA^{\Delta 2/\Delta 2}$ in P1–P3 products; and sequncing confirmed in Fig. 1I); mRNA level (Fig. 1J–L) and

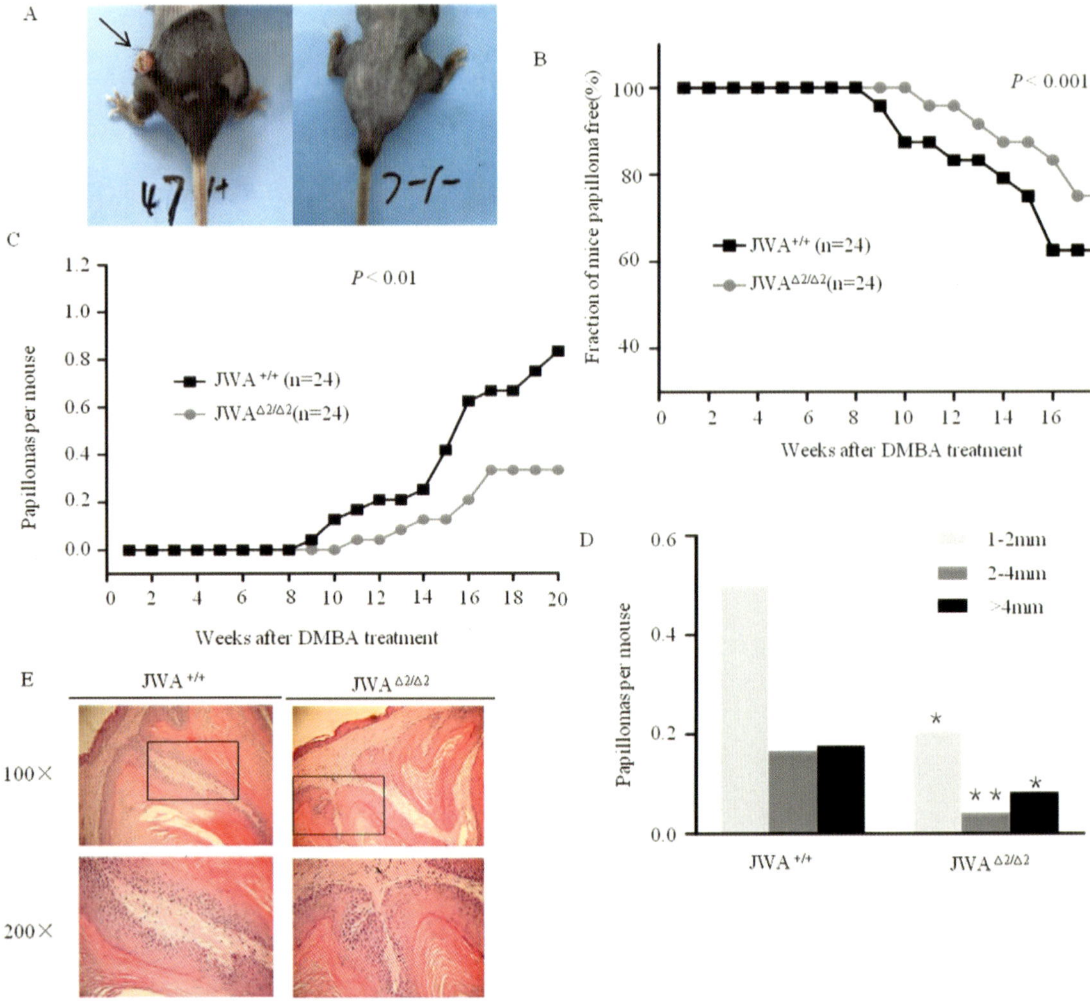

Figure 2. Mouse skin papillomas induced by DMBA/TPA. (A) Papillomas induced by DMBA/TPA treatment in $JWA^{+/+}$ mouse skin (left). Arrow indicates the papilloma. (B) Comparison of the percentage of papilloma-free mice between $JWA^{+/+}$ and $JWA^{\Delta 2/\Delta 2}$ groups after DMBA/TPA treatment. ***$P<0.001$. (C) Comparison of average numbers of papillomas per mouse between $JWA^{+/+}$ and $JWA^{\Delta 2/\Delta 2}$ groups. ***$P<0.001$. (D) Comparison of papilloma size distribution between $JWA^{+/+}$ and $JWA^{\Delta 2/\Delta 2}$ groups. The diameter of papillomas was used to represent the tumor size. *$P<0.05$, **$P<0.01$. (E) H&E staining for typical papillomas from both $JWA^{+/+}$ and $JWA^{\Delta 2/\Delta 2}$ mice.

protein level (Fig. 1M). Although the *JWA*$^{\Delta2/\Delta2}$ mice developed premature ageing like phenotypes such as decreased body weight, kyphosis, osteoporosis, and immune organ atrophy, we have not found any spontaneous tumors during their lifespan (described elsewhere).

JWA deficiency attenuates the development of mouse skin papillomas

As shown in Fig. 2A, skin papilloma was induced by DMBA/TPA treatment in both *JWA*$^{+/+}$ and *JWA*$^{\Delta2/\Delta2}$ mouse skin. In the present study, the first papilloma was observed after 8 weeks of TPA treatment in *JWA*$^{+/+}$ mouse and appeared 2 weeks later in *JWA*$^{\Delta2/\Delta2}$ mouse than in *JWA*$^{+/+}$ mouse (Fig. 2B). At the 19th week of TPA treatment, the end point of experiment, 11 *JWA*$^{+/+}$ mice and 6 *JWA*$^{\Delta2/\Delta2}$ mice developed skin papillomas. The ratio of tumor induction in *JWA*$^{+/+}$ mice was significantly higher than in *JWA*$^{\Delta2/\Delta2}$ mice ($P<0.001$). There were significantly fewer number and smaller sizes of papillomas occurred in *JWA*$^{\Delta2/\Delta2}$ mice than in *JWA*$^{+/+}$ mice ($P<0.05$ and $P<0.01$, respectively; Fig. 2 C and D). Skin specimens with H&E staining confirmed that the papillomas with no significant difference between the mice (Fig. 2E). These data suggest that JWA deficiency attenuates the initiation and development of mouse skin papillomas induced by DMBA/TPA treatment.

JWA deficiency inhibits DMBA/TPA induced cell proliferation

To understand whether reduced papillomas in JWA knockout mice was due to inhibition of cell proliferation, expression of PCNA in mouse papillomas and skin tissues nearby was analyzed. As we predicted, data showed the expressions of mRNA ($P<0.01$) (Fig. 3A), protein (Fig. 3B), and the amount of PCNA-positive cells in papillomas was significantly higher in *JWA*$^{+/+}$ than in *JWA*$^{\Delta2/\Delta2}$ mice ($P<0.05$) (Fig. 3C and D). Similar result was obtained from the expression of Ki67 in mouse papillomas (Fig. 3E and F). In addition, the expression levels of PCNA between mouse skin tissues and the papillomas have shown no difference (Fig. S1).

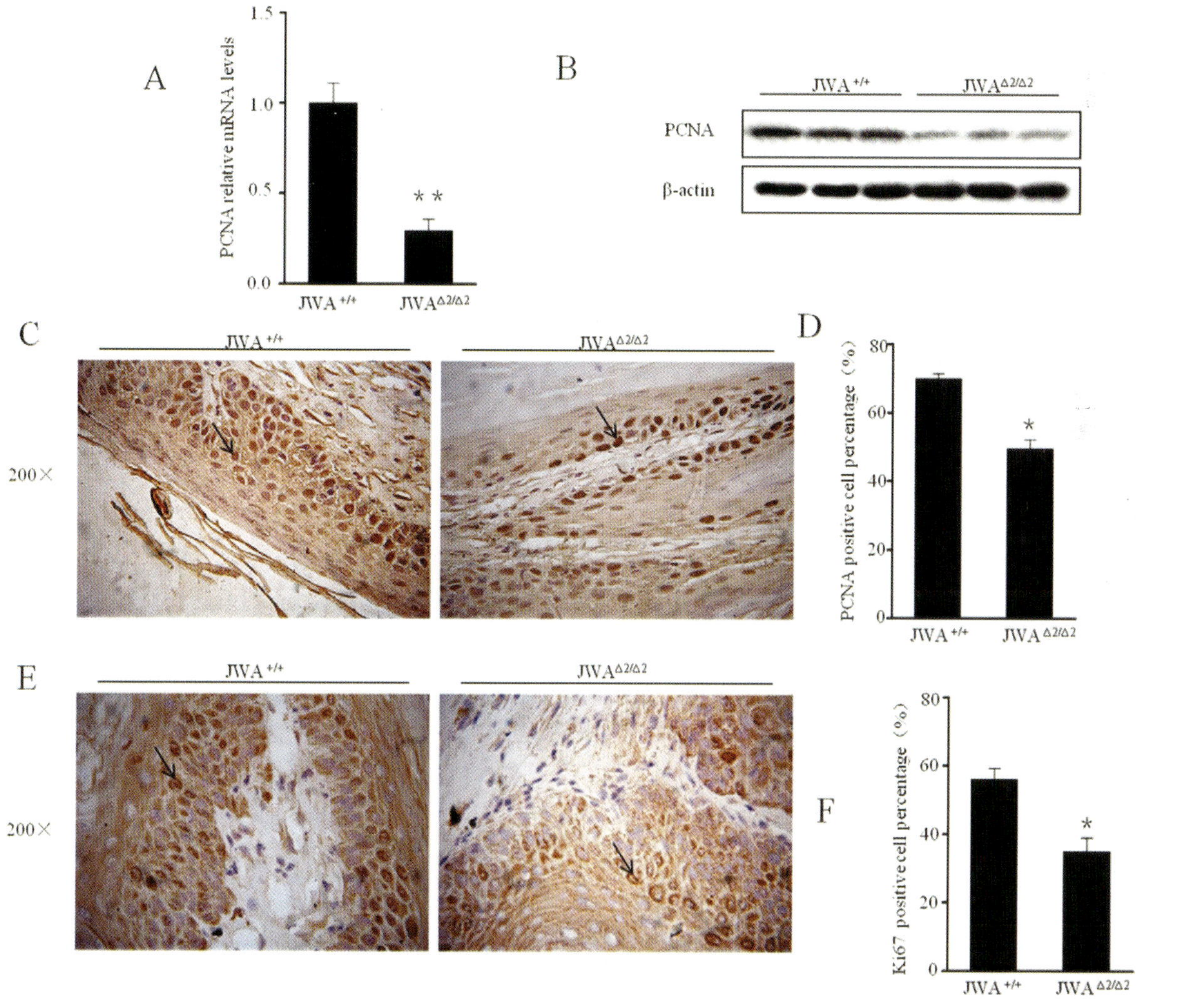

Figure 3. The expression of PCNA and Ki67 in mouse papillomas treated with DMBA/TPA. PCNA expression in the papillomas of *JWA*$^{+/+}$ and *JWA*$^{\Delta2/\Delta2}$ mice (n = 3) treated with DMBA/TPA was analyzed at mRNA level by real-time PCR (A) and protein level by Western blotting (B). * $P<0.05$. (C, E) Typical PCNA and Ki67 immunostaining in papillomas from *JWA*$^{+/+}$ and *JWA*$^{\Delta2/\Delta2}$ mice. Arrows indicate PCNA and Ki67 positive cells. (D, F) The numbers of PCNA and Ki67 positive epidermal cells were counted from at least 100 cells in five separate fields for each section respectively (n = 3). *$P<0.05$. Data were presented as means ± s.d. from three independent experiments.

JWA deficiency blocks TPA-mediated phosphorylations of MAPKs

Cellular proliferation can be mediated by the activation of MAPK signal pathway. We previously reported that JWA as critical activator of MAPK signal pathway involves in the regulation of cell migration [17]. ERK activity was essential for the development of skin papillomas induced by the classic DMBA/TPA skin carcinogenesis protocol [19,20]. To determine whether JWA deficiency attenuated papilloma formation was due to inactivation of MAPKs in mice; both papillomas and skin tissues nearby were extracted for Western blot analysis. As a result, compared to the *JWA*$^{+/+}$ mice, less activation of p-MEK and p-ERK in *JWA*$^{\Delta2/\Delta2}$ mice was found (Fig. 4A and B), although the total expressions of MEK and ERK were unaffected. Interestingly, both phosphorylation and expression of JNK and p38 proteins were also unaffected in papillomas of both *JWA*$^{+/+}$ and *JWA*$^{\Delta2/\Delta2}$ mice (Fig. S2A).

The primary keratinocytes of the both genotypes mice were isolated to verify if JWA deletion blocks the role of TPA on the activation of MAPKs. As shown in Fig. 4C, TPA treatment resulted in more intensive phosphorylations of MEK and ERK in *JWA*$^{+/+}$ keratinocytes, however, this effect was obviously reduced and did not last in *JWA*$^{\Delta2/\Delta2}$ keratinocytes. Furthermore, our data also confirmed *in vivo* result that TPA had no effect on JNK and p38 proteins in both *JWA*$^{+/+}$ and *JWA*$^{\Delta2/\Delta2}$ keratinocytes (Fig. S2B).

JWA regulates transcription factor Elk1 via MEK/ERK pathway

It has been reported that transcription factors Elk1, c-fos and c-myc are all highly related to cell proliferation, and regulated by MEK/ERK pathway [21,22]. We investigated if the role of JWA on PCNA was mediated by any of these transcription factors. As a result, compared to *JWA*$^{+/+}$mice, only expressions of Elk1 at both mRNA ($P<0.05$) (Fig. 5A and Fig. S3A) and protein (Fig. 5B and Fig. S3B) levels were significantly down-regulated in *JWA*$^{\Delta2/\Delta2}$ mouse papillomas and skin tissues.

To investigate if TPA treatment would affect Elk1 expression via activation of MAPKs, we treated *JWA*$^{+/+}$ and *JWA*$^{\Delta2/\Delta2}$ keratinocytes with TPA and found that Elk1 expression was only increased in *JWA*$^{+/+}$ keratinocytes (Fig. 5C). There was no significant difference in protein level of c-fos and c-myc in keratinocytes of both genotypes after treatment with TPA alone or with the MEK inhibitor U0126. Similarly, TPA induced Elk1

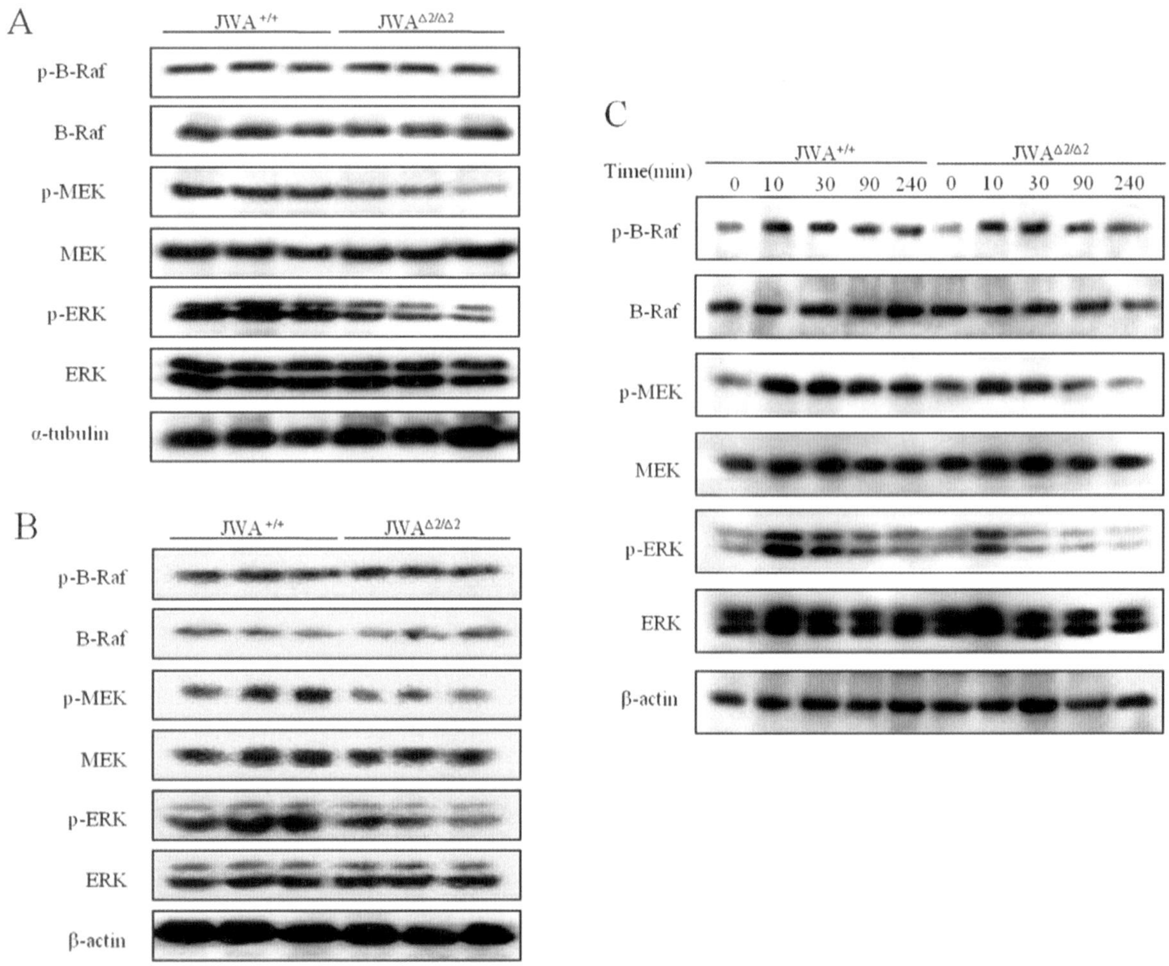

Figure 4. TPA-stimulated phosphorylations of MAPKs in *JWA*$^{+/+}$ and *JWA*$^{\Delta2/\Delta2}$mouse papillomas, skin tissue and keratinocytes. (A–B) Epidermal lysates were prepared in tissue protein extraction buffer from *JWA*$^{+/+}$ and *JWA*$^{\Delta2/\Delta2}$ mouse papillomas (A) and skin (B) treated with DMBA/TPA at the end point of experiment. Total protein (60 μg per well) from paired samples (n = 3) was run on SDS-PAGE and probed with antibodies for phosphorylated or total amounts of B-Raf, MEK and ERK. (C) *JWA*$^{+/+}$ and *JWA*$^{\Delta2/\Delta2}$ keratinocytes were treated with 100 ng/ml TPA at indicated time points. Phosphorylations or total amounts of B-Raf, MEK and ERK were determined by Western blotting. β-actin was used as the loading control. Each experiment was performed in triplicate.

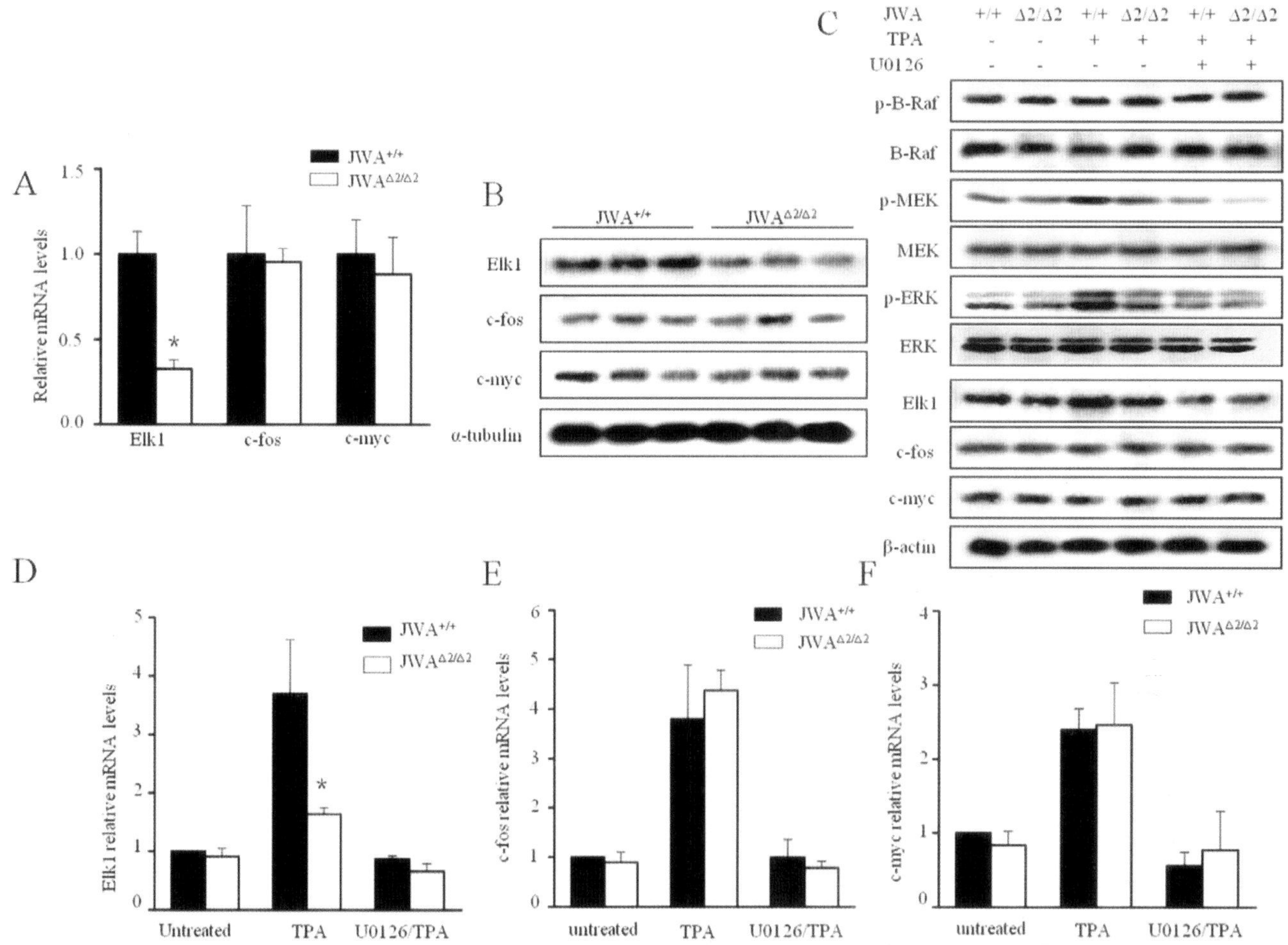

Figure 5. Transcription factor Elk1 was regulated by JWA. (A–B) Elk1, c-fos and c-myc expression in the papillomas from $JWA^{+/+}$ and $JWA^{\Delta2/\Delta2}$ mice (n = 3) were analyzed at mRNA level by real-time PCR (A) and at protein level by Western blotting (B). (C) $JWA^{+/+}$ and $JWA^{\Delta2/\Delta2}$ keratinocytes were treated with or without 100 ng/ml TPA for 30 min or with 5 μg/ml U0126 (MEK inhibitor) for 6 h to silent MEK/ERK signaling, and then treated with 100 ng/ml TPA for 30 min. Related protein expressions were shown. (D–F) The mRNA expression of Elk1 (D), c-fos (E) and c-myc (F) in $JWA^{+/+}$ and $JWA^{\Delta2/\Delta2}$ keratinocytes were analyzed by real-time PCR after TPA and/or U0126 treatment. *$P<0.05$. Data were presented as means ± s.d. from three independent experiments.

mRNA expression ($P<0.05$), and no effects on c-fos and c-myc (Fig. 5D–F). Similar results were obtained from MEFs (Fig. S3C–F). These data provide further evidence that JWA may regulate Elk1 transcription factor via MEK/ERK pathway.

JWA deficiency enhances DMBA-induced DNA damage

MAPK pathway was shown to be involved in DNA damage repair process [23,24]. To investigate if MAPK pathway is involved in DMBA-induced DNA damage repair, phosphorylations of MEK/ERK were examined and results indicated that DMBA does not cause significant change on MEK/ERK phosphorylation (Fig. S4).

Since JWA is a DNA damage repair associated protein, we further investigated if JWA deficiency enhances DMBA-induced DNA damage and genome instability. The neutral comet assay was used to detect DNA double strand breaks (DSBs) of keratinocytes induced by DMBA treatment. As a result, DMBA induced more DSBs in $JWA^{\Delta2/\Delta2}$ keratinocytes than in $JWA^{+/+}$ cells ($P<0.01$) (Fig. 6A and B). Consistent with the result from neutral comet assay, $JWA^{\Delta2/\Delta2}$ keratinocytes had more γ-H2AX positive foci than in $JWA^{+/+}$ cells after DMBA exposure ($P<0.05$) (Fig. 6C and D).

Discussion

JWA was initially isolated as an all-trans-retinoic acid responsive and cytoskeleton-associated gene [11]. Previously, we identified JWA as a novel mitogen activated protein, which binds to α- and β-tubulin and is essential for the rearrangement of F-actin cytoskeleton and activation of MAPK cascades induced by As_2O_3 and TPA [17]. Down-regulation of JWA accelerates melanoma cell migration and adhesion, and promotes cell invasion through matrigel-coated chamber *in vitro* [18]. On the other hand, JWA was regulated by environmental stressors such as heat shock and oxidative stress [14,25]. JWA also participated in the protection of cells from oxidative stress-induced DNA damage [15]. Therefore, JWA is precisely involved in both DNA damage repair process and regulation of MAPK pathway. In the present study, we examined whether combined treatment with DMBA and TPA will affect the development of skin papillomas in $JWA^{\Delta2/\Delta2}$ mice. The data showed that although JWA deficiency enhanced DMBA-induced DNA damage *in vitro*, TPA promotion on the development of skin papillomas was reduced in $JWA^{\Delta2/\Delta2}$ mice compared with $JWA^{+/+}$ mice. These results verified the unique role of MEK/ERK in TPA tumor promotion model and

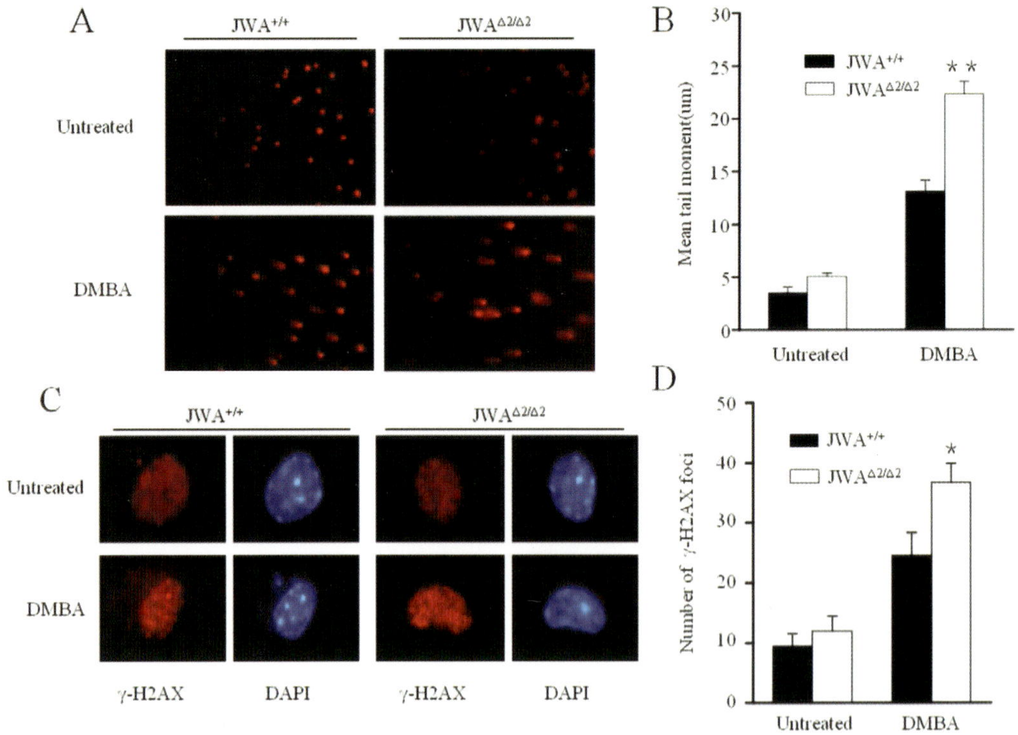

Figure 6. JWA deficiency enhances the DMBA-induced DNA damage. (A) DNA strand breaks in $JWA^{+/+}$ and $JWA^{\Delta 2/\Delta 2}$ keratinocytes after DMBA treatment. Cells were either treated with or without 0.15 μg/ml DMBA for 24 h, and DNA strand breaks were detected by neutral comet assay. (B) Quantification of comet tail movement in (A) from 50 cells in each sample in three independent experiments. $^{**}P<0.01$. (C) γ-H2AX staining in $JWA^{+/+}$ and $JWA^{\Delta 2/\Delta 2}$ keratinocytes after DMBA treatment. Cells were treated with or without 0.15 μg/ml DMBA for 24 h, and DNA strand breaks were detected with γ-H2AX labeling. (D) Quantification of γ-H2AX foci. Foci were counted in at least 50 cells for each sample, and the results were presented as the mean ± s.d. $^{*}P<0.05$.

also indicated for the first time that JWA controls the process as an important checkpoint.

It has been understood for many years that skin carcinogenesis is a multistep process of several separable genetic alterations [26]. The results of mouse skin chemical carcinogenesis studies have provided a conceptual framework for malignant progression. The oxidation of DMBA by P450 enzymes produces metabolites that form covalent adducts with DNA and the formation within DNA of depurinated abasic sites and induces genetic alteration whereby normal cells are converted to a premalignant state. Several DNA repair genes are involved in this step, such as Sirt1, Rad1, Rad9, etc. Rad1 and Rad9 are important for preventing tumor development, probably through maintaining genomic integrity [27,28], while Sirt1 does not behave like a classical tumor-suppressor but partly participates the antitumor activity of resveratrol [29]. Our present study suggests that JWA, as a DNA repair protein, actively responds to DMBA-induced cell stress, which is consistent with the previous studies [15,16]. JWA deficiency cells acquired more severe injury than JWA wild type cells, suggesting JWA deletion increased the susceptibility to tumor induction might be due to reduced DNA repair capacity of cells. This seems to be contradictory to the results from skin carcinogenesis animal model showing that JWA deficiency attenuated tumor formation induced by DMBA/TPA treatment. However, further evidences indicate that JWA deficiency effectively inhibits TPA promotion step. TPA is considered to promote DNA damaged cells to enter hyper-proliferative state via activating transcriptional factors. This step results in clonal expansion of cells to form benign premalignant lesions called papillomas. This promotion step is always involved in the activation of B-Raf/MEK/ERK pathway [19,30], since this pathway is identified to regulate fundamental processes in normal and malignant cells, including proliferation and cell survival [31]. In response to tumor promotion induced by TPA, the inhibition of MEK/ERK is beneficial because it prevents skin tumor development [20,32,33]. We have previously shown that JWA is an upstream activator of MEK. Further analysis in JWA knockout keratinocytes and MEFs revealed that JWA is required for TPA-induced MEK and ERK phosphorylation. Consistent with this result, there was a remarkable decrease in the expression of PCNA in $JWA^{\Delta 2/\Delta 2}$ mice. Therefore, our data indicated that in DMBA/TPA two-stage skin papilloma induction model, MEK-ERK activation is critical for the second step. Without effective activation of MEK-ERK, the cells are less prone to papilloma development even they receive severe DNA damage.

AP-1, which consists of a family of Jun/Fos dimers, is a major positive regulator of cell proliferation and transformation and can be activated by TPA in the skin [34,35,36]. In this study, however, we did not find any positive role of AP-1 during DMBA/TPA papilloma induction. Elk1, as a member of ETS oncogene family, is an identified target of MAPK which has been reported to play a key role in cell proliferation [21,37,38]. We found reduced Elk1 expression in $JWA^{\Delta 2/\Delta 2}$ mouse skin tissues as well as in cultured $JWA^{\Delta 2/\Delta 2}$ MEFs, suggesting that Elk1 may be involved in TPA induced cell proliferation.

The other two MAP kinase pathways (JNK and p38) have observed to counteract malignant transformation under the stress response [31]. Consistent with those findings, we observed that, unlike the B-Raf/MEK/ERK proteins, TPA treatment increased phosphorylations of neither p38 nor JNK in both skin tissue and keratinocytes.

In this study, the reduced skin tumor formation observed in the *JWA*$^{\Delta2/\Delta2}$ mice might be also partially contributed by the similar mechanisms of premature ageing like phenotype, however, the exact molecular evidences need to be further provided. To exclude the contribution of non cell autonomous effects in skin tumor phenotypes observed in the full knockout mice, future studies should include the conditional deletion of this gene from the skin.

In summary, we demonstrate for the first time that JWA deficiency enhances DNA damage in epidermal cells induced by DMBA, however, suppresses TPA-induced MEK-ERK activation, cell proliferation, and formation of skin papillomas. These data has potential clinical implications for targeting JWA in chemoprevention and therapy of skin tumors.

Supporting Information

Figure S1 The expression of PCNA in mouse skin treated with DMBA/TPA. PCNA expression in the skin of *JWA*$^{+/+}$ and *JWA*$^{\Delta2/\Delta2}$ mice (n = 3) treated with DMBA/TPA was analyzed at mRNA level by real-time PCR (A) and protein level by Western blotting (B). * $P<0.05$. (C) Typical PCNA immunostaining in skin from *JWA*$^{+/+}$ and *JWA*$^{\Delta2/\Delta2}$ mice. Arrows indicate PCNA-positive cells. (D) The numbers of PCNA positive epidermal cells were counted from at least 100 cells in five separate fields for each section (n = 3). *$P<0.05$. Data were presented as means ± s.d. from three independent experiments.

Figure S2 TPA-stimulated phosphorylations of MAPKs in *JWA*$^{+/+}$ and *JWA*$^{\Delta2/\Delta2}$ mouse skin and keratinocytes. (A) Skin lysates were prepared in tissue protein extraction buffer from *JWA*$^{+/+}$ and *JWA*$^{\Delta2/\Delta2}$ mouse skin treated with DMBA/TPA at the end point of experiment. Total protein (60 µg per well) from paired samples (n = 3) was run on SDS-PAGE and probed with antibodies for phosphorylated or total amounts of JNK and p38. (B) *JWA*$^{+/+}$ and *JWA*$^{\Delta2/\Delta2}$ keratinocytes were treated with 100 ng/ml TPA for the time period indicated, and phosphorylated or total amounts of JNK and p38 were detected by Western blotting. Each experiment was performed in triplicate.

Figure S3 Transcription factor Elk1 was regulated by JWA. (A, B) Elk1, c-fos and c-myc expression in the skin of *JWA*$^{+/+}$ and *JWA*$^{\Delta2/\Delta2}$ mice (n = 3) were analyzed at mRNA level by real-time PCR (A) and at protein level by Western blotting (B). (C) *JWA*$^{+/+}$ and *JWA*$^{\Delta2/\Delta2}$ MEFs were treated with or without 100 ng/ml TPA for 30 min or with 5 µg/ml U0126 (MEK inhibitor) for 6 h to silent MEK/ERK signaling, and then treated with 100 ng/ml TPA for 30 min. Related protein expressions were shown. (D–F) mRNA expression of Elk1 (D), c-fos (E) and c-myc (F) in *JWA*$^{+/+}$ and *JWA*$^{\Delta2/\Delta2}$ MEFs were analyzed by real-time PCR after TPA and/or U0126 treatment. * $P<0.05$. Data were presented as means ± s.d. from three independent experiments.

Figure S4 The effect of DMBA on phosphorylation of MEK and ERK. *JWA*$^{+/+}$ and *JWA*$^{\Delta2/\Delta2}$ keratinocytes were treated with or without 100 ng/ml DMBA for 30 min or with 5 µg/ml U0126 for 6 h, then by 100 ng/ml DMBA for further 30 min. Phosphorylated or total MEK, ERK expression was determined by Western blotting. β-actin was used for loading control.

Acknowledgments

The authors thank Dr. Yihong Zhong in Department of Pathology, the Safety Assessment and Research Center for Drugs, Jiangsu Province, Nanjing Medical University for the assistance of immunohitochemistry analysis.

Author Contributions

Conceived and designed the experiments: ZG GL J. Zhou. Performed the experiments: ZG ZZ YS XL YY J. Zhang AL. Analyzed the data: ZG ZZ XL J. Zhang. Contributed reagents/materials/analysis tools: ZG ZZ AL. Wrote the paper: ZG GL J. Zhou.

References

1. Carrano AV, Minkler JL, Dillehay LE, Thompson LH (1986) Incorporated bromodeoxyuridine enhances the sister-chromatid exchange and chromosomal aberration frequencies in an EMS-sensitive Chinese hamster cell line. Mutat Res 162: 233–239.
2. Dominguez I, Daza P, Natarajan AT, Cortes F (1998) A high yield of translocations parallels the high yield of sister chromatid exchanges in the CHO mutant EM9. Mutat Res 398: 67–73.
3. Caldecott KW (2008) Single-strand break repair and genetic disease. Nat Rev Genet 9: 619–631.
4. Hanahan D, Weinberg RA (2000) The hallmarks of cancer. Cell 100: 57–70.
5. Denhardt DT (1996) Signal-transducing protein phosphorylation cascades mediated by Ras/Rho proteins in the mammalian cell: the potential for multiplex signalling. Biochem J 318(Pt 3): 729–747.
6. Marshall CJ (1995) Specificity of receptor tyrosine kinase signaling: transient versus sustained extracellular signal-regulated kinase activation. Cell 80: 179–185.
7. Schaeffer HJ, Weber MJ (1999) Mitogen-activated protein kinases: specific messages from ubiquitous messengers. Mol Cell Biol 19: 2435–2444.
8. Hao D, Gao P, Liu P, Zhao J, Wang Y, et al. (2011) AC3-33, a novel secretory protein, inhibits Elk1 transcriptional activity via ERK pathway. Mol Biol Rep 38: 1375–1382.
9. Ely HA, Mellon PL, Coss D (2011) GnRH induces the c-Fos gene via phosphorylation of SRF by the calcium/calmodulin kinase II pathway. Mol Endocrinol 25: 669–680.
10. Pawelczyk T, Sakowicz M, Podgorska M, Szczepanska-Konkel M (2003) Insulin induces expression of adenosine kinase gene in rat lymphocytes by signaling through the mitogen-activated protein kinase pathway. Exp Cell Res 286: 152–163.
11. Zhou J, Di Y, Zhao D, Wu R (1999) Investigation on Cell Modulation: Signal Transduction, Apoptosis and Gene Expression. Military Medical Sciences Press: Beijing. pp 110–119.
12. Butchbach ME, Lai L, Lin CL (2002) Molecular cloning, gene structure, expression profile and functional characterization of the mouse glutamate transporter (EAAT3) interacting protein GTRAP3-18. Gene 292: 81–90.
13. Schweneker M, Bachmann AS, Moelling K (2005) JM4 is a four-transmembrane protein binding to the CCR5 receptor. FEBS Lett 579: 1751–1758.
14. Zhu T, Chen R, Li AP, Liu J, Liu QZ, et al. (2005) Regulation of a novel cell differentiation-associated gene, JWA during oxidative damage in K562 and MCF-7 cells. J Biomed Sci 12: 219–227.
15. Chen R, Qiu W, Liu Z, Cao X, Zhu T, et al. (2007) Identification of JWA as a novel functional gene responsive to environmental oxidative stress induced by benzo[a]pyrene and hydrogen peroxide. Free Radic Biol Med 42: 1704–1714.
16. Wang S, Gong Z, Chen R, Liu Y, Li A, et al. (2009) JWA regulates XRCC1 and functions as a novel base excision repair protein in oxidative-stress-induced DNA single-strand breaks. Nucleic Acids Res 37: 1936–1950.
17. Chen H, Bai J, Ye J, Liu Z, Chen R, et al. (2007) JWA as a functional molecule to regulate cancer cells migration via MAPK cascades and F-actin cytoskeleton. Cell Signal 19: 1315–1327.
18. Bai J, Zhang J, Wu J, Shen L, Zeng J, et al. (2009) JWA regulates melanoma metastasis by integrin alphaVbeta3 signaling. Oncogene 29: 1227–1237.
19. Cheepala SB, Yin W, Syed Z, Gill JN, McMillian A, et al. (2009) Identification of the B-Raf/Mek/Erk MAP kinase pathway as a target for all-trans retinoic acid during skin cancer promotion. Mol Cancer 8: 27.
20. Bourcier C, Jacquel A, Hess J, Peyrottes I, Angel P, et al. (2006) p44 mitogen-activated protein kinase (extracellular signal-regulated kinase 1)-dependent signaling contributes to epithelial skin carcinogenesis. Cancer Res 66: 2700–2707.
21. Fukuda K, Tsuchihara K, Hijikata M, Nishiguchi S, Kuroki T, et al. (2001) Hepatitis C virus core protein enhances the activation of the transcription factor, Elk1, in response to mitogenic stimuli. Hepatology 33: 159–165.

22. Atanasova GN, Isaeva AR, Zhelev N, Poumay Y, Mitev VI (2007) Effects of the CDK-inhibitor CYC202 on p38 MAPK, ERK1/2 and c-Myc activities in papillomavirus type 16 E6- and E7-transformed human keratinocytes. Oncol Rep 18: 999–1005.
23. Wood CD, Thornton TM, Sabio G, Davis RA, Rincon M (2009) Nuclear localization of p38 MAPK in response to DNA damage. Int J Biol Sci 5: 428–437.
24. Yacoub A, McKinstry R, Hinman D, Chung T, Dent P, et al. (2003) Epidermal growth factor and ionizing radiation up-regulate the DNA repair genes XRCC1 and ERCC1 in DU145 and LNCaP prostate carcinoma through MAPK signaling. Radiat Res 159: 439–452.
25. Zhu T, Chen R, Li A, Liu J, Gu D, et al. (2006) JWA as a novel molecule involved in oxidative stress-associated signal pathway in myelogenous leukemia cells. J Toxicol Environ Health A 69: 1399–1411.
26. Zoumpourlis V, Solakidi S, Papathoma A, Papaevangeliou D (2003) Alterations in signal transduction pathways implicated in tumour progression during multistage mouse skin carcinogenesis. Carcinogenesis 24: 1159–1165.
27. Hu Z, Liu Y, Zhang C, Zhao Y, He W, et al. (2008) Targeted deletion of Rad9 in mouse skin keratinocytes enhances genotoxin-induced tumor development. Cancer Res 68: 5552–5561.
28. Han L, Hu Z, Liu Y, Wang X, Hopkins KM, et al. (2010) Mouse Rad1 deletion enhances susceptibility for skin tumor development. Mol Cancer 9: 67.
29. Boily G, He XH, Pearce B, Jardine K, McBurney MW (2009) SirT1-null mice develop tumors at normal rates but are poorly protected by resveratrol. Oncogene 28: 2882–2893.
30. Cheepala SB, Syed Z, Trutschl M, Cvek U, Clifford JL (2007) Retinoids and skin: microarrays shed new light on chemopreventive action of all-trans retinoic acid. Mol Carcinog 46: 634–639.
31. Dhillon AS, Hagan S, Rath O, Kolch W (2007) MAP kinase signalling pathways in cancer. Oncogene 26: 3279–3290.
32. Scholl FA, Dumesic PA, Barragan DI, Harada K, Charron J, et al. (2009) Selective role for Mek1 but not Mek2 in the induction of epidermal neoplasia. Cancer Res 69: 3772–3778.
33. Johansen C, Vestergaard C, Kragballe K, Kollias G, Gaestel M, et al. (2009) MK2 regulates the early stages of skin tumor promotion. Carcinogenesis 30: 2100–2108.
34. Greenhalgh DA, Welty DJ, Player A, Yuspa SH (1990) Two oncogenes, v-fos and v-ras, cooperate to convert normal keratinocytes to squamous cell carcinoma. Proc Natl Acad Sci U S A 87: 643–647.
35. Angel P, Szabowski A, Schorpp-Kistner M (2001) Function and regulation of AP-1 subunits in skin physiology and pathology. Oncogene 20: 2413–2423.
36. Murray AR, Kisin ER, Kommineni C, Vallyathan V, Castranova V, et al. (2007) Pro/antioxidant status and AP-1 transcription factor in murine skin following topical exposure to cumene hydroperoxide. Carcinogenesis 28: 1582–1588.
37. Yung Y, Yao Z, Aebersold DM, Hanoch T, Seger R (2001) Altered regulation of ERK1b by MEK1 and PTP-SL and modified Elk1 phosphorylation by ERK1b are caused by abrogation of the regulatory C-terminal sequence of ERKs. J Biol Chem 276: 35280–35289.
38. Kilanczyk E, Filipek S, Jastrzebska B, Filipek A (2009) CacyBP/SIP binds ERK1/2 and affects transcriptional activity of Elk-1. Biochem Biophys Res Commun 380: 54–59.

6

Up-Regulated Dicer Expression in Patients with Cutaneous Melanoma

Zhihai Ma[1], Helen Swede[2], David Cassarino[3], Elizabeth Fleming[4], Andrew Fire[1], Soheil S. Dadras[4,5]*

1 Department of Genetics, Stanford University School of Medicine, Stanford, California, United States of America, **2** Department of Community Medicine and Health Care, University of Connecticut Health Center, Farmington, Connecticut, United States of America, **3** Department of Pathology, Southern California Permanente Medical Group, Los Angeles, California, United States of America, **4** Department of Genetics/Developmental Biology, University of Connecticut Health Center, Farmington, Connecticut, United States of America, **5** Department of Dermatology, University of Connecticut Health Center, Farmington, Connecticut, United States of America

Abstract

Background: MicroRNAs (miRNAs) are small non-coding RNAs (18–24 nucleotides) that have recently been shown to regulate gene expression during cancer progression. Dicer, a central enzyme in the multi-component miRNA biogenesis pathway, is involved in cutting precursor miRNAs to functionally mature forms. Emerging evidence shows that Dicer expression is deregulated in some human malignancies and it correlates with tumor progression, yet this role has not yet been investigated in skin cancers.

Methods and Findings: Using an anti-human monoclonal antibody against Dicer and immunohistochemistry, we compared the expression of Dicer protein among 404 clinically annotated controls and skin tumors consisting of melanocytic nevi (n = 71), a variety of melanomas (n = 223), carcinomas (n = 73) and sarcomas (n = 12). Results showed a cell-specific up-regulated Dicer in 81% of cutaneous, 80% of acrolentiginous and 96% of metastatic melanoma specimens compared to carcinoma or sarcoma specimens ($P<0.0001$). The expression of Dicer was significantly higher in melanomas compared to benign melanocytic nevi ($P<0.0001$). In patients with cutaneous melanomas, Dicer up-regulation was found to be significantly associated with an increased tumor mitotic index ($P = 0.04$), Breslow's depth of invasion ($P = 0.03$), nodal metastasis ($P = 0.04$) and a higher American Joint Committee on Caner (AJCC) clinical stage ($P = 0.009$). Using western blot analysis, we confirmed the cell-specific up-regulation of Dicer protein *in vitro*. A pooled-analysis on mRNA profiling in cutaneous tumors showed up-regulation of Dicer at the RNA level in cutaneous melanoma, also showing deregulation of other enzymes that participate in the biogenesis and maturation of canonical miRNAs.

Conclusions: Increased Dicer expression may be a clinically useful biomarker for patients with cutaneous melanoma. Understanding deregulation of Dicer and its influence on miRNA maturation is needed to predict the susceptibility of melanoma patients to miRNA-based therapy in the future.

Editor: Chun-Ming Wong, University of Hong Kong, Hong Kong

Funding: This work was supported by 2008 Melanoma Research Foundation Career Development Award (SSD), Seed Grant from Stanford University Cancer Center (SSD) and research funds from the department of Pathology, Stanford University (SSD). The funders had no role in study design, data collection and analysis, decision to publish, or preparation of the manuscript.

Competing Interests: The authors have declared that no competing interests exist.

* E-mail: dadras@uchc.edu

Introduction

Small (18–24 nucleotides) non-coding RNAs, including microRNAs (miRNAs), regulate gene expression in many biological processes [1] and in human cancers [2]. miRNAs down-regulate expression of specific target genes, in part drawing specificity from seed sequence pairing within the 3′-untranslated region of target mRNAs leading to translational repression and/or mRNA degradation [3]. Specific miRNAs can function as tumor suppressor genes or oncogenes (oncomirs) [4] where deregulated miRNA expression has been demonstrated in a variety of human cancers including chronic lymphocytic leukemia [5], lung cancer [6], colorectal neoplasia [7] and pancreatic endocrine and acinar tumors [8]. Global miRNA expression profiling has provided some evidence that the expression of certain miRNAs is deregulated during melanoma progression. While these studies are limited to cell lines [9,10,11] and metastatic lesions [12], little is known about the role of miRNAs or their biogenesis pathway in clinical primary melanoma [13,14].

Dicer, a member of the RNase III family of double-stranded RNases, is a central enzyme in a multi-component miRNA biogenesis pathway where the Drosha/DGCR8 complex and Dicer act sequentially to crop long primary and precursor miRNAs into functionally mature miRNAs [15]. The expression levels of the processing components themselves are certainly candidates for deregulation in the development and the progression of human cancers. For example, high dicer expression is a poor prognostic factor in patients with prostate adenocarcinoma [16], whereas low Dicer expression is a poor prognostic factor in lung [17] and ovarian [18] carcinoma.

Although changes in the expression level of Dicer, and possibly other miRNA processing enzymes, are of clinical significance in some cancers, these alterations or their clinical consequences in melanoma or other skin cancers remain unknown.

We demonstrate herein that Dicer protein is specifically up-regulated in melanoma compared to other skin cancers such as carcinomas and sarcomas. This up-regulation is further specific to melanoma subtype and is significantly associated with clinical stage in patients with cutaneous melanoma. Additional analyses of Dicer levels in tissue culture cells support a general up-regulation of Dicer in melanoma and suggest an autonomous up-regulation in the absence of supporting cells.

Materials and Methods

Clinical Profile of Tissue Microarrays and Cases

We used seven different tissue microarray (TMA) slides, prepared from formalin-fixed paraffin embedded (FFPE) specimens, representing a wide variety of human skin tumors, both benign and malignant, from 404 different patients arrayed onto slides at 80 to 100 cores per slide (in duplicates or triplicates). This set also included complete tumor FFPE sections. The TMA slides included normal tissue (skin and other organs), melanocytic nevi (compound, intradermal and blue), primary melanomas (acrolentiginous, cutaneous, desmoplastic, mucosal, ocular), metastatic melanomas, squamous cell carcinoma, adenocarcinoma (eccrine, sebaceous and metastatic), basal cell carcinoma, sarcomas (dermatofibrosarcoma protuberans and fibrosarcomas), neurofibromas, and benign and malignant schwannomas. We purchased TMA slides ME1001, ME801, SK803 and BC21011 from US Biomax, Inc. (Rockville, MD) and CS38-01-001 from Cybrdi (Rockville, MD). The squamous or melanocytic differentiation of tumors was confirmed by immunohistochemical staining for cytokeratins or HMB-45, respectively, by the manufacturers. DC-1 and DC-2 TMAs were built at Stanford University Pathology Department (DC). For most TMAs, the information on age, sex and anatomic sites were available. For primary melanomas arrayed on DC-1 and DC-2 TMAs, the information on age, tumor thickness (Breslow's depth, Clark's level of invasion and histological type were available. Complete tumor sections were also examined that included cutaneous melanomas ($n = 19$), metastatic melanomas to lymph node ($n = 5$) and common nevi ($n = 9$). At least two pathologists/dermatopathologists (SSD and/or DC) confirmed all diagnoses. The institutional review boards of the Stanford University Medical Center and the University of Connecticut Health Center approved this protocol.

Patients

Out of 95 patients diagnosed with primary cutaneous melanoma, we had complete clinical follow-up information for 19 patients (mean = 26.6 month, range 7 to 64 months). The majority of cases were obtained from the Stanford University Pathology archive from 1997-2006. Clinical information included gender, age, anatomic site of the primary tumor, relapse-free survival, American Joint Committee on Cancer (AJCC) pathological (tumor, node, metastasis) stage [19], site of first metastasis, sentinel (SLN) and non-sentinel lymph node (NSLN), distant metastasis and overall survival. Distant metastasis was defined as either distant nodal or visceral. Histological information included tumor thickness (mm), Clark's level of invasion, ulceration, histological subtype, regression, and mitotic index (mitoses per square millimeter) as previously described [20]. At least two pathologists confirmed all the diagnoses of primary and metastatic melanomas. The institutional review board of the Stanford University Medical Center approved this protocol.

Immunohistochemistry and Statistical Analysis

Immunostaining for all cases (TMAs and complete sections) was performed on 4-mm-thick FFPE sections mounted on charged slides and incubated at 60°C overnight. All slides were incubated with the anti-human Dicer monoclonal antibody through Clonegene (1:100, clone mab 13D6, Hartford, CT), generously provided by Dr. Henry Furneaux. We performed antigen retrieval using DakoCytomation Target Retrieval Solution (High pH, Catalogue No. S-3308) and biocare digital decloaking chamber (Biocare Medical, Concord, CA) at 100°C for 10 minutes, followed by treatment of 3% H_2O_2 to block the endogenous peroxidase activity. The slides were incubated at room temperature for 1 hour with anti-Dicer antibodies at 1:100 dilution. Hematoxylin was used for counterstaining. Following the manufacturer's instructions, we developed the immunohistochemical stain using EnVision^{TM}+ kit (DAKO, Carpinteria, CA).

The expression of Dicer was examined in normal skin and other organs; Dicer immunoreactivity was seen in the cytoplasm without nuclear staining. A semi-quantitative, four-point ordinal immunoreactivity score was established: "0" reflected the lack of Dicer immunoreactivity and was the most common pattern in normal skin, carcinomas and sarcomas. Weakly positive ("1") staining was observed in epidermal keratinocytes and melanocytic nevi. Moderately positive ("2") staining was assigned to modest granular staining. Strongly positive ("3") staining consisted of diffuse and homogenous staining. Basal levels of Dicer were detected in epidermal keratinocytes. Only staining of tumor cells was scored in comparison to adjacent keratinocytes (internal positive control). Melanophages, specialized macrophages containing dark, brown coarse melanin pigment were not scored. Two investigators scored the stained slides independently. Scores for multiple cores from one case were averaged, and final Dicer scores were categorized into a three-level grouping of Negative, Low (>0 and ≤ 1.5) or High (>1.6) for analyses that included all 404 patients. For the exploratory analyses ($n = 19$), a dichotomous breakdown of Negative or Positive (>0) Dicer expression was used. These analyses included the following clinical and histopathological variables: AJCC Stage (I, II, III, IV); Distant Metastases, Non-Sentinel Node Metastases, Organ Metastases, Evidence of Regression, and Ulceration, which were treated as dichotomous variables; Melanoma Histology (Superficial Spreading, Nodular, Acrolentiginous or Lentigo Maligna); Vital status (alive, dead); and, Mitotic Index (mm^2), Clark's Level and Breslow's depth of invasion, i.e. Tumor Thickness (mm) were treated as continuous variables. Pearson Chi-Square tests were employed to assess categorical levels of Dicer status. Kruskal-Wallis ($k = 3$) or Mann-Whitney ($k = 2$) non-parametric tests were used for analyses when Dicer expression was treated as a continuous value as well as for analyses of Mitotic Index, Clarks Level and Breslow's depth of invasion. SPSS version 18.0 was used, and tests were two-sided in all analyses.

Bioinformatic Pooled Analysis on Gene Expression Profiling

Using NextBio (nextbio.com), we mined and pooled publically available gene expression profiling data interrogating the mRNA levels of the genes encoding all of the known enzymes involved in the canonical miRNA biogenesis and maturation pathway (Table S1). This analysis included 25,135 genes profiled from 20 disease groups consisting of 139 total excision specimens of cutaneous melanoma in various stages (Clark level I and II-radial growth phase, Clark level III, IV and V-vertical growth phase), melanoma metastases to skin and lymph node, common acquired melanocytic nevi, dysplastic nevi with low and high atypia, normal skin, basal cell carcinoma and squamous cell carcinoma. These two studies used whole genome oligo-microarray platforms: GPL1708 Agilent-012391 Whole Human Genome Oligo Microarray G4112A [21] and GPL570 Affymetrix GeneChip Human Genome U133 Plus 2.0 Array [22]. This analysis examined the 5,023 genes (out of 25,135) significantly altered based on the following criteria: overall gene score (top ranking genes), disease group score (significance among disease groups) and *P*-value specific to the gene and the disease group. For example, Dicer1 ranked among the top 20% most significantly altered genes, appeared in 11 out of 20 disease groups and it was expressed 2.54-fold higher than basal cell carcinoma (*P*-value = 0.0055) (Table S1). Color specified direction of regulation (red = up, green = down and orange = no direction), while size indicates magnitude of change.

Cell Lines and Cell Culture

The detailed summary of cell lines is shown (Table S2). TE 354.T cell line was purchased from the American Type Culture Collection (Manassas, VA) and cultured in Dulbecco's modified Eagle's medium with 10% fetal bovine serum (Gibco, Sydney, Australia) and 1% penicillin/streptomycin (Invitrogen). A2058, A375P, C32, A375SM and HEK 293 cells (embryonic kidney 293) were kindly provided by Dr. Stanley N. Cohen, Stanford school of medicine, CA. These cells were cultured in Dulbecco's modified Eagle's medium supplemented with 10% FCS and 2 mM glutamine. WM983A (Coriell), WM278 (Coriell), WM35 and WM1552C were purchased (Wistar institute, Philadelphia, PA) and cultured in 80% MCDB153 (Sigma), 20% Leibovitz's L15 (Mediutech), 2% fetal bovine serum, 5 ug/ml insulin (Sigma) and 1.68 mM $CaCl_2$. Three types of epidermal primary melanocytes isolated from 3 individuals with light, medium and dark skin were purchased from ScienCell (Carlsbad, CA) and cultured in melanocyte medium as specified by ScienCell. All cell cultures, except for TE 354.T (at 37°C and 10% CO_2), were incubated at 37°C in a 5% CO_2 completely humidified incubator.

Western Blot Detection of Dicer

Cultured cells were lysed in NP40 Cell Lysis Buffer (Invitrogen, Carlsbad, CA) and spun at 16,000×g to extract soluble proteins. Twenty microgram of total protein was resolved on a 4-20% Tris-Glycine gradient gel (BioRad) and blotted onto a nitrocellulose membrane. The membrane was blocked with 5% powdered nonfat milk in TBST buffer for 1 hour, then incubated with 1:500 dilution of anti-Dicer or 1:50,000 dilution of anti-SDHA antibody (Abcam) or 1:1000 dilution of α-tubulin antibody overnight at 4°C. The membrane was then washed three times with TBST buffer and incubated with anti mouse HRP conjugated secondary antibody, washed thrice with TBST, developed with the ECL Western Blotting Substrate (Pierce, Rockford, IL) and imaged and analyzed on a Kodak Image Station 4000 MM Pro (Carestream Health, Rochester, NY). Relative band intensity for Dicer was normalized against SDHA or α-tubulin as a loading control and quantified according to pixel intensity using Adobe Photoshop.

Quantitative real-time reverse transcription-PCR (qRT-PCR)

For measuring mRNA levels, total RNA was extracted from cultured cells with TRIzol and the reverse transcription of purified RNA was performed using oligo(dT) priming and superscript II reverse transcription according to the manufacturer's instructions (Invitrogen). The quantification of Dicer and GAPDH transcripts by Real-time quantitative PCR amplification of a cDNA template corresponding to 15 ng total RNA was performed using TaqMan Universal PCR Master Mix and TaqMan gene expressions assay probes (Applied Biosystems, Foster City, CA, USA). As previously described [13], for all miRNAs, 5 ng total RNA was used as a template for TaqMan® miRNA assays (Applied Biosystems, Foster City, CA, USA). All reactions were run in an ABI 7500 Fast system (Applied Biosystems). Cycle threshold (Ct) values for each miRNA were normalized to a small nuclear RNA RNU6 and for Dicer mRNA Ct values were normalized to GAPDH (ΔCt) and represented as $2^{-\Delta CT}$.

Results

Dicer Up-regulation in Cutaneous Malignancies Is Specific to Melanoma

We initially sought to determine if Dicer is expressed in any of the major categories of human cutaneous malignancies, namely

Table 1. Dicer expression in relation to tumor type (n = 404).

		Dicer Immunoreactivity									
			Negative		Low (≤1.5)		High (>1.6)		*P*-Value[1]	Mean ± SD	*P*-Value
		Total	n	%	n	%	n	%			
Tumor Type	Normal Tissue	12	11	91.7%	1	8.3%	0	-		0.04±0.14	
	Melanocytic Nevus	71	13	18.3%	48	67.6%	10	14.1%		0.83±0.60	
	Cutaneous Melanoma	95	18	18.9%	33	34.7%	44	46.4%		1.40±0.96	
	Acrolentiginous Melanoma	40	4	10.0%	14	35.0%	22	55.0%		1.61±0.92	
	Mucosal Melanoma	24	8	33.3%	13	54.2%	3	12.5%		0.79±0.65	
	Ocular Melanoma	4	0	-	2	50.0%	2	50.0%		1.50±0.58	
	Desmoplastic Melanoma	8	5	62.5%	2	25.0%	1	12.5%		0.44±0.73	
	Metastatic Melanoma	52	2	3.8%	21	40.4%	29	55.8%		1.71±0.83	
	Carcinoma	73	45	61.6%	24	32.9%	4	5.5%		0.39±0.59	
	Sarcoma	12	11	91.7%	1	8.3%	0	-		0.08±0.29	
	Neural Tumors	13	9	69.2%	4	30.8%	0	-	**<0.0001**	0.23±0.39	**<0.0001**[2]

[1]Pearson Chi-Square test for proportions.
[2]Kruskal-Wallis (k = 3 or more) non-parametric test for continuous values.

melanoma, carcinoma or sarcoma. To this end, we tested a large clinical sample set of formalin-fixed paraffin-embedded (FFPE) benign and malignant tumors (n = 404) including melanocytic nevi (benign melanocytic hyperplasia), a variety of melanoma subtypes (cutaneous, acrolentiginous, mucosal, ocular and desmoplastic), a variety of carcinomas (squamous, basal cell and eccrine) and sarcomas (Table 1) using a monoclonal anti-human Dicer antibody and immunohistochemistry on tissue microarrays (TMAs) (Fig. 1A) and full tumor sections (Fig. S1A-F). After determining the immunostaining pattern for Dicer in normal skin and other organs, we established a semi-quantitative, four-point ordinal immunoreactivity scoring scale: negative (0), weakly positive (1), moderately positive (2) and strongly positive (3). Scores for multiple cores from one case were averaged, and final Dicer scores were categorized into a three-level grouping of Negative, Low (>0 and ≤1.5) or High (>1.6) for analyses that included all 404 patients (Table 1). In normal skin, epidermal keratinocytes expressed Dicer consistently at low levels (Fig. 1B). Carcinoma cells of skin (basal and squamous), adenocarcinoma cells (primary or metastatic) and sarcoma cells expressed none to very low levels of Dicer (Fig. 1C-E). In contrast, the cytoplasm of primary cutaneous and metastatic melanoma cells exhibited high levels of Dicer immunoreactivity (Fig. 1F-G). The majority of carcinomas (94.5%), sarcomas (100%) and tumors with neural differentiation (100%) of the skin was negative for Dicer or expressed it at low levels (Table 1). Among tumors with melanocytic differentiation, we observed low levels of Dicer immunoreactivity in the cytoplasm of melanocytic nevus cell

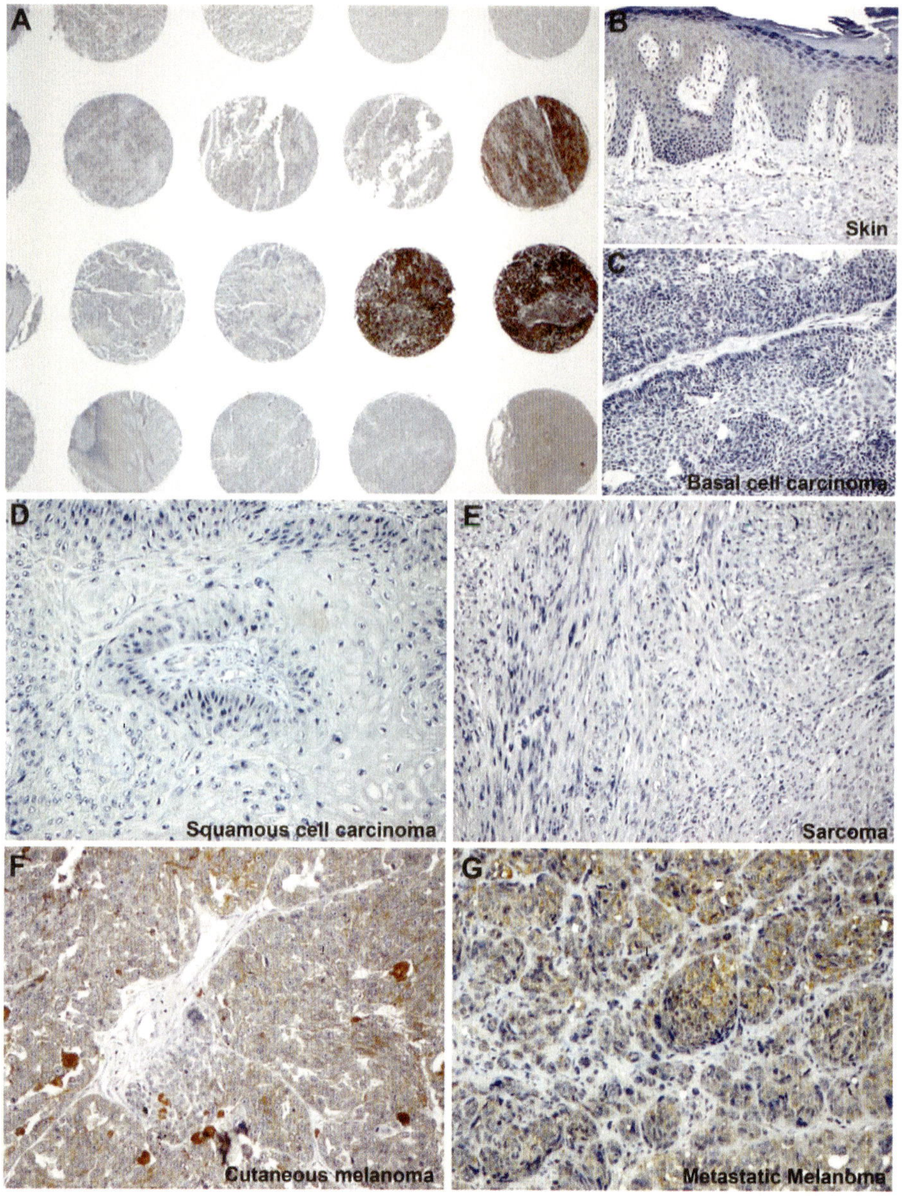

Figure 1. Dicer was specifically expressed in melanoma cells and not carcinoma or sarcoma cells. A) Dicer immunoreactivity was variable across different types of skin cancer by immunohistochemistry using tissue microarrays. B) Normal epidermal keratinocytes exhibited low, basal level of Dicer expression. C–E) The cytoplasm of basal cell carcinoma, squamous cell carcinoma and sarcoma cells were negative for Dicer, respectively. In contrast, melanoma cells strongly and diffusely expressed Dicer in both primary cutaneous (F) and metastatic (G) melanoma. Original magnification: A, 20X; B–C, 100X and D–G, 200X.

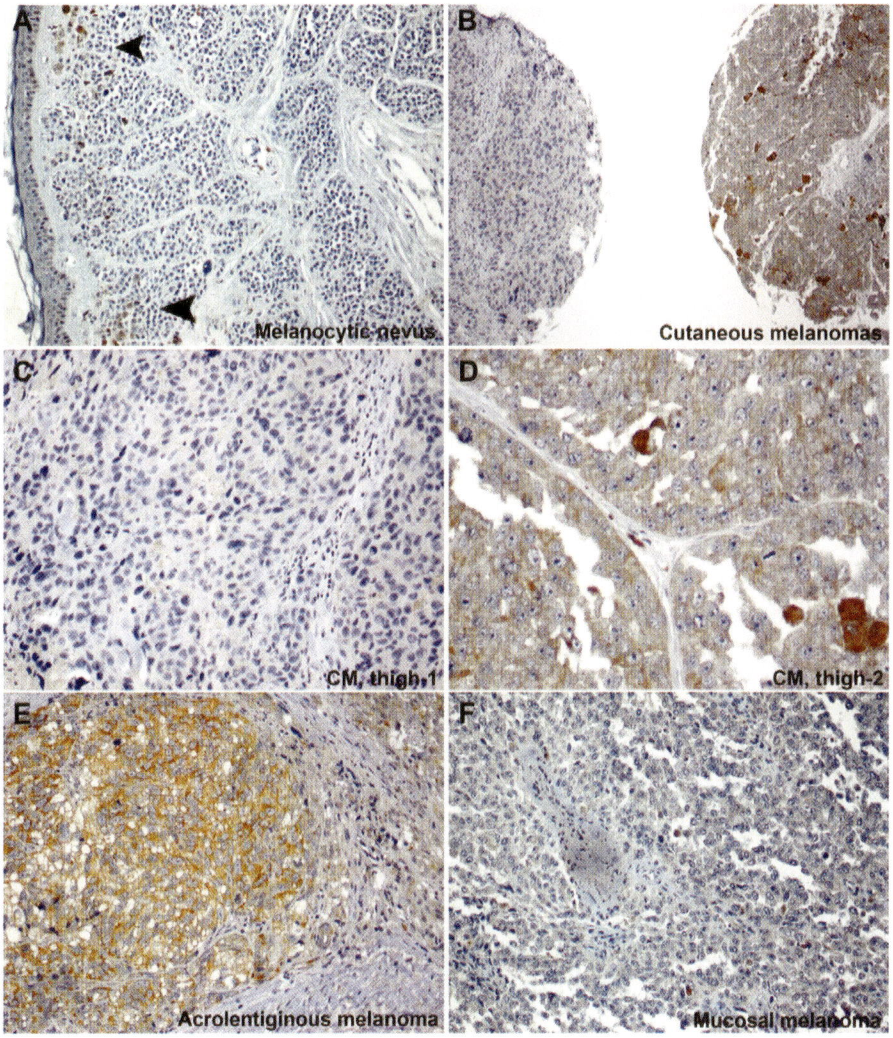

Figure 2. Dicer was expressed at higher levels in cutaneous and acrolentiginous melanomas. A) Intradermal melanocytic nevus cells weakly expressed Dicer in a small group of cells in the superficial dermis (arrowheads) whereas melanoma cells diffusely expressed Dicer at higher levels (B). However, two independent individuals with cutaneous melanoma (CM), both excised from the thigh, expressed Dicer at different levels (B, left and right cores). C–D) Both tissue cores are shown at a higher magnification (CM, thigh-1 and CM, thigh-2). The immunoreactivity for Dicer in melanoma cells was granular and cytoplasmic. E) Cancer cells strongly expressed Dicer in an acrolentiginous melanoma while they were negative for Dicer in a mucosal melanoma (F). Original magnification: A–B, 100X; C, E–F, 200X and D, 400X.

(Fig. 2A) compared to the high levels seen in cutaneous and acrolentiginous melanomas (Fig. 2B-E). The cytoplasm of mucosal melanoma cells was devoid of Dicer immunoreactivity (Fig. 2F). Dicer was consistently expressed at high levels in the majority of metastatic (55.8%), acrolentiginous (55.0%) and cutaneous (46.4%) melanomas compared to mucosal melanoma (12.5%), conferring further cancer-cell specificity among different types of melanomas (Table 1). The remainder of Dicer-positive cutaneous melanomas expressed Dicer either at low levels (34.7%) or exhibited no expression (18.9%). Two different patients with cutaneous melanoma (both excised from the thigh) exemplified this variability in expression Dicer. The melanoma from patient 1 expressed Dicer at low levels (Fig. 2B and C) compared to that in patient 2 who expressed Dicer at high levels (Fig. 2B and D). Dicer expression was not associated with differences in gender (n = 328) or age (n = 335) in the examined cutaneous tumors (Table S3). Among the cutaneous (n = 93) and acrolentiginous (n = 40) melanomas examined, there was no statistically significant association between Dicer expression and the anatomic site (head and neck, trunk, upper and lower extremities or genital skin) (Table S4).

Overall, when compared among all examined cutaneous malignancies, Dicer up-regulation was tumor-type specific by immunostaining, as Dicer was highly expressed by melanomas (metastatic and cutaneous) compared to carcinomas or sarcomas ($P<0.0001$, Fig. 3A). Furthermore Dicer up-regulation was specific to the melanoma subtype, i.e. cutaneous and acrolentiginous compared to mucosal and desmoplastic melanomas ($P<0.0001$, Fig. 3B). Importantly, higher Dicer levels were detected in cutaneous, acrolentiginous and metastatic melanomas compared to common melanocytic nevi. To confirm the up-regulation of Dicer in melanoma, we performed a pooled analysis by mining published whole genome oligo-microarray dataset on two recent large studies that profiled gene expression pattern in excisional specimens of cutaneous tumors (n = 139) [21,22]. The combined dataset included 20 different disease groups consisting of

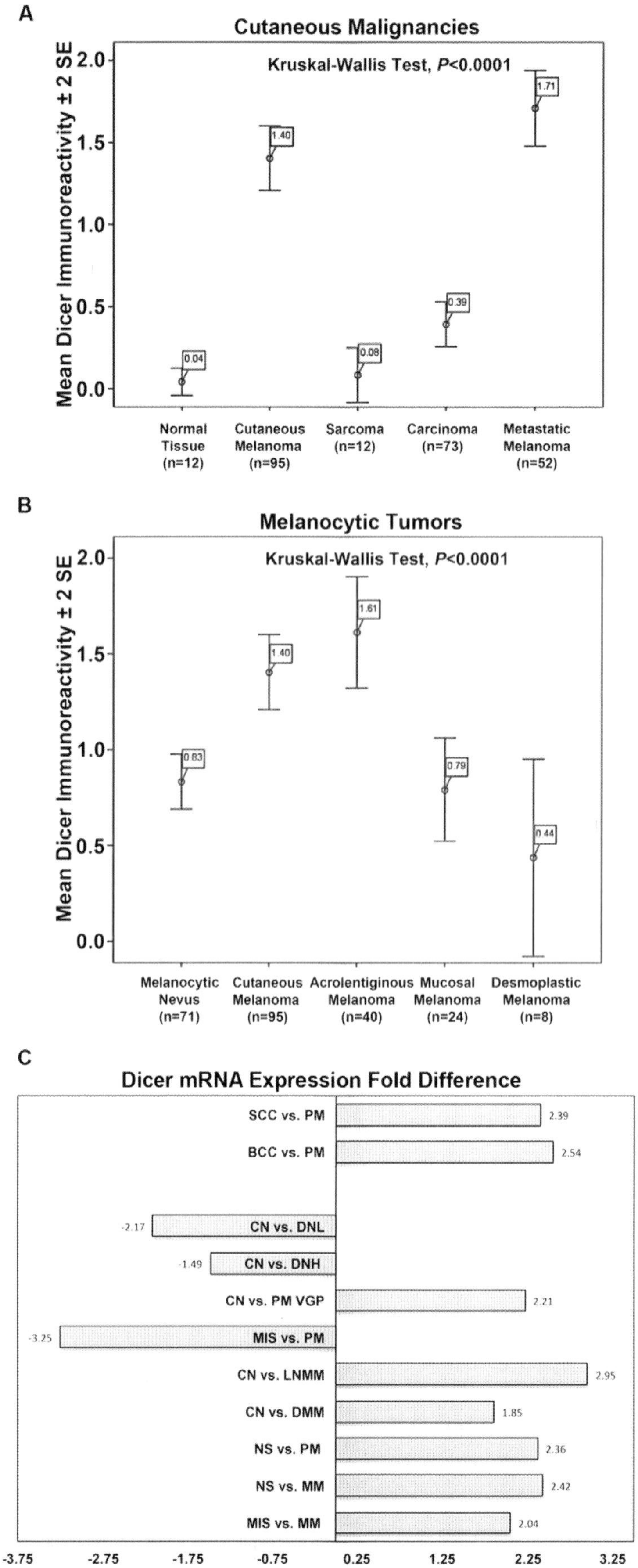
A
Cutaneous Malignancies
Kruskal-Wallis Test, P<0.0001
Mean Dicer Immunoreactivity ± 2 SE
2.0
1.5
1.0
0.5
0.0
0.04
1.40
0.08
0.39
1.71
Normal Tissue (n=12)
Cutaneous Melanoma (n=95)
Sarcoma (n=12)
Carcinoma (n=73)
Metastatic Melanoma (n=52)
B
Melanocytic Tumors
Kruskal-Wallis Test, P<0.0001
Mean Dicer Immunoreactivity ± 2 SE
2.0
1.5
1.0
0.5
0.0
0.83
1.40
1.61
0.79
0.44
Melanocytic Nevus (n=71)
Cutaneous Melanoma (n=95)
Acrolentiginous Melanoma (n=40)
Mucosal Melanoma (n=24)
Desmoplastic Melanoma (n=8)
C
Dicer mRNA Expression Fold Difference
SCC vs. PM
2.39
BCC vs. PM
2.54
CN vs. DNL
-2.17
CN vs. DNH
-1.49
CN vs. PM VGP
2.21
MIS vs. PM
-3.25
CN vs. LNMM
2.95
CN vs. DMM
1.85
NS vs. PM
2.36
NS vs. MM
2.42
MIS vs. MM
2.04
-3.75
-2.75
-1.75
-0.75
0.25
1.25
2.25
3.25

Figure 3. Dicer expression was cancer-cell specific among cutaneous malignancies and was significantly higher in primary and metastatic melanoma compared to common melanocytic nevus. A) Primary cutaneous (n = 95) and metastatic (n = 52) melanomas had the highest levels of Dicer immunoreactivity vs. carcinomas (n = 73) and sarcomas (n = 12). B) Cutaneous (n = 95) and acrolentiginous (n = 40) melanomas had the highest levels of Dicer immunoreactivity vs. melanocytic nevi (n = 71), mucosal (n = 24) and desmoplastic (n = 8) melanomas. Dicer immunoreactivity is shown as mean (boxed) ±2 standard error (SE). The statistical significance was measured for all independent samples comparing to each other (Kruskal-Wallis Test, $P<0.0001$). C) Pooled analysis performed on publically available transcriptional profiling data showed significant changes in Dicer mRNA levels during melanoma progression. This analysis included 25,135 genes from 20 disease groups and 139 individual specimens of squamous cell carcinoma (SCC), basal cell carcinoma (BCC), primary melanoma (PM), common nevus (CN), dysplastic nevus with low (DNL), dysplastic nevus with high atypia (DNH), primary melanoma vertical growth phase (PM VGP), melanoma in situ (MIS), lymph node melanoma metastases (LNMM), dermal melanoma metastases (DMM), normal skin (NS) and melanoma metastases (MM) [21,22]. Dicer1 ranked among the top 20% most significantly altered genes.

cutaneous melanoma in various stages (in situ, Clark level I and II-radial growth phase, Clark level III, IV and V-vertical growth phase), melanoma metastases to skin and lymph node, common acquired melanocytic nevi, dysplastic nevi with low and high atypia, normal skin, basal cell carcinoma and squamous cell carcinoma (Table 2). The combined dataset provided 25,135 genes, which we interrogated for Dicer mRNA expression levels. Comparing cutaneous melanoma to other skin cancers, squamous and basal cell carcinoma, or normal skin (mostly consisting of keratinocytes) showed significantly higher levels Dicer mRNA in melanoma (Fig. 3C, Table 2), confirming our immunostaining results (Fig. 3A) and indicating an up-regulation at the level of mRNA accumulation. Furthermore, invasive and metastatic melanomas had significantly higher levels of Dicer mRNA than common melanocytic nevi (Fig. 3C, Table 2), again confirming our immunostaining results (Fig. 3B). Interestingly, the Dicer mRNA levels are decreased in dysplastic when compared common melanocytic nevi and in melanoma in situ when compared to invasive (Fig. 3C, Table 2). Overall, these results showed that Dicer up-regulation, at both the protein and the RNA levels, is specific to melanoma subtypes and that Dicer levels are higher in primary cutaneous and metastatic melanomas compared to common melanocytic nevi.

Table 2. Pooled analysis performed on Dicer mRNA expression in publically available gene expression profiling studies (clinical sample size = 139, disease groups = 20).

	DICER1	
	P-value	Fold change
NS vs. BCC	NS	NS
NS vs. SCC	NS	NS
SCC vs. BCC	NS	NS
SCC vs. PM	0.0108	+2.39
BCC vs. PM	0.0055	+2.54
CN vs. DNL	0.0006	−2.17
CN vs. DNH	0.0074	−1.49
CN vs. C I RGP	NS	NS
CN vs. C II RGP	NS	NS
CN vs. C III VGP	NS	NS
CN vs. C IV VGP	NS	NS
CN vs. C V VGP	0.0323	+2.21
MIS vs. PM	0.0391	−3.25
CN vs. LNMM	0.0244	+2.95
CN vs. DMM	0.0242	+1.85
NS vs. MIS	NS	NS
NS vs. PM	0.0082	+2.36
NS vs. MM	0.0045	+2.42
MIS vs. MM	1.70E-06	+2.04
PM vs. MM	NS	NS

To stay consistent with the direction of disease progression, the sign (+ or −) was changed appropriately. Fold changes with a (−) sign are lower and those with a (+) sign are higher than the disease group to which it was compared. For example, PM showed 2.36-fold increase in Dicer mRNA levels when compared to NS. The abbreviations of disease groups are as follows: DNL-dysplastic nevus low-grade atypia; DNH-dysplastic nevus high-grade atypia; CN-common nevus; C I RGP-Clark's level I radial growth phase; C II RGP-Clark's level II radial growth phase; C III VGP-Clark's level III vertical growth phase; C IV VGP-Clark's level IV vertical growth phase; C V VGP-Clark's level V vertical growth phase; LNMM-lymph node metastatic melanoma; DMM-dermal metastatic melanoma; MIS-melanoma in situ; PM-primary melanoma invasive; MM-metastatic melanoma; NS-normal skin; BCC-basal cell carcinoma; SCC-squamous cell carcinoma. NS-not significant.

Clinical Features Associated with Dicer Up-regulation

To characterize Dicer expression pattern and distribution, we immunostained melanocytic nevi, cutaneous and metastatic melanomas in complete sections (n = 33). In 30% of cutaneous melanomas, the intratumoral expression of Dicer varied where immunoreactivity was focally high compared no expression in other areas within the same lesion (Fig. S1A). Dicer was expressed both in the intraepidermal (*in-situ*) and dermal (invasive) melanoma cells (Fig. S1B-D). The majority of cutaneous melanomas, TMAs and complete sections, expressed Dicer either at high (44 of 95, 46.3%) or low (33 of 95, 34.7%) levels; however a minority of the cases (18 of 95, 18.9%) was negative for expression. This finding prompted us to investigate whether this difference might be associated with clinical outcome in cutaneous melanomas patients with available clinical information. For 19 patients, tumor pathological features, clinical stage and clinical follow-up (rage 7.1 to 69.7 months; median = 22.4 months; mean = 26.6 months) were available. Dicer expression level was significantly associated with tumor mitotic index ($P=0.04$, n = 19) and Breslow's depth of invasion ($P=0.03$, n = 19) (Fig. 4A-B-D, Tables 3-4), two of three most important parameters currently used in staging and predicting prognosis for melanoma patients by the American Joint Committee on Cancer (AJCC) [19]. Dicer expression was not significantly associated with other tumor pathological features such as histological subtype, inflammation (tumor infiltrating lymphocytes), regression, ulceration or Clark's level (Table 4). Most important, Dicer expression significantly correlated with metastasis to the non-sentinel lymph node (SLN, $P=0.04$, n = 16) (Fig. 4C, Table 4) and the AJCC clinical stage ($P=0.009$, n = 19) (Fig. 4D). Melanoma patients with positive Dicer expression did demonstrate a trend towards higher rates of SLN, organ and distant metastases (Table 4); however this association did not reach a statistical significance.

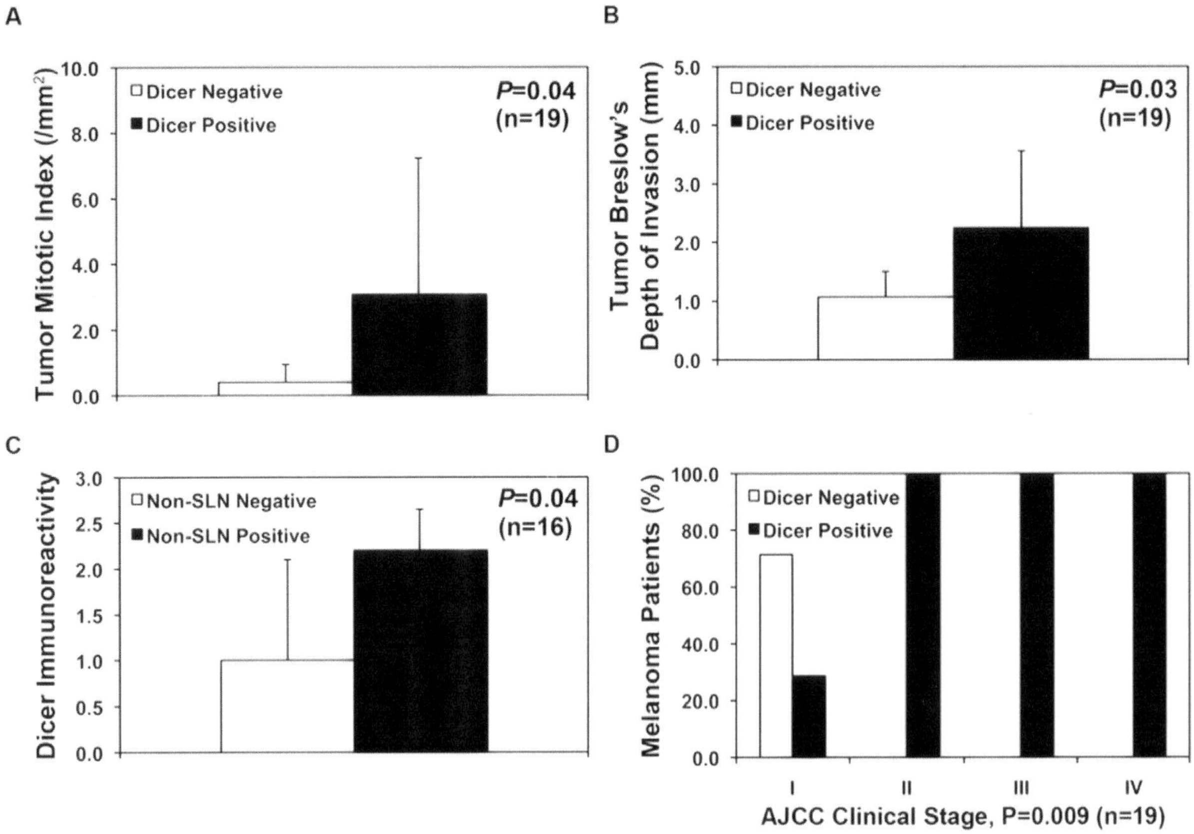

Figure 4. Dicer expression significantly correlated with clinical outcome in patients with cutaneous melanoma. A–B) The mean values for melanoma mitotic index (per mm^2) and Breslow's depth of invasion significantly correlated with Dicer expression ($P = 0.04$ and $P = 0.03$, respectively). C) Dicer immunoreactivity score was significantly associated with metastasis to non-sentinel lymph node (SLN) in patients with cutaneous melanoma ($P = 0.04$). D) The American Joint Commission on Cancer (AJCC) staging was significantly associated with Dicer expression ($P = 0.009$).

Expression of Dicer and let-7 miRNA family *in vitro*

Our findings in clinical melanoma specimens raised the question of whether Dicer up-regulation might be intrinsic to the tumor cells. We compared Dicer protein levels between primary melanocytes, primary (n = 3) and metastatic (n = 3) melanoma cell lines. Western blot analysis combined with measured relative band intensity, normalized against succinate dehydrogenase (SDHA), showed >2 to 4-fold higher Dicer levels in melanoma cell lines (WM278, WM1552C and A375P) when compared to melanocyte-L or other melanoma cell lines (WM35 and A375M) (Fig. 5A-B). Furthermore, we tested additional cell lines; combined western blot analysis and measured relative band intensity showed >2-fold higher Dicer levels in melanoma cell lines (WM1552C and A2058) compared to basal cell carcinoma (BCC), primary melanocytes (n = 3) or other melanoma cell lines (WM35 and C32) (results not shown). The melanocytes were derived from three different individuals with light, medium and dark skin color. Dicer levels were comparable among the three melanocytes, despite the skin color. Overall, Dicer expression in cell lines recapitulated the observed deregulation in clinical specimens, confirming higher Dicer immunostaining in melanomas when compared to melanocytic nevi or carcinomas of the skin (Figs. 1, 2 and 3).

Given the differential levels of Dicer expression in melanoma cell lines and the prior finding of let-7a miRNA exerting a negative feedback loop on Dicer expression in lung and pancreatic cell lines [23], it was conceivable that the differences in let-7a miRNA levels might be associated with Dicer regulation via such mechanism in melanoma. We compared the relative expression of the entire let-7 family to Dicer mRNA levels using quantitative real-time reverse transcription-PCR (qRT-PCR). Neither Dicer mRNA nor Dicer protein levels correlated with any of the mature miRNAs tested (let-7a, let-7b, let-7c, let-7d, let-7e, let-7f, left-7g or let-7i). Interestingly, we found that let-7b expression levels are significantly down-regulated in metastatic (A375P, A375SM and A2058) compared to primary (WM35, WM1552C and C32) melanoma

Table 3. Dicer expression in relation to melanoma mitotic activity and depth of invasion (n = 19).

	Dicer Immunoreactivity		
	Negative n = 5	**Positive n = 14**	***P*-Value**[1]
	Mean ± SD	Mean ± SD	
Mitotic Index	0.40±0.55	3.07±4.16	**0.04**
Breslow's Depth (mm)	1.07±0.43	2.25±1.31	**0.03**
Clark's Level	3.20±0.84	3.79±0.43	0.08

[1]Mann-Whitney (k = 2) non-parametric test for continuous values.

Table 4. Dicer expression in relation to melanoma clinicopathological features (n = 19).

		Dicer Immunoreactivity						
		Negative		Positive		*P*-Value[1]	Mean ± SD	*P*-Value
		n	%	n	%			
Subtype	Superficial spreading	5	29.4%	12	70.6%		1.35±0.99	
	Nodular	0	-	2	100%	0.99	2.00±1.41	0.43[2]
Tumor infiltrating lymphocytes	Absent	2	28.6%	5	71.4%		1.43±1.13	
	Present	3	25.0%	9	75.0%	0.99	1.41±0.99	0.96[2]
Regression	Absent	4	25.0%	12	66.7%		1.50±1.03	
	Present	1	50.0%	1	50.0%	0.49	0.50±0.71	0.18[2]
Ulceration	Absent	5	38.5%	8	61.5%		1.23±1.09	
	Present	0	-	6	100%	0.13	1.83±0.75	0.28[2]
Stage	I	5	71.4%	2	28.6%		0.71±1.25	
	II	0	-	4	100%		1.75±0.50	
	III	0	-	2	100%		1.50±0.71	
	IV	0	-	6	100%	**0.009**	2.00±0.63	0.17[3]
Sentinel Lymph Node Metastases	Negative	5	38.5	8	61.5%		1.23±1.09	
	Positive	0	-	6	100%	0.12	1.83±0.75	0.28[2]
Non-Sentinel Node Metastases[4]	Negative	5	45.5%	6	54.5%		1.00±1.10	
	Positive	0	-	5	100%	0.12	2.20±0.45	**0.04**[2]
Organ Metastases	Absent	5	33.3%	10	66.7%		1.33±1.11	
	Present	0	-	4	100%	0.53	1.75±0.50	0.52[2]
Distant Metastases	M0	5	38.5%	8	61.5%		1.15±1.07	
	M1	0	-	6	100%	0.13	2.00±1.41	0.10[2]
Vital Status	Alive	0	-	4	100%		1.75±0.50	
	Dead	5	33.3%	10	66.7%	0.53	1.33±1.11	0.52[2]

[1]Pearson Chi-Square test for Stage and Tumor Thickness (Table 3); Fisher's Exact Test for all other variables.
[2]Mann-Whitney (k = 2) non-parametric test for continuous values.
[3]Kruskal-Wallis (k = 3 or more) non-parametric test for continuous values.
[4]Three cases with unknown nodal status.

cell lines; while let-7d levels are significantly down-regulated in all six melanoma cell lines (metastatic and primary) compared to primary melanocytes (Fig. S2).

Perturbed miRNA Biogenesis Pathway during Melanoma Progression

Since the expression of Dicer is significantly altered from common to dysplastic nevi to melanoma in situ to invasive and to metastatic melanoma, we interrogated the same combined dataset, which included 20 different disease groups and 25, 135 genes, for the mRNA levels of all the known enzymes involved in canonical miRNA biogenesis by performing a pooled analysis mining published whole genome oligo-microarray dataset [21,22]. Enzymes tested in the canonical miRNA biogenesis pathway included Drosha, DGCR8, RAN, XPO5, Dicer1, GEMIN3, GEMIN4, EIF2C2, Ago2 and TRBP (Table S1). Dicer1, DGCR8 and Gemin4 ranked among the top ~20 percentile of most significantly altered genes. We represent this data with respect to a linear, step-wise progression model for melanomagenesis, plotting changes in the expression level of the enzyme detected in our own immunostaining (protein) and in microarray pooled analysis (mRNA) (Fig. 6). This analysis suggests that the biogenesis of mature miRNAome maybe enhanced in the early steps of melanocyte transformation and melanoma formation raising the possibility that Dicer may play a central role in the melanocyte transformation and metastasis. Surprisingly, Dicer, Drosha and Gemin4 are down-regulated in melanoma in situ compared to invasive melanoma; in addition, Dicer is down-regulated in dysplastic nevi compared to common nevi, suggesting a global repression of miRNA biogenesis in these steps.

Discussion

In this study, we examined the expression and the clinical relevance of Dicer in cutaneous melanoma. We showed that a large portion of cutaneous melanomas exhibited up-regulation of Dicer significantly associated with aggressive cancer features. We demonstrated definitive evidence that Dicer up-regulation is specific to the malignant proliferation of melanocytes (melanoma) and not keratinocytes (carcinoma) or fibroblasts (sarcoma) in 404 human skin tumors. Given that the "melanoma disease group" is a heterogeneous cancer, to have a complete representation, we compared Dicer expression among the various subtypes of melanomas occurring in glabrous (subungual, palm and sole) skin, non-glabrous skin, eye, mucosal sites (e.g. oral, urothelial and anal mucosa) and metastatic sites (variety of organs) to melanocytic

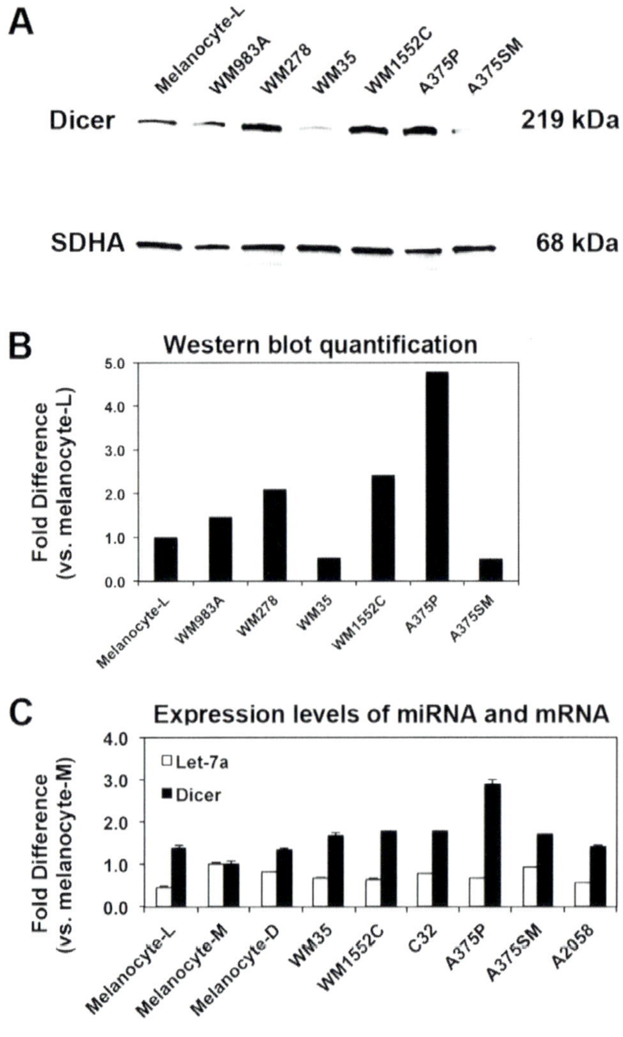

Figure 5. Dicer expression in cell lines recapitulated the observed deregulation in clinical specimens. A) Western blot analysis of Dicer shows a 219-kDa band. Relative band intensity was compared to succinate dehydrogenase (SDHA, 68 kDa) as a loading control. B) Western blot quantification showed >2 to 4-fold change in Dicer levels in melanoma cell lines (WM278, WM1552C and A375P) when compared to melanocyte-L or other melanoma cell lines (WM35 and A375M). C) Dicer mRNA expression did not correlate with mature let-7a expression *in vitro*. Using qRT-PCR, the relative expression levels of let-7a miRNA and Dicer mRNA were compared to show no significant correlation. All qRT-PCRs were performed in triplicates. Data were normalized to small nuclear RNA RNU6 for let-7a and GAPDH mRNA for Dicer. The samples are: Primary melanocytes were cultured from individuals with light (Melanocyte-L), medium (Melanocyte-M) and dark (Melanocyte-D) skin color, WM983A (primary melanoma), WM278 (primary melanoma), WM35 (primary melanoma), WM1552C (primary melanoma), C32 (amelanotic primary melanoma), A375P (metastatic melanoma), A375SM (metastatic melanoma) and A2058 (metastatic melanoma).

nevi. These immunostaining results clearly showed that Dicer up-regulation was specific to cutaneous, acrolentiginous and metastatic melanomas. To complement the immunostaining, we carried out a pooled analysis using two recent large studies that profiled gene expression pattern in cutaneous tumors. This analysis corroborated our immunostaining data and indicated that at least a component of Dicer up-regulation in melanoma is due to differences in mRNA accumulation.

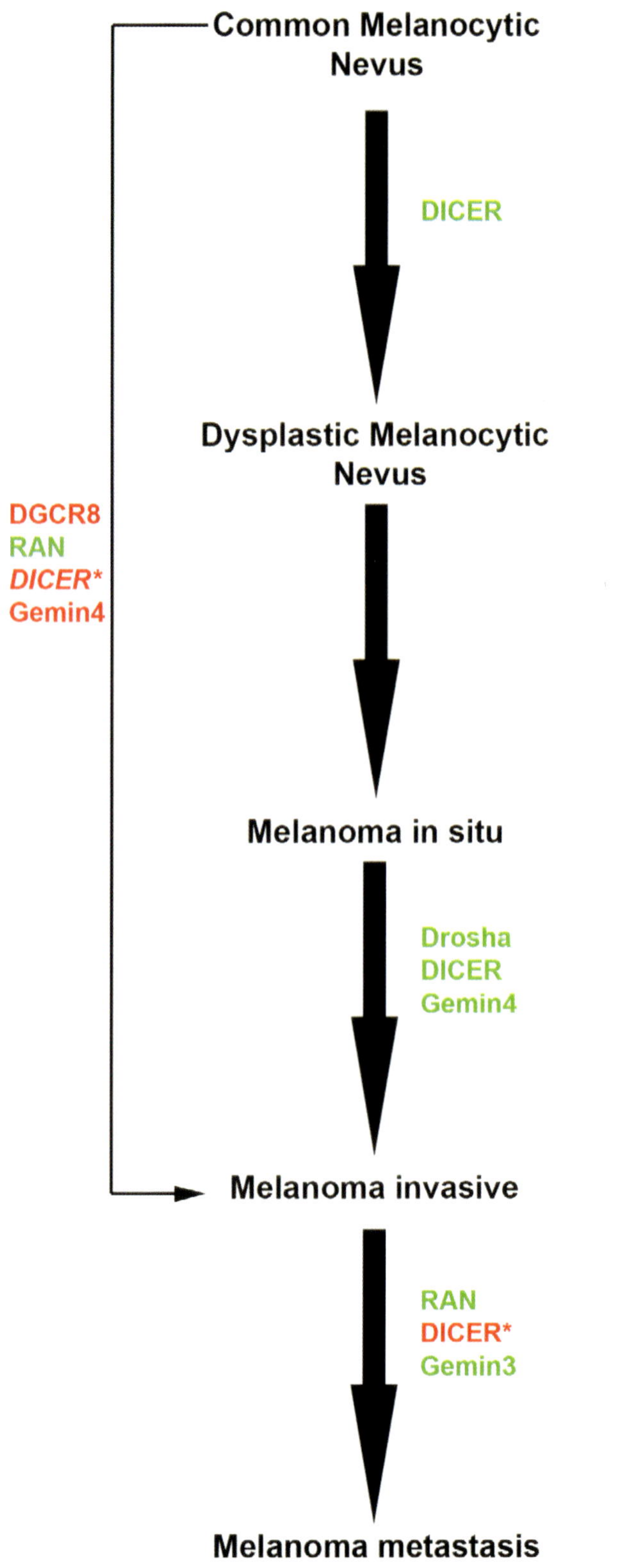

Figure 6. Enzymes involved in the canonical miRNA biogenesis are deregulated during melanoma progression. Combined Dicer immunoreactivity, presented herein (denoted by asterisk '*'), and mRNA transcriptional profiling [21,22] examined for Dicer and other enzymes in the miRNA biogenesis showed a global change in their expression levels during tumor progression. Enzymes shown in red are up-regulated and those in green are down-regulated. Up-regulation of Dicer (italicized) from common melanocytic nevus to invasive

melanoma was found both in our study and others [21,22]. Dicer, DGCR8 and Gemin4 ranked among the top 20 percentile of most significantly altered genes.

Although our results provide strong evidence that up-regulated Dicer was tumor-cell specific and reflective of mRNA levels, these results provided little mechanistic explanation. Given the involvement of Dicer, Dicer products, and associated components of the RNAi machinery in diverse cellular processes [24] there are certainly numerous mechanisms both for the potential regulation of Dicer in melanoma and for the effects of this regulation in the context of the tumor. Further analysis of both questions will certainly be warranted. Here, we provide a number of (not necessarily exclusive) connections between Dicer functions and other factors that may regulate or depend on these.

First, the presence of cell-specific transcription factors might be expected to partially explain the difference in Dicer expression between melanocytes vs. keratinocytes or fibroblasts. Recently, it has been shown that Dicer is a direct transcriptional target of microphthalmia-associated transcription factor (MITF); tissue-restricted master transcriptional regulator of melanocytes; and that targeted KO of Dicer is lethal to melanocytes [25]. MITF targeting Dicer in melanocytes may partially explain our findings of up-regulated Dicer in melanoma and not carcinoma or sarcoma. As for the underlying mechanisms of increased Dicer expression in melanoma, one class of conceivable mechanisms would occur if human *Dicer* were amplified through gains in DNA copy number by genomic instability. *Dicer* is mapped to chromosome 14 (14q32.13); a genetic locus altered in other human malignancies: esophageal carcinoma [26], nasopharygeal carcinoma [27] and urothelial carcinoma [28]. From a set of primary melanoma cell lines, *Dicer1* locus showed 19.6% gain and 8.7% loss of DNA copy number [29]. Finally, it has been demonstrated that let-7a enforces a negative feedback loop on Dicer expression in lung and pancreatic carcinoma cell lines [23]. Despite the potential of this feedback loop, our measurements of levels for let-7a (or other members of let-7 family) and Dicer do not support a let-7 regulatory loop as the key element of Dicer up-regulated expression in melanoma cell lines.

We found that the expression of Dicer was variable among cutaneous melanomas (n = 95) where, the great majority (81%) of cases expressed it while 19% of cases demonstrated an absence of immunoreactivity. Postulating that this difference could be clinically relevant, we examined correlations with other clinical features, observing a statistically significant association between Dicer expression and melanoma mitotic index and Breslow's depth of invasion, both indicative of a more aggressive cancer (these are two of the three most important AJCC staging parameters) currently used to determine prognosis for melanoma patients [19]. Dicer expression significantly correlated with non-SLN metastasis and AJCC stage but not disease-specific survival. Given the small patient population with available clinical follow-up information in this study (n = 19), our findings need to be validated in larger melanoma cohorts. Our results suggest analogy to prostate adenocarcinoma where up-regulated Dicer correlated with metastasis to regional lymph nodes and clinical stage [16]. Deregulation of Dicer, or other enzymes in the miRNA biogenesis pathway, maybe a common central feature shared by several solid cancers [16,17,18,30,31,32,33,34] to globally regulate the biogenesis of oncomirs. From our pooled analysis focusing on all known enzymes that participate in the biogenesis and maturation of canonical miRNAs, we also propose the possibility of a more general phenomenon where several deregulated RNAi enzymes, in addition to Dicer, may influence the various steps in melanoma progression (Fig. 6).

Overall, our results show definitive up-regulation of Dicer in cutaneous melanoma, compared to other skin cancer types, which correlated with a more aggressive behavior. When confirmed by independent studies in larger cohorts, increased Dicer expression may serve as a clinically useful prognostic biomarker for cutaneous melanoma patients. Beyond this, a combined understanding of deregulated Dicer and its influence on the expression pattern of mature miRNAs may lead to indications of directions in which small RNA modulations may contribute therapeutically in melanoma treatment. During the revision of this manuscript, we noted an abstract for a small pilot study [35] comparing Dicer immunostaining pattern among cutaneous melanomas, melanocytic nevi and dysplastic nevi. The abstract suggested that a significantly higher Dicer immunostaining was detected in melanoma cells than in nevus cells.

Supporting Information

Figure S1 Expression of Dicer in primary cutaneous and metastatic melanomas by immunohistochemistry using complete tumor sections. A) Cancer cells focally expressed Dicer at high levels in the left margin (arrowhead) compared to the cancer cells in the center (asterisks) that were negative for Dicer in the same cutaneous melanoma (CM). B) In another CM, cancer cells expressed Dicer along the dermal-epidermal junction and follicular epithelium (*in situ*, arrowhead) as well as in the dermis (invasive, arrow). C) In an ulcerated CM, cancer cells, invading throughout the dermis, strongly and diffusely expressed Dicer. D) Cancer cells expressed Dicer in *in situ* and invasive components of another CM. E) Melanoma cells expressed Dicer in a subcapsular (arrowhead) location in the sentinel lymph node (SLN) of a patient with metastatic melanoma (MM) compared to the adjacent nodal tissue containing mature lymphocytes (asterisk) that are negative for Dicer. F) In another patient with MM, cancer cells strongly and diffusely expressed Dicer in the SLN, where expanding tumor nodules obliterated the normal lymph node architecture. Under higher magnification, Dicer was localized to the cytoplasm of melanoma cells with a granular quality (inset D and F). Original magnification: A, 200X; B-D, 100X, E, 200X and F, 100X; insets: 400X.

Figure S2 Dicer mRNA expression did not correlate with the expression of any mature miRNA members in the let-7 family *in vitro*. Using qRT-PCR, the relative expression levels of let-7b, let-7c, let-7d, let-7d, let-7f and let-7g miRNAs and Dicer mRNA were compared to show no significant correlation. However, let-7b expression is significantly down-regulated in all three metastatic compared to three primary melanoma cell lines; whereas let-7d expression is significantly down-regulated in all 6 metastatic and primary melanoma cell lines compared to three melanocytes. All qRT-PCRs were performed in triplicates. Data were normalized to small nuclear RNA RNU6 for let-7 family and GAPDH mRNA for Dicer.

Table S1 Pooled analysis performed on enzymes in miRNA biogenesis pathway in publically available gene expression profiling studies (clinical sample size = 139, disease groups = 20).

Table S2 Summary of cell lines, source and type.

Table S3 Dicer expression in relation to cutaneous tumors, sex (n = 328) and age (n = 335).

Table S4 Dicer expression in relation to melanoma type and anatomic site (n = 133).

Acknowledgments

We acknowledge Dr. Stanley N. Cohen for the gift of melanoma cell lines (A2058, A375P, C32 and A375SM).

Author Contributions

Conceived and designed the experiments: SSD AF. Performed the experiments: ZM EF. Analyzed the data: SSD ZM HS EF. Contributed reagents/materials/analysis tools: SSD. Wrote the paper: SSD. Confirmed histological diagnoses and build TMA: DC.

References

1. Bartel DP (2004) MicroRNAs: genomics, biogenesis, mechanism, and function. Cell 116: 281–297.
2. Ryan BM, Robles AI, Harris CC (2010) Genetic variation in microRNA networks: the implications for cancer research. Nat Rev Cancer 10: 389–402.
3. Doench JG, Petersen CP, Sharp PA (2003) siRNAs can function as miRNAs. Genes Dev 17: 438–442.
4. Esquela-Kerscher A, Slack FJ (2006) Oncomirs - microRNAs with a role in cancer. Nat Rev Cancer 6: 259–269.
5. Calin GA, Liu CG, Sevignani C, Ferracin M, Felli N, et al. (2004) MicroRNA profiling reveals distinct signatures in B cell chronic lymphocytic leukemias. Proc Natl Acad Sci U S A 101: 11755–11760.
6. Takamizawa J, Konishi H, Yanagisawa K, Tomida S, Osada H, et al. (2004) Reduced expression of the let-7 microRNAs in human lung cancers in association with shortened postoperative survival. Cancer Res 64: 3753–3756.
7. Michael MZ, SM OC, van Holst Pellekaan NG, Young GP, James RJ (2003) Reduced accumulation of specific microRNAs in colorectal neoplasia. Mol Cancer Res 1: 882–891.
8. Roldo C, Missiaglia E, Hagan JP, Falconi M, Capelli P, et al. (2006) MicroRNA expression abnormalities in pancreatic endocrine and acinar tumors are associated with distinctive pathologic features and clinical behavior. J Clin Oncol 24: 4677–4684.
9. Mueller DW, Rehli M, Bosserhoff AK (2009) miRNA expression profiling in melanocytes and melanoma cell lines reveals miRNAs associated with formation and progression of malignant melanoma. J Invest Dermatol 129: 1740–1751.
10. Stark MS, Tyagi S, Nancarrow DJ, Boyle GM, Cook AL, et al. (2010) Characterization of the Melanoma miRNAome by Deep Sequencing. PLoS One 5: e9685.
11. Caramuta S, Egyhazi S, Rodolfo M, Witten D, Hansson J, et al. (2010) MicroRNA expression profiles associated with mutational status and survival in malignant melanoma. J Invest Dermatol 130: 2062–2070.
12. Segura MF, Belitskaya-Levy I, Rose AE, Zakrzewski J, Gaziel A, et al. (2010) Melanoma MicroRNA signature predicts post-recurrence survival. Clin Cancer Res 16: 1577–1586.
13. Ma Z, Lui WO, Fire A, Dadras SS (2009) Profiling and discovery of novel miRNAs from formalin-fixed, paraffin-embedded melanoma and nodal specimens. J Mol Diagn 11: 420–429.
14. Jukic DM, Rao UN, Kelly L, Skaf JS, Drogowski LM, et al. (2010) Microrna profiling analysis of differences between the melanoma of young adults and older adults. J Transl Med 8: 27.
15. Hammond SM (2005) Dicing and slicing: the core machinery of the RNA interference pathway. FEBS Lett 579: 5822–5829.
16. Chiosea S, Jelezcova E, Chandran U, Acquafondata M, McHale T, et al. (2006) Up-regulation of dicer, a component of the MicroRNA machinery, in prostate adenocarcinoma. Am J Pathol 169: 1812–1820.
17. Chiosea S, Jelezcova E, Chandran U, Luo J, Mantha G, et al. (2007) Overexpression of Dicer in precursor lesions of lung adenocarcinoma. Cancer Res 67: 2345–2350.
18. Merritt WM, Lin YG, Han LY, Kamat AA, Spannuth WA, et al. (2008) Dicer, Drosha, and outcomes in patients with ovarian cancer. N Engl J Med 359: 2641–2650.
19. Balch CM, Gershenwald JE, Soong SJ, Thompson JF, Atkins MB, et al. (2009) Final version of 2009 AJCC melanoma staging and classification. J Clin Oncol 27: 6199–6206.
20. Dadras SS, Paul T, Bertoncini J, Brown LF, Muzikansky A, et al. (2003) Tumor lymphangiogenesis: a novel prognostic indicator for cutaneous melanoma metastasis and survival. Am J Pathol 162: 1951–1960.
21. Scatolini M, Grand MM, Grosso E, Venesio T, Pisacane A, et al. (2010) Altered molecular pathways in melanocytic lesions. International journal of cancer Journal international du cancer 126: 1869–1881.
22. Riker AI, Enkemann SA, Fodstad O, Liu S, Ren S, et al. (2008) The gene expression profiles of primary and metastatic melanoma yields a transition point of tumor progression and metastasis. BMC medical genomics 1: 13.
23. Tokumaru S, Suzuki M, Yamada H, Nagino M, Takahashi T (2008) let-7 regulates Dicer expression and constitutes a negative feedback loop. Carcinogenesis 29: 2073–2077.
24. Nakagawa A, Shi Y, Kage-Nakadai E, Mitani S, Xue D (2010) Caspase-dependent conversion of Dicer ribonuclease into a death-promoting deoxyribonuclease. Science 328: 327–334.
25. Levy C, Khaled M, Robinson KC, Veguilla RA, Chen PH, et al. (2010) Lineage-specific transcriptional regulation of DICER by MITF in melanocytes. Cell 141: 994–1005.
26. Ihara Y, Kato Y, Bando T, Yamagishi F, Minamimura T, et al. (2002) Allelic imbalance of 14q32 in esophageal carcinoma. Cancer Genet Cytogenet 135: 177–181.
27. Shao J, Li Y, Wu Q, Liang X, Yu X, et al. (2002) High frequency loss of heterozygosity on the long arms of chromosomes 13 and 14 in nasopharyngeal carcinoma in Southern China. Chin Med J (Engl) 115: 571–575.
28. Tzai TS, Chen HH, Chan SH, Ho CL, Tsai YS, et al. (2003) Clinical significance of allelotype profiling for urothelial carcinoma. Urology 62: 378–384.
29. Zhang L, Huang J, Yang N, Greshock J, Megraw MS, et al. (2006) microRNAs exhibit high frequency genomic alterations in human cancer. Proc Natl Acad Sci U S A 103: 9136–9141.
30. Karube Y, Tanaka H, Osada H, Tomida S, Tatematsu Y, et al. (2005) Reduced expression of Dicer associated with poor prognosis in lung cancer patients. Cancer Sci 96: 111–115.
31. Sugito N, Ishiguro H, Kuwabara Y, Kimura M, Mitsui A, et al. (2006) RNASEN regulates cell proliferation and affects survival in esophageal cancer patients. Clin Cancer Res 12: 7322–7328.
32. Muralidhar B, Goldstein LD, Ng G, Winder DM, Palmer RD, et al. (2007) Global microRNA profiles in cervical squamous cell carcinoma depend on Drosha expression levels. J Pathol 212: 368–377.
33. Chiosea SI, Barnes EL, Lai SY, Egloff AM, Sargent RL, et al. (2008) Mucoepidermoid carcinoma of upper aerodigestive tract: clinicopathologic study of 78 cases with immunohistochemical analysis of Dicer expression. Virchows Arch 452: 629–635.
34. Jakymiw A, Patel RS, Deming N, Bhattacharyya I, Shah P, et al. (2010) Overexpression of dicer as a result of reduced let-7 MicroRNA levels contributes to increased cell proliferation of oral cancer cells. Genes Chromosomes Cancer 49: 549–559.
35. Sand M, Gambichler T, Sand D, Altmeyer P, Stuecker M, Bechara FG. Immunohistochemical expression patterns of the microRNA processing enzyme Dicer in cutaneous malignant melanomas, benign melanocytic nevi and dysplastic melanocytic nevi. Eur J Dermatol. 2011 1–2 1;21(1):18–21.

7

Ethnicity and Cutaneous Melanoma in the City of Sao Paulo, Brazil: A Case-Control Study

Olinda C. Luiz[1]*, Reinaldo José Gianini[2,3], Fernanda T. Gonçalves[4], Guilherme Francisco[5], Cyro Festa-Neto[6], José Antonio Sanches[6], Gilka J. F. Gattas[4], Roger Chammas[5], José Eluf-Neto[1]

1 Laboratório de Epidemiologia e Imunobiologia – LIM38, Departamento de Medicina Preventiva da Faculdade de Medicina da Universidade de São Paulo, Sao Paulo, Brazil, **2** Laboratório de Processamento de Dados Biomédicos – LIM39, Departamento de Medicina Preventiva da Faculdade de Medicina da Universidade de São Paulo, Sao Paulo, Brazil, **3** Pontifícia Universidade Católica de São Paulo, Sorocaba, Brazil, **4** Laboratório de Imuno-hematologia e Hematologia Forense – LIM40, Departamento de Medicina Legal, Ética Médica, Medicina Social e do Trabalho, Faculdade de Medicina da Universidade de São Paulo, Sao Paulo, Brazil, **5** Laboratório de Oncologia Experimental – LIM24, Departamento de Radiologia, Faculdade de Medicina da Universidade de São Paulo, Sao Paulo, Brazil, **6** Departamento de Dermatologia, Faculdade de Medicina da Universidade de São Paulo, Sao Paulo, Brazil

Abstract

Background: Over the last century the incidence of cutaneous melanoma has increased worldwide, a trend that has also been observed in Brazil. The identified risk factors for melanoma include the pattern of sun exposure, family history, and certain phenotypic features. In addition, the incidence of melanoma might be influenced by ethnicity. Like many countries, Brazil has high immigration rates and consequently a heterogenous population. However, Brazil is unique among such countries in that the ethnic heterogeneity of its population is primarily attributable to admixture. This study aimed to evaluate the contribution of European ethnicity to the risk of cutaneous melanoma in Brazil.

Methodology/Principal Findings: We carried out a hospital-based case-control study in the metropolitan area of Sao Paulo, Brazil. We evaluated 424 hospitalized patients (202 melanoma patients and 222 control patients) regarding phenotypic features, sun exposure, and number of grandparents born in Europe. Through multivariate logistic regression analysis, we found the following variables to be independently associated with melanoma: grandparents born in Europe—Spain (OR = 3.01, 95% CI: 1.03–8.77), Italy (OR = 3.47, 95% CI: 1.41–8.57), a Germanic/Slavic country (OR = 3.06, 95% CI: 1.05–8.93), or ≥2 European countries (OR = 2.82, 95% CI: 1.06–7.47); eye color—light brown (OR = 1.99, 95% CI: 1.14–3.84) and green/blue (OR = 4.62; 95% CI 2.22–9.58); pigmented lesion removal (OR = 3.78; 95% CI: 2.21–6.49); no lifetime sunscreen use (OR = 3.08; 95% CI: 1.03–9.22); and lifetime severe sunburn (OR = 1.81; 95% CI: 1.03–3.19).

Conclusions: Our results indicate that European ancestry is a risk factor for cutaneous melanoma. Such risk appears to be related not only to skin type, eye color, and tanning capacity but also to others specific characteristics of European populations introduced in the New World by European immigrants.

Editor: Yury E. Khudyakov, Centers for Disease Control and Prevention, United States of America

Funding: 1. Fundação de Amparo à Pesquisa do Estado de São Paulo – FAPESP (process 06-52041-9, 5-56069-2) www.fapesp.br. 2. Conselho Nacional de Desenvolvimento Científico e Tecnológico - Brasil (National Counsel of Technological and Scientific Development - Brazil) - CNPq (process n°478239/03-3)- www.cnpq.br. The funders had no role in study design, data collection and analysis, decision to publish, or preparation of the manuscript

Competing Interests: Roger Chammas, co-author, is an academic editor for PLoS ONE. This does not alter the authors' adherence to all the PLoS ONE policies on sharing data and materials.

* E-mail: olinda@usp.br

Introduction

Populations on different continents vary considerably in their predisposition to disease, probably as a result of adaptation to local selective factors such as climate and available nutrients but also as a result of genetic ancestry.

The population of Brazil is a diverse mix of ethnic groups. After Brazil was discovered in 1500, Portuguese settlers and (later) African slaves intermarried with the indigenous peoples of Brazil. In the 19th and 20th centuries, there were waves of immigration to Brazil from various European countries. Between 1872 and 1975, Brazil received more than 5.4 million immigrants [1]: 34% from Italy; 29% from Portugal; 14% from Spain; 5% from Japan; 4% from Germany; 2% from Syria or Lebanon; and 12% from other countries. Because of extensive admixture among these various groups, the Brazilian population shows great variability in terms of skin pigmentation, phenotypic features, and genomic structure [2].

Cutaneous melanoma is associated with high mortality rates. Worldwide, its incidence has increased progressively over the last century, as have the levels of exposure to ultraviolet (UV) radiation, a well-known risk factor, and it has been suggested that certain environmental and genetic factors also increase melanoma risk [3]. Recent increases in the incidence of melanoma have also been observed in Brazil [4]. These increases are probably related to changes in individual habits, including the pursuit of recreational activities in the sun [4].

The identified risk factors for melanoma include the pattern of sun exposure [5], a family history of melanoma, a high number of nevi, and certain phenotypic features, such as skin type, hair color, and eye color [6,7]. Some studies have suggested that ethnicity influences the occurrence of melanomas. The European phenotype, characterized by blue or green eyes, together with light-colored hair, pale skin, and low tanning ability, has consistently been associated with an increased risk of malignant melanoma [7,8]. It seems reasonable that the increased risk associated with European ethnicity should be attributed to lighter skin pigmentation. However, European ethnicity as predictor of melanoma independent of skin pigmentation has been poorly investigated. Most studies of melanoma have been carried out in Europe, North America, or Australia, mainly involving White populations in geographic regions where there is little admixture. Ethnicity has been investigated in only a few studies and for limited approaches [9–13].

It seems logical that admixture between European immigrants and indigenous peoples would have increased susceptibility to melanoma in the population of Brazil.

The aim of this case-control study was to assess the importance of ethnicity as a risk factor for melanoma in an admixed population. Our main hypothesis was that European ethnicity is predictor for cutaneous melanoma independent of phenotype.

Methods

Participants

Patients with melanoma were recruited from among those diagnosed between October 2004 and July 2008 at one of three facilities in the city of Sao Paulo, Brazil: *Hospital das Clínicas da Faculdade de Medicina da Universidade de São Paulo*; *Hospital do Câncer Antônio Cândido Camargo*; and *Instituto Brasileiro de Controle do Câncer*. The inclusion criteria were having received histopathological confirmation of cutaneous melanoma, being White, and being a resident of the metropolitan area of Sao Paulo. Patients were recruited during the pre-treatment phase. Age and sex frequency-matched controls were recruited from among cancer-free White patients hospitalized on the orthopedic or gastroenterology ward of the *Hospital das Clínicas*, who were confirmed as being melanoma-free upon recruitment. Controls also had to be residents of the metropolitan area of Sao Paulo. In both groups, only patients between 15 and 75 years of age were included.

The study was designed to detect a 1.9-fold increase in risk with a type I error of 0.05 and a type II error of 0.2 (80% statistical power). Assuming a 20% exposure rate in the control population and a 1:1 control to case ratio, the minimum sample size was determined to be 420 (210 cases and 210 controls).

Investigations Undertaken

During hospitalization, interviews were conducted by one of the three trained interviewers. Using a standardized questionnaire, we collected data related to sociodemographic characteristics (sex, age, income, and level of education); self-reported characteristics, including natural eye/hair color at 15 years of age, Fitzpatrick sun-reactive skin type [14], also known as skin phototype; and the history of UV exposure (use of tanning beds, use of sunscreen from birth to 9 years, number of sunburns during childhood/adolescence, and lifetime history of severe sunburn).

Participants were asked to classify the distribution of freckles on their face in childhood as either sparse or dense. Skin phototypes were defined as follows [14]: type I (always burns, never tans); type II (often burns, tans minimally); type III (rarely burns, tans well); and type IV (never burns, always tans). Cases and controls were asked if they had previously had moles or other pigmented lesions removed. The parental history of cancer was classified as negative if neither the mother nor the father had had cancer, and as positive if either or both parents had had cancer. The family history of skin cancer was classified as positive if one or more brothers, sisters, sons, or daughters had had any type of skin cancer.

Sunscreen use was categorized as follows: often; occasionally; or modified (e.g., changed from "never" in infancy or adolescence to "often" in adult life or from "often"/"occasionally" to "never"). Severe sunburn was defined as event of sun exposure resulting in skin redness and discomfort for at least two days. The frequency of sunburn in infancy and adolescence was classified as less than once/year, one to six times/year, or more than seven times/year.

On the basis of the American Joint Committee on Cancer T-category criteria and Breslow thickness [15], the case group tumors were categorized, by diameter, as follows: ≤1.0 mm (T1); 1.01–2.00 mm (T2); 2.01–4.00 mm (T3); and >4.0 mm (T4). We also classified the tumors by Clark level of invasion [16]: level I - lesions involving only the epidermis (in situ melanoma); level II - invasion of the papillary dermis; level III - invasion filling and expanding the papillary dermis; level IV - invasion into the reticular dermis; level V -invasion through the reticular dermis into the subcutaneous tissue.

Ethnic background was determined by the origin of the grandparents and was assessed by four approaches in terms of the frequency of migration to Brazil. Individuals with four Brazilian grandparents were used as the reference for all comparisons of ethnicity.

In the first approach, we considered the following European countries as a set: Spain, France, Italy, Portugal, Germany, Austria, Hungary, Yugoslavia, Lithuania, Poland, Romania,

Table 1. Socio-demographic characteristics of participants.

Risk factors	Cases* (%)	Controls* (%)
Sex		
Male	100 (49.5)	110 (49.5)
Female	102 (50.5)	112 (50.5)
Age		
15–29	12 (5.9)	25 (11.3)
30–39	28 (13.9)	35 (15.8)
40–49	51 (25.3)	58 (26.1)
50–59	51 (25.3)	50 (22.5)
60–69	35 (17.3)	30 (13.5)
70–79	25 (12.4)	24 (10.8)
Age Average (SD)	51.7 (14.3)	48.2 (14.8)
Educational level		
Until incomplete elementary	40 (19.2)	32 (14.9)
Elementary/Junior high school	24 (11.9)	57 (26.6)
Senior high school	48 (23.8)	78 (36.4)
College	89 (44.9)	47 (22.0)
Income (Real)**		
Less than 720	23 (11.4)	43 (20.4)
721 a 1,200	25 (12.4)	37 (17.5)
1,201 a 2,400	32 (15.9)	48 (22.7)
Above 2,401	121 (60.2)	83 (39.3)

*Totals may vary because of missing value.
**One real is approximately U.S. dollar 0.59.

Table 2. Odds ratios of melanoma associated with phenotypic features and family history of cancer.

Risk factor	Cases[a] (%)	Controls[a] (%)	OR (95% CI)[b]
Hair color			
Black or dark brown	60 (29.9)	114 (51.8)	1
Light brown	98 (48.8)	89 (40.5)	2.11 (1.36–3.26)
Blond or red	43 (21.4)	17 (7.7)	4.49 (2.32–8.70)
p trend			<0.0001
Eye color			
Black or dark brown	47 (23.5)	113 (51.1)	1
Light brown	100 (50.0)	79 (35.8)	2.90 (1.82–4.60)
Blue or green	53 (26.5)	29 (13.1)	4.51 (2.50–8.15)
p trend			<0.0001
Childhood freckle distribution			
Sparse	123 (62.1)	175 (81.0)	1
Dense	75 (37.9)	41 (19.0)	2.40 (1.52–3.81)
Skin phototype[c]			
IV	22 (10.9)	58 (28.0)	1
III	60 (29.7)	68 (32.9)	1.95 (1.05–3.63)
II	97 (48.0)	60 (29.0)	4.13 (2.27–7.51)
I	23 (11.4)	21 (10.1)	2.42 (1.10–5.29)
p trend			0.001
History of pigmented lesion removal			
No	86 (42.8)	179 (81.4)	1
Yes	115 (57.2)	41 (18.6)	5.38 (3.42–8.48)
Parental history of cancer			
No	121 (62.7)	122 (65.9)	1
Yes	72 (37.3)	63 (34.1)	1.02 (0.66–1.58)
Family history of skin cancer[d]			
No	191 (94.6)	208 (97.7)	1
Yes	11 (5.4)	5 (2.3)	1.93 (0.65–5.73)

[a]Totals may vary because of missing values.
[b]Adjusted for age, sex and educational level by unconditional logistic regression analysis. Statistical significance: likelihood ratio test.
[c]I: always burns, never tans; II: often burns, tans minimally; III: rarely burns, tans well; IV: never burns, always tans.
[d]Brothers, sisters, sons, and daughters.

Table 3. Exposure to UV radiation, use of sunscreen, and history of sunburn.

Risk factor	Cases[a] (%)	Controls[a] (%)	OR (95% CI)[b]
Use of tanning bed			
No	185 (93.4)	201 (93.1)	1
Yes	13 (6.6)	15 (6.9)	1.03 (0.62–2.14)
Use of sunscreen at 0–9 years of age			
Often	8 (4.1)	18 (8.8)	1
Occasionally	2 (1.0)	3 (1.5)	0.99 (0.13–7.58)
Never/almost never	185 (94.9)	184 (89.8)	1.69 (0.67–4.25)
Lifetime sunscreen use			
Often	9 (4.5)	27 (12.7)	1
Occasionally	9 (4.5)	7 (3.3)	4.28 (1.12–16.39)
Never/almost never	85 (42.3)	101 (47.6)	2.02 (0.86–4.77)
Modified	98 (48.8)	77 (36.3)	2.62 (1.11–6.16)
Sunburn at 0–14 years of age			
<1 per year	72 (35.6)	126 (60.0)	1
1–6 per year	102 (50.5)	75 (35.7)	2.83 (1.78–4.50)
≥7 per year	28 (13.9)	9 (4.3)	6.22 (2.72–14.24)
p trend			<0.0001
Sunburn at 15–19 years of age			
<1 per year	55 (28.4)	126 (60.9)	1
1–6 per year	85 (43.8)	62 (30.0)	3.99 (2.35–6.79)
≥7 per year	54 (27.8)	19 (9.2)	8.48 (4.35–16.54)
p trend			<0.0001
Severe sunburn (lifetime)			
No	50 (24.8)	101 (48.3)	1
Yes	152 (75.2)	108 (51.7)	3.11 (1.99–4.87)

[a]Totals may vary because of missing values.
[b]Adjusted for age, sex and educational level by unconditional logistic regression analysis. Statistical significance: likelihood ratio test.

Russia, Switzerland, and Czechoslovakia. In this approach, cases and controls were distributed according to the total number of grandparents born in any of those countries.

In the second approach, we considered a smaller subgroup of European countries, including only Spain, France, Italy and Portugal. In this approach, cases and controls were also distributed according to the total number of grandparents born in any of these countries.

In the third approach, we considered a different subgroup, including Germany, Austria, Hungary, Yugoslavia, Lithuania, Poland, Romania, Russia, Switzerland, and Czechoslovakia. In this approach, cases and controls were also distributed according to the total number of grandparents born in any of these countries.

In the fourth approach, the countries with the highest rates of migration to Brazil were analyzed separately, whereas those with lower rates of migration to Brazil were grouped. Cases and controls were distributed as follows: those having one or more grandparents born in Spain (category 1); those having one or more grandparents born in Italy (category 2); those having one or more grandparents born in Portugal (category 3); those having one or more grandparents born in a Germanic or Slavic country (category 4); and those having one or more grandparents born in one European country and one or more grandparents born in a different European country (category 5).

Ethics

The study protocol was approved by the Research Ethics Committee of all three facilities (*Hospital das Clínicas da Faculdade de Medicina da Universidade de São Paulo*; *Hospital do Câncer Antônio Cândido Camargo*; and *Instituto Brasileiro de Controle do Câncer*). All participating patients gave written informed consent. Participants under eighteen years old also had written informed consent from parents or legal guardians.

Table 4. Odds ratios of melanoma associated with European ethnicity.

Country of grandparent birth	Number of Grandparents	Cases[a] (%)	Controls[a] (%)	OR (95% CI)[b]	OR (95% CI)[c]
Brazil (reference)	Four	71 (35.9)	132 (62.0)	1	1
European group 1[d]					
	One	16 (8.1)	15 (7.0)	1.87 (0.87–4.00)	1.68 (0.74–3.81)
	Two	34 (17.2)	35 (16.4)	1.94 (1.31–3.23)	1.47 (0.78–2.77)
	Three or four	77 (38.9)	31 (14.5)	4.45 (2.53–7.82)	3.46 (1.87–6.41)
	p trend			<0.0001	<0.0001
European group 2[e]					
	One	12 (6.7)	11 (5.5)	1.43 (0.66–3.06)	1.46 (0.64–3.31)
	Two	30 (17.1)	31 (15.4)	2.03 (1.12–3.66)	1.51 (0.77–2.94)
	Three or four	62 (35.4)	27 (13.4)	4.24 (2.30–7.80)	3.52 (1.81–6.83)
	p trend			<0.0001	<0.0001
European group 3[f]					
	One	4 (4.2)	4 (2.8)	1.89 (0.45–7.92)	0.99 (0.19–5.15)
	Two	4 (4.2)	4 (2.8)	1.63 (0.38–7.07)	1.37 (0.30–6.20)
	Three or four	15 (16.0)	4 (2.8)	5.89 (1.82–19.08)	3.71 (0.94–14.61)
	p trend			0.01	0.07
Spain[g]	One or more	19 (9.6)	14 (6.6)	4.45 (1.78–11.14)	3.32 (1.24–8.92)
Italy[g]	One or more	46 (23.5)	29 (13.6)	4.62 (2.20–9.68)	3.34 (1.47–7.58)
Portugal[g]	One or more	18 (9.1)	17 (8.0)	3.01 (1.27–7.14)	2.65 (1.05–6.65)
Germanic/Slavic subset[f,g]	One or more	19 (9.6)	9 (4.2)	4.94 (1.94–12.57)	3.31 (1.15–9.48)
≥2 European countries	Two or more	24 (12.2)	12 (5.6)	4.63 (2.05–10.47)	3.44 (1.44–8.24)

[a]Totals may vary because of missing values.
[b]Adjusted for age, sex and educational level by unconditional logistic regression analysis. Statistical significance: likelihood ratio test.
[c]Adjusted for age, sex, level of education, eye color, hair color, freckle density, and skin phototype by unconditional logistic regression analysis. Statistical significance: likelihood ratio test.
[d]Spain, France, Italy, Portugal, Germany, Austria, Hungary, Yugoslavia, Lithuania, Poland, Romania, Russia, Switzerland, or Czechoslovakia.
[e]Spain, France, Italy, or Portugal.
[f]Germany, Austria, Hungary, Yugoslavia, Lithuania, Poland, Romania, Russia, Switzerland, or Czechoslovakia.
[g]Adjusted further for the number of European grandparents.

Statistical Methods

To estimate the risk of melanoma associated with selected factors, we calculated odds ratios (ORs) and 95% confidence intervals (95% CIs) using unconditional logistic regression analysis. Because cases and controls were frequency-matched according to age and sex, all ORs were adjusted for age and sex. Level of education was also included, in order to control for socioeconomic status. Statistical significance was assessed using the likelihood ratio test. For ordered categorical variables, we employed tests for linear trend, categorizing the exposure variables and entering the scores as continuous values. Variables with a $p<0.20$ after adjustment for age, sex, and level of education were included in the multivariate models and were selected by backward stepwise regression. All four approaches to determining ethnicity presented a $p<0.20$. However, to avoid collinearity, only the fourth approach (because it was the most detailed approach) was included in multivariate analysis.

The STATA statistical program, version 10 (Stata Corp., College Station, TX, USA), was used for statistical analysis. All tests were two-tailed, and the level of statistical significance was set at $p\leq0.05$.

Results

A total of 212 patients with cutaneous melanoma were admitted to the three hospitals during the study period. Of those 212 melanoma patients, 6 (2.8%) declined to participate in the study and 4 (1.9%) died before the questionnaire was applied. The remaining 202 patients were included in the case group. We identified 230 eligible inpatient controls among inpatients on the orthopedics and gastroenterology wards. Of those 230 patients, 8 (3.5%) declined to participate in the study. Therefore, the control group comprised 222 patients. Proportion (%) of males in cases and controls were 49.5. The mean (SD) age in the case and control groups was 51.7 (14.3) years and 48.2 (14.8) years, respectively (Table 1).

On the basis of the American Joint Committee on Cancer T-category criteria and Breslow thickness [15], we categorized the tumors as T1 in 61% of the cases, T2 in 16%, T3 in 14%, and T4 in 9%. When we classified the tumors by Clark level [16], 5% of the cases were level I (in situ), 23% level II, 49% level III, 20% level IV, and 3% level V.

Table 2 shows the distribution of cases and controls by hair/eye color, density of childhood freckling, skin phototype, history of pigmented lesion removal, and family history of skin cancer. Risk factors such as eye color (blue, green, or light brown), hair color (blond, red, or light brown), density of childhood freckling, skin phototype, and history of pigmented lesion removal were associated with an overall increase in melanoma risk. Blond/red hair color and blue/green eye color were associated with a 4-fold increase in the

Table 5. Factors associated with melanoma in the multivariate logistic regression analysis.

Ethnicity	OR (95% CI)[a]
Brazilian	1
Spanish	3.01 (1.03–8.77)
Italian	3.47 (1.41–8.57)
Portuguese	2.32 (0.82–6.61)
Germanic or Slavic	3.06 (1.05–8.93)
Mixed European	2.82 (1.06–7.47)
Eye color	
Black or dark Brown	1
Light Brown	1.99 (1.14–3.84)
Blue or Green	4.62 (2.22–9.58)
p trend	<0.0001
History of pigmented lesion removal	
No	1
Yes	3.78 (2.21–6.49)
Lifetime sunscreen use	
Often	1
Occasionally	3.53 (0.59–21.21)
Never/almost never	3.08 (1.03–9.22)
Modified	2.74 (0.93–8.12)
Sunburn at 15–19 years of age	
<1 per year	1
1–6 per year	3.47 (1.83–6.59)
≥7 per year	4.60 (2.22–9.50)
p trend	<0.0001
Severe sunburn (lifetime)	
No	1
Yes	1.81 (1.03–3.19)

[a]Adjusted for age, sex, education level and the other factors shown in the table.

risk of melanoma. Family history of skin cancer or parental history of any cancer were not associated with melanoma risk.

As can be seen in Table 3, neither tanning bed use nor the use of sunscreen from birth to 9 years age was associated with occurrence of melanoma. A frequency of sunburn in childhood and adolescence was associated with a 4- to 8-fold increase in the risk of melanoma. A lifetime history of severe sunburn was also strongly associated with melanoma risk.

Table 4 presents the ethnicity of the sample, based on the four approaches taken. The first approach (analyzing 14 European countries as a set) and second approach (analyzing 4 southern European countries as a set) showed a trend, with a strong gradient, toward an association with the number of grandparents. Having 3 or 4 European grandparents was found to increase melanoma risk by approximately 4 times compared with having four Brazilian grandparents. When adjusting for phenotypic features (eye color, hair color, childhood freckle density, and skin phototype) the trend remained strong, indicating that the increased risk related to ethnicity is not solely attributable to specific physical features. The fourth approach produced a result similar to that of the first two approaches. For countries with higher rates of immigration to Brazil (Spain, Italy, and Germanic/Slavic countries), adjusting for phenotypic features reduced the magnitude of the risk but did not negate the statistical significance of this association. In the multivariate logistic regression (Table 5), the following variables were identified as independent predictors of melanoma: European ethnicity (Spanish, Italian, Germanic/Slavic, or mixed); eye color (green, blue, or light brown); history of pigmented lesion removal; lifetime history of no sunscreen use; sunburn in adolescence; and lifetime history of severe sunburn.

Discussion

Summarizing our findings, data suggest that European ethnicity is a risk factor for cutaneous melanoma, with a strong trend toward greater risk associated with the number of European grandparents. This increased risk might be related not only to skin phototype but also to genetic polymorphisms introduced into the New World by European immigrants.

In this case-control study, we also corroborated the findings of other authors in relation to the role that certain phenotypic features play in increasing susceptibility to melanoma in an admixed population [5–8].

The history of Brazil involved waves of immigration and minimal social stigma associated with interethnic marriage [2]. The heterogeneity of its population is therefore the product of five centuries of admixture between and among individuals native to Brazil and those of African, Portuguese, German, Italian, Spanish, Middle Eastern or Asian descent.

In the present study, we found that European ethnicity was associated with an increased risk of cutaneous melanoma in Brazil, as previously suggested in a relatively small study conducted in the southern region of the country [12]. Very little has been published regarding cutaneous melanoma in other admixed populations [13]. Acton et al., analyzing the population of the American state of Alabama, found that being of Northern European descent was associated with the risk of cutaneous melanoma, although being of Mediterranean descent was not [9]. Loria et al. studied a sample of individuals born in Argentina and found a higher risk of cutaneous melanoma among those with four European grandparents [10]. Bakos et al. found that being a member of an indigenous population in Brazil was protective against melanoma and that being of European descent was an independent factor for the occurrence of melanoma [12]. To our knowledge, there have been no studies conducting a detailed investigation of European ethnicity in relation to melanoma, as we have done here.

Certain phenotypic features, such as light-colored hair, pale skin, and light eye color, are specific to Europe. The European population shows small genetic distances and few differences in population structure when compared with populations on other continents, suggesting a relatively homogenous continental population [17]. It seems reasonable that the increased risk associated with European ethnicity should be attributed to skin phototype [6–8]. However, European ethnicity persisted as an independent risk factor for melanoma, even after adjustment for phenotypic features. Phenotypic features are genetically determined by a relatively small number of genes [2] that were evolutionarily selected by environment, especially the amount of UV exposure [18]. The melanoma risk associated with European ethnicity might be related to factors that have yet to be extensively researched. This association might be explained by the influence of combinations of genetic polymorphisms related to ancestry rather than by phenotypic features. Various studies have found positive associations between genetic polymorphisms and the risk of cutaneous melanoma [19–23].

Studies carried out in other regions of the world have reported that certain phenotypic features increase the risk of melanoma

[6,7,24]. In fact, there is strong evidence that melanoma development is associated with the UV index and latitude [24,25]. In addition, a study conducted in the city of Sao Paulo during the 2005–2008 period showed that the UV index ranged from very high to extreme (according to the World Health Organization classification) on 65% of the days in the summer and in 40% of the days in the winter [27]. Therefore, Sao Paulo residents are continually exposed to high-intensity solar radiation and high UV indices, critical factors for the development of skin cancers, including melanoma [27].

We found that individuals with a history of sunburn were at an increased risk of developing melanoma. This was probably related to skin phototype. Individuals with skin phototype I or II produce less melanin, especially eumelanin, which acts as a physical barrier, scattering the incident UV light, and as a filter to reduce its penetration into the epidermis [28,29]. Multiple episodes of sunburn can damage the genetic material, causing mutations that accumulate throughout life and promote the process of skin carcinogenesis. Recent studies indicate that increased sensitivity to sun exposure is also associated with polymorphisms and mutations in genes involved in skin pigmentation [30,31].

All epidemiology studies are subject to limitations. Population controls, though preferable for reasons of validity, present more information bias than that affecting cases. Response of individuals selected from the general population tends to be worse than that from other types of controls because they are often less cooperative. We chose hospital-controls because they are more suitable when hospital cases are studied [32]. A case-control design is susceptible to confounders if there is differential ascertainment of risk factors between cases and controls. We minimized this aspect by standardizing our methods of data collection. In addition, the interviewers were blinded to the status (case or control) of the subjects. Non-differential misclassification could have occurred if subjects not truly having melanoma were included as cases, independent of their exposure status. This could result in an underestimation of the risk of cutaneous melanoma. To avoid this problem, we included only cases in which there was histopathological confirmation of the diagnosis. In case-control studies such as ours, there is a potential for recall bias. It is unlikely that ancestry was misclassified, because the birthplace of grandparents is relatively objective information. To address potential problems with recall for others self-reported variables, we enrolled only untreated cases, so that their responses were less likely to be influenced by changes that occurred after diagnosis. Therefore the associations with skin phototype, hair color, and history of pigmented lesion removal were comparable to those reported in previous studies. Nevertheless, some residual confounding cannot be completely ruled out. No association was found between melanoma risk and tanning bed exposure, a variable for which the occurrence of recall bias is more likely. Therefore, the degree of tanning bed exposure might may have been underreported [33]. Additionally caution is advised due to a relatively small sample that can result in lower precision with larger confidence interval.

Our results open new perspectives for research into the etiology of melanoma. The population of Brazil differs from those of other countries with high rates of immigration because of the admixture of various ethnicities. Therefore, we cannot assume that European ethnicity plays a similar role in the etiology of melanoma in other regions of the world. However, to determine whether the role of European ethnicity in other admixed populations is similar to that observed for Brazil, it would be useful to conduct new studies in countries such as the United States, Australia and other Latin America countries. In addition, the identification of genetic polymorphisms specific to a given ethnicity could form the basis for investigations of molecular markers of cutaneous melanoma. Such studies should consider the diversity of European ethnicity

Author Contributions

Conceived and designed the experiments: OCL RJG FTG GF GJFG RC JEN. Performed the experiments: OCL FTG GF GJFG RC JEN CF JAS. Analyzed the data: OCL RJG FTG GF GJFG RC JEN CFN JAS. Wrote the paper: OCL RJG FTG GF GJFG RC JEN CFN JAS. Contributed to conception and design: OCL RJG FTG GF CF JAS GJFG RC JEN. Interpreted the data: OCL RJG FTG GF CF JAS GJFG RC JEN. Revised the article critically and approved the final version to be published: OCL RJG FTG GF CF JAS GJFG RC JEN.

References

1. IBGE (2000) Brasil: 500 anos de povoamento. Rio de Janeiro: IBGE. 231 p.
2. Pena SDJ, Di Pietro G, Fuchshuber-Moraes M, Genro JP, Hutz MH, et al. (2011) The Genomic Ancestry of Individuals from Different Geographical Regions of Brazil Is More Uniform Than Expected. PLoS ONE 6(2): e17063.
3. MacKie RM, Hauschild A, Eggermont AM (2009) Epidemiology of invasive cutaneous melanoma. Ann Oncol 20: 1–7.
4. Mendes GL, Koifman RJ, Koifman S (2010) Mortality Frequency and Trends Attributed to Melanoma in Brazil from 1980–2005. J Toxicol Environ Health 73: 850–857.
5. Chang YM, Barrett JH, Bishop DT, Armstrong BK, Bataille V, et al. (2009) Sun exposure and melanoma risk at different latitudes: a pooled analysis of 5700 cases and 7216 controls. Int J Epidemiol 38: 814–830.
6. Gilchrest BA, Eller MS, Geller AC, Yaar M (1999) The pathogenesis of melanoma induced by ultraviolet radiation. N Engl J Med 340: 1341–1348.
7. Gandini S, Sera F, Cattaruzza MS, Pasquini P, Zanetti R, et al. (2005) Meta-analysis of risk factors for cutaneous melanoma: III. Family history, actinic damage and phenotypic factors. Eur J Cancer 41: 2040–2059.
8. Nijsten T, Leys C, Verbruggen K, Verlinden V, Drieghe J, et al. (2005) Case-control study to identify melanoma risk factors in the Belgian population: the significance of clinical examination. J Eur Acad Dermatol Venereol 19: 332–339.
9. Acton RT, Barton EH, Hollowell WW, Dreibelbis AL, Go RC, et al. (2004) Ancestry reported by white adults with cutaneous melanoma and control subjects in central Alabama. BMC Cancer 4: 47.
10. Loria D, Matos E (2001) Risk factors for cutaneous melanoma: a case-control study in Argentina. Int J Dermatol 40: 108–114.
11. Lascano AR, Kuznitzky R, Cuestas E, Mainardi C, Albertini R, et al. (2004) Factores de riesgo para melanoma cutaneo. Estudio de casos y controles em Córdoba, Argentina. Medicina (B Aires) 64: 504–508.
12. Bakos L, Masiero NC, Bakos RM, Burttet RM, Wagner MB, et al. (2009) European ancestry and cutaneous melanoma in Southern Brazil. J Eur Acad Dermatol Venereol 23: 304–307.
13. Swan MC, Hudson DA (2003) Malignant melanoma in South Africans of mixed ancestry: a retrospective analysis. Melanoma Res 13: 415–419.
14. Fitzpatrick TB (1988) The validity and practicality of sun-reactive skin types I through VI. Arch Dermatol 124: 869–871.
15. Edge SB, Byrd DR, Compton CC, Fritz AG, Greene FL, et al. (2010) AJCC (American Joint Committee on Cancer) Cancer Staging Manual. 7th ed. New York: Springer-Verlag. 646 p.
16. Clark WH, From L, Bernardino EA, Mihm MC (1969) The histogenesis and biologic behavior of primary human malignant melanomas of the skin. Cancer Res 29: 705–726.
17. Bauchet M, McEvoy B, Pearson LN, Quillen EE, Sarkisian T, et al. (2007) Measuring European population stratification with microarray genotype data. Am J Hum Genet 80: 948–956.
18. Sturm RA, Box NF, Ramsay M (1998) Human pigmentation genetics: the difference is only skin deep. Bioessays 20: 712–721.
19. Li C, Hu Z, Liu Z, Wang LE, Strom SS, et al. (2006) Polymorphisms in the DNA repair genes XPC, XPD, and XPG and risk of cutaneous melanoma: a case-control analysis. Cancer Epidemiol Biomark Prev 15: 2526–2532.
20. Tomescu D, Kavanagh G, Ha T, Campbell H, Melton DW. Nucleotide excision repair gene XPD polymorphisms and genetic predisposition to melanoma. Carcinogenesis 22: 403–408.
21. Millikan RC, Hummer A, Begg C, Player J, de Cotret AR, et al. (2006) Polymorphisms in nucleotide excision repair genes and risk of multiple primary melanoma: the Genes Environment and Melanoma Study. Carcinogenesis 27: 610–618.
22. Khan SG, Muniz-Medina V, Shahlavi T, Baker CC, Inui H, et al. (2002) The human XPC DNA repair gene: arrangement, splice site information content and

influence of a single nucleotide polymorphism in a splice acceptor site on alternative splicing and function. Nucleic Acids Res 30: 3624–3631.
23. Gonçalves FT, Francisco G, Souza SP, Luiz OC, Festa-Neto C, et al. (2011) European ancestry and polymorphisms in DNA repair genes modify the risk of melanoma: A case-control study in a high UV index region in Brazil. J Dermatol Sci 64: 59–66.
24. Cust AE, Schmid H, Maskiell JA, Jetann J, Ferguson M, et al. (2009) Population-based, case-control-family design to investigate genetic and environmental influences on melanoma risk: Australian Melanoma Family Study. Am J Epidemiol 170: 1541–1554.
25. Hu S, Ma F, Collado-Mesa F, Kirsne RS (2004) UV radiation, latitude, and melanoma in US Hispanics and blacks. Arch Dermatol 140: 819–824.
26. Eide MJ, Weinstock MA (2005) Association of UV index, latitude, and melanoma incidence in nonwhite populations- US Surveillance, Epidemiology, and End Results (SEER) Program, 1992 to 2001. Arch Dermatol 141: 477–481.
27. de Paula-Correa M, Ceballos JC (2010) Solar ultraviolet radiation measurements in one of the most populous cities of the World: Aspects related to skin cancer cases and vitamin D availability. Photochem Photobiol 86: 438–444.
28. Slominski A, Tobin DJ, Shibahara S, Wortsman J (2004) Melanin pigmentation in mammalian skin and its hormonal regulation. Physiol Rev 84: 1155–1228.
29. Ou-Yang H, Stamatas G, Kollias N (2004) Spectral responses of melanin to ultraviolet A irradiation. J Invest Dermatol 122: 492–496.
30. Gruber F, Kastelan M, Brajac I, Saftić M, Peharda V, et al. (2008) Molecular and genetic mechanisms in melanoma. Coll Antropol 32: 147–152.
31. Sturm RA (2009) Molecular genetics of human pigmentation diversity. Hum Mol Genet 18: 9–17.
32. Breslow NE, Day NE (1980) Statistical methods in cancer research: the analysis of case-control studies. Lyon, v. 1 (IARC Scient. Publ. n. 32).
33. de Vries E, Boniol M, Severi G, Eggermont AM, Autier P, et al. (2005) Public awareness about risk factors could pose problems for case-control studies: the example of sunbed use and cutaneous melanoma. Eur J Cancer 41: 2150–2154.

8

Time Course and Pattern of Metastasis of Cutaneous Melanoma Differ between Men and Women

Liljana Mervic[1,2]*

1 Department of Dermatology, Center of Dermatooncology, University of Tüebingen, Germany, **2** Department of Dermatovenereology, University Medical Centre Ljubljana, Slovenia

Abstract

Background: This study identified sex differences in progression of cutaneous melanoma.

Methodology/Principal Findings: Of 7,338 patients who were diagnosed as an invasive primary CM without clinically detectable metastases from 1976 to 2008 at the University of Tuebingen in Germany, 1,078 developed subsequent metastases during follow up. The metastatic pathways were defined in these patients and analyzed using the Kaplan-Meier method. Multivariate survival analysis was performed using Cox modeling. In 18.7% of men and 29.2% of women ($P<0.001$) the first metastasis following diagnosis of primary tumor was locoregional as satellite/in-transit metastasis. The majority of men (54.0%) and women (47.6%, $P=0.035$) exhibited direct regional lymph node metastasis. Direct distant metastasis from the stage of the primary tumor was observed in 27.3% of men and 23.2% of women ($P=0.13$). Site of first metastasis was the most important prognostic factor of survival after recurrence in multivariate analysis (HR:1.3; 95% CI: 1.0–1.6 for metastasis to the regional lymph nodes vs. satellite/in-transit recurrence, and HR:5.5; 95% CI: 4.2–7.1 for distant metastasis vs. satellite/in-transit recurrence, $P<0.001$). Median time to distant metastasis was 40.5 months (IQR, 58.75) in women and 33 months (IQR, 44.25) in men ($P=0.002$). Five-year survival after distant recurrence probability was 5.2% (95% CI: 1.4–2.5) for men compared with 15.3% (95% CI: 11.1–19.5; $P=0.008$) for women.

Conclusions/Significance: Both, the pattern of metastatic spread with more locoregional metastasis in women, and the time course with retracted metastasis in women contributed to the more favorable outcome of women. Furthermore, the total rate of metastasis is increased in men. Interestingly, there is also a much more favorable long term survival of women after development of distant metastasis. It remains a matter of debate and of future research, whether hormonal or immunologic factors may be responsible for these sex differences.

Editor: Andrzej T. Slominski, University of Tennessee, United States of America

Funding: Parts of this work were funded by Deutsche Krebshilfe, Bonn, Germany. The funders had no role in study design, data collection and analysis, decision to publish, or preparation of the manuscript. No additional external funding was received for this study.

Competing Interests: The author has declared that no competing interests exist.

* E-mail: liljana.mervic@kclj.si

Introduction

Cutaneous melanoma (CM) is considered to have a high malignant potency. Metastatic spread may arise from very small tumors. At a time when the incidence of many tumor types is decreasing, melanoma incidence continues to increase. Mortality figures over the past decades show trends that differ from those for incidence, with a much lower rate of mortality increase than that recorded for incidence [1]. Nevertheless, at the start of the 21st century, CM remains a potentially fatal malignancy. The most important factor for successful management of melanoma is early diagnosis, allowing treatment to be undertaken at a stage when cure is readily achievable. Malignant melanoma in its advanced stage of metastatic disease has a poor prognosis with a median survival time of approximately 8 months [2].

Significant differences exist between male and female patients in melanoma incidence, presentation of primary tumor, and mortality [3–5]. Despite differences in incidence between sexes across continents with a greater incidence among woman in Europe and predominance of men in Australia and United States, the survival advantage for women is consistently observed independently of the incidence pattern [3–6]. It has been shown that men have worse primary tumors and experience shorter survival than women [3–5]. The differences in tumor thickness, ulceration and body site distribution between sexes can explain the sex differences in survival of melanoma to a certain degree, however, large body of evidence observed sex to remain an independent significant predictor of survival after adjusting for these factors [4–8].

Melanoma can metastasize either by the lymphatic or by the hematogenous route. Melanoma metastases develop via three main metastatic pathways, beginning with either satellite or in-transit metastases, up to 2 cm from the primary tumor or in the skin between the site of the primary tumor and the first lymph node, respectively, with regional lymph node metastasis, or with distant metastasis. About half of all patients with tumor progression develop regional lymph node metastasis as first metastasis. In about one third primary development of distant metastasis is observed and in the remaining patients, satellite or in-transit metastases are the site of the first recurrence [9,10]. Little is currently known of factors that might influence which type of recurrence occurs.

The primary objective of this study was to analyze the time course of melanoma progression and three different metastatic pathways for the spread of CM, divided into satellite or in-transit metastasis, regional lymph node metastasis, and distant metastasis, with a particular emphasis on the differences between sexes. A research of sex-related differences in progression of CM may contribute to our understanding of the observed differences in survival between men and women.

Methods

From 1976 to 2008, the German Central Malignant Melanoma Registry (CMMR) recorded the data of 9,044 melanoma patients (4,221 men and 4,823 women) treated at the Tübingen University Department of Dermatology in southern Germany. For this study, only the patients from the Center in Tübingen were included, because in this region the registration of patients reaches the completeness of population based registries [11]. All patients had given their written informed consent to have their data on primary tumor and follow-up recorded within the CMMR. Approval for this retrospective analysis was obtained by the Ethics commitee Tübingen, Germany (approval number 655/2011A). Patient data were analyzed anonymously. Approval for this study was gained retrospectively.

The CMMR is a hospital-based registry. Written informed consent was obtained from all patients in this study. The aims and methods of data collection by the CMMR have previously been reported in detail [12,13]. Data obtained for each patient included sex, date of birth, date of diagnosis, anatomical location and histopathological characteristics of the primary tumor, date of diagnosis and site of recurrence, date of the last follow-up examination, and (if a patient died) the date and cause of death. The patient sample was divided into three different age groups: 43 years or younger, 44–60 years old, and more than 60 years old. The anatomical sites of the primary tumors were divided into four groups: head and neck, trunk, upper extremities, and lower extremities. The tumor thickness was divided into four groups according to the Tumor Node Metastasis classification of the American Joint Committee on Cancer: less than or equal to 1, 1.01–2, 2.01–4, and more than 4 mm. The level of invasion was classified according to the system described by Clark. The following histopathological subtypes were distinguished: superficial spreading melanoma, nodular melanoma, lentigo maligna melanoma, and acral lentiginous melanoma. The site of recurrence was categorized into three groups: satellite or in-transit recurrence, metastasis to the regional lymph nodes, and metastasis to distant anatomical sites. Satellite metastasis is defined as the development of metastatic nodules within 2 cm of the primary tumor. In-transit metastasis develops within the metastatic drainage area before the first regional lymph node basin. Different metastatic pathways in the progression of CM were analyzed. A metastatic pathway was taken to be the first pathway of spread in disease progression. Three pathways were defined: satellite/in-transit metastases, regional lymph node metastasis, and distant metastasis. The decades of diagnosis were classified as follows: 1970–1979, 1980–1989, 1990–1999, and 2000–2008.

All patients underwent a physical examination, blood tests, abdominal ultrasound scans, and chest X-rays at the time of the initial diagnosis and were thereafter regularly followed. The analysis included only patients with an invasive primary CM without clinically detectable metastases after all investigations performed at the time of primary diagnosis who later on developed metastases. Patients with ocular, mucosal, and in-situ melanomas, patients younger than 14, and those with a follow-up of less than 3 months were excluded from the analysis. 7,338 patients (3,347 men and 3,991 women) were diagnosed as an invasive primary CM without clinically detectable metastases (Stages I and II, American Joint Committee on Cancer). Among these patients, 517 women and 561 men developed subsequent metastases during 10-year follow up and were included into the analysis.

Statistical analysis

A χ^2 test was used to compare the distribution of categorical variables between groups. The Mann-Whitney test was used to compare continuous variables between groups. The follow-up times were defined. Recurrence-free survival (RFS) time was defined as the date of diagnosis of first recurrence minus the date of diagnosis of primary tumor. Distant recurrence-free survival (DRFS) time was defined as the date of diagnosis of distant metastasis minus the date of diagnosis of primary tumor. Survival-after-recurrence (SAR) time was defined as the date of the last follow-up or death minus date of diagnosis of first recurrence, and survival after distant recurrence (SADR) time as the date of the last follow-up or death minus date of diagnosis of first distant metastasis. Follow-up time was cut to a maximum of 10 years because in this period patients usually participate in the CM follow-up program. Only deaths caused by CM were considered in the analysis of SAR and SADR, and deaths from other causes were regarded as censored events. In the analysis of RFS and DRFS, deaths due to melanoma were regarded as recurrence if no other event had been documented. The patients who died from melanoma were nearly all treated at the Tuebingen University Department of Dermatology and melanoma deaths are very unlikely to be under-reported. Deaths of causes not otherwise specified were regarded not to be caused by melanoma and regarded as censored. The follow-up time was described as a median value with an interquartile range (IQR). All 1,078 patients with an invasive primary CM at the time of diagnosis (clinically and histopathologically staged) who developed metastases during follow up were included in survival analysis. Probability of metastasis in the group comparison and melanoma-specific survival curves and estimated survival rates with relative 95% confidence intervals (CIs) were generated using the Kaplan-Meier method and were compared using a two-sided log-rank test. In the multivariate analysis, age, tumor thickness, SAR time, and the decades of diagnosis were entered as continuous variables. Categorical variables were dummy-coded. The Cox model was described by means of hazard ratios (HRs) together with 95% CIs, and P values were based on the Wald test.

Throughout the analyses, two-sided P values of less than 0.05 were considered statistically significant. Statistical analyses were carried out using the Statistical Package for the Social Sciences (SPSS) V.15.0.1 (SPSS, Chicago, Illinois, USA).

Results

Natural course of melanoma

During follow-up of 7,338 patients who were diagnosed at a stage of an invasive primary CM without clinically detectable metastases, disease progression was noted in 1,078 patients. More men (561, 16.8%) than women (517, 13.0%, $P<0.001$) with primary CM at diagnosis developed metastases. A total of 414 (12.4%) men and 348 (8.7%, $P<0.001$) women in our study group had developed distant metastasis by the time of the analysis. Various clinical and histopathological characteristics of the 1,078 melanoma patients who progressed from the stage of primary

Table 1. Clinical and histopathological characteristics.

	Pathway 1		Pathway 2		Pathway 3		P*
	Men %	Women %	Men %	Women %	Men %	Women %	
	n = 105	n = 151	n = 303	n = 246	n = 153	n = 120	
Anatomical site							<0.001 between sexes in pathways 1 and 2; 0.003 between sexes in pathway 3
Head and neck	15.2	15.2	17.5	12.2	17.8	23.3	
Trunk	42.9	13.2	52.1	25.6	64.1	42.5	
Upper extremities	10.5	9.3	10.6	16.7	7.8	12.5	
Lower extremities	31.4	62.3	19.8	45.5	10.5	21.7	
Histological type							NS between sexes
SSM	45.7	46.4	57.1	50.8	54.2	52.5	
NM	38.1	26.5	27.7	28.9	30.7	29.2	
LMM	5.7	9.9	5.3	5.7	4.6	7.5	
ALM	5.7	9.3	4.0	10.2	4.6	4.2	
Other	4.8	7.9	5.9	4.5	5.9	6.7	
Tumor thickness in mm							0.017 between sexes in pathway 1; NS between sexes in pathways 2 and 3
≤1.00	12.4	11.9	23.4	19.9	19.0	21.7	
1.01–2.00	29.5	35.8	29.7	29.3	32.0	35.8	
2.01–4.00	26.7	37.1	32.8	35.8	32.0	25.8	
>4.00	31.4	15.2	14.2	15.0	20.3	16.7	
Median (IQR)	2.6 (3.6)	2.1 (1.9)	2.0 (2.1)	2.1 (1.9)	2.2 (2.4)	1.7 (2.0)	†NS between sexes
Ulceration							NS between sexes
Yes	30.5	24.5	20.5	17.1	25.5	16.7	
No	69.5	75.5	79.5	82.9	74.5	83.3	
Age							NS between sexes in pathways 1 and 2; 0.002 between sexes in pathway 3
≤43 years	21.0	14.6	27.4	28.5	19.0	35.0	
44–60 years	28.7	29.8	40.6	36.2	45.1	27.5	
>60 years	52.4	55.6	32.0	35.4	35.9	37.5	

1,078 patients (561 male and 517 female) diagnosed from 1976 to 2008 as invasive primary cutaneous melanoma who developed metastases during follow up stratified by sex and metastatic pathway.

The funders had no role in study design, data collection and analysis, decision to publish, or preparation of the manuscript. No additional external funding was received for this study.

ALM, acral lentiginous melanoma; IQR, interquartile range; LMM, lentigo maligna melanoma; NM, nodular melanoma; NS, not significant; SSM, superficially spreading melanoma.

Pathway 1, primary tumor, then satellite/in-transit metastases; Pathway 2, primary tumor, then regional lymph node metastasis; Pathway 3, primary tumor, then distant metastasis.

*Pearson's χ^2 test.

†Mann-Whitney test.

invasive CM at the time of diagnosis to the stage of regional or distant metastases stratified by sex and metastatic pathway is presented in Table 1.

Using the Kaplan Meier method, probabilities for developing metastasis over a period of ten years was calculated, taking censored observations into account. The 10-year probability for developing metastases after the diagnosis of primary tumor was 22.8% (95% CI: 20.9–24.7) for men compared with 16.9% (95% CI: 15.4–18.4; $P<0.001$) for women (Figure 1A). The 10-year probability for developing distant metastases after the diagnosis of primary tumor was 17.8% (95% CI: 16.0–19.6) for men compared with 11.7% (95% CI: 10.4–13.1; $P<0.001$) for women (Figure 1B).

Women developed their first metastasis significantly later compared with men ($P=0.048$). Median time to first metastasis was 25 months (IQR, 53) in women and 23 months (IQR, 38.5) in men (Figure 2A). Similarly, women developed distant metastasis significantly later compared with men ($P=0.002$). Median time to distant metastasis was 40.5 months (IQR, 58.75) in women and 33 months (IQR, 44.25) in men (Figure 2B).

Metastatic pathways

The most frequent site for the first metastasis was the regional lymph nodes (50.9%), followed by distant sites (25.3%). Satellite or/and in-transit metastases were the least frequent (23.7%). The metastatic pathways of the progression of CM were analyzed according to sex. A metastatic pathway was taken to be the first pathway of spread in disease progression. Three pathways were defined and are summarized in Figure 3: pathway 1 (primary

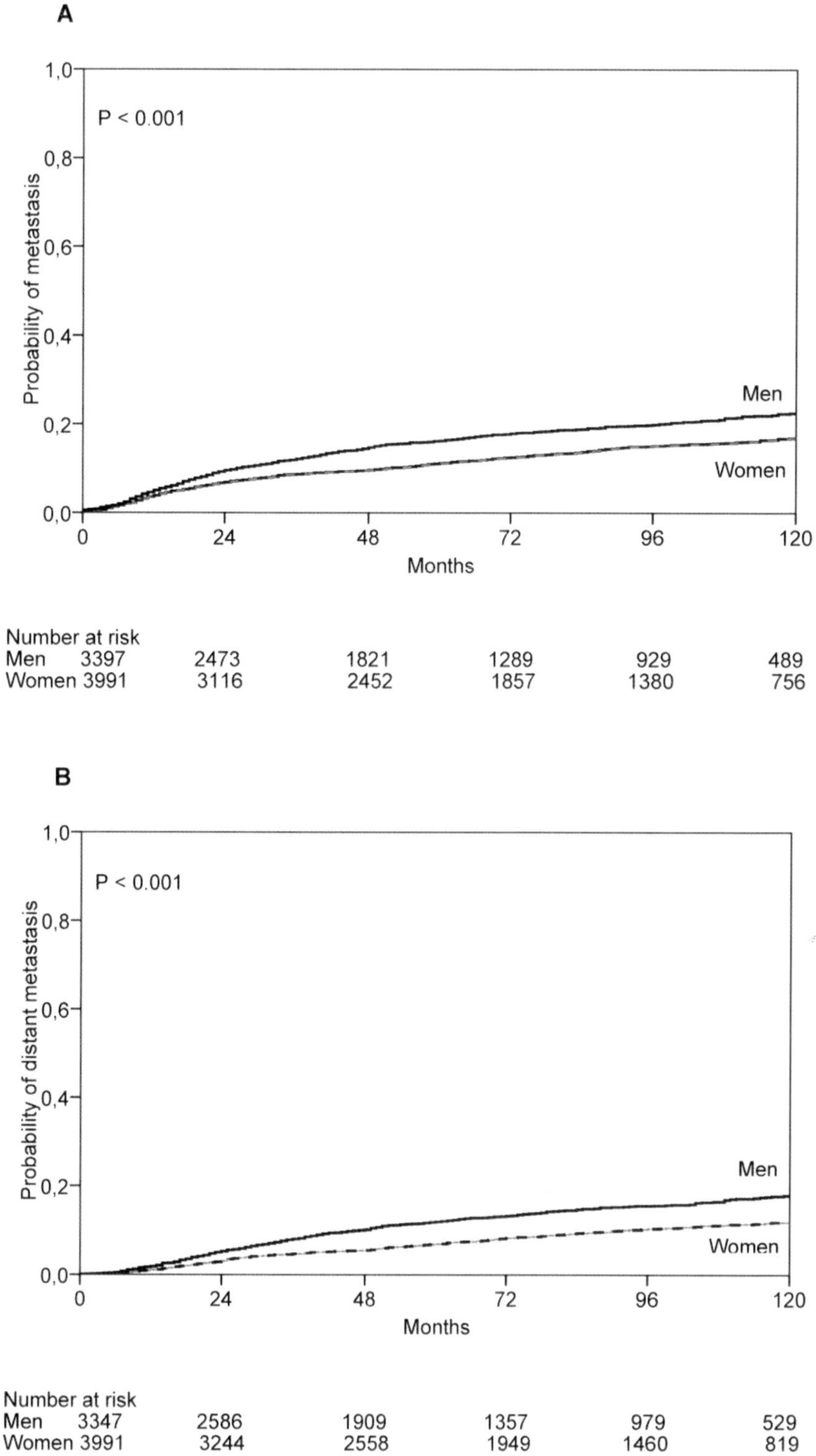

Figure 1. Probability for developing metastases. Probability for developing metastases (**A**), and distant metastases (**B**) after the diagnosis of primary cutaneous melanoma in 7,338 patients, 3,347 men and 3,991 women. *P* values are based on the log-rank test.

tumor, then satellite/in-transit metastases), pathway 2 (primary tumor, then regional lymph node metastasis), and pathway 3 (primary tumor, then distant metastasis).

Development of satellite and in-transit metastasis was analyzed in detail. In 105 (18.7%) men and 151 (29.2%, $P<0.001$) women this was the first metastasis following diagnosis of primary tumor (Pathway 1). Of these patients 9 (8.6%) men and 17 (11.3%) women later on developed regional lymph node metastases, and 37 (35.2%) men and 38 (25.2%) women progressed first to regional lymph node and then to distant metastases. In 28 (26.7%) men and 38 (25.1%) women, distant metastases occurred directly after satellite or/and in-transit metastases. Men developed distant

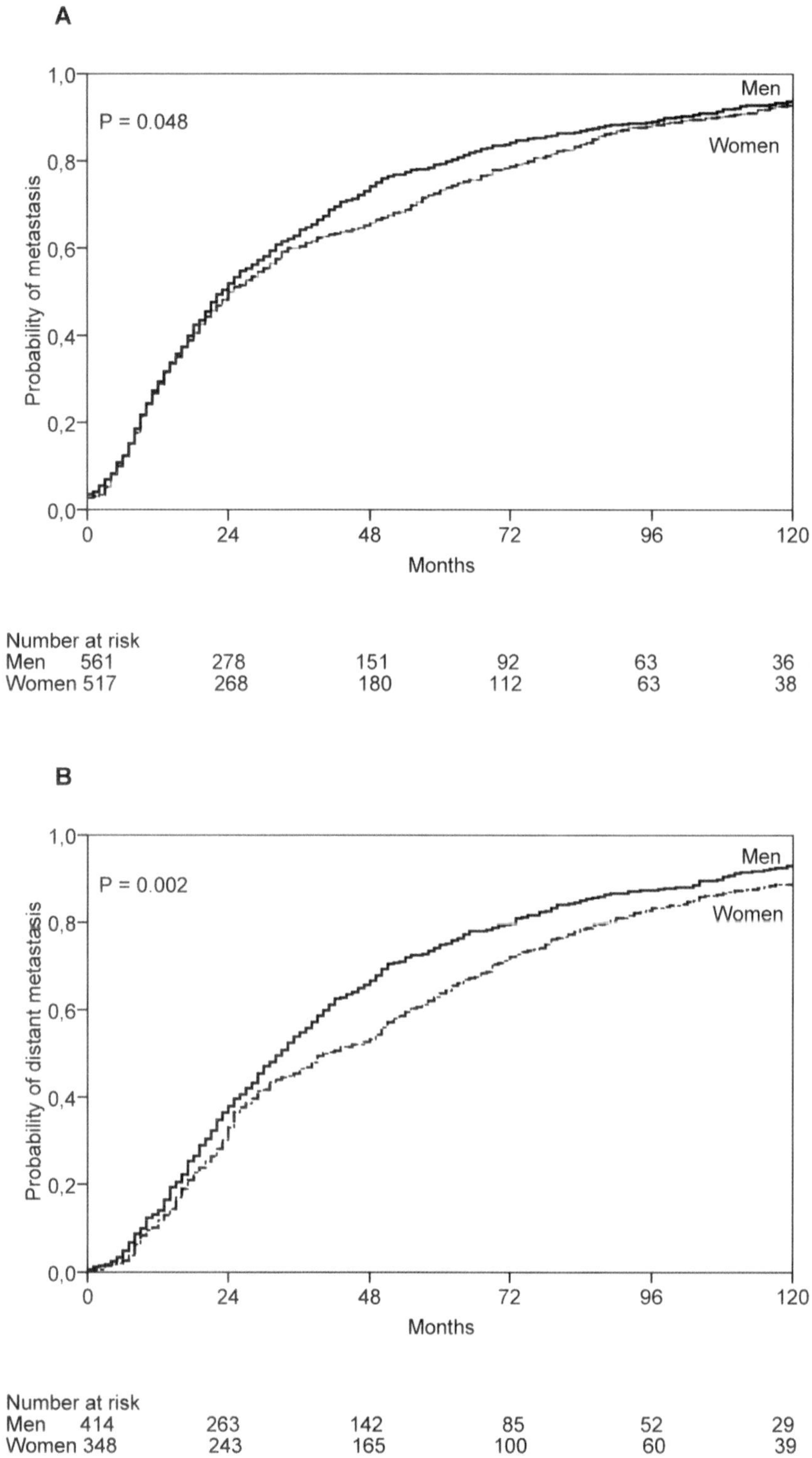

Figure 2. Probability for developing metastases. Probability for developing metastases (**A**), and distant metastases (**B**) in 1,078 patients (561 men and 517 women) who were diagnosed at the stage of primary cutaneous melanoma and then progressed by the time of analysis. *P* values are based on the log-rank test.

metastasis following pathway 1 after a median time of 29 months (IQR 39) compared to 52 months (IQR 67) in women (P=0.002).

Direct regional lymph node metastasis developed in the majority of patients. This was observed in the majority of men (303, 54.0%) and women (246, 47.6%, P=0.035; Pathway 2). Further progression of the tumor from this stage to the stage of distant metastasis was found in 196 (64.7%) men and 152 (61.8%) women. Men developed distant metastasis following pathway 2 after a median time of 30 months (IQR 43) compared to 32 months (IQR 51) in women (P=0.1).

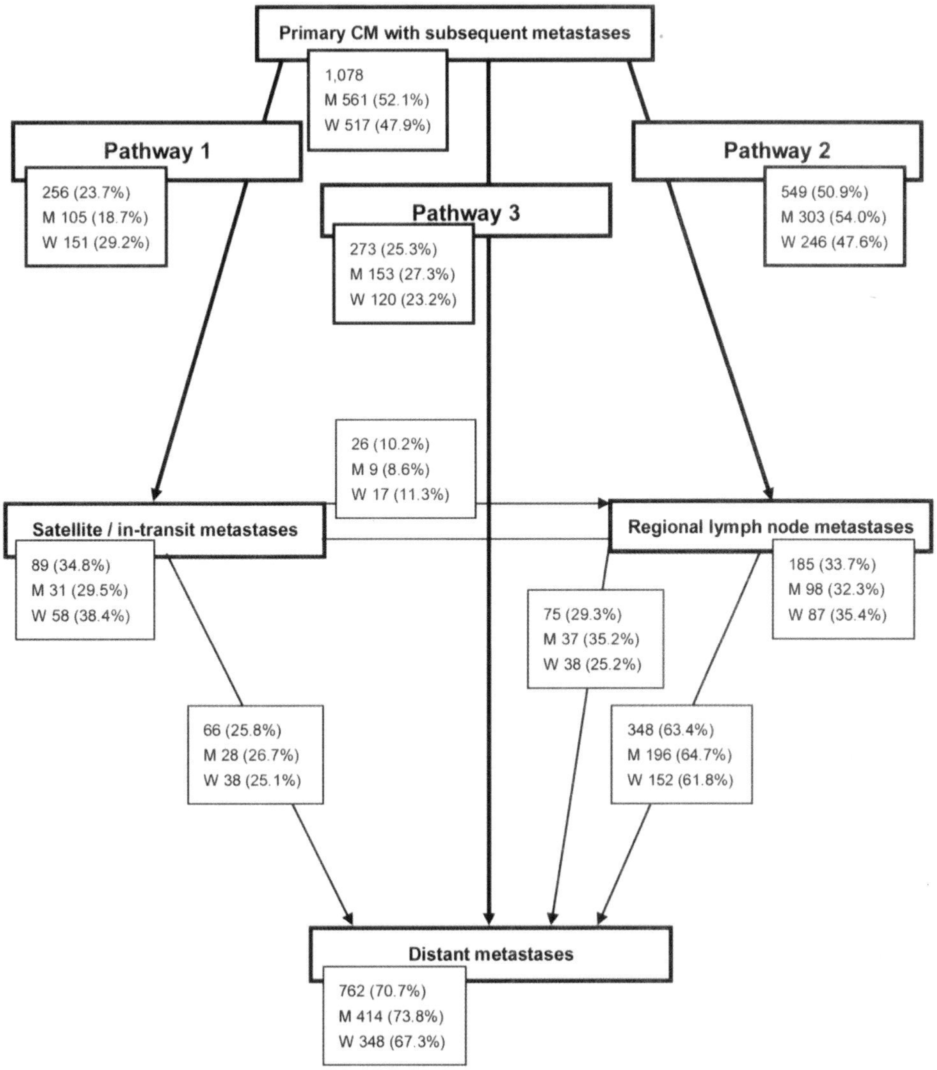

Figure 3. Three metastatic pathways of melanoma. Pathway 1 – primary tumor, then satellite/in-transit metastases, pathway 2 – primary tumor, then regional lymph node metastasis, and pathway 3 – primary tumor, then distant metastasis. M, men; W, women.

Direct distant metastasis from the stage of the primary tumor was observed in 153 (27.3%) men and 120 (23.2%, $P = 0.13$) women (Pathway 3). Men developed direct distant metastasis after a median time of 38 months (IQR 44) and women after a median time of 49 months (IQR 57, $P = 0.4$).

The anatomical site of tumor was the most important factor in the pattern of progression of the disease and there were significant differences between sexes ($P < 0.001$ in pathways 1 and 2, and $P = 0.003$ in pathway 3). The primary melanoma was located on the lower-extremity in almost two thirds of women and one third of men who first progressed to satellite or in-transit metastases and only in 22% of women and 11% of men who first progressed to distant disease. Patients who progressed directly to distant sites had most frequently their primary tumors located on the trunk (64% of men and 43% of women). The second most frequent location of the primary melanoma in the case of direct distant metastases was head and neck. We did not observe any significant differences between sexes in the distribution of metastatic pathways for the different histological types, tumor thicknesses and presence of ulceration.

Survival analysis

Patients with primary CM, who subsequently developed satellite/in-transit, regional lymph node or distant metastases as the first site of recurrence, were included into the survival analysis and were stratified by sex.

In 105 males and 151 females first metastasis occurred in local anatomical sites as satellite or/and in-transit metastasis. In these patients, five-year SAR probability differed significantly between sexes. It was 28.5% (95% CI: 17.0–39.9) for men and 63.0% (95% CI: 54.1–71.8; $P < 0.001$) for women (Figure 4A). Median survival time of these patients was 19 months (IQR 22) for men and 33 months (IQR 69.75) for women.

In 302 male and 246 female patients their first metastasis developed in the regional lymph nodes. Five-year SAR probability in these patients was 36.8% (95% CI: 30.6–43.1) for men and 42.8% (95% CI: 35.9–49.7, $P = 0.1$) for women, and the difference was not statistically significant (Figure 4B). Median survival time of these patients was 23 months (IQR 37) for men and 27.5 months (IQR 53) for women.

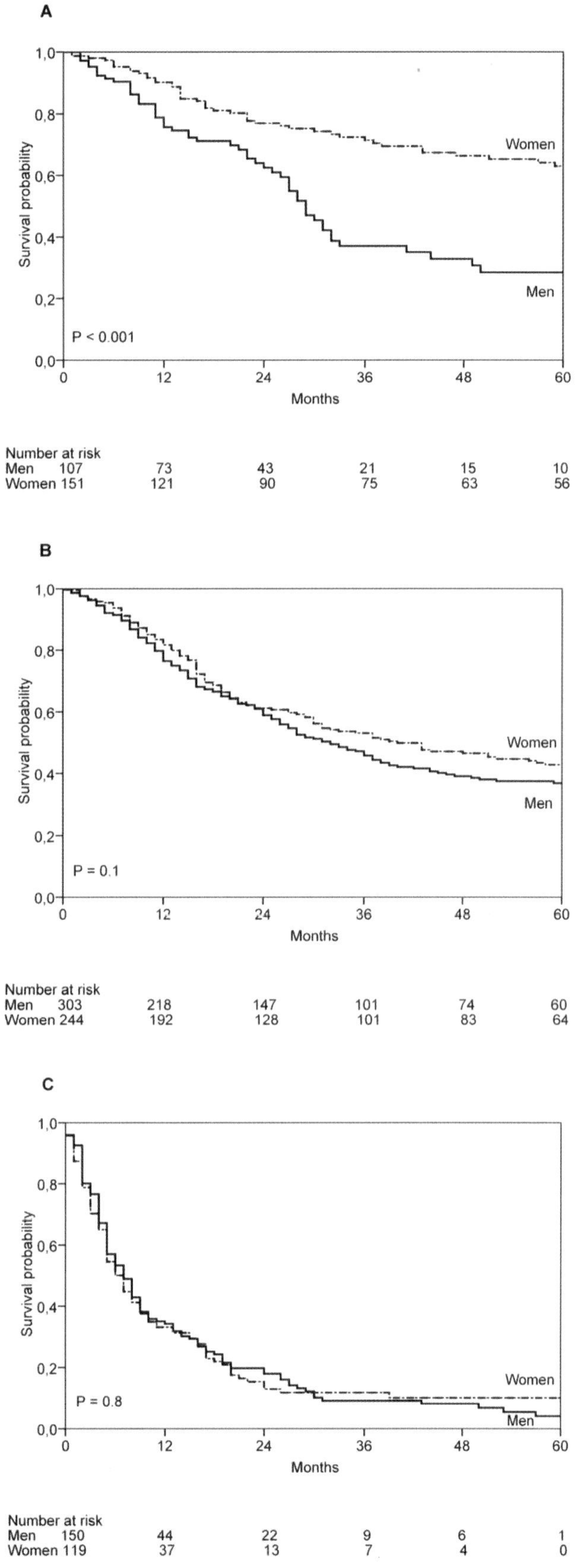

Figure 4. Survival after recurrence. Survival after recurrence in patients who progressed first to satellite/in-transit (**A**), regional lymph node (**B**), and distant metastases (**C**). *P* values are based on the log-rank test.

In 153 men and 120 women their first metastasis developed at distant sites. Five-year SAR probability in these patients was 4.1% (95% CI: 0.1–8.2) for men and 10.1% (95% CI: 3.8–16.4, $P = 0.8$) for women, and this difference was likewise not statistically significant (Figure 4C). Median survival time of these patients was 6 months (IQR 11) for men, the same as for women (IQR 13).

During follow up, altogether 414 male and 348 female patients with primary CM at diagnosis eventually developed distant metastases in the course of the disease following all three metastatic pathways. SADR time was significantly longer in women compared with men. Male patients had 5.2% (95% CI: 1.4–2.5) five-year SADR probability compared with 15.3% (95% CI: 11.1–19.5; $P = 0.008$) for female patients. Median SADR-time was 7 months (IQR 11) for men and 8 months (IQR 14) for women. A total of 581 patients (322 men and 259 women) died of melanoma during the 10 years of follow-up time.

In the total cohort of 1078 patients who had developed metastasis, independent predictive factors for survival were analyzed. The results of the multivariate Cox regression analysis regarding SAR are presented in table 2. In the model showing the main effects of the variables, site of first metastasis was the most important prognostic factor (HR: 1.3; 95% CI: 1.0–1.6 for metastasis to the regional lymph nodes vs. satellite/in-transit recurrence and HR: 5.5; 95% CI: 4.2–7.1 for distant metastasis vs. satellite/in-transit recurrence, $P < 0.001$). Other independent prognostic factors were sex (HR: 1.2; 95% CI: 1.0–1.5; $P = 0.018$), time to relapse after primary diagnosis (HR: 0.996; 95% CI: 0.994–0.998; $P < 0.001$), and decade of diagnosis (HR: 0.8; 95% CI: 0.7–0.9; $P < 0.001$). Age, anatomical site of primary melanoma, tumor thickness, Clark's level of invasion, histological ulceration, and histological subtype were not important factors in the equation, and seemingly do not play any role once metastasis has developed.

Discussion

It is well established, that gender is an independent prognostic factor in primary invasive melanoma and that female patients have a more favorable outcome compared to male patients when other prognostic features of the primary tumor are comparable. This study addresses for the first time the differences in the natural course of cutaneous melanoma between men and women. The results of this study show that women metastasize less often and develop all kinds of metastases later as compared with men. Furthermore, women show a different pattern of metastasis with a strikingly higher percentage of the prognostically favorable satellite/in-transit metastasis. Finally, women have a significantly higher five-year survival probability once distant metastasis has developed.

The probability for developing metastasis and distant metastasis after the diagnosis of primary tumor in our series of patients was significantly higher for men compared with women. Additionally, if disease progression had taken place, women developed their first metastasis as well as distant metastasis significantly later compared with men.

It is well known that approximately two thirds of patients who develop clinical metastases following a primary CM initially present with locoregional metastases and one third initially present with distant metastases [10]. In our study group the most frequent site for the first metastasis was the regional lymph nodes (50.9%), followed by distant sites (25.3%) and satellite or/and in-transit metastases (23.7%). In significantly more women compared with men the first metastasis following diagnosis of primary tumor took the form of satellite or/and in-transit metastases. The majority of

Table 2. Multivariate predictors of survival after first recurrence.

	HR (95% CI)[a]	p[b]
Sex (male vs. female)	1.2 (1.0–1.5)	0.018
Age (years)	1.002 (0.996–1.008)	0.5
Anatomical site		
Head/neck	1.0	0.2
Trunk	1.3 (1.0–1.6)	0.09
Upper extremities	1.1 (0.8–1.5)	0.7
Lower extremities	1.0 (0.8–1.4)	0.9
Tumor thickness (mm)	1.0 (0,96–1.04)	0.9
Clark (II/III vs. IV/V)	0.9 (0.7–1.0)	0.1
Ulceration (yes vs. no)	1.1 (0.9–1,4)	0.3
Histological type		
SSM	1.0	0.5
NM	1.0 (0.8–1.3)	0.8
LMM	1.2 (0.8–1.8)	0.3
ALM	1.1 (0.7–1.6)	0.7
Other	0.8 (0.5–1.2)	0.2
Site of first metastasis		
Satellite/in-transit	1.0	<0.001
Regional lymph node	1.3 (1.0–1.6)	0.07
Distant	5.5 (4.2–7.1)	<0.001
Recurrence free survival time (months)	0.996 (0.994–0.998)	<0.001
Decade of diagnosis	0.8 (0.7–0.9)	<0.001

ALM, acral lentiginous melanoma; CI, confidence interval; HR, hazards ratio; LMM, lentigo maligna melanoma; NM, nodular melanoma; SSM, superficially spreading melanoma.
[a]HR with its 95% CI.
[b]Wald test significance; *P* values listed at the level of the reference categories (HR = 1.0) represent significance for the variable as a whole, all other *P* values represent significance of the category specified as compared to the reference category.

patients exhibited direct regional lymph node metastasis with significant predominance of men. We observed no difference between sexes in frequency of direct distant metastasis from the stage of the primary tumor. About one third of patients, who first developed satellite/in-transit or regional lymph node metastasis, remained at the stage of locoregional metastasis during follow up, while approximately two thirds of patients (more men than women) exhibited further progression to distant sites. Therefore, the pattern of metastasis differed between sexes. There was a clear tendency for women to recur locally and they experienced further progression to distant sites less often then men. Furthermore, time from primary tumor diagnosis to distant metastasis after satellite/in-transit metastases (Pathway 1) was significantly longer in female compared with male patients. There were no sex related differences in time appearance of distant metastasis in other two metastatic pathways, namely after lymph node metastasis as the first site of recurrence or direct distant metastasis after the primary tumor.

Interestingly, in several studies patients were reported to reach the stage of distant metastasis after a similar period of time (median approximately 25 months) irrespective of the metastatic pathway [10,14,15]. At present, there are several models that attempt to explain how melanoma spreads. The stepwise spread model, in which the melanoma spreads first by a lymphatic pathway towards the regional lymph nodes, from where systemic dissemination is initiated with a certain time lag does not explain the fact that about a third of patients progress directly to distant sites [16,17]. A model of simultaneous spread assumes that the primary tumor would metastasize simultaneously by lymphatic and hematogenous pathways, and lymph node involvement would therefore be a marker of systemic disease. This model does not fit with the fact that regional lymph node dissection is curative in about one third of cases [17,18]. The third model of differential spread is based on the assumption that some melanomas will not have the biological potential to metastasize, others will only be able to metastasize to regional lymph nodes or to metastasize to both regional lymph nodes and distant organs, or some melanomas will only be able to metastasize at the systemic level. Tumor progression in CM is a complex and multistep process including proliferation, neovascularization, lymphangiogenesis, invasion, circulation, embolism, and extravasation. This last model can explain some premises about the natural history of melanoma that cannot be explained by the other two models, namely that some melanoma patients can achieve complete and long-lasting remission following therapeutic lymph node resection, but not all of them because lymph node and distant metastases can develop at the same time. Furthermore, this model can explain why a negative finding in the sentinel lymph node biopsy does not provide an absolute guarantee of survival [17,19]. In our study group of patients women more frequently metastasized locally as satellite/in-transit metastasis and further progression to distant site was noted after a significant time lag as compared with men.

Analyzing the distribution of various clinical and histopathological characteristics of melanoma at the time of the first diagnosis in patients who progressed to the stage of locoregional or distant metastases, the anatomical site of tumor was the most important factor influencing the pattern of progression of the disease and there were significant differences between sexes. The primary melanoma was located on the lower-extremity in almost two thirds of women and one third of men who firstly progressed to satellite or/and in-transit metastases. Patients who progressed directly to distant sites most frequently had their primary tumors located on the trunk (64% of men and 43% of women). The second most frequent location of the primary melanoma in the case of direct distant metastases was head and neck. Sex-related differences in metastatic pathways could be related to sex-related differences in the site of the primary tumor. It is well known that melanomas on the lower extremities, which are more common in female, have a better prognosis than tumors located on the trunk, which are more commonly seen in male patients [9,10].

The prognostically unfavorable locations of primary tumors were proposed for classification as TANS (trunk, upper arm, neck, scalp) or BANS (back, upper arm, neck, scalp) regions [20,21]. It has been speculated that lymphatic drainage may be responsible for differences in the clinical course of melanomas at different anatomical sites. The length of the lymph tracts and the number of lymph nodes to be passed before the lymphatic fluid reaches the blood circulation at the venous angle in the upper thorax could be decisive factors for the defense of the immune system of the host against metastasizing tumor cells. Therefore, better prognosis for the lower extremity tumors might be due to the higher barrier to metastatic cells presented by the longer lymphatic vessels and greater number of lymph nodes before reaching systemic circulation [9,10].

Site of first metastasis was the most important prognostic factor of survival after recurrence in multivariate analysis in our series of patients, followed by sex, time to diagnosing the first metastasis and decade of diagnosis of the primary tumor. Hazard rate for dying of melanoma was 1.3 if the patient exhibited metastasis to the regional lymph nodes vs. satellite/in-transit recurrence, and 5.5 for distant metastasis vs. satellite/in-transit recurrence. Satellite or in-transit metastases after the primary tumor which are prognostically favorable were significantly more common in women. Furthermore, female patients had significantly longer time to diagnosing the first metastasis, also explaining their better survival. The finding that site of first metastasis is the most important prognostic factor of survival after first recurrence has been reported previously [22].

Five-year SAR probability for patients from our collective in whom first metastasis occurred in local anatomical sites as satellite or/and in-transit metastasis differed significantly between sexes. However, it did not reach statistical significance in patients who developed their first metastasis in the regional lymph nodes, neither in patients who developed their first metastasis at distant sites. Despite the finding that there were no differences between sexes in survival after first recurrence in the regional lymph nodes or at distant sites, SADR probability in patients who eventually developed distant metastases in the course of the disease following all three metastatic pathways was significantly higher in women compared with men.

Favorable natural course of melanoma in women with a lower chance of melanoma progression after the diagnosis of primary tumor and later development of metastases in the case of disease progression is crucial for better survival of female patients. Additionally, different pattern of metastasis with more frequent local recurrencies in the form of satellite/in-transit metastasis explains their better survival. Even women who eventually progress to the stage of distant disease have better five-year survival compared with men.

The molecular basis for sex differences in the natural course of melanoma remains undefined. Sex steroids have been suggested as playing a role in melanoma progression, but the majority of evidence now is that melanoma is not hormone dependent [23–25]. There may be sex differences in immunity, which could also explain the observed differences in melanoma progression. Sexual dimorphism in the immune system of female and male patients suggested by sex differences in the incidence of autoimmune diseases could be of relevance to natural course and surviving melanoma [26,27]. Another proposed explanation of the female advantage could be sex differences in oxidative stress caused by radical oxygen species, which are known to be able to promote metastasis through a wide variety of mechanisms. Worse outcome of male melanoma patients may be explained by the lower amounts of antioxidant enzymes expressed in men, resulting in more oxidative stress than in women [28].

Present study has several limitations. It was not planned in a statistical manner, but it is the evaluation of cancer registry data. Also the issue of multiple testing has to be acknowledged. On account of these limitations, an independent verification of this study results is required. Unfortunately, CMMR had no data regarding gynecological details and the mitotic rate of primary tumor, which was recently shown to be an independent prognostic variable in CM patients. The presence of ulceration may have been underreported during the early years of the study period. The sentinel lymph node status of our patients diagnosed during the early years of the study was not available. Patients with clinically undetectable lymph node micrometastasis were classified into stages I and II before 1996 and afterwards into stage III melanoma, and were therefore excluded from the present analysis. In addition, we had no details regarding the number of involved lymph nodes in patients that developed regional lymph node metastasis, about systemic treatments administered to our patients, and about socioeconomic factors that are known to influence the outcome. On the other hand, we had high-quality data with negligible rates of unknown or missing events and almost complete long-term follow-up data for our entire sample. Although our sample is not population based, it is largely representative of the situation in southern Germany.

In conclusion, men had higher probability for developing metastases and distant metastases after the diagnosis of primary tumor. Additionally, if disease progression took place, women developed their first metastasis as well as distant metastasis significantly later compared with men. When the metastatic pathways are taken into consideration, women more frequently progressed first to local sites in the form of satellite or in-transit metastases and men more frequently exhibited direct regional lymph node metastasis. About two thirds of these patients, more men than women, showed further progression to distant sites. There were no differences between sexes in the occurrence of direct distant metastasis after the primary invasive CM. Site of first metastasis was shown to be the most important prognostic factor of survival after recurrence in multivariate analysis. This analysis shows, that different factors like delay in the development of metastasis and different pathways of metastasis contribute to the more favorable survival of women, even when metastasis has already developed. These findings may stimulate further research concerning the potential role of molecular factors responsible for this sex differences and differences in survival of patients with cutaneous melanoma in general.

Acknowledgments

I thank my mentor, Professor Dr. Claus Garbe, from the University of Tübingen, Germany, and his team for allowing me to evaluate this comprehensive data bank of the Department of Dermatology in Tübingen and for his guidance through my scientific work. I also acknowledge the support from Dr. Tanja Planinšek Ručigaj, Head of the Department of Dermatovenereology in Ljubljana, Slovenia, for enabling this scientific cooperation.

Author Contributions

Conceived and designed the experiments: LM. Analyzed the data: LM. Wrote the paper: LM.

References

1. Mackie RM, Hauschild A, Eggermont AM (2009) Epidemiology of invasive cutaneous melanoma. Ann Oncol 20 Suppl 6: vi 1–7.
2. Lee ML, Tomsu K, Von Eschen KB (2000) Duration of survival for disseminated malignant melanoma: results of a meta-analysis. Melanoma Res 10: 81–92.
3. Kolmel KF, Kulle B, Lippold A, Seebacher C (2002) Survival probabilities and hazard functions of malignant melanoma in Germany 1972–1996, an analysis of 10433 patients. Evolution of gender differences and malignancy. Eur J Cancer 38: 1388–94.
4. Lasithiotakis K, Leiter U, Meier F, Eigentler T, Metzler G, et al. (2008) Age and gender are significant independent predictors of survival in primary cutaneous melanoma. Cancer 112: 1795–804.
5. Scoggins CR, Ross MI, Reintgen DS, Noyes RD, Goydos JS, et al. (2006) Gender-related differences in outcome for melanoma patients. Ann Surg 243: 693–8.
6. Balch CM, Soong SJ, Gershenwald JE, Thompson JF, Reintgen DS, et al. (2001) Prognostic factors analysis of 17,600 melanoma patients: validation of the American Joint Committee on Cancer melanoma staging system. J Clin Oncol 19: 3622–34.
7. Balch CM, Gershenwald JE, Soong SJ, Thompson JF, Atkins MB, et al. (2009) Final version of 2009 AJCC melanoma staging and classification. J Clin Oncol 27: 6199–206.
8. Mervic L, Leiter U, Meier F, Eigentler T, Forschner A, et al. (2011) Sex differences in survival of cutaneous melanoma are age dependent: an analysis of 7338 patients. Melanoma Res 21: 244–52.

9. Leiter U, Meier F, Schittek B, Garbe C (2004) The natural course of cutaneous melanoma. J Surg Oncol 86: 172–8.
10. Meier F, Will S, Ellwanger U, Schlagenhauff B, Schittek B, et al. (2002) Metastatic pathways and time courses in the orderly progression of cutaneous melanoma. Br J Dermatol 147: 62–70.
11. Lasithiotakis KG, Leiter U, Gorkievicz R, Eigentler T, Breuninger H, et al. (2006) The incidence and mortality of cutaneous melanoma in Southern Germany: trends by anatomic site and pathologic characteristics, 1976 to 2003. Cancer 107: 1331–9.
12. Garbe C, Mcleod GR, Buettner PG (2000) Time trends of cutaneous melanoma in Queensland, Australia and Central Europe. Cancer 89: 1269–78.
13. Lasithiotakis KG, Leiter U, Eigentler T, Breuninger H, Metzler G, et al. (2007) Improvement of overall survival of patients with cutaneous melanoma in Germany, 1976–2001: which factors contributed? Cancer 109: 1174–82.
14. Dong XD, Tyler D, Johnson JL, DeMatos P, Seigler HF (2000) Analysis of prognosis and disease progression after local recurrence of melanoma. Cancer 88: 1063–71.
15. Meyskens FL, Jr., Berdeaux DH, Parks B, Tong T, Loescher L, et al. (1988) Cutaneous malignant melanoma (Arizona Cancer Center experience). I. Natural history and prognostic factors influencing survival in patients with stage I disease. Cancer 62: 1207–14.
16. Leong SP (2004) Paradigm of metastasis for melanoma and breast cancer based on the sentinel lymph node experience. Ann Surg Oncol 11: 192S–7S.
17. Tejera-Vaquerizo A, Barrera-Vigo MV, Fernandez-Canedo I, Blazquez-Sanchez N, Mendiola-Fernandez M, et al. (2007) Longitudinal study of different metastatic patterns in the progression of cutaneous melanoma. Actas Dermosifiliogr 98: 531–8.
18. Medalie N, Ackerman AB (2004) Sentinel node biopsy has no benefit for patients whose primary cutaneous melanoma has metastasized to a lymph node and therefore should be abandoned now. Br J Dermatol 151: 298–307.
19. Fidler IJ (2003) The pathogenesis of cancer metastasis: the 'seed and soil' hypothesis revisited. Nat Rev Cancer 3: 453–8.
20. Bernengo MG, Reali UM, Doveil GC, Cappello N, Lisa F, et al. (1992) BANS: a discussion of the problem. Melanoma Res 2: 157–62.
21. Garbe C, Buttner P, Bertz J, Burg G, d'Hoedt B, et al. (1995) Primary cutaneous melanoma. Prognostic classification of anatomic location. Cancer 75: 2492–8.
22. Fusi S, Ariyan S, Sternlicht A (1993) Data on first recurrence after treatment for malignant melanoma in a large patient population. Plast Reconstr Surg 91: 94–8.
23. Holman CD, Armstrong BK, Heenan PJ (1984) Cutaneous malignant melanoma in women: exogenous sex hormones and reproductive factors. Br J Cancer 50: 673–80.
24. Miller JG, Gee J, Price A, Garbe C, Wagner M, et al. (1997) Investigation of oestrogen receptors, sex steroids and soluble adhesion molecules in the progression of malignant melanoma. Melanoma Res 7: 197–208.
25. Richardson B, Price A, Wagner M, Williams V, Lorigan P, et al. (1999) Investigation of female survival benefit in metastatic melanoma. Br J Cancer 80: 2025–33.
26. Miller JG, Mac NS (1997) Gender and cutaneous melanoma. Br J Dermatol 136: 657–65.
27. Paharkova-Vatchkova V, Maldonado R, Kovats S (2004) Estrogen preferentially promotes the differentiation of CD11c+ CD11b(intermediate) dendritic cells from bone marrow precursors. J Immunol 172: 1426–36.
28. Joosse A, de Vries E, van Eijck CH, Eggermont AM, Nijsten T, et al. (2010) Reactive oxygen species and melanoma: an explanation for gender differences in survival? Pigment Cell Melanoma Res 23: 352–64.

Loss of *Hairless* Confers Susceptibility to UVB-Induced Tumorigenesis via Disruption of NF-kappaB Signaling

Hyunmi Kim[1,3]¶, Alexandre Casta[2]¶, Xiuwei Tang[3], Courtney T. Luke[3], Arianna L. Kim[3], David R. Bickers[3], Mohammad Athar[3], Angela M. Christiano[1,3]*

1 Department of Genetics & Development, Columbia University, College of Physicians & Surgeons, New York, New York, United States of America, **2** Institute of Human Nutrition, Columbia University, College of Physicians & Surgeons, New York, New York, United States of America, **3** Department of Dermatology, Columbia University, College of Physicians & Surgeons, New York, New York, United States of America

Abstract

In order to model squamous cell carcinoma development *in vivo*, researchers have long preferred hairless mouse models such as SKH-1 mice that have traditionally been classified as 'wild-type' mice irrespective of the genetic factors underlying their hairless phenotype. The work presented here shows that mutations in the *Hairless* (*Hr*) gene not only result in the hairless phenotype of the SKH-1 and $Hr^{-/-}$ mouse lines but also cause aberrant activation of NFκB and its downstream effectors. We show that in the epidermis, *Hr* is an early UVB response gene that regulates NFκB activation and thereby controls cellular responses to irradiation. Therefore, when *Hr* expression is decreased in *Hr* mutant animals there is a corresponding increase in NFκB activity that is augmented by UVB irradiation. This constitutive activation of NFκB in the *Hr* mutant epidermis leads to the stimulation a large variety of downstream effectors including the cell cycle regulators cyclin D1 and cyclin E, the anti-apoptosis protein Bcl-2, and the pro-inflammatory protein Cox-2. Therefore, *Hr* loss results in a state of uncontrolled epidermal proliferation that promotes tumor development, and *Hr* mutant mice should no longer be considered merely hairless 'wild-type' mice. Instead, *Hr* is a crucial UVB response gene and its loss creates a permissive environment that potentiates increased tumorigenesis.

Editor: Amanda Ewart Toland, Ohio State University Medical Center, United States of America

Funding: The following National Institutes of Health grants supported this work: R01AR47338 (AMC), T32AR007605 (HK and CTL), Research Supplement for Underrepresented Minorities (CTL), P30AR044535 (Columbia University SDRC and R01ES015323 (MA). The funders had no role in the study design, data collection and analysis, decision to publish, or preparation of the manuscript.

Competing Interests: The authors have declared that no competing interests exist.

* E-mail: amc65@columbia.edu

¶ These authors contributed equally to this work.

Introduction

As a group, non-melanoma skin cancers (NMSC) are the most common type of cancer in the US with a combined incidence of over 2 million new cases annually [1]. Squamous cell carcinoma (SCC) is the second most common form of NMSC and is the most likely type to lethally metastasize, which makes understanding SCC development crucially important to human health [2]. In recent years, several genetic pathways have been implicated in the development of SCCs, particularly the ras and NFκB pathways ([3,4], reviewed in [5]), but despite these advances, the molecular events leading to SCC development and progression remain poorly understood. Current research strategies utilize mice strains that lack hair to model carcinogenesis using either UV irradiation or chemical carcinogenesis since researchers prefer not to perform repeated shaving or depilation to visualize tumor development. Particularly favored strains feature mutations in the *Hairless* (*Hr*) gene (Entrez Gene ID 15460) that result in almost complete hair loss early in life [6].

Hairless mutant mice first appeared in the literature in the 1930's when they were described as having a striking wave of hair loss that occurs in a rostral to caudal manner starting at 3 weeks of age [6,7,8,9]. Some fifty years later, *Hr* mutant mice were widely adopted as a convenient model for skin carcinogenesis studies and were discovered to be uniquely susceptible to both UV induced and chemical carcinogenesis [10,11,12]. Since then, the molecular basis of the Hairless phenotype has been established as either a proviral insertion into exon 6, as in the case of Hr^{hr} and SKH-1 animals [13,14], or point mutations, as is the case of the Hr^{rh} animals [15,16,17]. Despite the knowledge that these strains have a mutated *Hr* gene, many carcinogenesis studies continue to use them and refer to unirradiated/untreated animals as 'wild-type hairless' mice.

Two early experiments using different *Hairless* mutant animals suggested that the increased susceptibility to carcinogenesis was, in fact, due to disruption of *Hr*. First, Iversen and Iversen (1976) showed increased tumorgenesis in *Hairless* mice bearing the *Hr/Hr* Oslo mutation as compared to wild-type, hairy littermates when both cohorts were exposed to a chemical carcinogenesis protocol. Secondly, Stoye *et al.* (1988) described the appearance and propagation of a revertant, hairy mouse (Hr^{hr+}) that spontaneously lost the proviral insertion in the *Hr* allele. When used in both chemical and UV induced carcinogenesis protocols, the Hr^{hr+} mice were found to have develop less tumors as compared to their Hr^{hr} counterparts [11,18]. Taken together, these genetic data suggested that *Hairless* is a key determinant of skin tumorigenesis.

Due to the overall phenotype of *Hairless* mutant mice, it has long been hypothesized that *Hairless* plays crucial roles in both the interfollicular epidermis and hair follicle. Supporting this hypothesis is the fact that *Hr* has been shown to be abundantly expressed in the suprabasal layers of the interfollicular epidermis, the matrix region of the hair follicle in catagen, and other follicular compartments such as the dermal papillae [19]. We (and others) have established a role for *Hairless* in the regressing catagen hair follicle [20,21,22], yet its function in the interfollicular epidermis has remained elusive. What has been deduced so far is that Hairless functions as a transcriptional co-factor that interacts with several nuclear hormone receptors such as the Vitamin D receptor (VDR) and thyroid hormone receptor (TR) (reviewed in [23]). In addition to a VDR/TR binding domain, Hr also contains a zinc finger domain, a nuclear localization signal and a putative Jumonji C domain (reviewed in [23]). Altogether, the presence of these multiple domains raises the possibility that Hr regulates multiple pathways thereby having pleotropic effects in the epidermis and influencing tumor susceptibility.

UV induced tumorigenesis occurs, in part, through the activation of the NFκB pathway and subsequent cellular stress and inflammation, therefore, one of the key UV response mechanisms is regulation of the NFκB pathway (reviewed in [24]). Furthermore, constitutive activation of the NFκB pathway is a hallmark of several types of tumors including SCCs [25,26,27] while its inhibition is a known chemoprevention for several tumor types (reviewed in [28]). Recent work from our lab has shown that in primary human keratinocytes *HR* is an early UVB response gene that regulates UVB induced NFκB activation thereby modulating cell cycling [29]. Due to these *in vitro* results and the clear role of the NFκB pathway in UV induced carcinogenesis, we postulated a connection between Hr and the NFκB pathway *in vivo*. Here, we present multiple lines of evidence demonstrating that disruption of the *Hr* gene leads to constitutive activation of the NFκB pathway, uncovering the molecular mechanism of the skin tumorigenesis susceptibility of *Hairless* mutant mice for the first time.

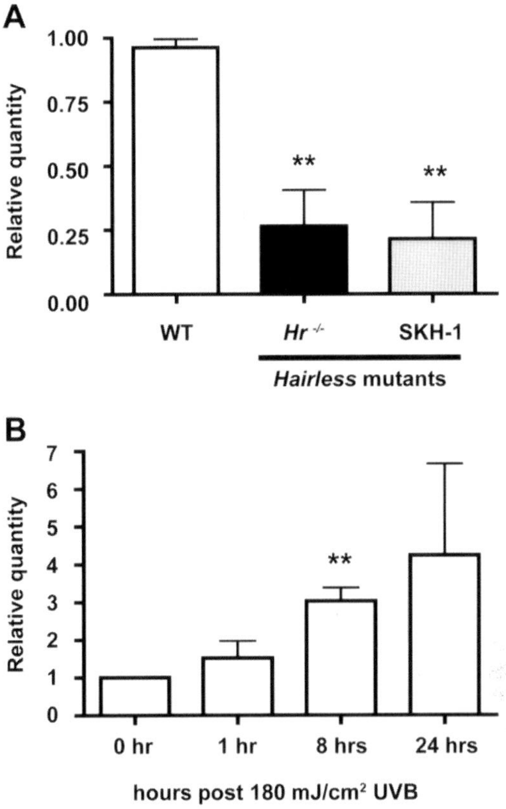

Figure 1. *Hairless* mutants have lower levels of *Hr*, an early a UVB response gene. A) *Hr* expression was measured in whole skin extracts by quantitative RT-PCR using primers designed to several locations in the *Hr* coding sequence. The $Hr^{-/-}$ and SKH-1 *Hairless* mutant strains have significantly decreased levels of *Hr* compared to WT. B) *Hr* expression was also measured in WT ($Hr^{+/+}$) epidermis before and after UVB (100 mJ/cm^2) exposure at 1, 8 and 24 hrs. *Hr* expression significantly increased at the 8 hr time point.

Results

Hr is rapidly upregulated in response to UVB and loss of *Hr* increases susceptibility to UVB induced tumorigenesis

In order to place our studies in the context of earlier work, we first confirmed that the mouse lines SKH-1 and Hr^{hr} (hereafter referred to as $Hr^{-/-}$) both contained the mutation, a proviral insertion disrupting the open reading frame of *Hr* (Figure S1). We then quantified and compared the level of *Hr* mRNA from whole skin extracts of $Hr^{-/-}$, SKH-1, and WT littermates. Both $Hr^{-/-}$ and SKH-1 animals exhibited significantly lower levels of *Hr* mRNA that equaled an ~70% decrease in expression (Figure 1). Our previous work showed that *Hr* is expressed in suprabasal kerationcytes [19,20] and is involved in the early UV response mechanism in primary human kerationcytes [29]. Therefore, we decided to focus our future experiments on the epidermis. In order to implicate Hr in the UV response pathway *in vivo*, we used real time PCR to evaluate *Hr* levels in the WT ($Hr^{+/+}$) epidermis at baseline as compared to 1, 8, and 24 hrs after a single, acute UVB dose. We observed a three-fold increase in epidermal *Hr* mRNA transcript levels from baseline (3.028±0.6147) as early as 8 hrs post UVB exposure (Figure 1B). Thus, *Hr* is rapidly transcriptionally activated in response to acute UVB suggesting that Hr plays a role in the immediate UVB response.

To assess the impact of *Hr* mutations to UVB response, we performed a long-term UVB tumorigenesis protocol [180 mJ/cm^2, the equivalent of 2 MEDS [30,31], three times a week for a total of 50 weeks] using $Hr^{-/-}$ mutants and strain-matched WT ($Hr^{+/+}$) animals. Neither WT ($Hr^{+/+}$) nor $Hr^{-/-}$ animals showed any signs of papilloma formation at 22 weeks, however by week 30, $Hr^{-/-}$ animals began to develop small papillomas (Figure S2). 50 weeks into the protocol, the $Hr^{-/-}$ animals had an average of 22 tumors that necessitated the termination of the study (Figure 2). In contrast, WT ($Hr^{+/+}$) animals showed no sign of tumor or papilloma formation at any time during the study.

Histological analysis of tissues obtained from the tumors in $Hr^{-/-}$ animals at 50 weeks indicated that they were highly aggressive SSCs, while there was no evidence of even microscopic tumor formation in WT ($Hr^{+/+}$) skin (Figure 2B). Since the only known genetic difference between $Hr^{-/-}$ animals and WT ($Hr^{+/+}$) littermates was the *Hairless* mutation (Figure 1), these results demonstrate that the disruption of *Hairless* was directly responsible for conferring tumor susceptibility.

The *Hairless* mutant epidermis is hyperproliferative both basally and in response to UVB

Given the evidence in the literature and the results of our long-term UVB study, we next investigated the molecular role of *Hr* in the UVB response pathways. For these studies we used a single, acute UVB dose (180 mJ/cm^2) and assessed early time points (1, 8,

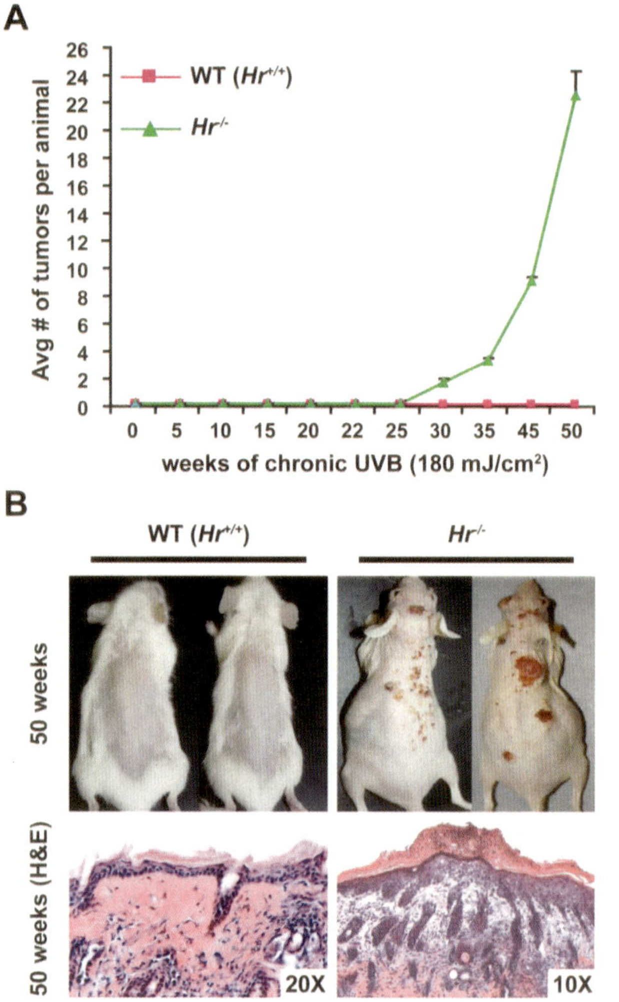

Figure 2. Mutations in *Hr* render animals susceptible to UVB-induced tumorigenesis. A) Female $Hr^{-/-}$ (n = 10) and age/sex matched WT littermates ($Hr^{+/+}$) were irradiated using 180 mJ/cm^2 UVB three times a week for a total of 50 weeks and the number of tumors per animal were recorded on a weekly basis. WT littermates never developed tumors or papillomas, while $Hr^{-/-}$ animals developed tumors by 30 weeks. B) After 50 weeks of irradiation, $Hr^{-/-}$ mice had obvious tumors and histological analysis revealed that the majority of the tumors were aggressive SSCs. In contrast, WT animals did not develop any tumors even at the microscopic level.

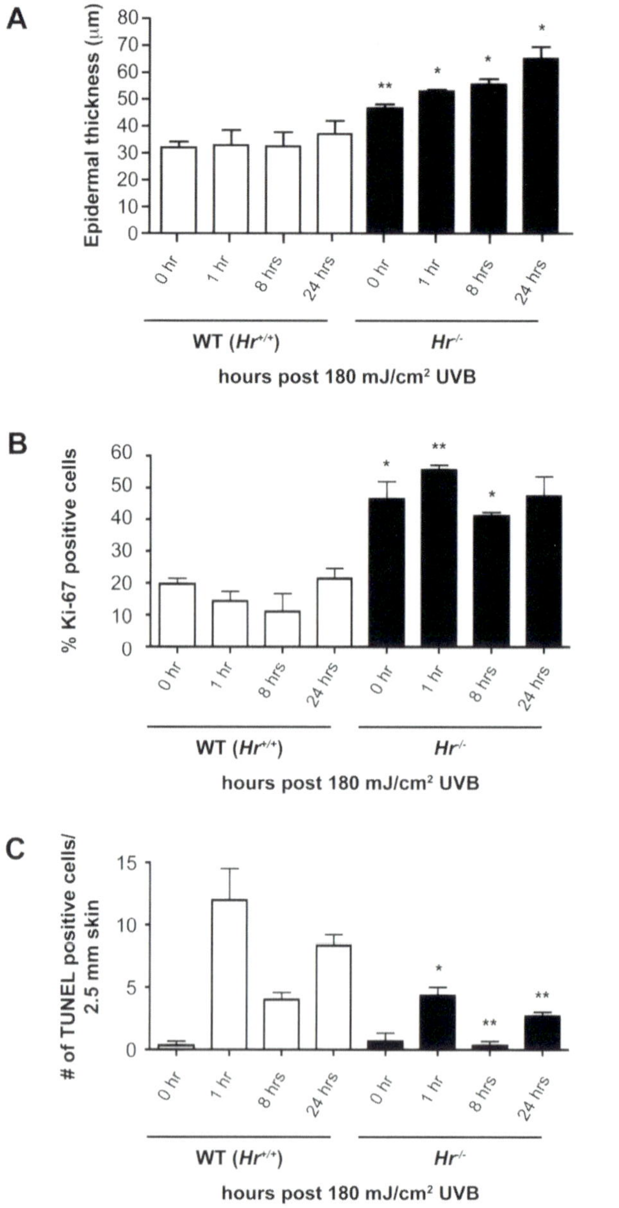

Figure 3. *Hairless* mutant epidermis is highly proliferative and exhibits a defective UVB response. A) Assessment of epidermal thickness using epidermal morphometry on H&E stained sections indicates that $Hr^{-/-}$ mice have significantly greater thickness prior to UVB (180 mJ/cm^2) as compared to WT controls. Epidermal thickness remains elevated after UVB exposure. B) Skin sections were stained with Ki-67 to identify proliferating basal keratinocytes both at baseline and after UVB exposure at the specified time points. $Hr^{-/-}$ mice had a significantly higher percentage of Ki-67 positive cells at baseline as compared to WT and continued to have an elevated amount of Ki-67 positive cells after UVB. C) Skin sections were stained with TUNEL to identify apoptotic cells both at baseline and at the designated time points. The number of TUNEL positive cells was plotted per 2.5 mm section of skin. $Hr^{-/-}$ mice have a significantly lower number of TUNEL positive cells at 1 hr and 24 hr post UVB compared to WT.

and 24 hrs post-irradiation) without the variable of secondary effects of a long term UVB protocol.

Using epidermal morphometry, we found a significant increase in epidermal thickness both before and after UVB in $Hr^{-/-}$ mice as compared to wildtype conterparts (Figure 3A). At baseline, $Hr^{-/-}$ mice have a significantly thicker epidermis indicating the possibility of a hyperproliferative phenotype. Increased epidermal thickness in $Hr^{-/-}$ skin is maintained after UVB exposure with gradual increases at the indicated timepoints. We hypothesized that such an increase in epidermal thickness was due to either increased numbers of proliferating keratinocytes or a defect in apoptosis.

Therefore, we investigated the amount of proliferation found in the *Hairless* mutant epidermis by staining skin sections from $Hr^{-/-}$ and their respective WT littermates with the proliferation marker Ki67. As seen in Figure 3B, the percent of Ki67 positive cells found in the non-irradiated $Hr^{-/-}$ epidermis was significantly higher than in the WT epidermis [0.1969 ± 0.0246 (WT) vs 0.4649 ± 0.0772 ($Hr^{-/-}$) as measured by the amount of Ki67 positive basal cells as a percentage of total basal cells). Throughout the time points sampled, the $Hr^{-/-}$ epidermis continued to exhibit a higher amount of proliferation than WT epidermis. Altogether this data indicated that the epidermal thickening seen in Figure 3A may, in part, be due to increased proliferation in the *Hairless* mutant epidermis.

In order to determine if the epidermal thickening could be partially attributed to defects in apoptosis, TUNEL staining was also performed (Figure 3C). We found that at homeostasis both WT and $Hr^{-/-}$ epidermis contained a low level of apoptosis that increased 1 hr after UVB exposure. However, the amount of apoptosis found in the $Hr^{-/-}$ epidermis was approximately 3 times less than in WT controls. This trend continued at 8 and 24 hrs with the level of apoptosis in the $Hr^{-/-}$ epidermis always being significantly less than that found in WT epidermis. When taken together with the proliferation data, this suggests that apoptosis may be impaired by loss of *Hr*, perhaps due to signals favoring proliferation or possibly because of the increased epidermal thickness partially shielding the keratinocytes from UVB irradiation.

Loss of *Hr* leads to constitutively activated NFκB

NFκB has long been known to play a role in UVB induced tumorigenesis and forms a nexus of proliferative and apoptotic pathways; additionally, our previous work shows that HR regulates NFκB *in vitro* [29]. We therefore theorized that Hr and NFκB may be mechanistically related in a similar fashion *in vivo*. To investigate a possible connection between the two proteins, we examined p65 protein levels in $Hr^{-/-}$ and matching WT ($Hr^{+/+}$) littermate epidermis with and without acute UVB irradiation using Western blotting (Figure 4A). Prior to irradiation, $Hr^{-/-}$ epidermis had a significantly higher amount of the p65 subunit of NFκB. $Hr^{-/-}$ epidermis continued to express higher levels of p65 at 1 hr, 8 hrs, and 24 hrs post-UVB irradiation. Altogether this indicates that the lack of *Hr* in the $Hr^{-/-}$ epidermis results in a constitutively upregulated NFκB pathway.

In order to determine if the increase in p65 protein levels correlated with activation of the NFκB signaling pathway following acute UVB exposure, we examined $Hr^{-/-}$ and WT ($Hr^{+/+}$) skin sections using an antibody against the phosphorylated inhibitor of NFκB signaling, IκBα. Activation of the NFκB complex is dependent on IκBα phosphorylation (p-IκBα) and subsequent degradation that allows nuclear translocation of the NFκB complex [32]. In addition to being upstream of NFκB, IκBα is also a known target gene that is transcriptionally regulated by NFκB [32]. Therefore, NFκB and IκBα form a positive feedback loop and p-IκBα, when assessed in conjunction with the overall increased levels of p65, can be used as an indicator to specifically localize the activated NFκB pathway [33].

Staining of non-irradiated $Hr^{-/-}$ skin showed the presence of p-IκBα throughout all the epidermal layers, including the basal layer, while in WT ($Hr^{+/+}$) skin IκBα expression was restricted to the differentiated, suprabasal layers (Figure 4B). This clear demarcation of p-IκBα expression suggests that perturbation of NFκB signaling in basal keratinocytes may be responsible for the dysregulated proliferation and apoptosis observed in *Hairless* mutants. In response to acute UVB, we observed a gradual increase in the levels of p-IκBα in WT ($Hr^{+/+}$) skin, with signaling in the basal keratinocytes beginning at 8 hrs post-UVB irradiation (Figure 4B). This expression pattern coincides with the time point previously observed to have a significantly higher amount of *Hr* mRNA in the WT epidermis after acute irradiation (Figure 1B). As expected, the intensity of p-IκBα signaling increased in response to UVB exposure in both the WT ($Hr^{+/+}$) and $Hr^{-/-}$ mutant skin and by 24 hrs post UVB irradiation, both genotypes showed uniform p-IκBα staining in all layers of the epidermis with comparable intensity.

To study the role of NFκB activation in the increased susceptibility of *Hairless* mutant mice to tumorigenesis, we returned to the non-tumor bearing skin samples generated in the long-term irradiation study described in Figure 2. Interestingly, p-IκBα staining appeared in the basal and suprabasal layer of the mutant epidermis by week 25, a time point prior to tumor development (Figure 4C). In contrast, at the same timepoint, the WT ($Hr^{+/+}$) epidermis continued to show only suprabasal localization of p-IκBα. By week 30 (when tumors were first observed on $Hr^{-/-}$ mice) the staining pattern remained the same in both sets of animals, though the $Hr^{-/-}$ epidermis had a higher intensity of staining. The intensity of the p-IκBα staining in the $Hr^{-/-}$ epidermis continued to increase at week 42 and plateaued at week 50, while the WT ($Hr^{+/+}$) epidermis only began to show staining in the basal layer of the epidermis at week 42 which increased at week 50.

Pharmacological inhibition of NFκB signaling reduces UVB induced tumorigenesis in *Hairless* mutant mice

We next reasoned that blockade of NFκB signaling *in vivo* should inhibit tumor formation in *Hairless* mutant mice. Therefore, we performed chronic UVB tumor induction studies while simultaneously treating the mice with a pharmacological inhibitor of NFκB, pyrrolidinedithiocarbomate (PDTC), which was given *ad libitum* the mice's drinking water. PDTC suppresses NFκB DNA-binding activity and IκBα degradation thereby inhibiting NFκB activation [34]. 60 SKH-1 mice were divided into two groups: group-I mice received tap water and group-II mice received PDTC (0.5%) supplemented drinking water. All mice were irradiated with UVB, 180 mJ/cm^2 twice a week for 35 weeks, which was sufficient to induce tumorigenesis both with and without PDTC treatment (Figure 5A and B).

PDTC and its concomitant reduction in NFκB activity significantly reduced tumorigenesis by approximately 60%, as measured in average tumor number, throughout the duration of the irradiation protocol (Figure 5A). Average tumor volume was also significantly decreased in the animals treated with PDTC (Figure 5B). Inhibition of the NFκB pathway altered gross tumor morphology suggesting that the tumors that formed on the PDTC treated animals were more likely to be papillomas than SCCs. In contrast, the animals given only tap water developed signs of aggressive SCCs (Figure S3A). Taken together, these results demonstrate that the tumor susceptibility of the SKH-1 animals is dependent on the overactivation of the NFκB pathway that is a downstream result of *Hairless* mutation.

We next performed a detailed molecular analysis of the NFκB pathway in the PDTC treated SKH-1 animals (Figure 5C-F). For this analysis we used the non-tumor bearing skin and the tumors from the PDTC treated and control SKH-1 animals that had been irradiated for 35 weeks. In addition to analyzing whole tumors in this study, the epidermis was isolated from non-tumor bearing skin in order to localize the biochemical effects of the PDTC treatment. Our initial hypothesis was that non-tumor bearing skin of the PDTC treated animals would exhibit reduced NFκB signaling thereby indicating less tumor promotion when NFκB activation is blocked. Furthermore, we hypothesized that tumors from both untreated and PDTC treated animals would show similar levels of NFκB activity. We reasoned that any tumors formed despite PDTC treatment would suggest the occurance of other molecular events occurred thereby allowing specific cells to bypass PDTC-mediated inhibition and develop into tumors. Therefore, we expected the effects of PDTC and NFκB inhibition in UVB

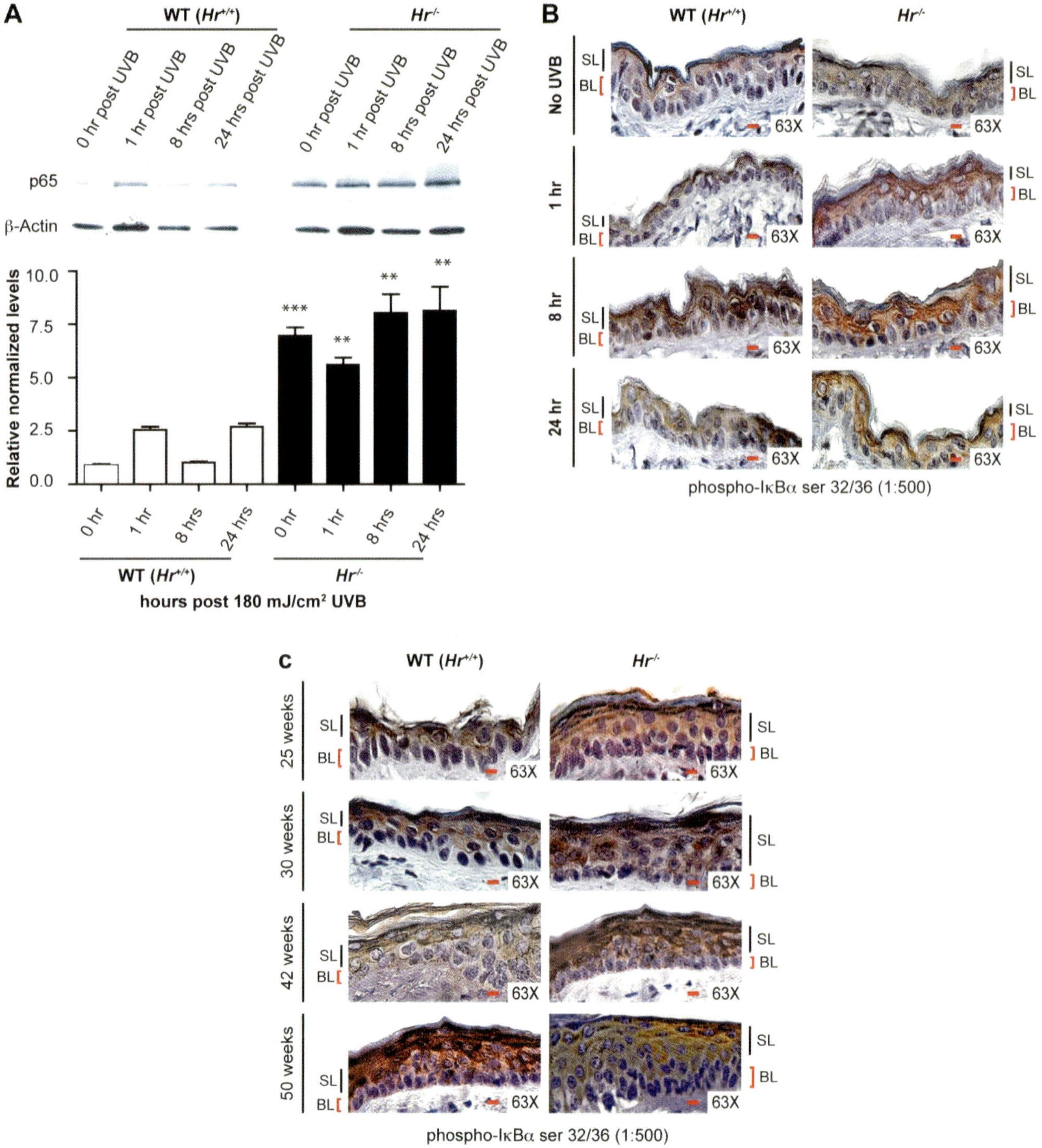

Figure 4. ***Hairless*** **mutant epidermis shows constitutive activation of the NFκB signaling pathway.** A) Western Blot and ImageJ densitometry analysis using anti-p65 antibody on isolated $Hr^{-/-}$ epidermal extracts after 1, 8 and 24 hrs post UVB (180 mJ/cm^2) irradiation. B) Immunohistochemistry using p-IκBα antibody to determine the extent of NFκB signaling activity in the epidermis of WT ($Hr^{+/+}$) and $Hr^{-/-}$ animals before and after a single, acute UVB (180 mJ/cm^2) irradiation. IκBα is increased constitutively and after irradiation throughout the epidermal layer. C) Immunohistochemistry using p-IκBα antibody to determine the extent of NFκB signaling activity in the epidermis of WT ($Hr^{+/+}$) and $Hr^{-/-}$ animals at the indicated time points during chronic UVB irradiation (180 mJ/cm^2 UVB three times a week for a total of 50 weeks). IκBα is increased constitutively and after irradiation throughout the epidermal layer.

irradiated SKH-1 animals to be more prominent in the non-tumor bearing skin compared to non-treated SKH-1 animals.

PDTC inhibition of NFκB blocks downstream target genes in chronically UVB exposed *Hairless* mutant skin

We began by assessing NFκB activation by Western blot analysis of nuclear extracts; we found decreased nuclear localiza-

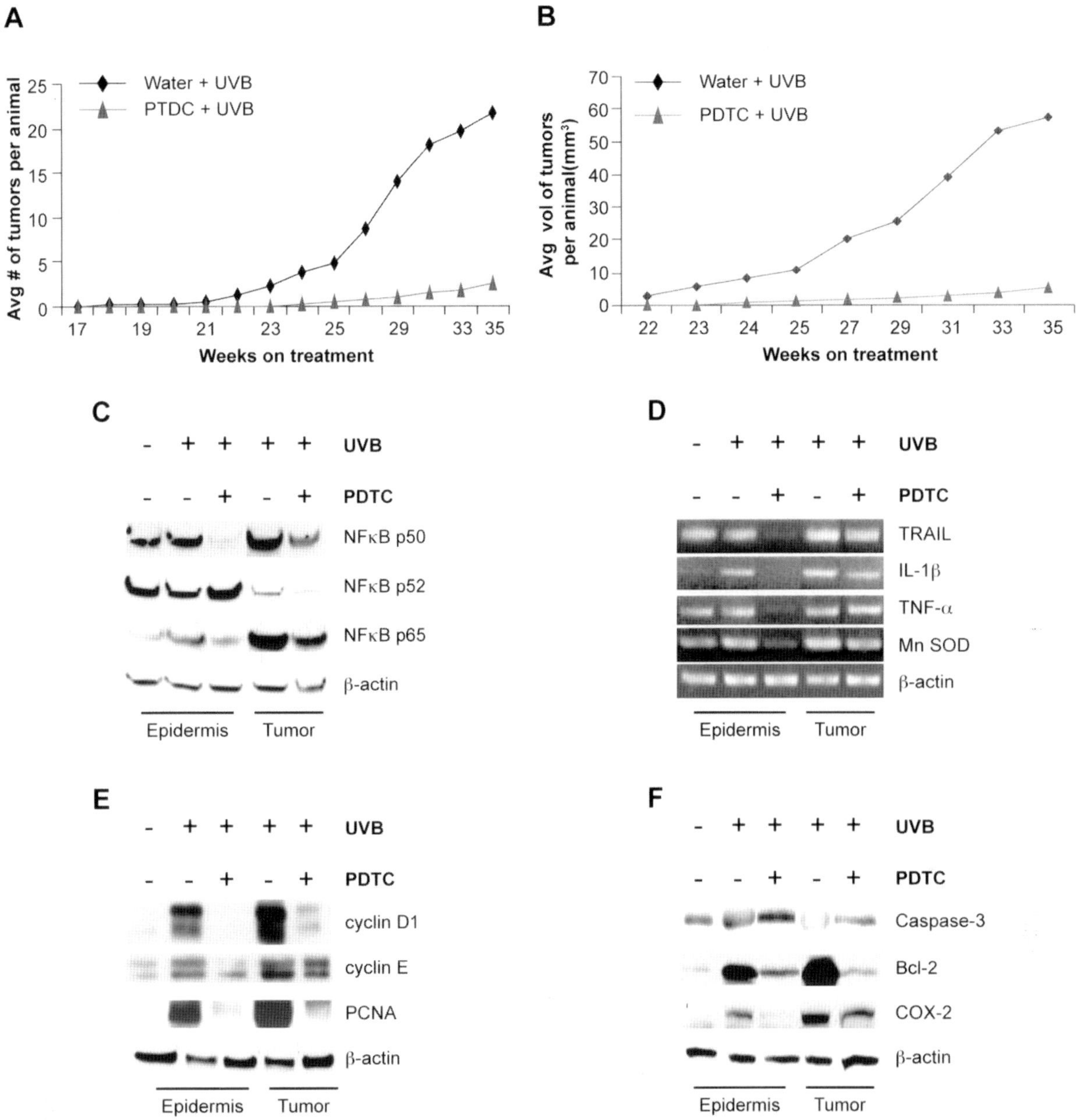

Figure 5. Administration of the NFκB inhibitor PDTC abrogates UVB-induced skin carcinogenesis in SKH-1 mice. SKH-1 mice (n = 30 per treatment) were chronically irradiated with UVB (180 mJ/cm^2, twice a week for 35 weeks) and either given PDTC (0.5%) or no treatment in drinking water (*ad libitum*). Non-irradiated SKH-1 mice (n = 12) were used as controls. A) PDTC treatment decreased the average number of tumors per mouse. B) PDTC treatment decreased the average tumor volume per mouse. C) Western blot analysis for the p50, p52, and p65 subunits of NFκB were performed on nuclear extracts prepared from non-irradiated epidermal samples and chronically irradiated epidermal and tumor samples from mice treated with PDTC or untreated. While PDTC treatment prevented the upregulation of p50 in both skin and tumor samples, it had no effect on the p52 expression in either sample. PDTC treatment specifically abrogated upregulation of p65 in non-tumor bearing epidermis. D) RT-PCR for the NFκB transcriptional targets TRAIL, IL-1β, TNF-α and Mn SOD was performed on non-irradiated epidermal samples and chronically irradiated epidermis and tumor samples from mice treated with PDTC or untreated. PDTC prevented upregulation of the NFκB targets in irradiated skin samples but not in tumor samples. E) Western blot analysis for cyclin D1, cyclin E, and PCNA (which are involved in cell cycle regulation) was performed on non-irradiated epidermal samples and chronically irradiated epidermis and tumor samples from either untreated mice or mice treated with PDTC. PDTC treatment abrogates the overexpression of these proteins in non-tumor bearing skin samples. F) Western blot analysis of caspase-3 (pro-apoptosis), Bcl-2 (anti-apoptosis), and COX-2 (inflammation) was performed on non-irradiated epidermal samples and chronically irradiated epidermis and tumor samples from mice treated with PDTC or untreated. PDTC inhibited Bcl-2 and COX-2 in both epidermis and tumor samples while it did not affect caspase-3.

tion of the NFκB subunits p65 and p50 in non-tumor bearing epidermis and tumors but no change in p52 (Figure 5C). This indicated that as expected, PDTC specifically blocked nuclear translocation of the p65/p50 heterodimer and the canonical NFκB pathway. We also found that PDTC treated epidermis exhibited decreased NFκB activation as measured by direct binding of NFκB to consensus binding sites, electrophoretic mobility shift assay (EMSA)(Figure S3B). Total and phosphorylated IκBα protein levels were measured by Western blot in non-tumor bearing epidermis and tumors; it was found that PDTC treatment specifically abrogated increases in phophorylated IκBα in non-tumor bearing skin suggesting a functional blockade of the NFκB signaling pathway (Figure S3C). Taken together, the data indicates an overall reduction in NFκB signaling activity in the non-tumor bearing skin of SKH-1 animals subjected to chronic UVB exposure and treated with PDTC.

In order to assess the downstream consequences of NFκB regulation by PDTC in SKH-1 animals, we analyzed the mRNA expression of various NFκB target genes in epidermal extracts and tumors using semi-quantitative PCR. As shown in Figure 5D, we found that PDTC treatment significantly reduced the expression of TRAIL [35], IL-1β [36], TNFα [37], and MnSOD [38] in the non-tumor bearing epidermis with a less appreciable decrease in tumors. This data confirms that NFκB activation is crucial for tumor development in chronically UVB irradiated SKH-1 skin, and that PDTC efficiently blocked NFκB activation in non-tumor bearing skin, thus attenuating the susceptibility of SKH-1 animals to tumor development.

To further investigate the PDTC-dependent repression of tumor susceptibility in chronically irradiated *Hairless* mutant mice, we studied its effects on the expression of genes that regulate cell cycle progression, proliferation, and apoptosis. As shown in Figure 5E, PDTC treatment inhibited the expression of the key cell cycle regulators cyclin D1 [39], cyclin E1 [40], and PCNA [41] in both tumors and in non-tumor bearing epidermis. When combined with the increased Ki67 staining seen in Figure 3B, increased expression of these proteins in irradiated SKH-1 skin and tumors is yet another indication of a hyperproliferative state that can be abrogated by blockade of the NFκB pathway.

We then examined the expression of two proteins involved in apoptotic response pathways, the pro-apoptotic caspase 3 and the anti-apoptotic Bcl-2. Caspase 3 has not been implicated in the NFκB pathway so as expected, we saw no significant change in expression with PDTC treatment (Figure 5F). Bcl-2, however, is a known NFκB target gene and its expression is decreased with PDTC treatment in both non-tumor bearing epidermis and tumors (Figure 5F) [42]. This is consistent with the TUNEL and Ki67 results in Figures 3B and 3C that show increased proliferation and decreased apoptosis, which together with the data presented here, illustrates that repression of NFκB restores the normal apoptotic response in the irradiated *Hr* mutant epidermis.

To further understand the mechanism behind increased tumor promotion in the context of NFκB activation, we assessed the expression of the pro-inflammatory protein COX-2. COX-2 is known to be downstream of NFκB and is strongly implicated in squamous cell carcinoma progression [43,44,45]. In agreement with the expression pattern of the other pro-inflammatory NFκB target genes TNFα and IL-1β, we found that COX-2 levels were dramatically decreased with PDTC treatment in non-tumor bearing skin but not in tumors. Therefore, we theorize that in the *Hr* mutant epidermis, increased COX-2 levels in conjunction with TNFα and IL-1β create an pro-inflammatory environment that promotes tumor growth [46].

Discussion

Hairless mice, particularly the SKH-1 line, have long been a favorite animal model used for skin carcinogenesis studies because of their convenience, however, researchers have not generally taken into consideration the underlying mechanism for their lack of hair and whether this may be linked to their tumor susceptibility. To address this issue, we show for the first time that $Hr^{-/-}$ and SKH-1 mouse lines are allelic mutants of one another that have significantly lower amounts of *Hr*, a crucial early UVB response gene, and are thus predisposed to UVB induced carcinogenesis. The results detailed above indicate that Hr plays a crucial role in cell cycle kinetics by functioning as an inhibitor of the NFκB pathway in the epidermis; therefore, loss of *Hr* results in altered cell cycling, increased proliferation and subsequent tumorigenesis.

We found that both $Hr^{-/-}$ and SKH-1 animals exhibit similar decreases of *Hr* expression throughout the skin that amounts to approximately 30% of that found in WT animals; this allowed them to be used interchangeably in our experiments. We further determined that *Hr* is significantly upregulated in the WT epidermis 8 hours after a single, acute dose of UVB. Furthermore, when $Hr^{-/-}$ mice were used in chronic UVB carcinogenesis studies they developed papillomas by week 30, and these papillomas progressed into aggressive SCCs by the end of the protocol 20 weeks later. In contrast, WT mice with normal *Hr* expression failed to show even microscopic signs of tumorigenesis by week 50.

Together, these findings led us to postulate that Hr is an essential component of the epidermal response to UVB insult and perturbation of *Hr* levels causes a genetic predisposition to tumorigenesis due to a dysregulated UVB response in the *Hr* mutant epidermis. Under normal conditions, a tightly regulated signaling cascade is triggered by UVB irradiation leading to the apoptosis of severely damaged cells and proliferation of undamaged and/or repaired cells (reviewed in [47]). Therefore, we examined the epidermis of $Hr^{-/-}$ animals and found that at homeostasis *Hr* loss results in a significantly thicker epidermis that is sustained after UVB exposure. We then investigated the contribution of both proliferation and apoptosis to this thicker epidermis and found both increased proliferation at all time points and decreased apoptosis in response to UVB irradiation. This indicated that the thicker epidermis found in *Hr* mutant mice was the result of uncontrolled proliferation and decreased apoptosis, factors which when combined together contribute to the increased tumorigenesis seen during the chronic UVB exposure protocol. It should be noted that the thicker epidermis in and of itself might contribute to the decreased apoptosis due to possible UVB shielding.

One of the key mechanistic links between proliferation and apoptosis is the NFκB signaling pathway and we have previously established a regulatory loop between Hr and NFκB *in vitro* [29,46]. Thus we investigated a possible mechanistic connection between NFκB and Hr *in vivo*. While there are many NFκB hetero- and homo-dimers that can activate NFκB-mediated transcription and regulate cell proliferation, we began by focusing on the canonical p65/p50 hetero-dimer complex since it is known to be an important UVB response factor in both mouse and human skin [24]. We found that at homeostasis, *Hairless* mutant epidermis exhibits constitutive activation of the NFκB pathway as indicated by increased expression of both the p65 subunit and p-IκBα. Unlike in the WT epidermis, p-IκBα activation in the $Hr^{-/-}$ skin is not confined to the superbasal layer; instead p-IκBα is expressed throughout the epidermis both basely and in response to UVB thererby indicating aberrant upregulation of NFκB in $Hr^{-/-}$ skin.

We postulate that Hr regulates tumor promotion via regulation of NFκB activation and thereby modulates proliferation and apoptosis following UVB irradiation. Therefore, when Hr expression is decreased, there is an increased likelihood of the survival and proliferation of UVB damaged basal keratinocytes and subsequent tumorigenesis. As we also show here, blockade of the NFκB pathway by the pharmacological inhibitor PDTC decreases both tumor burden and tumor volume in the *Hairless* mutant mouse line SKH-1.

In the non-tumor bearing skin irradiated SKH-1 mice, PDTC treatment specifically decreased NFκB activity in the *Hairless* mutant epidermis as reflected by attenuated expression of the NFκB subunits p50 and p65, decreased NFκB binding to target sequences, and decreased expression of p-IκBα. Additionally, the non-tumor bearing skin of PDTC treated mice also exhibited decreases in the expression of downstream NFκB targets such as TRAIL, IL-1β, TNFα, and MnSOD as well as the inhibition of cell cycling proteins such as cyclin D1, cyclin E, PCNA, and BCL-2 thereby indicating a return to normal proliferation. We also show that in non-tumor bearing skin, *Hr* influences inflammation via COX-2 expression which decreases with PDTC treatment. The combination of decreased TNFα, IL-1β, and COX-2 found in the PDTC treated epidermis provides compelling evidence that *Hr* is capable of modulating epithelial inflammation via regulation of the NFκB pathway and thereby further contributes to tumor promotion. Therefore, the data provides evidence that the decreases in *Hr* expression result in gross epithelial dysregulation that can be ameliorated by inhibition of the NFκB pathway.

We hypothesize that since NFκB is the nexus of proliferative and inflammatory signals [46], the lack of *Hr* allows the proliferation of UVB damaged cells and eventual tumor development. Previous work in our laboratory has shown that after UVB insult, cells lacking *Hr* have decreased amounts of cells in the G2/M phase [29] which is a key cell cycle checkpoint for DNA damage [48,49]. Attenuation of the G2/M checkpoint after UVB insult increases genomic instability which when combined with increased proliferation and inflammation found in the *Hairless* mutant epidermis creates an ideal cellular environment for tumor development. Thus, loss of *Hr* and subsequent overactivation of NFκB provide all the components necessary for increased tumorigenesis.

While it is possible that Hr-mediated repression of the NFκB pathway could occur at multiple junctures due to the inherent complexities of the NFκB pathway, the evidence presented here suggests the involvement of Hr in two possible regulatory mechanisms. One is through the control of the kinase cascade leading to IκBα phosphorylation and subsequent degradation. This then allows the canonical NFκB heterodimer to translocate to the nucleus, bind to target DNA sequences, and modulate downstream gene transcription. This possibility is seen in the increased IκBα staining seen in $Hr^{-/-}$ epidermis both prior to and after irradiation. The other possible regulatory mechanism is through direct transcriptional regulation of the p65 subunit. Evidence for this regulation is seen in the increased expression of p65 in epidermal extracts from unirradiated and irradiated $Hr^{-/-}$ mice. Since IκBα is also downstream of NFκB activation, direct transcriptional regulation of the NFκB subunits would also result in the increased IκBα phosphorylation seen in the *Hr* mutant epidermis. Therefore either hypothesis fits the data presented here and further work will be necessary to clarify the method of Hr regulation of NFκB.

While non-tumor bearing skin showed significant changes with PDTC, there were less obvious effects in the tumor samples. We postulate that specific keratinocyte populations escaped PDTC-mediated inhibition of NFκB and developed into tumors despite PDTC treatment. We further postulate that this escape may be due to other molecular events such as DNA damage in other genes downstream of PDTC inhibition of the NFκB pathway. Therefore, the effects of PDTC are more prominent in the non-tumor bearing skin and a small number of tumors develop despite PDTC treatment.

Altogether, we provide here multiple lines of evidence that Hr plays an essential role in the regulation of NFκB signaling in the epidermis and thereby effects keratinocyte apoptosis and proliferation. Hr mediated NFκB regulation occurs during epidermal homeostasis but it is particularly important during the keratinocyte response to UVB irradiation where it is essential to the proper apoptosis of damaged keratinocytes. Thus, we postulate that Hr plays a crucial regulatory role in SCC development via inhibition of NFκB pathway after UVB irradiation. We conclude that *Hr* mutant mouse strains, including SKH-1, exhibit qualities associated with increased proliferation and cellular dysregulation, providing a molecular mechanism for their inherent tumor susceptibility.

Materials and Methods

Animals

SKH-1 mice were purchased from Charles River Laboratories (Kingston, NY). HRS/J ($Hr^{-/-}$) were purchased from Jackson Laboratory (Bar Harbor, ME). This study was carried out in strict accordance with the recommendations in the Guide for the Care and Use of Laboratory Animals of the National Institutes of Health. The protocol was approved by the Institutional Animal Care and Use Committee of Columbia University (IACUC Protocol Number: AC-AAAA5875).

RNA and Protein Extraction

Dorsal skin was harvested from mutant and WT animals and divided into two parts; one portion was kept intact for histological analysis and RNA extraction (see below) and the other was used for epidermal isolation and subsequent RNA and protein extraction. Briefly, dorsal whole skin was scraped to remove excess subcutaneous fat and divided into small strips and incubated in 0.25% trypsin with EDTA (Invitrogen, Grand Island, NY) for 2 hrs at 37°C. The epidermis was mechanically separated from the dermis by scraping and incubated in SMEM with 10% FBS, 1% PS (Invitrogen) at room temperature with shaking for 30 min to separate the keractinoyctes. Keratinocyte clumps were then filtered out using a 70 μM cell strainer (BD Biosciences, San Diego, CA) and the remaining single cell filtrate was pelleted by centrifugation. The cells were then resuspended in either RLT Buffer for RNA Extraction (Qiagen, Valencia, CA) or the Flag-Lysis Buffer (50 mM Tris-HCl pH 7.8, 137 mM NaCl, 10 mM NaF, 1 mM EDTA, 1% Triton X-100, 0.2% Sarkosyl, 1 mM DTT, 10 % glycerol and fresh proteinase inhibitors) for protein extraction.

A portion of the whole skin was also homogenized in RLT Buffer and RNA was isolated from either the epidermis or the whole skin using an RNeasy Mini Kit (Qiagen) followed by DNase treatment. 2 μg of total RNA was used for the cDNA synthesis using Superscript III (Invitrogen) and a 2:1 ratio of random hexamers: oligo (dT) primers according to manufacturer's instructions.

Protein was extracted from either epidermal extracts or whole tumors homogenized in Flag-Lysis buffer. Proteins were quantified using RD DC protein assay protocol as instructed by the manufacturer (BioRad, Hercules, CA). Relative band intensity was measured using ImageJ software.

Quantitative RT-PCR

Real time PCR was performed on a ABI 7300 (Applied Biosystems, Carlsbad, CA) using the Relative Quantification Assay and software. Primers (Invitrogen) were designed according to ABI guidelines.

All are written 5′ to 3′:

m*Hr* ex 6 FTTCCACATTGCTGCAGTCAT
m*Hr* ex 6/7 RGTTCTCAGG AACAGCA
m*Hr* ex15 FCTGGTATCGAGCACAGAAAG
m*Hr* ex 16 FCTTTCTCCAGATGGTGTGC
m*B2M* FACTGACCGGCCTGTATGCTA
m*B2M* RTAGAGATGTCAGATATGTCCTTCA
mTNF-α FTGCCTATGTCTCAGCCTCTT
mTNF-α RGGAAGACTCCTCCCAGGTAT
mIL-1β FATAACCTGCTGGTGTGTGAC
mIL-1β RTGAGGTGCTGATGTACCAGTT
mMnSOD FGACCTGCCTTACGACTATGG
mMnSOD R GACCTTGCTCCTTATTGAAGC
mTRAIL FTCACCAACGAGATGAAGCAGC
mTRAIL RCTCACCTTGTCCTTTGAGACC

All reactions were performed using ABI Power Sybr Master Mix, 200nM primers and 200ng cDNA. The following protocol was used: step 1 −50°C 2 min, step 2 −95°C 10 min, step 3 −95°C 15 sec, step 4 −60°C 1 min, repeat step 2–4 for 40 cycles. All samples were run on a 1.5% agarose gel to confirm amplicon size. The data output was imported into the GraphPad Prism 4 software (GraphPad Software, Inc., La Jolla, CA), plotted, and the error calculated as standard error of the mean (SEM). Statistical analysis was performed between time points and samples as indicated using Student's T-test.

UV irradiation protocol

For all protocols, irradiation was performed using eight FS72T12-UVB-HO lamps (Daavlin, Bryan, OH) and all animals were irradiated at 180 mJ/cm^2 UVB which has been established as approximately equivalent to 2 MEDs [30,31]; UVC was eliminated by a Kodacel filter (TA401/407) (Kodak, Rochester, NY). The UVB dose was measured with a UVB Spectra 305 Dosimeter (Daavlin) and calibrated with a secondary radiometer (IL1700) (International Light, Peabody, MA).

Chronic UVB protocol. Female 9–11 week old HRS/J and shaved WT counterparts (n = 10 for each) were irradiated three times a week for a total of 50 weeks. Tumors were counted when they reached 2 mm in diameter on a weekly basis. After 25 and 30 weeks of irradiation mice were randomly selected for euthanization. At 42 weeks of irradiation mice were chosen for sacrifice based on their tumor size; any animal with an average tumor diameter greater than 7.5 mm was euthanized. After 50 weeks of irradiation the remaining mice were sacrificed. At all timepoints skin and tumor samples were embedded in both paraffin and frozen blocks.

Chronic UVB protocol with PDTC treatment. 60 9–11 week old SKH-1 mice were split into two groups of 30 animals each, one group received no treatment and the other group received 0.5% PDTC in their drinking water. PDTC treatment began 2 weeks prior to first irradiation and continued throughout irradiation protocol. Both groups were irradiated twice a week with for a total of 35 weeks. 12 SKH-1 mice served as non-irradiated, untreated, age matched controls. When tumor diameter reached 2 mm, the tumor number and size were recorded biweekly. All animals were sacrificed 24 hrs after last UVB exposure and dorsal skin and tumors were collected for Western blotting, EMSA and RT-PCR analysis. Three samples for each group was used per assay and each assay was repeated for a total of three times.

Acute UVB protocol. Female 9–11 week old HRS/J and shaved WT counterparts were irradiated once. Three animals of each group per post irradiation timepoint were used for 4 replicates (n = 12).

Immunohistochemistry

Skin samples for frozen blocks were prepared and embedded as previously described [50]. Sections were done at 4 μm, parallel to the paravertebral line, fixed in buffered 4% paraformaldehyde with 1% Triton-X and processed for H&E, TUNEL (Apo-Tag kit) (Chemicon, Billerica, MA) and Ki-67 (AbCam, Cambridge, MA) staining. Epidermal morphometry was measured on H&E stained sections using AdobePhotoshop. Approximately 20 measurements (from basement membrane to stratum corneum) were made per 2.5 mm section at 10X objective on a HRC Axiocam fitted onto an Axioplan2 fluorescent microscope (Carl Zeiss, Thornwood, NY). TUNEL and Ki67 positive cells were counted per 2.5 mm section of skin at 20X. For Ki67 analysis the total number of basal keratinocytes were also counted in the same field of view. Data was plotted and analyzed using GraphPad Prism 4 software. Error was calculated as standard error of the mean (SEM).

For phospho-IκBα staining, tissue was fixed in 10% formalin, embedded in paraffin blocks and sectioned at 4 μm parallel to paravetebral line following standard procedures. Sections were treated with Antigen Unmasking Solution (Vector Labs, Burlingame, CA) then probed with phospho-IκBα (ser32/36) (AbCam) followed by avidin-biotintylated HRP complex (ABC Elite system, Vector Labs). The antibody was detected with DAB and images were taken using a HRC Axiocam fitted onto an Axioplan2 fluorescent microscope.

Western Blots

Protein extracts were prepared as described above, while nuclear extracts were prepared using NE-PER Nuclear and Cytoplasmic Extractions kit (Pierce, Rockford, IL). All samples were used for Western blotting analysis using standard protocols and the following primary antibodies: p65 (AbCam), p50 (Santa Cruz, Santa Cruz, CA), and p52 (Santa Cruz). Western blotting was done using standard protocols and the following primary antibodies: IκBα (Santa Cruz) IκBα (ser32/36) (AbCam), PCNA (Santa Cruz), Bcl-2 (Enzo Life Sciences, Farmingdale, NY), active caspase 3 (AbCam), Cyclin D1 (Cell Signaling Technology, Boston, MA), Cyclin E (Santa Cruz), COX-2 (Santa Cruz), and β-actin (Sigma-Aldrich, St Louis, MO). Appropriate horseradish-peroxidase conjugated secondary antibodies (Jackson ImmunoResearch, West Grove, PA) were used at 1:1000 and visualized using SuperSignal West Dura Chemiluminescent Substrate (Pierce, Rockford, IL). Relative band intensity was measured using ImageJ (NIH, Bathesda, MD).

EMSA

3.5 pmol of NFκB consensus oligonucleotide (5′- AGTTGAGGGGACTTTCCCAGGC-3′) (Promega, San Louis Obispo, CA) was 5' labeled with [γ-32P] ATP using T4 polynucleotide kinase (Promega). Nuclear protein extracts were incubated in Gel Shift Binding Buffer (Promega) containing 20% glycerol (v/v), 5mM $MgCl_2$, 2.5mM EDTA, 2.5mM DTT, 250mM NaCl and 50mM Tris-HCl (pH 7.5) and labeled oligonucleotide. In competition experiments, a 100-fold molar excess of unlabeled probe was added before the labeled probe. Reaction products were separated on 4% a polyacrylamide gel, after which the gel was dried and exposed to X-ray film overnight at −70°C.

Supporting Information

Figure S1 SKH-1 and $Hr^{-/-}$ mice contain the same proviral insertion. A) Schematic layout of primer locations and insertion site. B) Using PCR primers designed to intron 5F and intron 6R1 (lane1) yields a product in all genotypes, while primers designed to intron6F, mid intron6R2 (lane2), and exon6/intron6F, intron6R3 (lane3) amplifies only in the WT samples indicating an insertion is present causing the PCR to fail. C) Using *Hairless* specific Hairless primer (ex6/intron6F) and viral specific reverse primers (lane3), products were observed only in the mutants indicating SKH-1 and $Hr^{-/-}$ have the same viral insertion. D) DNA sequencing was performed to confirm the insertion as the same as that found in $Hr^{-/-}$. Black arrow indicates the insertion site junctions.

Figure S2 $Hr^{-/-}$ animals are unaffected by chronic UVB irradiation until 30 weeks. A) At 22 weeks of chronic UVB irradiation, neither WT nor $Hr^{-/-}$ animals show any-signs of tumorigenesis. B) By 30 weeks of chronic UVB irradiation, $Hr^{-/-}$ animals begin to develop small papillomas.

Figure S3 PDTC treatment prevents tumorigenesis and activation of NFκB in SKH-1 animals. A) After 35 weeks of chronic UVB irradiation, SKH-1 animals given only tap water develop tumors with the gross morphology of aggressive SSCs. PDTC treated SKH-1 animals at the same time point develop significantly less tumors that appear to be less aggressive. B) EMSA using samples derived from unirradiated epidermis, non-tumor bearing epidermis from untreated and PDTC-treated animals, and tumors from untreated and PDTC-treated animals. PDTC treatment significantly decreases NFκB binding to target sequences (indicated by black arrow). C) Western blot of IκBα and p-IκBα from unirradiated epidermis, non-tumor bearing epidermis from untreated and PDTC-treated animals, and tumors from untreated and PDTC-treated animals. PDTC treatment decreased p-IκBα expression in the non-tumor bearing skin of irradiated animals.

Acknowledgments

The authors wish to thank Mr. Ming Zhang and the Skin Disease Research Center (SDRC) Core Facilities for excellent technical support.

Author Contributions

Conceived and designed the experiments: HK AC AMC. Performed the experiments: HK AC XT ALK. Analyzed the data: HK AC XT CTL ALK DRB MA AMC. Contributed reagents/materials/analysis tools: DRB MA AMC. Wrote the paper: HK AC CTL.

References

1. Rogers HW, Weinstock MA, Harris AR, Hinckley MR, Feldman SR, et al. (2010) Incidence estimate of nonmelanoma skin cancer in the United States, 2006. Arch Dermatol 146: 283–287.
2. Weinberg AS, Ogle CA, Shim EK (2007) Metastatic cutaneous squamous cell carcinoma: an update. Dermatol Surg 33: 885–899.
3. Kanoh M, Amoh Y, Sato Y, Katsuoka K (2008) Expression of the hair stem cell-specific marker nestin in epidermal and follicular tumors. Eur J Dermatol 18: 518–523.
4. Abbassi MS, Torres C, Achour W, Vinue L, Saenz Y, et al. (2008) Genetic characterisation of CTX-M-15-producing Klebsiella pneumoniae and Escherichia coli strains isolated from stem cell transplant patients in Tunisia. Int J Antimicrob Agents 32: 308–314.
5. Green CL, Khavari PA (2004) Targets for molecular therapy of skin cancer. Semin Cancer Biol 14: 63–69.
6. Brooke HC (1924) Hairless mouse. Journal of Heredity 17: 173–174.
7. Crew FAE, Mirskaia L (1931) The character "hairless" in the mouse. Journal of Genetics 25: 17–24.
8. Howard A (1940) "Rhino," an allele of Hairless in the house mouse. Journal of Heredity 31: 467–470.
9. Snell G (1931) Inheritence in the house mouse, the linkage relations of short-ear, hairless, and naked. Genetics 16: 42–74.
10. Forbes PD, Blum HF, Davies RE (1981) Photocarcinogenesis in hairless mice: dose-response and the influence of dose-delivery. Photochem Photobiol 34: 361–365.
11. Steinel HH, Baker RS (1988) Sensitivity of HRA/Skh hairless mice to initiation/promotion of skin tumors by chemical treatment. Cancer Lett 41: 63–68.
12. Iversen U, Iversen OH (1976) The sensitivity of the skin of hairless mice to chemical carcinogenesis. Cancer Res 36: 1238–1241.
13. Schaffer BS, Grayson MH, Wortham JM, Kubicek CB, McCleish AT, et al. (2010) Immune competency of a hairless mouse strain for improved preclinical studies in genetically engineered mice. Mol Cancer Ther 9: 2354–2364.
14. Stoye JP, Fenner S, Greenoak GE, Moran C, Coffin JM (1988) Role of endogenous retroviruses as mutagens: the hairless mutation of mice. Cell 54: 383–391.
15. Cachon-Gonzalez MB, Fenner S, Coffin JM, Moran C, Best S, et al. (1994) Structure and expression of the hairless gene of mice. Proc Natl Acad Sci U S A 91: 7717–7721.
16. Ahmad W, Panteleyev AA, Henson-Apollonio V, Sundberg JP, Christiano AM (1998) Molecular basis of a novel rhino (hr(rhChr)) phenotype: a nonsense mutation in the mouse hairless gene. Exp Dermatol 7: 298–301.
17. Ahmad W, Panteleyev AA, Sundberg JP, Christiano AM (1998) Molecular basis for the rhino (hrrh-8J) phenotype: a nonsense mutation in the mouse hairless gene. Genomics 53: 383–386.
18. Lan R, Greenoak GE, Moran C (1994) Pyrimidine dimer induction and removal in the epidermis of hairless mice: inefficient repair in the genome overall and rapid repair in the H-ras sequence. Photochem Photobiol 59: 356–361.
19. Panteleyev AA, Paus R, Christiano AM (2000) Patterns of hairless (hr) gene expression in mouse hair follicle morphogenesis and cycling. Am J Pathol 157: 1071–1079.
20. Panteleyev AA, Botchkareva NV, Sundberg JP, Christiano AM, Paus R (1999) The role of the hairless (hr) gene in the regulation of hair follicle catagen transformation. Am J Pathol 155: 159–171.
21. Panteleyev AA, Paus R, Ahmad W, Sundberg JP, Christiano AM (1998) Molecular and functional aspects of the hairless (hr) gene in laboratory rodents and humans. Exp Dermatol 7: 249–267.
22. Zarach JM, Beaudoin GM, 3rd, Coulombe PA, Thompson CC (2004) The co-repressor hairless has a role in epithelial cell differentiation in the skin. Development 131: 4189–4200.
23. Thompson CC (2009) Hairless is a nuclear receptor corepressor essential for skin function. Nucl Recept Signal 7: e010.
24. Muthusamy V, Piva TJ (2010) The UV response of the skin: a review of the MAPK, NFkappaB and TNFalpha signal transduction pathways. Arch Dermatol Res 302: 5–17.
25. Hudson LG, Gale JM, Padilla RS, Pickett G, Alexander BE, et al. (2010) Microarray analysis of cutaneous squamous cell carcinomas reveals enhanced expression of epidermal differentiation complex genes. Mol Carcinog 49: 619–629.
26. Yan M, Xu Q, Zhang P, Zhou XJ, Zhang ZY, et al. (2010) Correlation of NF-kappaB signal pathway with tumor metastasis of human head and neck squamous cell carcinoma. BMC Cancer 10: 437.
27. Loercher A, Lee TL, Ricker JL, Howard A, Geoghegen J, et al. (2004) Nuclear factor-kappaB is an important modulator of the altered gene expression profile and malignant phenotype in squamous cell carcinoma. Cancer Res 64: 6511–6523.
28. Prasad S, Ravindran J, Aggarwal BB (2010) NF-kappaB and cancer: how intimate is this relationship. Mol Cell Biochem 336: 25–37.
29. Casta A, Kim H, Luke CT, Bachelor MA, Engelhard A, et al. (2012) Hairless and NFkappaB Form a Positive Feedback Loop After UVB and TNFalpha Stimulation. Photochem Photobiol.
30. Kim AL, Athar M, Bickers DR, Gautier J (2002) Stage-specific alterations of cyclin expression during UVB-induced murine skin tumor development. Photochem Photobiol 75: 58–67.
31. Zhao J, Jin X, Yaping E, Zheng ZS, Zhang YJ, et al. (1999) Photoprotective effect of black tea extracts against UVB-induced phototoxicity in skin. Photochem Photobiol 70: 637–644.
32. Sun SC, Ganchi PA, Ballard DW, Greene WC (1993) NF-kappa B controls expression of inhibitor I kappa B alpha: evidence for an inducible autoregulatory pathway. Science 259: 1912–1915.
33. Tracey L, Perez-Rosado A, Artiga MJ, Camacho FI, Rodriguez A, et al. (2005) Expression of the NF-kappaB targets BCL2 and BIRC5/Survivin characterizes small B-cell and aggressive B-cell lymphomas, respectively. J Pathol 206: 123–134.

34. Schreck R, Meier B, Mannel DN, Droge W, Baeuerle PA (1992) Dithiocarbamates as potent inhibitors of nuclear factor kappa B activation in intact cells. J Exp Med 175: 1181–1194.
35. Qin JZ, Bacon P, Chaturvedi V, Nickoloff BJ (2001) Role of NF-kappaB activity in apoptotic response of keratinocytes mediated by interferon-gamma, tumor necrosis factor-alpha, and tumor-necrosis-factor-related apoptosis-inducing ligand. J Invest Dermatol 117: 898–907.
36. Hiscott J, Marois J, Garoufalis J, D'Addario M, Roulston A, et al. (1993) Characterization of a functional NF-kappa B site in the human interleukin 1 beta promoter: evidence for a positive autoregulatory loop. Mol Cell Biol 13: 6231–6240.
37. Falvo JV, Tsytsykova AV, Goldfeld AE (2010) Transcriptional control of the TNF gene. Curr Dir Autoimmun 11: 27–60.
38. Xu Y, Kiningham KK, Devalaraja MN, Yeh CC, Majima H, et al. (1999) An intronic NF-kappaB element is essential for induction of the human manganese superoxide dismutase gene by tumor necrosis factor-alpha and interleukin-1beta. DNA Cell Biol 18: 709–722.
39. Guttridge DC, Albanese C, Reuther JY, Pestell RG, Baldwin AS Jr., (1999) NF-kappaB controls cell growth and differentiation through transcriptional regulation of cyclin D1. Mol Cell Biol 19: 5785–5799.
40. Feng B, Cheng S, Hsia CY, King LB, Monroe JG, et al. (2004) NF-kappaB inducible genes BCL-X and cyclin E promote immature B-cell proliferation and survival. Cell Immunol 232: 9–20.
41. Chen H, Yang S, Yang Z, Ma L, Jiang D, et al. (2007) Inhibition of GSK-3beta decreases NF-kappaB-dependent gene expression and impairs the rat liver regeneration. J Cell Biochem 102: 1281–1289.
42. Catz SD, Johnson JL (2001) Transcriptional regulation of bcl-2 by nuclear factor kappa B and its significance in prostate cancer. Oncogene 20: 7342–7351.
43. Kaur G, Athar M, Alam MS (2010) Eugenol precludes cutaneous chemical carcinogenesis in mouse by preventing oxidative stress and inflammation and by inducing apoptosis. Mol Carcinog 49: 290–301.
44. Tang X, Kim AL, Kopelovich L, Bickers DR, Athar M (2008) Cyclooxygenase-2 inhibitor nimesulide blocks ultraviolet B-induced photocarcinogenesis in SKH-1 hairless mice. Photochem Photobiol 84: 522–527.
45. Zhan H, Zheng H (2007) The role of topical cyclo-oxygenase-2 inhibitors in skin cancer: treatment and prevention. Am J Clin Dermatol 8: 195–200.
46. Sur I, Ulvmar M, Toftgard R (2008) The two-faced NF-kappaB in the skin. Int Rev Immunol 27: 205–223.
47. Van Laethem A, Garmyn M, Agostinis P (2009) Starting and propagating apoptotic signals in UVB irradiated keratinocytes. Photochem Photobiol Sci 8: 299–308.
48. Lobrich M, Jeggo PA (2007) The impact of a negligent G2/M checkpoint on genomic instability and cancer induction. Nat Rev Cancer 7: 861–869.
49. Deckbar D, Jeggo PA, Lobrich M (2011) Understanding the limitations of radiation-induced cell cycle checkpoints. Crit Rev Biochem Mol Biol 46: 271–283.
50. Paus R, Muller-Rover S, Van Der Veen C, Maurer M, Eichmuller S, et al. (1999) A comprehensive guide for the recognition and classification of distinct stages of hair follicle morphogenesis. J Invest Dermatol 113: 523–532.

Primary Cilium Depletion Typifies Cutaneous Melanoma In Situ and Malignant Melanoma

Jinah Kim[1,2], Salma Dabiri[1], E. Scott Seeley[1]*

1 Department of Pathology, Stanford University Medical Center, Stanford, California, United States of America, **2** Department of Dermatology, Stanford University Medical Center, Stanford, California, United States of America

Abstract

Cutaneous melanoma is a lethal malignancy that arises spontaneously or via in situ precursor neoplasms. While melanoma in situ and locally invasive malignant melanoma can be cured surgically, these lesions can sometimes be difficult to distinguish from melanocytic nevi. Thus, the identification of histolopathologic or molecular features that distinguish these biologically distinct lesions would represent an important advance. To this end, we determined the abundance of melanocytic primary cilia in a series of 62 cases composed of typical cutaneous melanocytic nevi, melanoma in situ, invasive melanoma, and metastatic melanoma. Primary cilia are sensory organelles that modulate developmental and adaptive signaling and notably, are substantially depleted from the neoplastic epithelium of pancreatic carcinoma at a stage equivalent to melanoma in situ. In this series, we find that while nearly all melanocytes in 22 melanocytic nevi possessed a primary cilium, a near-complete loss of this organelle was observed in 16 cases of melanoma in situ, in 16 unequivocal primary invasive melanomas, and in 8 metastatic tumors, each associated with a cutaneous primary lesion. These findings suggest that the primary cilium may be used to segregate cutaneous invasive melanoma and melanoma in situ from melanocytic nevi. Moreover, they place the loss of an organelle known to regulate oncogenic signaling at an early stage of melanoma development.

Editor: Cara Gottardi, Northwestern University Feinberg School of Medicine, United States of America

Funding: This study was supported by funding made available by the Stanford Department of Pathology (JK). The funders had no role in study design, data collection and analysis, decision to publish, or preparation of the manuscript.

Competing Interests: The authors have declared that no competing interests exist.

* E-mail: seeley@stanford.edu

These authors contributed equally to this work.

Introduction

Melanoma accounts for approximately 4% of skin neoplasms but 80-90% of skin cancer deaths. While the prognosis of disseminated melanoma is bleak, prospects for the cure of locally invasive and in situ melanoma by surgical approaches are excellent. Thus, improved recognition and understanding of the key biological steps that initiate melanomagenesis are critical. However, early stage melanomas can at times be challenging to distinguish morphologically from melanocytic nevi, which are also known aspigmented moles. Accordingly, diagnostic discordance rates as high as 25% have been reported when case series have been reviewed by multiple pathologists [1,2]. Moreover, because between 1 and 2 million biopsies are performed each year to evaluate for melanoma and there exist strong medicolegal incentives to overdiagnose this malignancy, a substantive cost-burden is placed on the heath care system and many patients are subjected to unnecessary treatment, surgical procedures, and disease monitoring. Conversely, missed melanoma diagnoses result in preventable morbidity and mortality. Thus, the continued development of ancillary testing modalities able to identify early events in melanomagenesis is a high priority.

Primary cilia are ubiquitous sensory organelles that coordinate adaptive and developmental signaling by recruiting, organizing, and mobilizing diverse classes of signaling molecules in response to extracellular ligands [3]. Indeed, the growing list of receptors known to localize to primary cilia includes those of the Hedgehog, Wnt, somatostatin, serotonin, PDGF, and EGF signaling pathways [4]. Structurally, the primary cilium is composed of a 9+0 microtubular axoneme ensheathed by a membrane that is contiguous with, but biochemically distinct from, the plasma membrane [5]. The microtubule doublets of the ciliary axoneme are assembled atop and continuous with two of the three triplet microtubules of the maternal centriole. Thus, primary cilia are always found in association with a maternal centriole. Moreover, because ciliary tubulins undergo extensive post-translational modification, antibodies directed towards modified tubulins, including acetylated, polyglutamylated, and detyrosinated forms, can be used in conjunction with antibodies recognizing centriolar proteins to identify primary cilia with a high degree of specificity [6,7].

Defects in primary cilium assembly and function are associated with profound developmental disorders including Bardet Biedl Syndrome, Alstrom Syndrome, and polycystic kidney disease [8]. However, relationships between this organelle, its associated transport machinery, and cancer are just beginning to be explored. In the first thorough study of the fate of this organelle during cancer development, we found that primary cilium assembly is actively suppressed by excessive Kras signaling in nearly all neoplastic epithelial cells during pancreatic ductal adenocarcinoma development, beginning with the appearance of its major in situ neoplasm [6]. However, more recent studies have shown variable frequencies of occurrence of primary cilia amongst the neoplastic cells of basal cell carcinoma, medulloblastoma, and renal carcinoma [9-11]. More historical accounts demonstrate that pituitary adenocarcinomas and ovarian Brenner tumors are ciliated and, indeed, there are examples in which cells appear to have acquired, rather than lost, the ability to ciliate following transformation [12]. Overall, the variation in the behavior of the primary cilium that follows neoplastic transformation may reflect variable requirements for the organelle in the oncogenic signaling pathways recruited by particular tumors and/or the particular cell type that has become transformed.

Interestingly however, pancreatic ductal adenocarcinoma and cutaneous melanoma have similar genetics, both exhibiting increased incidence in kindreds bearing heritable $p16^{Ink4a}$ and other mutations. Moreover, melanoma and pancreatic ductal adenocarcinoma are frequently driven by activating mutations in components of the Ras signaling pathway [13-16] and we have shown that excessive Ras signaling can actively suppress cilium assembly in pancreatic ductal adenocarcinoma cells [6]. Therefore, because primary cilia frequently appear on normal cutaneous melanocytes [17,18], we sought to determine whether a pattern of cilium loss analogous to that seen in pancreatic carcinoma development might permit the segregation of cutaneous melanoma and melanocytic nevi. In this study, we quantitated melanocytic primary cilia in a series of 62 cutaneous cases composed of typical melanocytic nevi, melanoma in situ, invasive melanoma, and metastatic melanoma of known cutaneous origin.

Results

To identify differences in the ciliation status of melanocytes present in distinct melanocytic lesions, we collected 22 cases of melanocytic nevi, 16 cases of melanoma in situ, and 16 cases of invasive melanoma and subjected them to immunofluorescence microscopy. These specimens were costained with antibodies directed towards Sox10, to detect melanocytes [19,20], acetylated or detyrosinated alpha tubulin, to detect the modified tubulins of the ciliary axoneme [21,22], and gamma tubulin or CP110, to detect centrioles and basal bodies [23]. To assess the abundance of primary cilia, we considered any elongated acetylated or detyrosinated tubulin -containing structure in association with CP110 or a gamma tubulin -positive puncta to be a primary cilium. Because cytoplasmic microtubules can also contain modified tubulins [21,22], this consideration ensured that primary cilia, and not cytoplasmic microtubules, were counted. Because tubulin acetylation is not obligate for axoneme assembly [24], it was also important to utilize multiple markers of the ciliary axoneme. Finally, because centriolar microtubules can also contain modified tubulins [25], we considered acetylated or detyrosinated tubulin puncta to represent centrioles and not primary cilia, though we appreciate that such structures may in fact represent extremely short ciliary axonemes. Nevertheless, this strategy was sufficient to identify unequivocal differences in the ciliation status of melanocytes present in the distinct types of lesions under study here.

When examined by immunofluorescence microscopy, we found that an average of 94% (range: 91% - 100%; SD: 3.06) of the Sox10 -positive melanocytes present in any of the 22 melanocytic nevi examined bore a primary cilium (figures 1 and S2). Identical

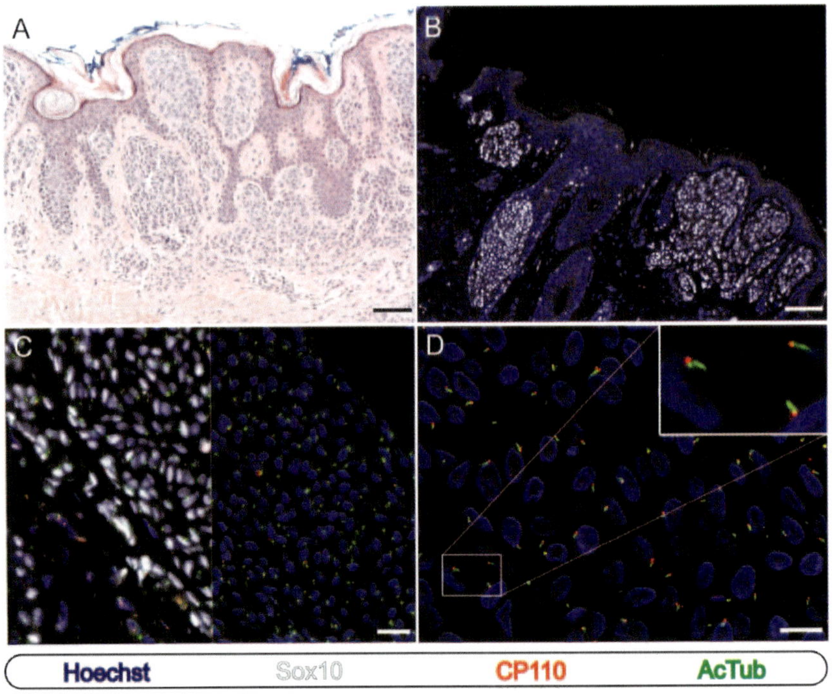

Figure 1. Primary cilia are retained by the melanocytes of typical compound and junctional cutaneous melanocytic nevi. Immunostaining as indicated. (A and B) Low-power images of cutaneous melanocytic nevi stained with hematoxylin and eosin (A) or for immunofluorescence microscopy (B). Scale bars: 100 μm. (C) Split image of nested melanocytes within a melanocytic nevus. Sox10 epifluorescence has been omitted from the right half of the image to enhance visualization of cilia and centriole staining. Scale bar: 50 μm. (D) High power image of nest shown in panel C. Scale bar: 25 μm.

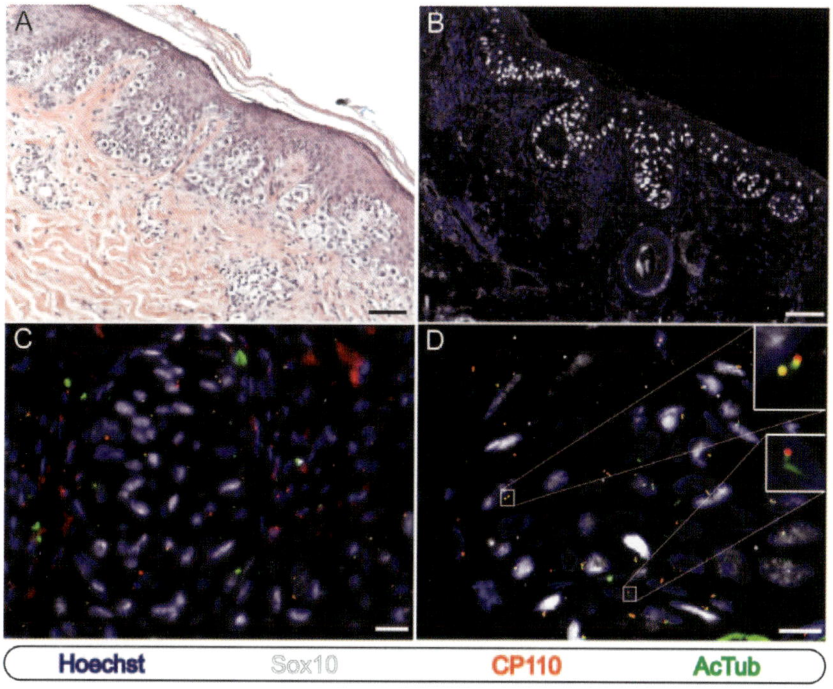

Figure 2. Melanocytes in melanoma in situ frequently fail to possess a primary cilium. Immunostaining as indicated. (A and B) Low-power images of cutaneous melanoma in situ stained with hematoxylin and eosin (A) or for immunofluorescence microscopy (B). Scale bars: 100 μm. (C) Melanoma in situ cells. Scale bar: μm. (D) High power image of melanoma. Upper inset: Sox10 positive melanoma in situ cell showing absence of ciliated centrioles. Lower inset: Sox10 negative cell with ciliated centriole.

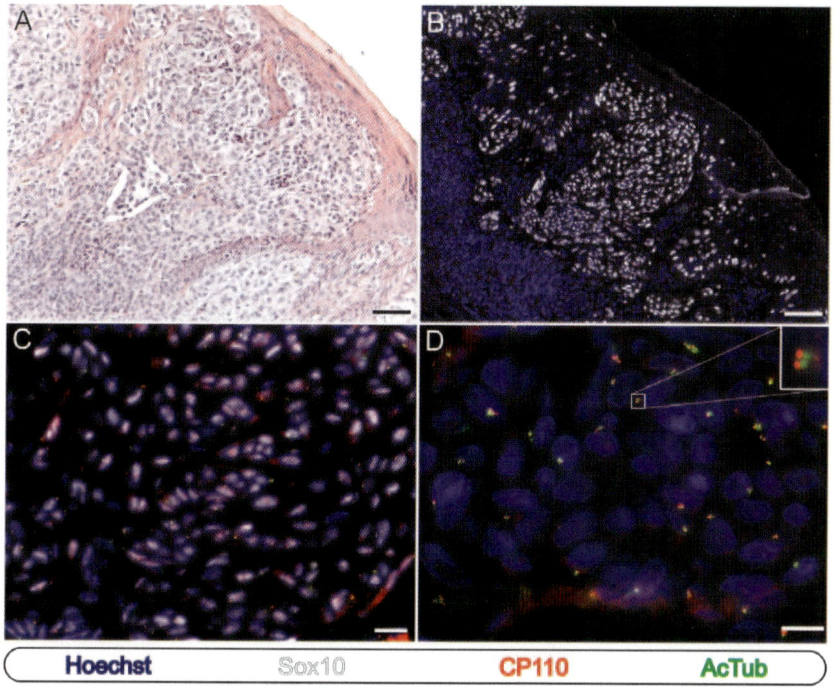

Figure 3. Melanocytes in invasive melanoma frequently fail to possess a primary cilium. Immunostaining as indicated. (A and B) Low-power images of invasive cutaneous melanoma stained with hematoxylin and eosin (A) or for immunofluorescence microscopy (B). Scale bars: 100 μm. (C) Invasive melanoma cells. Scale bar: 50 μm. (D) High power image of invasive melanoma. Upper inset: Invasive melanoma cell showing absence of ciliated centrioles.

results were obtained regardless of whether detyrosinated or acetylated tubulin antibodies were utilized (figure S1). We also identified primary cilia on non-melanocytic Sox10 -negative cells in regions adjacent to the melanocytic nevi in each specimen (not shown). In contrast, when dermal lymphocytes and other leukocyte populations were examined, detyrosinated and acetylated tubulin positive centrioles were observed but never a primary cilium, a finding consistent with the fact that leukocytes as a class have never been observed to ciliate (not shown). Together, these findings highlight the specificity of our staining and scoring system and demonstrate that benign melanocytes are ciliated.

We next examined a set of 32 cutaneous melanocytic proliferations comprised of 16 cases of cutaneous melanoma in situ and 16 primary invasive malignant melanomas. As seen in melanocytic nevi, we observed ciliated Sox10-negative cells (figure 2D, lower inset) and non-ciliated leukocytes (not shown) in all 16 cases, providing an internal positive control for each specimen. In contrast however, an average of 5% (range: 0%–9.5%; SD: 4.3) and 3% (range: 0%–9%; SD: 2.9) of the neoplastic Sox10 -positive melanoma in situ and invasive melanoma cells, respectively, were ciliated (figures 2, 3, and S2). Again, identical results were obtained regardless of whether detyrosinated or acetylated tubulin antibodies were utilized (figure S1). These findings demonstrate a uniform loss of the primary cilium amongst the neoplastic melanocytes of cutaneous melanoma in situ and malignant melanoma and suggest that primary cilium assembly is suppressed during the initiation of cutaneous melanoma.

Primary cilia can be either present or absent during progression through interphase [4]. Thus, we were interested in learning whether the observed loss of melanocytic primary cilia might be due to ongoing cell cycle progression or instead, as an alternative consequence of neoplastic transformation. To this end, we performed Ki67 staining to compare the proliferative and ciliation indices of the neoplastic melanocytes present in each case. Ki67 is a protein that is present in the nucleus throughout the cell cycle, including mitosis, but is absent during G0. Thus, were the loss of the primary cilium to occur as a consequence of ongoing proliferation we would expect the proportion of non-ciliated cells to closely match the proportion of Ki67 -positive cells. In agreement with prior reports documenting the highly variable proliferation indices of melanocytic neoplasms [26–28], we found average proliferative indices of 0.4% (range: 0%–3.2%; SD: 0.89), 8.4% (range: 2.4%–22.2%; SD: 7.0), and 37.4% (range: 11.6%–43.4%; SD: 8.3) amongst our cases of melanocytic nevi, melanoma in situ, and invasive melanoma, respectively (figures 4 and S2). Therefore, and similar to that observed in pancreatic ductal

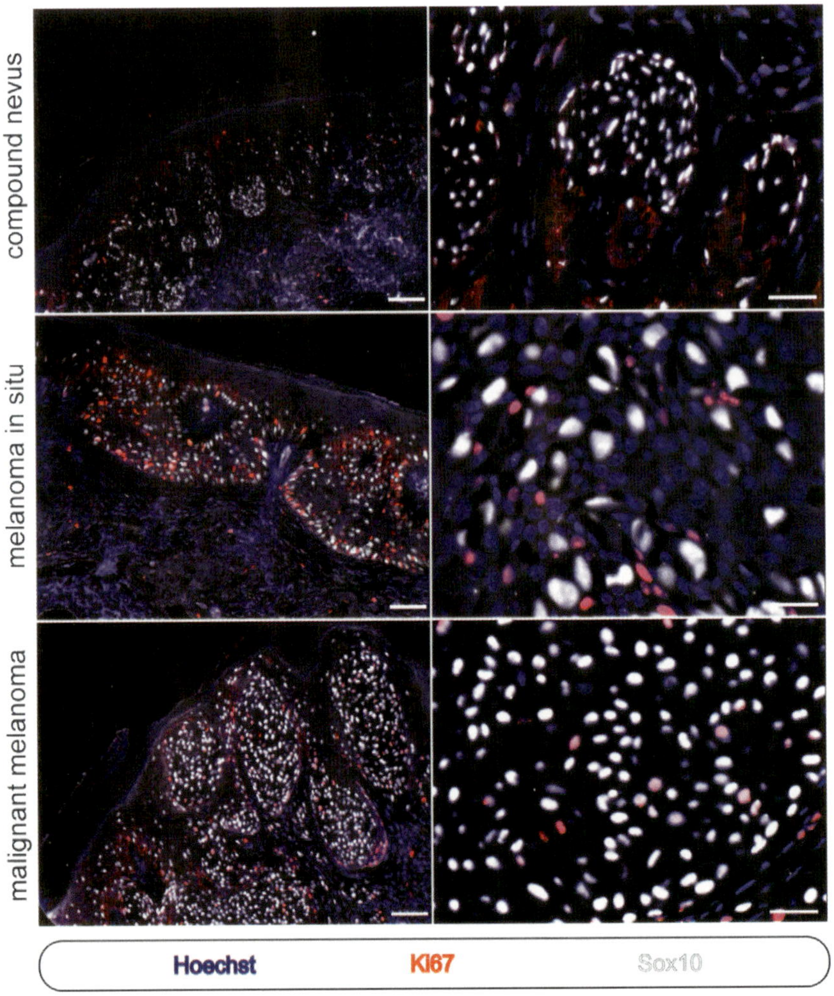

Figure 4. Cell cycle activity within melanocytic proliferations. See text for quantitation and further details. Immunostains and lesion types as indicated. Scale bars, left panels: 100 μm. Scale bars, right panels: 50 μm.

adenocarcinoma, the vast majority of the melanoma in situ and invasive melanoma cells failed to ciliate, while as few as 2% were actively progressing through the cell cycle. Thus, insofar as Ki67-negative cells are not actively progressing through the cell cycle, active cell cycle progression is unlikely to primarily account for the loss of primary cilia observed in melanoma. However, it remains formally possible that recent cell cycle activity could somehow exert a residual negative influence on cilium assembly or maintenance in melanoma cells.

Lastly, we were interested in learning whether the marked reduction in primary cilia seen in primary cutaneous melanocytic neoplasms might be seen in metastatic melanomas of known cutaneous origin. As such, we examined a series of involved lymph nodes from 8 patients with primary cutaneous invasive melanoma. Similar to the in situ and invasive cutaneous melanoma cases examined, we found that few metastatic melanocytes bore a cilium (figure 5). While we noted that primary cilia were slightly more apparent in metastatic lymph node deposits as compared to primary melanomas (figure 5), we did not encounter a metastatic deposit in which greater than 10% of the Sox10 positive cells were ciliated. Thus, primary cilia are substantially depleted from melanoma cells at all stages of cutaneous melanoma development and progression.

Discussion

This study adds an additional chapter to the growing literature describing the fate and function of primary cilia in cancer development. In this study, we determined that primary cilia are strikingly depleted during the development of cutaneous melanoma. By costaining for centriolar proteins and modified tubulins of the ciliary axoneme we have found that, while primary cilia are assembled by nearly all melanocytes contained within cutaneous melanocytic nevi, they are lost from the vast majority of those associated with cutaneous melanoma in situ, invasive melanoma, and metastatic melanoma of dermal origin. Moreover, insofar as at least 90% of the neoplastic melanocytes present in any single lesion studied here were not ciliated while only 2%–43% were actively progressing through the cell cycle as determined by Ki67 immunostaining, ongoing cell cycle progression does not account for the loss of the primary cilium during melanomagenesis. However, it remains formally possible that recent cell cycle activity may somehow exert a residual negative influence on cilium assembly or maintenance in melanoma cells.

Our findings provide an interesting parallel between pancreatic adenocarcinoma development and melanoma with regard to the ciliation status of in situ and malignant cell types and demonstrate clear differences between cutaneous melanocytic nevi and melanoma. However, several important questions remain.

One, at which stage during melanocyte transformation is the primary cilium lost? The natural histories of cutaneous melanocytic nevi and melanoma in situ have proven difficult to characterize and moreover, represent an area of ongoing controversy. Because it remains possible that melanoma in situ undergo a transient ciliated phase, it will be important to examine a larger case series of cutaneous nevi and melanoma in situ in order to determine whether ciliated melanoma in situ or unciliated cutaneous nevi occur. Such studies would help determine whether assays of primary cilium abundance may be developed and ultimately applied to the early diagnosis of melanoma.

Two, while we have examined typical cutaneous melanocytic nevi and melanoma, the more diagnostically challenging melanocytic proliferations include those with with ambiguous histopathological features. These lesions are of particular interest with regard to their ciliation status because they exhibit unpredictable malignant potential. Therefore, we are currently working to

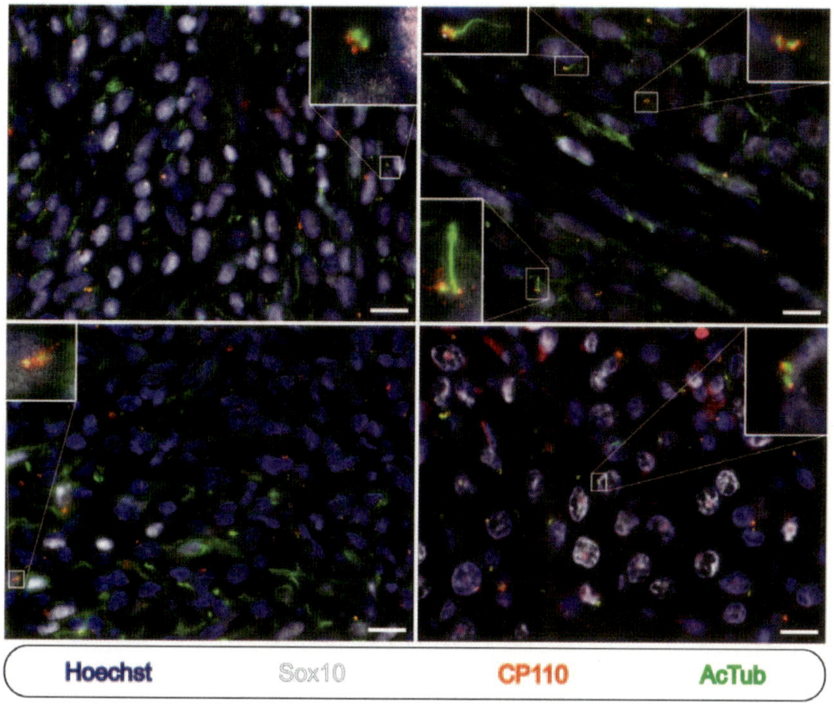

Figure 5. Metastatic melanoma cells of cutaneous origin frequently fail to possess a primary cilium. Immunostaining as indicated. Four separate lymph node metastases of distinct morphologies from 4 separate patients are shown. Insets show ciliated or unciliated centrioles of Sox10 positive metastatic melanoma cells. Scale bars: 50 μm.

determine whether quantitative or qualitative relationships exist between primary cilia, dysplasia, and clinical outcome in the setting of these lesions.

From a biological perspective, the implications of this study are less clear but certainly raise interesting questions regarding the initiation and progression of cutaneous melanoma. While biallelic deletion of genes required for the assembly and function of primary cilia dysregulates pathways important in cancer development [3] and can modify the tumorigenic potency of hedgehog pathway mutations [9,10], the relationship between the primary cilium and the development of cancers not bearing hedgehog mutations is unclear. In this regard, it is interesting that pancreatic carcinoma and cutaneous melanoma thus far appear to exhibit analogous patterns of cilium depletion during their development. While pancreatic carcinoma and cutaneous melanoma are of highly divergent embryologic origin, both are most frequently associated with mutations inducing constitutive Ras pathway activation and both are associated with frequent loss of function mutations or epigenetic silencing of the p16 tumor suppressor. It is likely that comparative analyses of these embryologically divergent cancers may hasten the discovery of the mechanisms by which cilium assembly is suppressed during their development and the isolation of key oncogenic or tumor suppressive functions of primary cilia.

Overall, while additional studies will be necessary to firmly establish diagnostic and biological roles for primary cilia in melanomagenesis, this study demonstrates that primary cilia are depleted from cutaneous melanoma in situ, invasive melanoma, and metastatic cutaneous melanoma cells and places the widespread loss of an important regulator of oncogenic signaling at an early phase of melanoma development.

Materials and Methods

Clinical Samples

All clinical samples were procured according to a protocol approved by the Stanford University Research Compliance Office Human Subjects Research Compliance Panel (FWA 00000935) from the archives of the Stanford Department of Pathology. All patient information associated with this study was obtained in de-identified format and, as such, study-specific patient consent was not obtained. All cases carried a prior pathological diagnosis rendered by a board-certified dermatopathologist and were verified histologically by J.K. and S.D.

Microscopy

7 µm-thick sections were cut, deparaffinized in xylene, rehydrated though graded ethanol dilutions, and subjected to hematoxylin and eosin staining according to standard procedures. Immunostaining was performed as described [6], with acetylated tubulin (Sigma), detyrosinated tubulin (Covance), gamma tubulin (Sigma), CP100 (gift from B.Dynlacht), Sox 10 (Santa Cruz Biotechnology), and Ki67 (AbCam) antibodies used at 1:2000, 1:500, 1:200, 1:200, 1:200, and 1:200, respectively. Alexafluor 488, 594, and 647 chicken anti -mouse, -rabbit, and -goat antibodies were used as secondary antibodies at a concentration of 1:300 each. Slides were then mounted using PermaFluor mounting medium (Thermo) and stored at room temperature. Imaging was performed as described in "Results" using a Zeiss LSM META confocal and an Olympus BX series upright fluorescence microscope.

Supporting Information

Figure S1 Detyrosinated tubulin antibodies show the same pattern of cilium loss in neoplastic melanocytes as do acetylated tubulin antibodies. Immunostaining and lesion types as shown. Scale bars: 20 µm.

Figure S2 Proliferative indices do not fully account for the loss of the primary cilium amongst neoplastic melanocytes. (L) Average ciliation indices of melanocytic proliferations expressed as the percent of lesional melanocytes that are ciliated. (R) Average Ki67 proliferation indices of melanocytic proliferations expressed as the percent of lesional melanocytes that exhibit nuclear Ki67 immunoreactivity. Error bars: Standard deviation of mean.

Author Contributions

Conceived and designed the experiments: JK SD ESS. Performed the experiments: JK SD ESS. Analyzed the data: JK SD ESS. Contributed reagents/materials/analysis tools: JK SD ESS. Wrote the paper: ESS. Edited and approved manuscript: JK SD.

References

1. Lodha S, Saggar S, Celebi JT, Silvers DN (2008) Discordance in the histopathologic diagnosis of difficult melanocytic neoplasms in the clinical setting. J Cutan Pathol 35: 349–352.
2. Farmer ER, Gonin R, Hanna MP (1996) Discordance in the histopathologic diagnosis of melanoma and melanocytic nevi between expert pathologists. Hum Pathol 27: 528–531.
3. Seeley ES, Nachury MV (2009) Constructing and deconstructing roles for the primary cilium in tissue architecture and cancer. Methods Cell Biol 94: 299–313.
4. Seeley ES, Nachury MV (2010) The perennial organelle: assembly and disassembly of the primary cilium. J Cell Sci 123: 511–518.
5. Nachury MV, Seeley ES, Jin H (2010) Trafficking to the ciliary membrane: how to get across the periciliary diffusion barrier? Annu Rev Cell Dev Biol 26: 59–87.
6. Seeley ES, Carrière C, Goetze T, Longnecker DS, Korc M (2009) Pancreatic cancer and precursor pancreatic intraepithelial neoplasia lesions are devoid of primary cilia. Cancer Res 69: 422–430.
7. Shida T, Cueva JG, Xu Z, Goodman MB, Nachury MV (2010) The major {alpha}-tubulin K40 acetyltransferase {alpha}TAT1 promotes rapid ciliogenesis and efficient mechanosensation. Proc Natl Acad Sci U S A.
8. Badano JL, Mitsuma N, Beales PL, Katsanis N (2006) The ciliopathies: an emerging class of human genetic disorders. Annu Rev Genomics Hum Genet 7: 125–148.
9. Wong SY, Seol AD, So P-LL, Ermilov AN, Bichakjian CK, et al. (2009) Primary cilia can both mediate and suppress Hedgehog pathway-dependent tumorigenesis. Nat Med.
10. Han Y-GG, Kim HJ, Dlugosz AA, Ellison DW, Gilbertson RJ, et al. (2009) Dual and opposing roles of primary cilia in medulloblastoma development. Nat Med.
11. Schraml P, Frew IJ, Thoma CR, Boysen G, Struckmann K, et al. (2009) Sporadic clear cell renal cell carcinoma but not the papillary type is characterized by severely reduced frequency of primary cilia. Mod Pathol 22: 31–36.
12. Wheatley DN (1995) Primary cilia in normal and pathological tissues. Pathobiology 63: 222–38.
13. Bartsch DK, Langer P, Habbe N, Matthäi E, Chaloupka B, et al. (2010) Clinical and genetic analysis of 18 pancreatic carcinoma/melanoma-prone families. Clin Genet 77: 333–341.
14. de Snoo FA, Bishop DT, Bergman W, van Leeuwen I, van der Drift C, et al. (2008) Increased risk of cancer other than melanoma in CDKN2A founder mutation (p16-Leiden)-positive melanoma families. Clin Cancer Res 14: 7151–7157.
15. Davies H, Bignell GR, Cox C, Stephens P, Edkins S, et al. (2002) Mutations of the BRAF.
16. Almoguera C, Shibata D, Forrester K, Martin J, Arnheim N, et al. (1988) Most human carcinomas of the exocrine pancreas contain mutant c-K-ras genes. Cell 53: 549–554.
17. Warfvinge K, Elofsson R (1988) Single modified cilia displayed by cells of human internal stratified epithelia (oral cavity, vagina). Cell Tissue Res 251: 237–41.
18. Warfvinge K (1995) Single cilia in human epidermis are susceptible to challenge. Acta Derm Venereol 75: 446–8.

19. Bakos RM, Maier T, Besch R, Mestel DS, Ruzicka T, et al. (2010) Nestin and SOX9 and SOX10 transcription factors are coexpressed in melanoma. Exp Dermatol 19: e89–e94.
20. Ramos-Herberth FI, Karamchandani J, Kim J, Dadras SS (2010) SOX10 immunostaining distinguishes desmoplastic melanoma from excision scar. J Cutan Pathol 37: 944–952.
21. Piperno G, LeDizet M, Chang XJ (1987) Microtubules containing acetylated alpha-tubulin in mammalian cells in culture. J Cell Biol 104: 289–302.
22. Cambray-Deakin MA, Burgoyne RD (1987) Acetylated and detyrosinated alpha-tubulins are co-localized in stable microtubules in rat meningeal fibroblasts. Cell Motil Cytoskeleton 8: 284–291.
23. Chen Z, Indjeian VB, McManus M, Wang L, Dynlacht BD (2002) CP110, a cell cycle-dependent CDK substrate, regulates centrosome duplication in human cells. Dev Cell 3: 339–350.
24. Roth KE, Rieder CL, Bowser SS (1988) Flexible-substratum technique for viewing cells from the side: some in vivo properties of primary (9+0) cilia in cultured kidney epithelia. J Cell Sci 89 (Pt 4): 457–466.
25. Singla V, Romaguera-Ros M, Garcia-Verdugo JM, Reiter JF (2010) Ofd1, a human disease gene, regulates the length and distal structure of centrioles. Dev Cell 18: 410–424.
26. Li LX, Crotty KA, McCarthy SW, Palmer AA, Kril JJ (2000) A zonal comparison of MIB1-Ki67 immunoreactivity in benign and malignant melanocytic lesions. Am J Dermatopathol 22: 489–495.
27. Nasr MR, El-Zammar O (2008) Comparison of pHH3, Ki-67, and survivin immunoreactivity in benign and malignant melanocytic lesions. Am J Dermatopathol 30: 117–122.
28. Ohsie SJ, Sarantopoulos GP, Cochran AJ, Binder SW (2008) Immunohistochemical characteristics of melanoma. J Cutan Pathol 35: 433–444.

Tumour Microenvironments Induce Expression of Urokinase Plasminogen Activator Receptor (uPAR) and Concomitant Activation of Gelatinolytic Enzymes

Synnøve Magnussen[1]*, Elin Hadler-Olsen[1], Nadezhda Latysheva[1], Emma Pirila[2], Sonja E. Steigen[1,4], Robert Hanes[1], Tuula Salo[2,3], Jan-Olof Winberg[1], Lars Uhlin-Hansen[1,4], Gunbjørg Svineng[1]

1 Department of Medical Biology, Faculty of Health Sciences, UiT - The Arctic University of Norway, Tromsø, Norway, **2** Department of Diagnostics and Oral Medicine, Institute of Dentistry, University of Oulu, and Medical Research Center, Oulu University Hospital, Oulu, Finland, **3** Institute of Dentistry, University of Helsinki, Helsinki, Finland, **4** Diagnostic Clinic - Department of Clinical Pathology, University Hospital of North Norway, Tromsø, Norway

Abstract

Background: The urokinase plasminogen activator receptor (uPAR) is associated with poor prognosis in oral squamous cell carcinoma (OSCC), and increased expression of uPAR is often found at the invasive tumour front. The aim of the current study was to elucidate the role of uPAR in invasion and metastasis of OSCC, and the effects of various tumour microenvironments in these processes. Furthermore, we wanted to study whether the cells' expression level of uPAR affected the activity of gelatinolytic enzymes.

Methods: The *Plaur* gene was both overexpressed and knocked-down in the murine OSCC cell line AT84. Tongue and skin tumours were established in syngeneic mice, and cells were also studied in an *ex vivo* leiomyoma invasion model. Soluble factors derived from leiomyoma tissue, as well as purified extracellular matrix (ECM) proteins, were assessed for their ability to affect uPAR expression, glycosylation and cleavage. Activity of gelatinolytic enzymes in the tissues were assessed by *in situ* zymography.

Results: We found that increased levels of uPAR did not induce tumour invasion or metastasis. However, cells expressing low endogenous levels of uPAR *in vitro* up-regulated uPAR expression both in tongue, skin and leiomyoma tissue. Various ECM proteins had no effect on uPAR expression, while soluble factors originating from the leiomyoma tissue increased both the expression and glycosylation of uPAR, and possibly also affected the proteolytic processing of uPAR. Tumours with high levels of uPAR, as well as cells invading leiomyoma tissue with up-regulated uPAR expression, all displayed enhanced activity of gelatinolytic enzymes.

Conclusions: Although high levels of uPAR are not sufficient to induce invasion and metastasis, the activity of gelatinolytic enzymes was increased. Furthermore, several tumour microenvironments have the capacity to induce up-regulation of uPAR expression, and soluble factors in the tumour microenvironment may have an important role in the regulation of posttranslational modification of uPAR.

Editor: Nikos K. Karamanos, University of Patras, Greece

Funding: This work was supported by grants from the North Norwegian Regional Health Authorities, The Norwegian Cancer Society, The Erna and Olav Aakre Foundation for Cancer Research, and The University of Tromsø. The funders had no role in study design, data collection and analysis, decision to publish, or preparation of the manuscript.

Competing Interests: The authors have declared that no competing interests exist.

* Email: synnove.magnussen@uit.no

Introduction

Oral squamous cell carcinoma (OSCC) is the most common malignancy of the oral cavity [1,2], with a poor 5-year survival rate [2–4]. Urokinase-type plasminogen activator (uPA), a member of the plasminogen activation (PA) system, and its receptor, the urokinase plasminogen activator receptor (uPAR), have both been linked to poor prognosis in several cancer types [5–7], including OSCC [8–10]. The PA system consists of plasminogen which is the precursor of the active serine protease plasmin, its two activators (tissue-type plasminogen activator (tPA) and uPA), uPAR, as well as the inhibitors plasminogen activator inhibitor-1 (PAI-1) and PAI-2. uPA is secreted in its inactive pro-form (pro-uPA), and is readily activated in a feed-back-loop by plasmin upon binding to uPAR. uPAR is a highly glycosylated protein consisting of three homologous domains (D1, D2, and D3) and is linked to the plasma membrane via a GPI-anchor [11]. Plasmin functions as a broad spectrum protease that is able to degrade several extracellular matrix (ECM) proteins including gelatin [12], and activate latent growth factors and matrix metalloproteases (MMPs)

[13]. Furthermore, plasmin, uPA, trypsin, chymotrypsin, cathepsin G, elastase and some MMPs are all able to cleave uPAR in the linker region between D1 and D2 [14–17]. This disrupts the receptor's ability to bind uPA [18] in what is thought to be a natural regulation of the uPA-mediated proteolytic activity [19]. Cleavage of human uPAR can also expose the chemotactic SRSRY peptide ($uPAR_{88-92}$) residing between D1 and D2 [20]. The SRSRY peptide can interact with the N-formyl peptide receptor (FPR), FPR-like 1 (FPRL1) and FPRL2 leading to directional cell migration [21–23]. Lastly, the GPI-anchor of uPAR may be cleaved by several phospholipases, releasing the soluble form of uPAR (suPAR), but also soluble uPAR D2+D3 either with or without the SRSRY peptide [17,19,24–26]. SuPAR and soluble cleaved forms of uPAR detected in either tissue and biological fluids may indicate an active PA-system and have been associated with poor prognosis in soft-tissue sarcoma, breast-, colorectal-, lung-, ovarian- and prostate cancer [27–38].

We previously observed that low expression of uPAR is associated with a favourable outcome in early stage OSCC [10]. Therefore, in the current study we wanted to elucidate the role of uPAR in invasive and metastatic tumour growth, and furthermore study how the tumour microenvironment participates in this process. To this end, tongue and skin tumours were established of the mouse OSCC cell line AT84 expressing either low uPAR levels or over-expressing uPAR. The cells were also analysed as they invaded the tissue of the leiomyoma invasion model [39]. Increased levels of uPAR did not lead to increased invasion or metastasis of these cells. However, the endogenous expression of uPAR was up-regulated in the initially low-uPAR expressing cells at the tumour stroma border *in vivo,* and as they invaded deep into the leiomyoma tissue. Analysis of gelatinolytic activity revealed that cells expressing high uPAR levels had an increased ability to activate gelatinolytic enzymes. When cells were stimulated *in vitro* with soluble factors derived from the leiomyoma stroma, an increase in the apparent molecular weight of the uPAR protein was observed, possibly due to increased glycosylation and/or an alteration in uPAR cleavage.

Together these results show that the tumour microenvironment can affect both the expression and posttranslational modifications of uPAR in the tumour cells, and thereby influence the activity of the gelatinolytic enzymes.

Results

Overexpression of uPAR in the murine AT84 cell line

uPAR expression is often increased in OSCCs at the invasive front [40], suggesting that it may have a role in invasion and metastasis. To better understand the role of uPAR in OSCC progression, cells expressing high and low levels of uPAR were generated. The murine OSCC cell line AT84 [41] was selected for this study, as it expresses low endogenous levels of uPAR in culture (figure 1a), and allowed the use of a syngeneic mouse model with immunocompetent mice. Single cell clones expressing high levels of uPAR were generated, and two clones were chosen for further study (uPAR1 expressing very high levels of uPAR, and uPAR2 expressing moderate levels of uPAR, figure 1a). Two single cell clones containing only the empty vector were selected as controls (EV1 and EV2), expressing low endogenous levels of uPAR as shown by Western blotting (figure 1a). Recombinant soluble His-tagged uPAR (rmuPAR) was loaded as a positive control, which (due to being produced in insect cells) is less glycosylated, and therefore has a lower MW than uPAR expressed by the AT84 cells (figure 1a). Cell surface localization of uPAR was verified by Western blotting of membrane fractions (figure 1b), and with flow cytometry on non-permeabilized cells (figure 1c). *Plaur* mRNA levels (figure 1d) reflected the uPAR protein expression levels (figure 1a), and all clones expressed *Plau* mRNA (figure 1e), as analysed by RT-qPCR. Bands with similar size to recombinant active high molecular weight (HMW)-uPA were detected when the conditioned medium was analysed by gelatin-plasminogen zymography, and not by gelatin zymography, indicating that the clones express similar levels of uPA (figure 1f - full gel images can be viewed in figure S1). *Plasminogen* mRNA levels varied among the clones, with EV1 displaying the highest expression, and EV2 the lowest (figure 1g).

Induction of endogenous uPAR expression *in vivo*

In order to analyse the effects of various levels of uPAR on tumour invasiveness and metastasis, cells expressing either high- (uPAR1 and uPAR2) or low endogenous- (EV1 and EV2) levels of uPAR were injected into the tongue of immunocompetent mice. Tumours were harvested already after 14 days due to rapid tumour growth, although not all mice developed tumours. None of the tumours displayed infiltrative growth and were rounded with clear and defined borders (figure 2a–b). No metastases were detected in lymph nodes, livers or lungs, showing that neither of these clones displayed aggressive behaviour *in vivo* within the limit of 14 days of tumour growth.

Tumours were ZBF-fixed and tissue sections were IHC stained and analysed for the presence of uPAR (figure 2c–h). uPAR staining was mostly seen in the tumour cells both at the cell membrane and in the cytoplasm. To verify the specificity of the uPAR antibody, control experiments were performed where the anti-uPAR antibody was pre-absorbed with recombinant uPAR. IHC staining using the pre-absorbed uPAR-antibody demonstrated that the staining was not due to unspecific binding of the antibody (file S1 and figure S2). Tongue tumours of uPAR1 cells, which in culture express high levels of uPAR, had an average staining index (SI) of 6.25 (out of max 9) and were more positive than tumours of uPAR2 cells (SI = 4.22) (figure 2i) that in culture expressed moderate levels of uPAR. Surprisingly, tumours generated from the EV-cells also displayed a moderately strong staining for uPAR. The EV1 (figure 2e) and EV2 (figure 2g) tongue tumours had an average SI of 3.25 and 4.60, respectively, and were therefore considered to have moderate expression of uPAR similar to uPAR2 (figure 2i). The staining was most prominent in the periphery of the EV-tumours (figure 2e), suggesting that the tumour microenvironment is involved in the up-regulation of uPAR expression.

A similar induction of uPAR expression was observed in the EV-cells when the cells were injected subcutaneously (figure S3), indicating that different types of tumour microenvironments can induce endogenous uPAR expression. The skin tumours, like the tongue tumours, also had clear and defined borders, displayed no infiltrative growth (see figure S3a–b) or metastases. The skin tumours generally displayed weaker uPAR staining in comparison to the tongue tumours with an average SI of 2.44 and 3.90 for the EV1 and EV2 tumours respectively (see figure S3i). This was similar to uPAR2 with an SI of 4.00. The uPAR1 tumours showed the highest SI of 6.38 (see figure S3i).

Knock-down of uPAR expression in AT84 cells

Due to the endogenous up-regulation of uPAR *in vivo*, shRNA was transfected into the cells to knock-down and keep uPAR levels low. Five different shRNA constructs were tested by transient transfection of uPAR1 (see figure S4a) cells. New single cell clones were generated based on the EV1 or uPAR1 cells as shown in the flow chart (figure 3a). As controls, EV1 and uPAR1 cells were

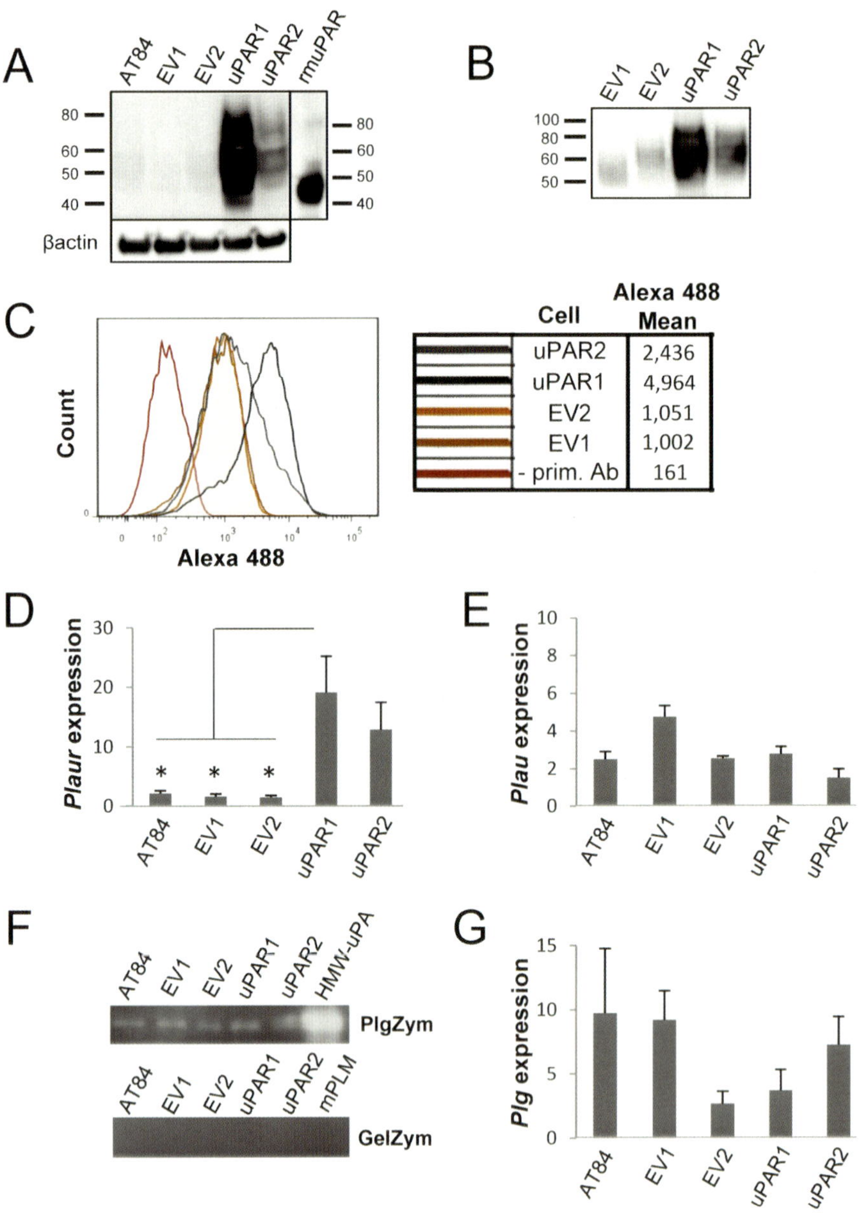

Figure 1. Expression of murine *Plaur* in AT84 cells. *In vitro* characterization of AT84 cells stably transfected with either empty vector (EV) or a vector containing cDNA encoding murine uPAR (*Plaur*). **A:** Western blot analysis of whole cell lysates using a polyclonal anti-murine uPAR antibody (AF534). A total of 7.5 ng of recombinant murine uPAR (rmuPAR) was loaded as a positive control. Re-probing for β-actin was used as a loading control. **B:** Western blot analysis of cellular membrane fractions using a polyclonal anti-murine uPAR antibody (AF534). Total protein was measured per sample and 53.5 μg of protein was loaded per lane. **A and B:** Images were cropped, as no additional bands were detectable. **C:** FACS analysis of non-permeabilized cells using a polyclonal anti-murine uPAR antibody (AF534). Alexa Fluor 488 anti-goat secondary antibody (A11055) was used as the secondary antibody. The quantified mean Alexa 488 fluorescence signal per cell line is presented in the panel to the right. **D and E:** Relative *Plaur* mRNA (uPAR) (**D**) or *Plau* mRNA (uPA) (**E**) expression levels as analysed using RT-qPCR. All expression levels were normalized to the expression of the reference genes *Trfc* and *β-actin*. Error bars represent the standard error of mean (+SEM) and N = 3. One-way ANOVA; $*p<0.05$. **F:** Plasminogen-gelatin (upper panel) and gelatin (lower panel) zymography analysis of conditioned medium of cells cultured for 24 hours in SFM. HMW-uPA and mPLM (mouse plasmin) were loaded as positive controls. The images were cropped to size. **G:** Relative *Plasminogen* mRNA (Plg) expression levels as analysed using RT-qPCR. Error bars represent standard error of mean (+SEM) and N = 3.

transfected with either empty vector (EV) or non-target shRNA (NT). The selected EV1-NT, EV1-sh3 and EV1-sh5 single cell clones all displayed low or undetectable levels of uPAR on Western blots (figure 3b). The selected control cells uPAR1-EV and uPAR1-NT displayed some reduction in uPAR levels when compared to the uPAR1 cells, but a much greater reduction was obtained in the uPAR1-sh3, uPAR1-sh4 and uPAR1-sh5 knock-down cells (figure 3b). A mixed population of shRNA bulk transfected cells (uPAR-sh-B) was also generated, though the efficiency of the uPAR knock-down was less than that obtained with single cell cloning (see figure S4b and file S2). Thus, the single cell clones were therefore chosen for the subsequent experiments.

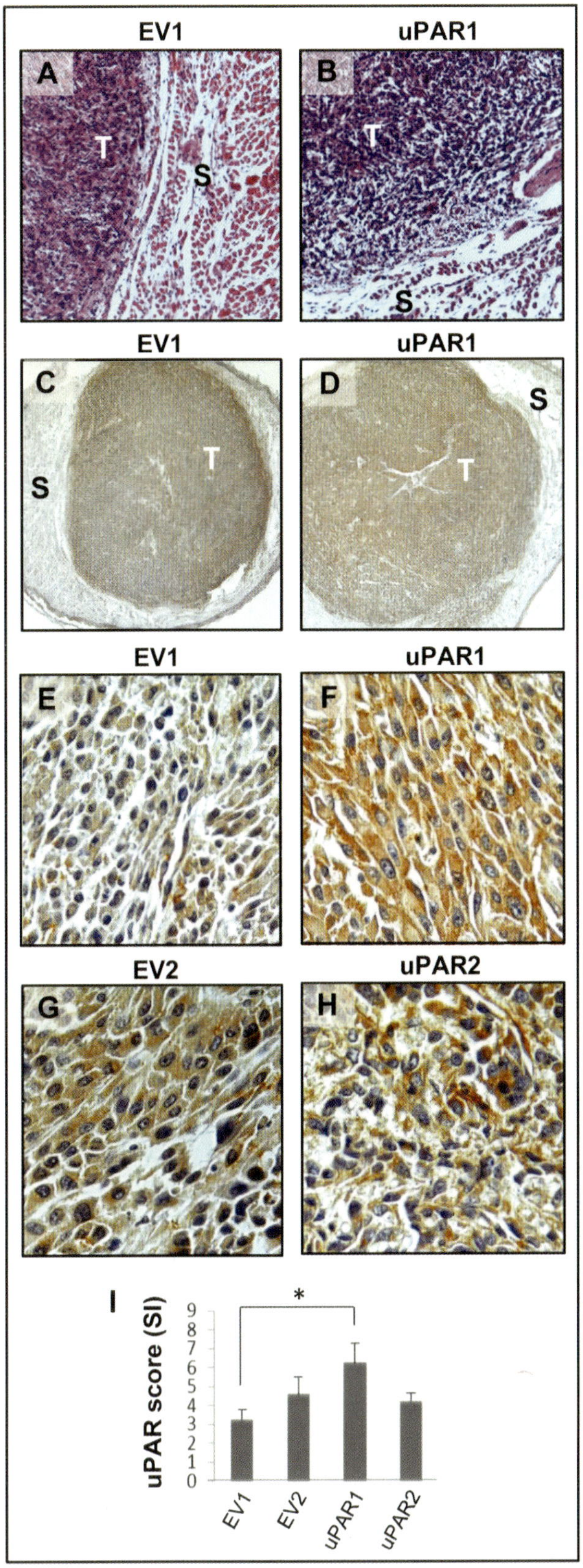

Figure 2. Tumour microenvironment induced uPAR protein expression in tongue tumours. Tumour growth pattern and uPAR protein levels in tongue tumours generated from the EV1, EV2, uPAR1 and uPAR2 cells. **A–B:** Representative images depicting the tumour growth pattern at the tumour-stroma interface in hematoxylin/eosin stained EV1 (**A**) and uPAR1 (**B**) tumours. Images were recorded at 10x magnification. **C–D:** Representative images depicting the IHC uPAR staining of the EV1 (**C**) or uPAR1 tumours (**D**). Images were recorded at 4x magnification. **E–H:** The images show high power magnification (20x magnifications) of the EV1 (**E**), uPAR1 (**F**), EV2 (**G**) and uPAR2 (**H**) tumours IHC stained for uPAR protein. Positive uPAR staining is seen as brown colour, and counterstaining was done with haematoxylin. **I:** The average staining index (SI) of the uPAR staining in the tumours. Maximum obtainable score is 9. The error bars shows the +SEM. N = number of tumours; EV1, N = 8/10; EV2, N = 5/10; uPAR1, N = 4/10; uPAR2 N = 9/10. One-way ANOVA; $^{**}p<0.01$, $^{*}p<0.05$. T = Tumours, S = Stroma.

In vivo tongue tumours of uPAR knock-down cells

Tongue tumours were generated with the new clones in order to analyse the effects on invasiveness and uPAR expression in the presence of *Plaur*-targeting shRNA. For the analysis of the tumours, the EV1-sh3 and EV1-sh5 tumours were grouped together as EV1-sh, and the uPAR1-sh4 and uPAR1-sh5 tumours were grouped together as uPAR1-sh. IHC staining revealed that the uPAR levels were kept low in the EV1-sh tumours (figure 4a). The average SI of the uPAR staining is presented in the graph in figure 4e. The EV1-sh tumours had an average SI of 1.55 and showed considerably lower levels of uPAR than the EV1 tumours (SI = 3.25), and a significantly lower expression than the uPAR1-NT tumours (figure 4b) which had an average SI of 7 (figure 4e). The uPAR1-sh tumours (figure 4c) displayed great variations in uPAR protein expression, resulting in a large standard error of mean (figure 4e). Tumours from the EV1-sh cells (figure 4d), as well as tumours from the control transfected cells (uPAR1-NT) (data not shown), displayed no signs of infiltrative or metastatic growth. Taken together, although shRNA mediated knock-down of uPAR enabled generation of tumours with significantly different levels of uPAR, no difference in tumour invasiveness or metastasis could be detected.

Leiomyoma stroma is a strong inducer of uPAR expression in invading cells

In order to more specifically analyse the effects of the tumour microenvironment on uPAR expression and invasive capacity, the leiomyoma invasion model was used [39]. The human neoplastic leiomyoma tissue is rich in collagen I, -III, -IV, and laminins, and this organotypic invasion model has proven to be a good model for local invasion, mimicking the hypoxic tumour environment [42]. Cells expressing either high- or low levels of uPAR were seeded on top of the leiomyoma tissue discs and incubated for 7 or 14 days, whereupon the leiomyoma tissue was ZBF-fixed. Tissue sections were stained with H/E and total invasion was scored (file S3). No differences in invasion that could be directly attributed to the uPAR expression status of the cells were found (figure S5). In order to determine the uPAR expression levels in the cells invading the leiomyoma tissue, they were IHC stained for uPAR (figure 5). Negative controls, with no added cells, gave no uPAR staining (results not shown). The high-uPAR expressing clones (uPAR1-EV and uPAR1-NT) remained uPAR positive throughout the experiment regardless of whether the cells were located on top or invading into the tissue (figure 5, right panels). In contrast, the low uPAR expressing cells (EV1-sh3 and EV1-sh5) located on top of the leiomyoma tissue remained uPAR negative for the duration of the experiment, while invasive cells gradually increased the uPAR protein levels with time despite the presence of shRNA constructs (figure 5, left panels). Thus, invading cells were strongly induced to express uPAR, further implicating the tumour microenvironment in regulation of uPAR expression.

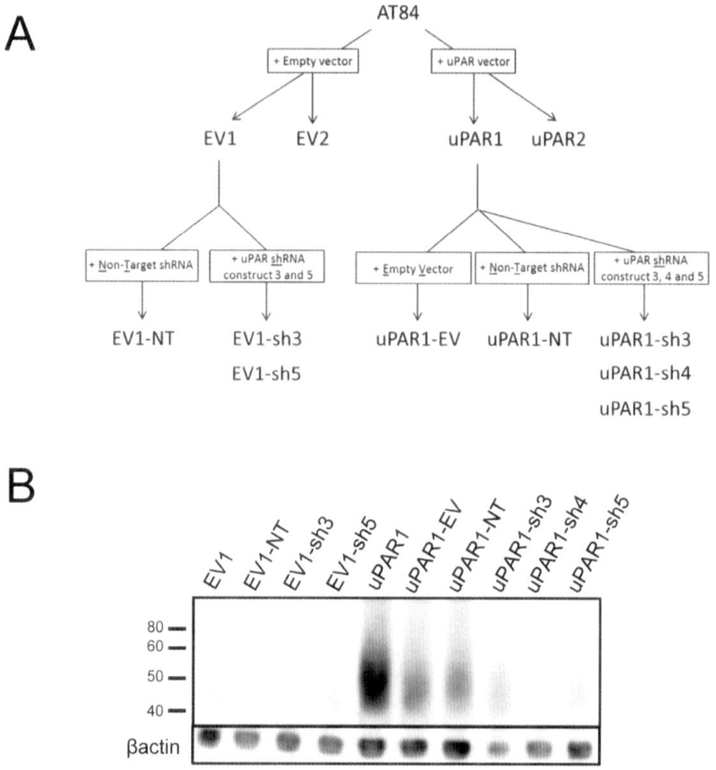

Figure 3. Knock-down of uPAR expression in AT84 cells. shRNA knock-down of *Plaur* in AT84 cells. **A:** Flow chart showing the generation of the single cell clones. **B:** Western blot analysis of whole cell lysates from the single cell clones stably transfected with either shRNA-constructs (shRNA 3 = sh3, shRNA 4 = sh4 or shRNA 5 = sh5) targeting *Plaur* or constructs containing non-target shRNA (NT) or the empty vector (EV). uPAR was detected using a polyclonal anti-murine uPAR antibody (AF534). Re-probing for β-actin was used as a loading control. Images were cropped, as no additional bands were detected in the blot.

Soluble factors from the leiomyoma tissue mediate a time dependent induction of uPAR levels

The up-regulated expression of uPAR seen in the EV-cells could be due to either soluble or insoluble factors present in the tumour microenvironment. Many different growth factors, cytokines and chemokines are known to up-regulate uPAR expression in various cell types [43–46]. To analyse whether soluble factors from the leiomyoma could explain the increased expression of uPAR, the freeze-dried leiomyoma tissue was rehydrated in serum free medium (SFM) which was subsequently used as conditioned growth medium for the cells in culture. After 24 (figure 6a) or 48 hours (figure S6), the cells were harvested and analysed for uPAR expression by Western blotting. uPAR levels were not notably increased in the uPAR1-EV and uPAR1-NT cells, although the size of the expressed uPAR was strikingly increased (figure 6a). Little uPAR could be detected in the low uPAR expressing clones (EV1-NT, EV1-sh3 and EV1-sh5) after 24 or 48 hours of incubation with leiomyoma conditioned medium (LCM). There was, however, a small induction of uPAR expression in the uPAR1-sh3 and uPAR1-sh5 clones after 24 hours (figure 6a). Incubating the cells in LCM for 48 hours induced a marked increase in uPAR expression levels in all the uPAR1-sh cells (figure S6), indicating that these cells more readily turn on the uPAR expression, as also seen *in vivo* (figure 4).

To further test whether ECM proteins known to be present in the tumour stroma could regulate the expression of uPAR, EV1-NT, EV1-sh3, uPAR1-NT and uPAR1-sh4 cells were seeded on different ECM substrates. Western blot analysis showed that none of the substrates induced detectable levels of uPAR in the EV1-NT, EV1-sh3 and uPAR1-sh4 cells (results not shown), whereas uPAR1-NT cells displayed equal levels of uPAR on all substrates tested (figure 6b).

To investigate whether the size change induced by the LCM was due to increased glycosylation, lysates of cells that had been treated with LCM or SFM were deglycosylated by PNGase F treatment (figure 6c). Western blot analysis using the polyclonal anti-uPAR antibody showed that cells treated with either SFM or LCM expressed three distinct bands after deglycosylation (figure 6c, indicated with the numbers 1, 2 and 3). Band no. 1 corresponds to the size previously reported for full length deglycosylated uPAR (approximately 35 kDa). Band no. 2 corresponds to the previously reported size of deglycosylated uPAR D2+D3 (approximately 25 kDa) [14]. Band no. 3 could possibly correspond to either D1 of uPAR or GPI-anchored D3 of uPAR (approximately 18 kDa) [16,19]. Hence, the increased size of uPAR after incubation with LCM was either due to increased glycosylation, or possibly due to less cleavage of full-length uPAR. Analysis of the bands by mass spectrometry revealed that uPAR-peptides were present in both band no. 1 as well as in band no. 2 (results not shown). No uPAR-peptides could be detected in the 18 kDa band. To verify that bands no. 1 and 2 represent full-length and cleaved uPAR, respectively, cells were incubated with the uPA inhibitor BC11 hydrobromide. uPA is reported to cleave the linker region between D1 and D2 of uPAR [14], hence producing uPAR D2+D3. Cells expressing high levels of uPAR were incubated in the presence of BC11 hydrobromide for 72 hours, harvested and analysed by Western blot using the anti-uPAR antibody (file S4 and figure S7). By inhibiting uPA, band

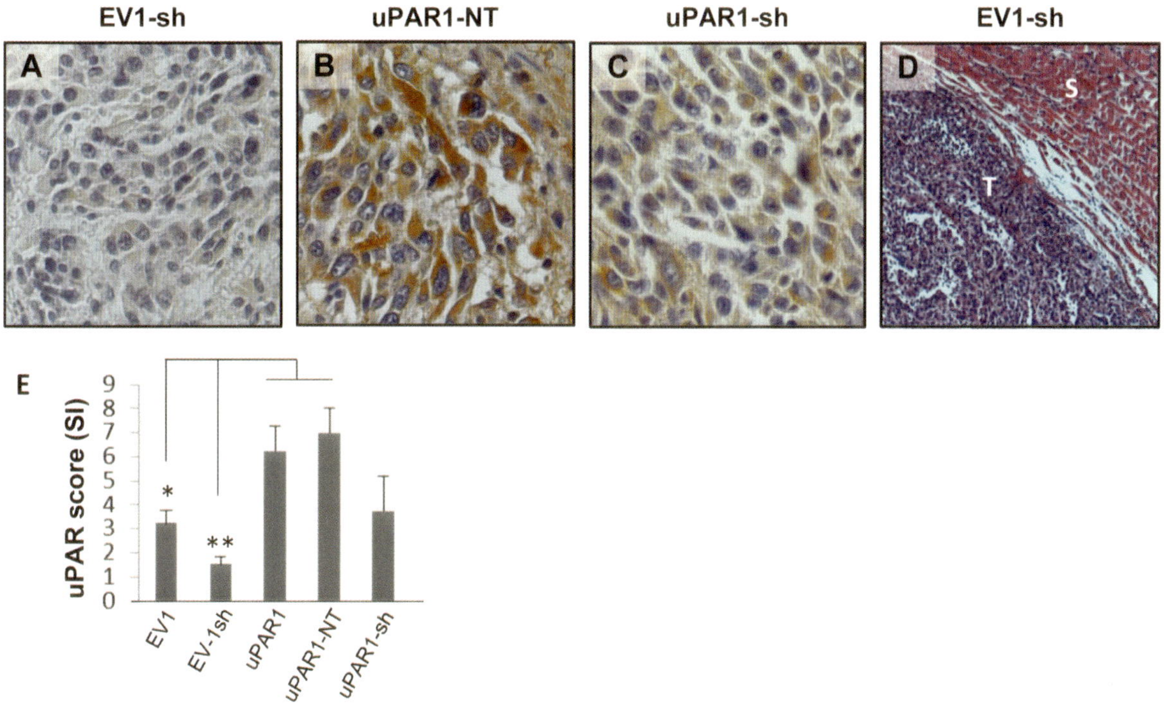

Figure 4. ***In vivo*** **tongue tumours of EV1 and uPAR1 knock-down cells.** IHC uPAR staining and growth pattern of tongue tumours generated from the EV1 and uPAR1 cells containing either shRNA targeting uPAR (EV1-sh and uPAR1-sh), or non-targeting shRNA (uPAR1-NT). **A–C:** IHC uPAR staining of EV1-sh (**A**), uPAR1-NT (**B**) and uPAR1-sh (**C**) tumours, respectively. Images were recorded at 20x magnifications. **D:** Representative image depicting the tumour growth pattern at the tumour-stroma interface in hematoxylin/eosin stained EV1-sh. **E:** The average SI of the uPAR staining in the tumours, with the maximum obtainable score of 9. The error bars shows the +SEM. N = number of tumours; EV1, N = 8/10; EV1-sh, N = 11/16; uPAR1, N = 4/10; uPAR1-NT, N = 3/8; uPAR1-sh, N = 4/16. One-way ANOVA; **$p < 0.01$, *$p < 0.05$. T = Tumour, S = Stroma.

no. 1 became stronger than band no. 2, indicating that the two bands indeed represent full-length and cleaved uPAR, respectively.

Taken together, soluble factors isolated from the leiomyoma tissue induced an increase in uPAR levels in a time dependent manner. In addition, the LCM induced an increase in the size of uPAR probably due to increased glycosylation, and possibly also altered the cleavage of uPAR.

Increased activity of gelatinolytic enzymes at the invasive front

Breakdown of surrounding stroma is a key step in the process of tumour invasion and metastasis. Plasmin, in addition to gelatinases such as MMP-2 and MMP-9, are known to be potent gelatin degrading enzymes. Furthermore, gelatinolytic enzymes have many non-ECM substrates which might have a role in cancer progression. To assess whether the regulation of uPAR expression affects the cell's ability to activate gelatinolytic enzymes, the tumours were analysed by *in situ* zymography. Sections of tongue tumours generated from EV1-sh3, EV1-sh5 and uPAR1-NT were incubated with dye quenched (DQ)-gelatin and analysed by confocal microscopy. The results showed a marked increase in active gelatinolytic enzymes in the tumours expressing high levels of uPAR (figure 7a). Auto-fluorescence was undetectable as assessed by incubating the sections at −20°C for 2 hours immediately after the substrate was added (results not shown). The gelatinolytic activity was quantified using Volocity software (figure 7b), and a statistically significant difference in gelatinolytic activity was found between the EV1-sh and the uPAR1-NT tumours. In order to distinguish between gelatinolytic activity of metalloproteases and activity from other gelatin degrading enzymes such as plasmin, the metalloprotease-inhibitor EDTA was added. EDTA reduced the activity to some extent, though with varying degrees from tumour to tumour (figure 7b). Thus the enzymes contributing to the gelatinolytic activity are a mixture of metalloproteases and non-metalloproteases. Tumours generated from uPAR1 and EV1 cells (figure 2) were also analysed by *in situ* zymography (figure S8). Also in these tumours the gelatinolytic activity was significantly increased in the uPAR1 tumours compared to the EV1 tumours though the difference was not as clear, possibly due to the up-regulation of uPAR in the EV1 cells *in vivo* (see figure 2a).

In addition, gelatinolytic activity was assessed in high- and low uPAR-expressing cells invading the leiomyoma tissue (figure 8). There was no significant difference between the clones, but the gelatinolytic activity was generally stronger in the invading cells compared to the non-invading cells. This is in accordance with the finding that all invading cells showed elevated uPAR expression regardless of the uPAR level of the clones *in vitro* (see figure 5). When EDTA was added, only the gelatinolytic activity of the non-invading cells, where uPAR levels were low, was reduced. Meanwhile, there was no inhibition seen in the gelatinolytic activity of the invading cells which had high uPAR expression. Taken together, tumour cells with increased uPAR levels also displayed increased ability to activate gelatinolytic enzymes.

Discussion

uPAR and uPA have both been linked to poor prognosis for several cancer types, where they are thought to play a role in invasion and metastasis [5–7]. In light of this, the main focus of the current study was to elucidate the role of uPAR expression in

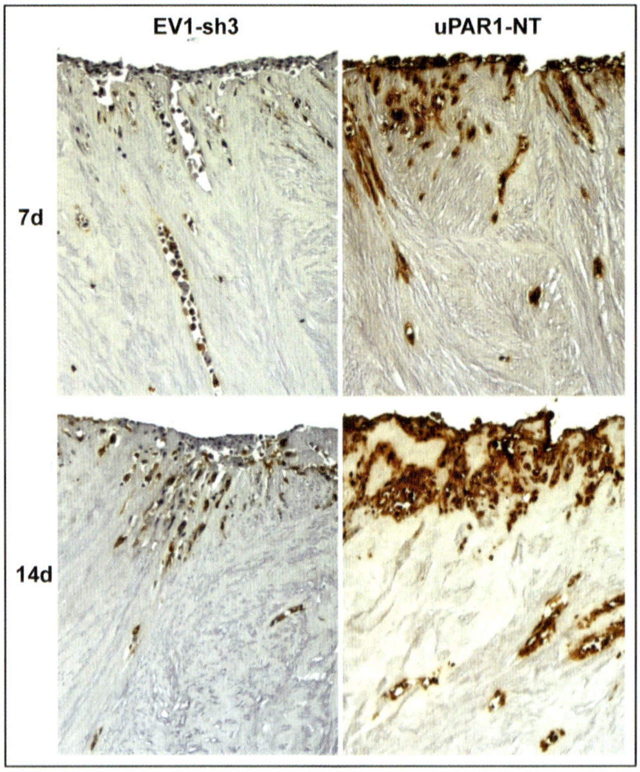

Figure 5. Leiomyoma stroma is a strong inducer of uPAR expression. Representative images of low- (EV1-sh3) and high- (uPAR1-NT) uPAR-expressing cells invading the *ex vivo* leiomyoma tissue. Cells were incubated for 7 and 14 days, as indicated. The tissue was IHC stained for uPAR. Positive uPAR staining is seen as brown colour, counterstained with haematoxylin. Images were recorded at 10x magnification.

OSCC. To this end, uPAR was first overexpressed in the murine OSCC cell line AT84 (figure 1), and cells were analysed *in vitro* in cell culture, *in vivo* as tongue and skin tumours (figure 2 and figure S3), and *ex vivo* when invading leiomyoma tissue (figure 5 and 8). The main finding was that the uPAR levels of the tumour cells did not affect the invasiveness, and that uPAR expression was readily up-regulated by the tumour microenvironment both *in vivo* in the tongue and *ex vivo* in the leiomyoma tissue. Furthermore, we observed that cells with high uPAR expression displayed increased gelatinolytic activity (figure 7 and 8).

Microenvironment induced uPAR expression

Analysis of the tongue- and skin tumours generated from cells expressing low endogenous levels of uPAR, revealed that these cells had up-regulated uPAR protein levels *in vivo* (EV1 and EV2 in figure 2). The IHC staining for uPAR was most prominent in the periphery of these tumours (figure 2c), where the cells were in contact with stromal cells including several types of immune cells. Furthermore, cells invading the tissue of the leiomyoma also showed enhanced uPAR expression (figure 5). These tumour microenvironments are potential storage depots of cytokines, chemokines and different growth factors such as transforming growth factor β (TGFβ), epidermal growth factor (EGF), basic fibroblast growth factor (bFGF) and vascular endothelial growth factor (VEGF) [47–49], many of which have been shown to up-regulate the expression of uPAR [43–46,50,51]. This could explain why the expression is stronger along the tumour-stroma interface, and in leiomyoma invading cells.

Specificity of the anti-uPAR antibody

The uPAR staining seen in the tumour cells was mostly located intracellularly (figure 2), which prompted analysis of the specificity of the anti-uPAR antibody used (file S1, figure S2). As the results showed that the antibody is highly specific for uPAR, the apparent lack of expected membrane staining could be explained by several factors, where uPAR cleavage either partially (inter-domain cleavage) or by complete shedding (cleavage of the GPI-anchor) from the cell surface is one option [17]. Both phospholipase C and D can cleave the GPI-anchor of uPAR [24,26], giving rise to soluble uPAR (suPAR). The proportion of cell surface located uPAR is also regulated by the rate of endocytosis. Both low-density lipoprotein (LDL) receptor-related protein 1 (LRP1) and Endo180/uPAR-associated protein (uPARAP) are involved in turnover of uPAR. Although most uPAR is recycled back to the cell surface, very active endocytosis could eventually deplete the fraction of uPAR at the plasma membrane [52,53]. Thus, the activity of both LRP1 and Endo180/uPARAP could very well influence the cell surface levels of uPAR.

Soluble factors induce altered posttranslational modifications of uPAR

To further investigate whether the soluble factors, such as growth factors in the leiomyoma tissue were involved in the regulation of uPAR expression, leiomyoma conditioned medium was used to stimulate the cells (figure 6a). Soluble factors present in the conditioned medium were able to override the shRNA in the uPAR1 knock-down cells, and gradually increase the expression of uPAR with time. Further experiments are needed to identify the molecular mechanisms for this effect. Interestingly

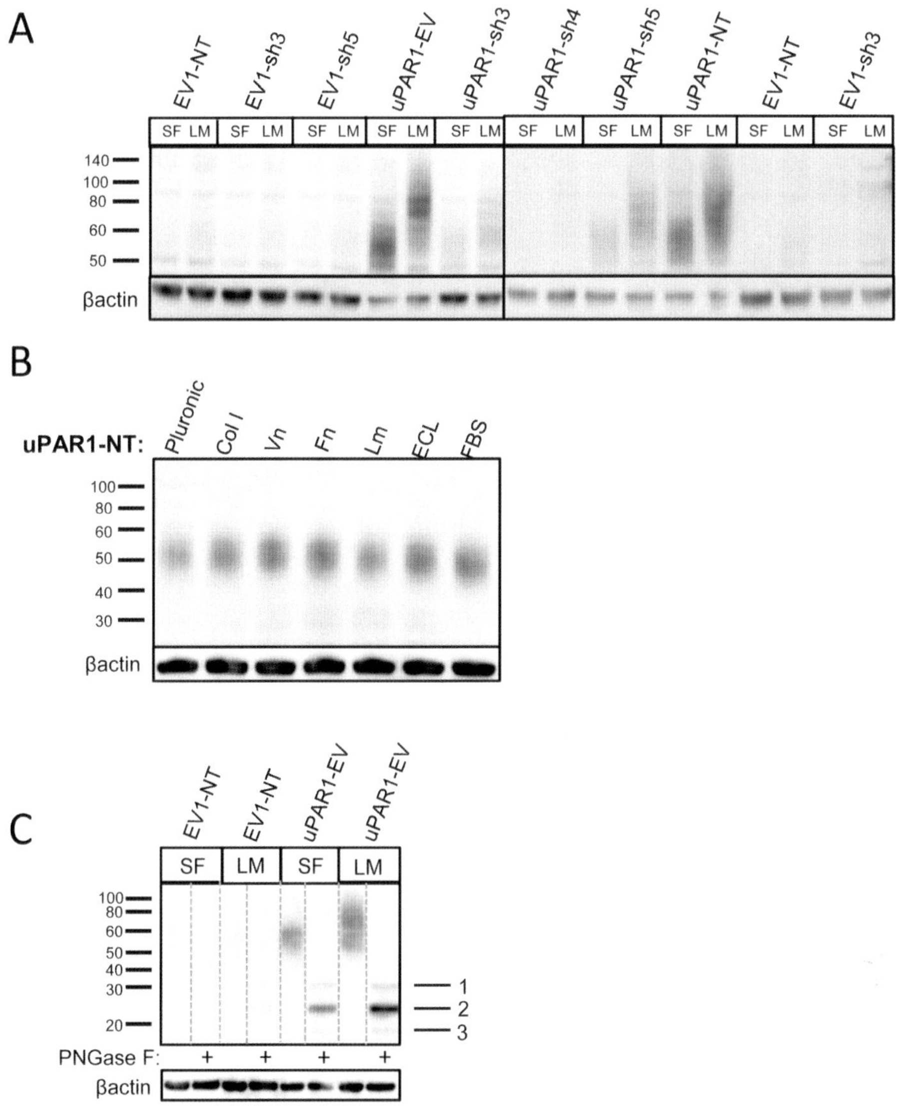

Figure 6. Leiomyoma conditioned medium induced uPAR expression. Analysis of uPAR expression induced by the LCM or purified ECM proteins in cultured uPAR knock-down cells. All Western blots were performed on whole cell lysates, and uPAR was detected using the polyclonal anti-murine uPAR antibody (AF534). **A:** Cells were either cultured in LCM (LM) or serum free medium (SF) for 24 hours. Cells were harvested with sample buffer and re-probing for β-actin was used as a loading control. **B:** uPAR1-NT cells were seeded on different ECM protein substrates, incubated for 24 hours and harvested using RIPA buffer. 7.5 μg of total protein was loaded per lane. Equal loading was verified by re-probing for β-actin. The poloxamer pluronic was used as a no-adhesion control. Col I = Collagen I, Vn = Vitronectin, Fn = Fibronectin, Lm = Laminin, ECL = Entactin, Collagen, Laminin, and FBS = Foetal Bovine Serum. **C:** Cells cultured in LCM (LM) or serum free medium (SF) for 24 hours were harvested using sample buffer and deglycosylated by PNGase F treatment (+) as indicated. Re-probing for β-actin was used as a loading control. The three bands detected by the anti-uPAR antibody are labelled 1, 2, and 3, respectively.

the conditioned medium induced a marked increase in the molecular weight of uPAR when compared to control cells treated with SFM. With five functional, and two potential, N-linked glycosylation sites reported for murine uPAR [54], an alteration in the glycosylation pattern could explain the increase in size. This is interesting as modifications of the glycosylation pattern can enhance uPAR's ability to bind and activate uPA [55,56]. In addition, more highly glycosylated variants of uPAR have been observed in malignant thyroid tumour cells when compared to normal thyroid cells [57]. Different cell types also express different glycosylated variants of uPAR, and the glycosylation pattern can be altered in response to different stimuli, such as PKC activation as shown by PMA stimulation [58]. Ragno et al. [59] also reported that the increased glycosylation of uPAR seen in the thyroid tumour cells rendered uPAR less susceptible to cleavage by uPA, plasmin and chymotrypsin. It has also been reported that cleavage-resistant uPAR is less efficiently cleared from the cell surface [60]. These are all events that could potentially increase the pericellular proteolysis of the tumour cells. Deglycosylation of the LCM treated and SFM treated cells revealed three distinct bands (figure 6c, band no. 1–3), indicating that uPAR was cleaved. Cells treated with LCM displayed more of uPAR D2+D3 (band no. 2), but also to some extent showed more of full-length uPAR (band no. 1). Thus, our finding that a large proportion of the expressed uPAR is cleaved is not consistent with the hypothesis that increased glycosylation protects uPAR against proteolytic cleavage. However, this might be cell type specific since N-linked glycans are known to be very heterogeneous in structure and that

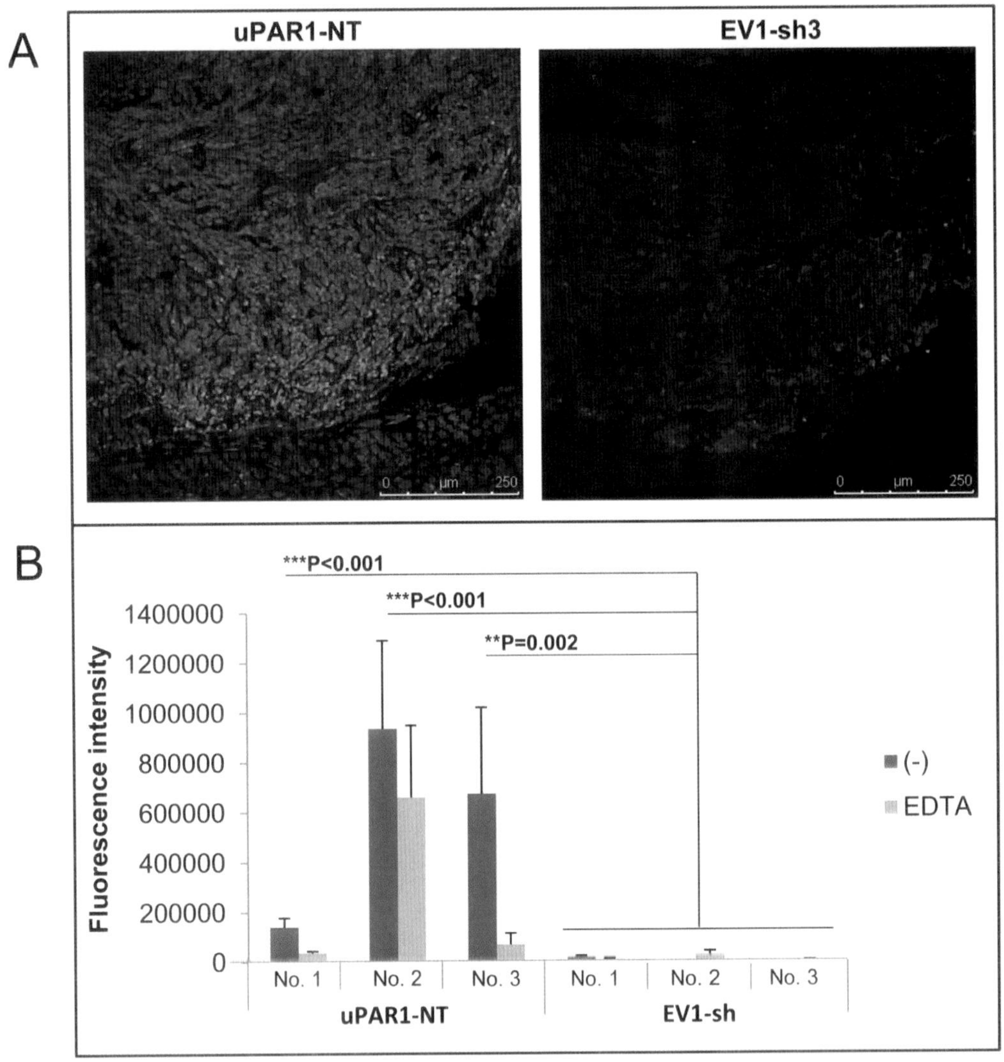

Figure 7. Gelatinolytic activity is enhanced in tumours expressing high levels of uPAR. ZBF-fixed tongue tumours were sectioned and analysed for the presence of gelatinolytic activity using DQ-gelatin *in situ* zymography. Gelatinolytic activity is seen as green fluorescence. **A:** Representative confocal images of tongue tumours generated from the uPAR1-NT cells (left panel) and EV1-sh3 cells (right panel). **B:** Quantification of fluorescence intensity (analysed using Volocity as described in materials and methods) for a minimum of 5 images per tumour, presented as mean values. Three individual uPAR1-NT tumours (No.1–No.3) and three EV1-sh tumours (No.1–No.3) were analysed. Error bars shows the standard deviation (+SD) between the five images analysed. Dark grey bars represents gelatinolytic activity in the tumour sections, light grey bars represents gelatinolytic activity in tumour sections treated with the metalloproteinase inhibitor EDTA. Mann-Whitney rank sum test; ***$p<0.001$, **$p<0.01$, *$p<0.05$.

many proteins exist in various glycoforms in different diseases [61]. Thus, it is therefore still uncertain whether the shift in the molecular weight of uPAR that we observed was due to a change in glycosylation, or whether it is due to increased levels of full length uPAR.

High uPAR levels increases the activity of gelatinolytic enzymes

A stromal-induced alteration in expression levels, glycosylation and/or cleavage of uPAR could potentially affect the pericellular proteolysis of tumour cells. Cleavage between D1 and D2 of uPAR renders it unable to bind pro-uPA, and may therefore represent a natural regulatory mechanism to avoid overactive proteolysis [7]. It might also reflect a highly active PA system, as uPA and plasmin can both cleave uPAR [14]. Whether the expressed uPAR in the tumours or the cells invading the leiomyoma tissue display altered glycosylation and/or cleavage has not been investigated. However, the results obtained using the LCM suggests that such modifications are plausible. When tongue tumours were examined for gelatinolytic activity, tumours expressing high levels of uPAR displayed a substantial ability to activate gelatinolytic enzymes compared to tumours with low uPAR levels (figure 7). Similar results were obtained when the cells invading the leiomyoma tissue were examined (figure 8). Cells invading deep into the tissue had up-regulated uPAR levels and displayed an increased ability to degrade gelatin, hence activate gelatinolytic enzymes. EDTA-treatment of leiomyoma tissue sections indicated that the activity seen in the invading cells mainly originates from non-metalloproteinases such as uPA and plasmin, underscoring a role for uPAR and the stroma in the regulation of gelatinolytic activity. On the other hand other enzymes such as trypsin and cathepsins could also cause the gelatin degradation seen in the tumours and the

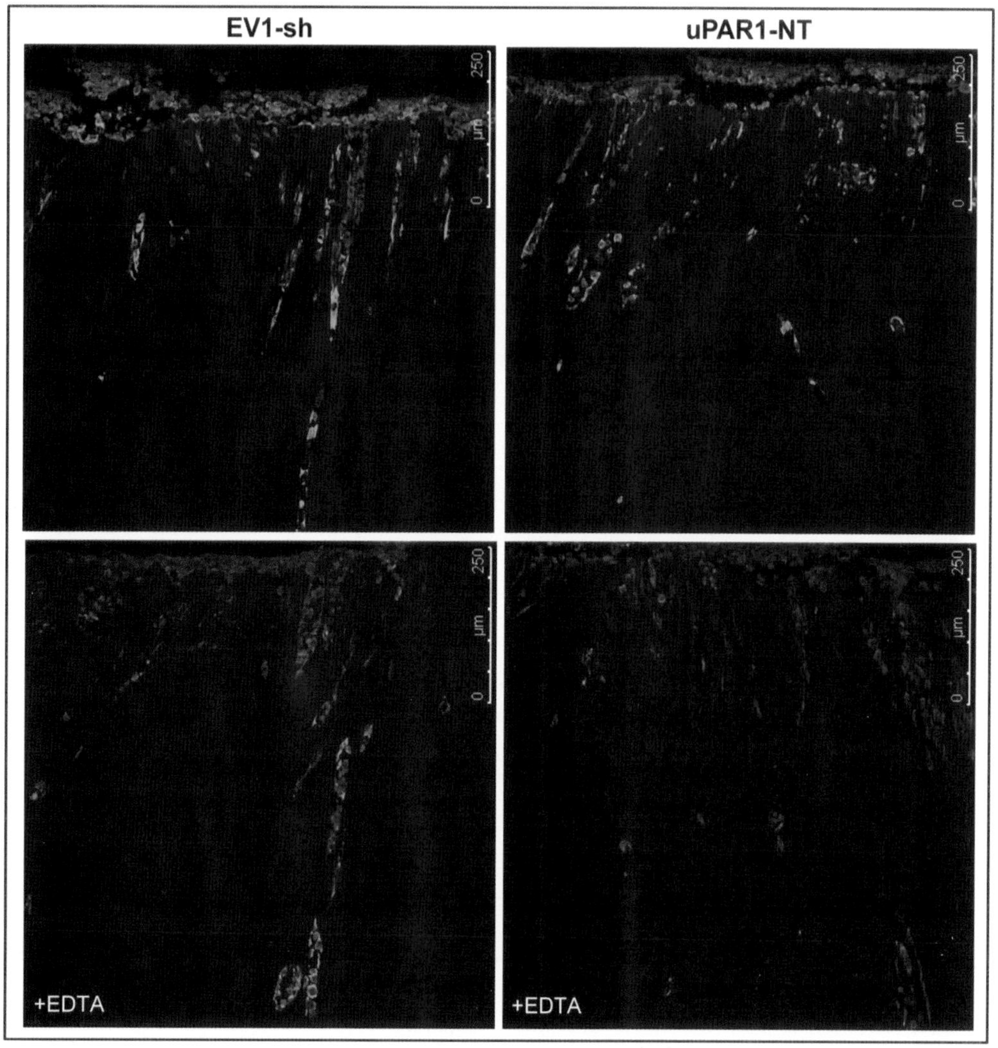

Figure 8. Gelatinolytic activity is enhanced in cells invading leiomyoma tissue. ZBF-fixed leiomyoma tissue was sectioned and analysed for the presence of gelatinolytic activity using DQ-gelatin *in situ* zymography. Gelatinolytic activity is seen as green fluorescence, nuclei are stained blue with DAPI. Representative confocal images of cells expressing either low- (EV1-sh3, left panels) or high (uPAR1-NT, right panels) levels of uPAR invading the *ex vivo* leiomyoma tissue. The upper panels show gelatinolytic activity in the tissue, while the lower panels show tissue sections treated with the metalloproteinase inhibitor EDTA.

invading cells, and further investigations are needed in order to reveal the identity of the proteolytic enzymes involved. Tumours expressing either high- or low levels of uPAR displayed similar growth patterns with few signs of aggressive behaviour. This indicates that the expression of uPAR and subsequent activation of gelatinolytic enzymes is not sufficient to induce infiltrative growth and metastatic behaviour of the AT84 cells in this *in vivo* tumour model. Several in vitro studies have suggested that suPAR could function as an inhibitor for tumour progression, scavenging the active uPA [62,63]. Whether this is the case in our tumour model is an interesting possibility. Thus, further studies on the role of uPAR cleavage and glycosylation in relation to tumour invasion and metastasis formation are warranted.

Conclusions

Taken together, we have observed that the tumour microenvironment is involved in the induction of uPAR expression. Furthermore the increased expression of uPAR, either by overexpression or by natural up-regulation, increased the activity of gelatinolytic enzymes in these cells, however this did not affect the tumour invasiveness in our mouse model. Further studies on the observed effects of the tumour microenvironment on expression and post-translational modifications of uPAR are warranted. Unravelling the biological significance of posttranslational modifications of uPAR, as well as the mechanisms regulating them, might provide answers to why uPAR is often associated with poor prognosis in many types of cancers.

Methods

Ethical statement

The experimental protocol was approved by the competent local authority reporting to the Norwegian National Animal Research Authority, project licence no. FOTS 2598 and 4020/ date of approval 27.04.2010 and 31.01.2012, respectively. All animal procedures were carried out in accordance with the Norwegian Regulations on Animal Experimentation (REG 1996-

01-15 no. 23) and in agreement with European Convention for the Protection of Vertebrate Animals used for Experimental and Other Scientific Purposes (Convention No. 123 Issued by the Council of Europe) [64]. Experimental applications included experimental set-up, rationale for the experiment, and efforts made to refine, replace and reduce the animal experiments. The work is reported according to the ARRIVE guidelines [65]. Use of patient material (leiomyoma tissue) was approved by the Northern Ostrobothnia Hospital District Ethics Committee (statement #8/ 2006 and amendment 19/10/2006), with written informed consent from the donors [66].

Cell culture

The mouse tongue SCC cell line AT84, originally isolated from a C3H mouse [41], was kindly provided by Professor Shillitoe, Upstate Medical University, Syracuse, NY [67]. AT84 has previously been reported as invasive and metastatic when injected into the floor of the mouth through an extra-oral route [67]. Cells were cultured at 37°C, 5% CO_2 in a humid environment in $NaHCO_3$-buffered RPMI-1640 (R8758, Sigma Aldrich, St. Louis, USA) supplemented with 10% FBS (F7524, Sigma Aldrich, St. Louis, USA). For AT84 cells overexpressing uPAR, the culture medium was supplemented with 5 µg/ml puromycin dihydrochloride (P9620, Sigma Aldrich, St. Louis, USA). uPAR shRNA knock-down cells were cultured in RPMI-1640 supplemented with 10% FBS, 5 µg/ml puromycin dihydrochloride (Sigma Aldrich, St. Louis, USA) and 300 µg/ml G418 (G8168, Sigma Aldrich, St. Louis, USA). Cells were also routinely checked for mycoplasma infections.

Cloning and overexpression of mouse *Plaur*

The mouse gene for uPAR, *Plaur*, was cloned using the Gateway cloning system (Invitrogen, CA, USA). RNA from mouse J774 macrophage cells was used as template and *Att*B-kozac-uPARmouse Fw primers (GGGGACAAGTTTGTACAAAAAAGCAGGCTTCGCCACCATGGGTCACCCGCCGCTGCTGCCG) and *Att*B-uPAR-mouse Rev primers (GGGGACCACTTTGTACAAGAAAGCTGGGTTTAGGTCCAGAGGAGAGTGCCTCCCCA) were used to make the Gateway *att*B-PCR product. Entry clones (pENTR/kozac/uPARmouse) were created by cloning the *att*B-PCR product into the pDONR-221 vector by BP clonase. The destination vector pcDNA5/FRT/TO (Invitrogen, Paisley, UK) was modified by replacing the FRT-site and the neomycin cassette with reading frame A (RfA) (Invitrogen, Paisley, UK) and the puromycin resistance gene controlled by the PGK promoter from the pLKO.1 vector (Thermo Scientific, Wilmington, USA), and termed pDest/TO/PGK-puro. The uPAR PCR-product was transferred to the destination vector by LR clonase and named pDest/TO/PGK-puro/uPAR. The pDest/TO/PGK-puro/uPAR, and pDest/TO/PGK-puro as control, were linearized by ScaI restriction enzyme digestion and transfected into AT84 cells using Lipofectamine LTX & Plus reagent (Invitrogen, Carlsbad, USA). Successfully transfected cells were selected in culture medium supplemented with 5 µg/ml puromycin dihydrochloride (Sigma Aldrich, St. Louis, USA), and single cell clones were expanded for further work. Two clones expressing high levels of uPAR were selected and named uPAR1 and uPAR2, and two clones containing only the empty vector and hence expressing low levels of uPAR were selected and named EV1 and EV2.

shRNA knock down of mouse *Plaur*

Constitutive knock-down of *Plaur* was achieved using MISSION shRNA Plasmid DNA (NM_011113, Sigma Aldrich, St. Louis, USA). Five different shRNA constructs TRCN0000088818 (construct 1), TRCN0000294900 (construct 2), TRCN0000294902 (construct 3), TRCN0000362694 (construct 4) and TRCN0000362760 (construct 5) under the control of the U6 promoter of the pLKO.1-neo vector were purchased from Sigma Aldrich (St. Louis, MO, USA). An empty pLKO.1-neo vector (EV) and a pLKO.1 vector containing non-target shRNA (NT) were used as controls. The constructs were stably transfected into uPAR1 and EV1 single cell clones using Lipofectamine 2000 (Cat# 11668-019, Invitrogen, Carlsbad, USA). Successfully transfected cells were selected in culture media supplemented with 5 µg/ml puromycin dihydrochloride and 1 mg/ml G418, and single cell clones were expanded for further work. The selected clones were given names as listed in the flow chart in figure 3b.

Antibodies

Antigen affinity-purified polyclonal goat anti-mouse uPAR antibody (AF534) was from R&D Systems (Minneapolis, MN, USA) and used at 1:100 in flow cytometer analysis, 1:200 in immunohistochemistry (IHC) for 1 hour at room temperature, and 1:1000 in Western blotting. For flow cytometery, the Alexa Fluor 488 donkey anti-goat antibody (A11055) from Invitrogen (Carlsbad, USA) was used at 1:500. For Western blotting, HRP-conjugated anti-goat/sheep (A9452) was used at 1:100.000, and HRP-conjugated anti-β-actin (A3854) at 1:25000 (Sigma Aldrich, St. Louis, USA).

Western blotting

Cells were detached using trypsin (0.25% in PBS with 0.05% Na_2EDTA), counted and seeded according to the specific assay. Untreated cells were seeded in serum-containing medium and incubated for 24 hours. For the ECM protein assay, plates were coated for 1 hour at 37°C with either Pluronic F108NF Prill Poloxamer 338 (BASF Corporation, Florham Park, NJ, USA) and fibronectin which was a kind gift from Professor Staffan Johansson, Uppsala University Sweden, collagen I (#C3867-1VL, Sigma Aldrich, St. Louis, MO, USA), vitronectin was purified from human blood as previously described [68], laminin (Lm) (#08–125, Upstate, Lake Placid, NY, USA), entactin, collagen and laminin (ECL) cell attachment matrix (#08–110, Upstate, Lake Placid, NY, USA), 10% FBS in RPMI-1640 medium, 1:5 dilution of Matrigel (#BS6234) and growth factor reduced (GFR) Matrigel (#BS354230) (BD Biosciences, Bedford, MA, USA). Cells were seeded in serum-free RPMI-1640 medium (SFM) and incubated for 24 hours. For the urokinase inhibitor experiment, cells were seeded in serum-containing medium and incubated for 24 hours. Media was replaced with fresh serum-containing medium with either 10 µM, 20 µM or 30 µM BC11 hydrobromide (#4372, Trocris Bioscience, Ellisville, MO, USA), or no added inhibitor as a control. Cells were incubated for 72 hours and fresh medium containing inhibitor was added every 24 hours. For the LCM-experiment, cells were seeded in serum containing medium. After 24 hours the medium was exchanged either for SFM or conditioned medium (see "organotypic invasion model"). Cell lysates were prepared by removing the culture medium and adding either RIPA buffer (25 mM Tris-HCl pH 7.6, 150 mM NaCl, 1% Triton, 1% sodium dexycholate, 0.1% SDS) with added 1x SIGMAFAST Protease inhibitor (S8830, Sigma Aldrich, St.Louis, MO, USA), or samples buffer (0.05 M Tris-HCl pH 6.8, 2% SDS, 10% glycerol, 0.1% bromphenol blue) and cells were harvested by scraping. Cells harvested with RIPA buffer were added 1x samples buffer. All cell lysates were sonicated and boiled before the samples were loaded onto NuPAGE Novex 4%–

12% Bis-Tris gels (Invitrogen, Eugene, USA), and subjected to reducing (PNGase F treated cells) or non-reducing SDS-PAGE. Recombinant mouse soluble His-tagged uPAR was loaded as a positive control in some experiments (CSI20008, Cell Sciences, Canton, MA, USA). Proteins were blotted onto PVDF membranes (Millipore Corp., Bedford, MA, USA). Blocking was done with 5% non-fat dry milk in Tris-buffered saline (150 mM NaCl, 20 mM Tris, pH 7.4) supplemented with 0.1% Tween 20. Membranes were incubated with primary antibody recognizing mouse uPAR (AF534). For some experiments the total protein concentration was measured using the Direct Detect Spectrometer (Millipore corp., Bedford, MA, USA), and equal protein amounts were loaded per lane. For all experiments, equal loading was controlled by re-probing for β-actin (A3854). Western blotting Luminol Reagent (Santa Cruz Biotechnology Inc., USA) was used for antibody detection, and images were obtained using the Fujifilm LAS-4000 imaging system (Fujifilm, Tokyo, Japan).

Isolation of cell membrane fractions

Cells were harvested using 10 ml ice cold 1×PBS by scraping and spun at 2021×g for 10 minutes. The pellet was re-suspended in 3 ml buffer A (50 mM Tris-HCl, pH 8.0, 5 mM $CaCl_2$, containing 1x SIGMAFAST Protease Inhibitor cocktail (S8830-20TAB, Sigma Aldrich, St. Louis, USA) and 10 mM EDTA). The cell suspension was then homogenized using a Dounce homogenizer, ultra-centrifuged at 50 000×g for 1 hour at 4°C. The pellet was re-suspended in 1.5 ml buffer B (20 mM Tris-HCl, pH 7.4, 8.7% sucrose containing 1x SIGMAFAST and 10 mM EDTA). The suspension was loaded atop a 37.5% sucrose solution and ultra-centrifuged at 100 000×g for 1 hour 4°C. The interface layer was collected and added to 8 ml of buffer B. The suspension was ultra-centrifuged at 100 000×g for 1 hour 4°C, and the pellet containing the cell membrane fraction, was re-suspended in 100 µl buffer A. The total protein concentration was determined using the DC Protein Assay (Bio-Rad Laboratories, Hercules, USA), and a total of 53.3 µg protein was loaded per lane and analysed by Western blotting as described above.

Flow cytometery

Cultured cells were detached with 1 mM EDTA and washed once in RPMI-1640 ^{w}/10% FBS. All subsequent washing steps were performed with Opti-MEM (#31985-047, Gibco, Paisley, UK) containing 1% BSA, and blocking was done with Opti-MEM ^{w}/5% BSA. Non-permeablized cells were labelled using anti-mouse uPAR antibody (AF534) and Alexa Fluor 488 donkey anti-goat secondary antibody (A11055). Cells were subsequently analysed using a BD FACSAria (BD Biosciences, San Jose, USA).

Reverse transcriptase quantitative PCR (RT-qPCR)

Cells cultured in SFM (1.71×10^5 cells) for 24 hours were harvested using RTL buffer (Qiagen, Hilden, Germany) containing 75 mM dithiothreitol (DTT) (Sigma Aldrich, St. Louis, USA). Samples were homogenized using the QIAshredder kit (Qiagen, Hilden, Germany) followed by total RNA extraction using the RNeasy kit (Qiagen, Hilden, Germany). Quantity and purity of the extracted RNA was determined using the NanoDrop spectrophotometer (Thermo Scientific, Wilmington, DE, USA), and RNA integrity was assessed using the Experion automated electrophoresis system (Bio-Rad Laboratories, Hercules, USA). mRNA expression levels were analysed using reverse transcription quantitative PCR (RT-qPCR) on a Stratagene Mx3000P instrument (Stratagene, La Jolla, USA). cDNA was synthesized from 1 µg total RNA using the QuantiTect Reverse Transcription Kit (Qiagen, Hilden, Germany). Target cDNA, corresponding to 10 ng RNA, was amplified through 40 cycles in a 25 µl qPCR mix (RT2 SYBR Green/ROX, SA Biosciences, USA) containing 1 µl Qiagen primer mix (uPAR: QT00102984, uPA: QT00103159, Plasminogen: QT01053332, β-actin: QT00095242, and TRFC: QT00122745). A dissociation curve was routinely run at the end of every PCR to verify sample purity, primer specificity and absence of primer dimers. qPCR cycling conditions: Step 1: 95°C for 10 min. Step 2: 95°C for 30 sec, 55°C for 1 min and 72°C for 30 sec was repeated 40 times. Step 3 (dissociation curve): 95°C for 1 min, 55°C for 30 sec and 95°C for 30 sec. Absence of genomic DNA and contaminants was confirmed by performing no reverse transcriptase (NoRT) controls with every round of RNA purification, and non-template controls (NTC) on each primer set, respectively. For each experiment RNA was purified from at least three biological replicates (N≥3). Reverse transcription was performed on all biological replicates, and each biological replicate was loaded as two technical replicates per RT-qPCR run. When needed, an inter-plate calibrator was used to enable comparisons of different runs. The delta-delta Cq method [69] was used to determine the relative amount of target mRNA in samples normalized against the average expression of the two reference genes *Trfc* and β-*actin*. The numbers are presented as fold differences where the lowest value is set to 1.

Gelatin and plasminogen zymography

Cells were seeded in 96-well plates at 30.000 cells per well. They were incubated overnight and washed three times in PBS before the medium was exchanged for SFM. The medium was harvested after 24 hours and spun down to remove any cells. uPA levels were assessed by gelatin and combined gelatin-plasminogen zymography respectively, as previously described [70]. When analysing plasminogen activators, a final concentration of 10 µg/ml of plasminogen (#528175, Merck KGaA, Darmstadt, Germany) was added to the gel. As controls, purified mouse HMW-uPA (Mr 44 kDa) (MUPA), mouse plasmin (MPLM) (Molecular Innovations, Peary Court, Novi, USA) and a mixture of human proMMP-9 monomer (Mr 92 kDa) and human proMMP-2 (Mr 72 kDa) were used.

Syngeneic mouse model for OSCC tumours

From a pilot study, 10 000 cells were found to be sufficient to produce tumours in both tongue and skin and were therefore chosen for the subsequent experiments, and all efforts were made to minimize suffering. To enable a realistic study of uPAR expressing tumours, compatible with host expression of plasminogen activators, the immune competent mouse strain C3H/HeNHsd (Harlan, Netherlands) was chosen for this study. Cells were detached from culture flasks using trypsin, washed once in serum containing media, and twice in PBS. Cells were re-suspended in 0.9% NaCl to a final concentration of 4×10^5 cells/ml and 25 µl of cell suspension containing 10 000 cells was injected into the anterior part of the tongue or subcutaneously into the flank of six week old female mice (mean 20 g). Mice were anaesthetized with 100–150 µl of hypnorm (Vetapharma, Leeds, UK)/dormicum (B. Braun Medical A/S, Oslo, Norway) depending on bodyweight. A total of 80 mice were used; EV1 and EV2 groups (10 mice per group), uPAR1 and uPAR2 groups (10 mice per group), EV1-sh group (16 mice), uPAR1-NT (8 mice), uPAR1-sh group (16 mice). The control group consisted of 5 mice of which 4 received saline injections, and one received no injection. Mice were euthanized using CO_2 to enable recovery of proximal lymph nodes, at the endpoint of 14 days, or earlier if more than 10% of the body weight was lost during the experimental period. Tongues, liver, lungs as well as proximal and distal lymph nodes were harvested from the mice. In the pilot study, the mandible was analysed for metastasis as this had been reported previously [67], but since no metastases were found here, they were not analysed in subsequent experiments. Lungs, liver and mandibles were fixed using 4% neutral buffered formalin (NBF), while tongues and lymph nodes were fixed using a zinc-based fixative (ZBF) (36.7 mM $ZnCl_2$, 27.3 mM $ZnAc_2 \times 2H_2O$ and 0.63 mM $CaAc_2$ in 0.1 mol/L Tris pH 7.4). Lymph nodes were paraffin embedded, sectioned and hematoxylin & eosin (H/E) stained to screen for metastasis. Lungs and livers were sliced and examined under a dissecting microscope. The invasive growth of the tumour was assessed by a pathologist via microscopic evaluation of H/E stained sections.

Organotypic invasion assay

Leiomyoma discs were prepared as previously described [39]. The discs were subsequently freeze-dried and stored at 4°C until use. All experiments were performed on discs originating from the same leiomyoma. Before use, four leiomyoma discs were placed in 20 ml SFM, and rehydrated overnight at 4°C on rotation. This medium was sterile filtered and kept for further experiments, termed "leiomyoma conditioned-medium" (LCM). A total of 0.4×10^6 cells suspended in 50 μl SFM were seeded on top of the discs, and three discs were used per cell line (N = 3). Cells were allowed to attach and invade the tissue over a 7 or 14 day period, using 10% FBS containing medium as attractant. Discs were then fixed in ZBF, dehydrated and paraffin-embedded. Discs where HSC-3 cells had been added were used as positive controls for invasion, as these are known to invade the leiomyoma tissue [39]. Tissue section of the leiomyoma discs were analysed by immunohistochemistry (IHC). Sections of leiomyoma tissue without added cells were used as negative controls. Images were recorded using the Leica DCF425 camera (Leica Microsystems, Heerburg, Switzerland) and the Leica Application Suite (LAS version 3.7.0, Leica Microsystems, Heerburg, Switzerland).

Immunohistochemistry (IHC)

For analysis of uPAR expression the ZBF fixed leiomyoma discs and mouse tongue- and skin tumours were IHC stained as previously described [70]. The primary antibody was diluted in 5% BSA in PBS. For visualization of the uPAR primary antibody, the Polink-2 Plus HRP Detection kit for goat primary antibody from GBI Labs (GBI Labs, Mukilteo, USA) was used. The chromogen diaminobenzidine (DAB) was used to visualize the secondary HRP-linked antibody. Sections in which the primary antibody was replaced with 5% BSA were used as negative controls and showed no staining. The specificity of the anti-uPAR antibody was verified by pre-absorbing the antibody with recombinant histidine-tagged mouse uPAR (His-uPAR) (see file S1 and figure S2). Tumour sections were scored for uPAR expression, where staining intensity of the tumour cells was set as follows: non-existent (0), weak (1), moderate (2) and strong (3). The score for number of positive cells was set as follows: 0% (0), less than 10% (1), 10–50% (2) and more than 50% (3). The two variables were multiplied giving the final staining index (SI).

In situ zymography

The gelatinolytic activity in the tongue tumours established from the different uPAR expressing clones, and the different uPAR expressing clones invading the leiomyoma tissue for 7 days were assessed by *in situ* zymography. Four μm sections of ZBF-fixed and paraffin embedded tumours were analysed as previously described [70]. The contribution of enzymatic activity from gelatinolytic enzymes that were not metal dependent was assessed by incubating the sections in 20 mM of EDTA (a metalloproteinase inhibitor). Auto-fluorescence was assessed by incubating the sections at −20°C for 2 hours immediately after the substrate was added. Images were recorded using a Leica TSC SPS confocal laser microscope and the Leica Application Suite Advanced Fluorescence software (Leica, Wetzlar, Germany). Confocal images were analysed using the Volocity software (Improvision, PerkinElmer Inc., Waltham, USA). A minimum of 5 images were analysed per section, where a standard protocol was made and used for all images. To avoid background signalling from the fluorescing epithelia, images containing epithelia were cropped so that only tumour cells were analysed. The lower cut-off for intensity was set at 100 and the upper cut-off at 255. The minimum object size was set to 21 μm^2. Read out numbers of mean intensity of the objects and sum of the area (μm^2) were collected. These numbers were multiplied and are presented in graphs as averages per section.

Deglycosylation by PNGase F treatment

Lysates of cells treated with either LCM or SFM for 24 hours was treated with PNGase F (P0704S, New England BioLabs, Beverly, MA, USA) to remove all N-linked glycosylations. The procedure was performed according to the manufacturer's protocol. In brief, 10 μl of cell lysate (see "Western blotting" and LCM-treatment) were added 1x denaturing buffer and boiled for 10 minutes. 1x G7 reaction buffer, 1% NP40 and 0.5 μl PNGase F were added in a total volume of 20 μl and incubated for 1 hour at 37°C. Samples were then analysed by SDS-PAGE and either Western blotting or mass spectrometry.

Statistical analysis

Data are presented as mean values + standard error of mean (+ SEM) or + standard deviation (+SD), specified in the figure legend. The differences between groups were assessed by one-way analysis of variance (ANOVA), followed by Tukey's multiple comparisons post-test. In some cases Mann-Whitney rank sum test was performed, indicated in the figure legend. P-values$<$0.05 were accepted as statistically significant. Graphics were made using Excel, and statistical analysis were performed using SPSS Statistics 19 for Windows or SigmaPlot (SPSS Corp., Chicago, Il, USA). Independent replicates (N) for the different data are presented in the figure legends.

Mass spectrometry

Gel pieces were subjected to in gel reduction, alkylation, and tryptic digestion using 6 ng/μl trypsin (V511A, Promega, Wisconsin, USA) [71]. OMIX C18 tips (Varian, Inc., Palo Alto, CA, USA) was used for sample clean-up and concentration. Peptide mixtures containing 0.1% formic acid were loaded onto a Thermo Fisher Scientific EASY-nLC1000 system and EASY-Spray column (C18, 2 μm, 100 Å, 50 μm, 15 cm). Peptides were fractionated using a 2–100% acetonitrile gradient in 0.1% formic acid over 50 min at a flow rate of 250 nl/min. The separated peptides was analysed using a Thermo Scientific Q-Exactive mass spectrometer. Data was collected in data dependent mode using a Top10 method. The raw data was processed using the Proteome Discoverer 1.4 software. The fragmentation spectra were searched against the Swissprot SwissProt_2011_12 database using an in-house Mascot server (Matrix Sciences, UK). Peptide mass tolerances used in the search were 10 ppm, and fragment mass tolerance was 0.02 Da. Peptide ions were filtered using a false discovery rate (FDR) set to 2% for peptide identifications.

Supporting Information

Figure S1 Full gel images of gelatin- and plasminogen-gelatin zymography. Full version of the cropped images presented in figure 1f. PlgZym = plasminogen gelatin zymography, GelZym = gelatin zymography, mPLM = mouse plasmin, std = standard containing human proMMP-9 and human proMMP-2.

Figure S2 Specificity of the anti-uPAR antibody (AF534). The polyclonal anti-murine uPAR antibody was preabsorbed with recombinant His-tagged mouse uPAR (His-uPAR) before IHC. The antibody-His-uPAR-complexes were removed by precipitation and serial sections of mouse skin tumour tissue expressing high levels of uPAR (uPAR1) were stained. IHC staining with **A**) untreated antibody, **B**) antibody pre-absorbed without His-uPAR, **C**) antibody pre-absorbed with His-uPAR. Sections were counterstained with haematoxylin. Images were recorded at 20x magnification.

Figure S3 Tumour microenvironment induced uPAR protein expression in skin tumours. Tumour growth pattern and uPAR protein levels in skin tumours generated from the EV1, EV2, uPAR1 and uPAR2 cells. **A–B:** Representative images depicting the tumour growth pattern at the tumour-stroma interface in hematoxylin/eosin stained EV1 (**A**) and uPAR1 (**B**) tumours. Images were recorded at 10x magnification. **C–D:** Representative images depicting the IHC uPAR staining of the EV1 (**C**) or uPAR1 tumours (**D**). Images were recorded at 4x magnification. **E–H:** The images show high power magnification (20x magnifications) of the EV1 (**E**), uPAR1 (**F**), EV2 (**G**) and uPAR2 (**H**) tumours IHC stained for uPAR. Positive uPAR staining is seen as brown colour, and counterstaining was done with haematoxylin. **I:** The average staining index (SI) of the uPAR staining in the tumours. Maximum obtainable score is 9. The error bars shows the +SEM. EV1, N = 9; EV2, N = 10; uPAR1, N = 8; uPAR2, N = 4. One-way ANOVA; $^{**}p<0.01$, $^{*}p<0.05$. T = Tumours, S = Stroma.

Figure S4 Knock-down of *Plaur*. shRNA knock down of uPAR in uPAR1 cells. **A:** Western blot analysis of whole cell lysates from uPAR1 cells transiently transfected with five different shRNA constructs. The positive control (pos. ctrl) is non-transfected uPAR1 cells. **B:** Western blot analysis of whole cell lysates from uPAR1 bulk transfected (mixed clones) cells. Cells were transfected with shRNA construct 3, 4 and 5, empty vector or non-target shRNA. **A–B:** Cells were harvested with sample buffer and analysed by Western blotting using the polyclonal anti-murine uPAR antibody (AF534). Equal loading was controlled by re-probing for β-actin.

Figure S5 Quantification of leiomyoma invasion. Cells invading the leiomyoma tissue were recorded for three individual discs per cell line and one invasion "hot spot" was counted per disc. The average value is presented, and error bars show the standard error of mean (+SEM).

Figure S6 Leiomyoma conditioned medium induced uPAR expression. Cells were cultured in LCM (LM) or serum free medium (SF) for 48 hours. All Western blots were performed on whole cell lysates, and uPAR was detected using the polyclonal anti-murine uPAR antibody (AF534). Re-probing for β-actin was used as a loading control.

Figure S7 Inhibition of uPA hinders cleavage of uPAR expressed by AT84 cells. A: Cultured cells were treated with increasing concentrations of the uPA inhibitor BC11 hydrobromide for 72 hours. As a control, cells were cultured without the inhibitor. Cells were harvested using RIPA buffer and total protein was measured in whole cell lysates. A total protein amount equal to 10 µg was either deglycosylated by PNGase F treatment (+), or received the same treatment without addition of PNGase F (−). uPAR was detected using the polyclonal anti-murine uPAR antibody (AF534), and equal loading was verified by re-probing for β-actin. **B**: Different combinations of HMW-uPA (uPA), plasmin (Plm), plasminogen (Plg) and BC11 hydrobromide (BC11) were mixed and incubated for 1 hour at room temperature. The activity of the proteins was subsequently assessed using either gelatin-plasminogen zymography (top panel) or gelatin zymography (lower panel). Lane 1: Standard (std) containing human proMMP-9 and human proMMP-2. Lane 2: Not in use. Lane 3: HMW-uPA. Lane 4: Plasminogen. Lane 5: Plasmin. Lane 6: BC11 hydrobromide. Lane 7: Plasmin and BC11 hydrobromide. Lane 8: HMW-uPA and BC11 hydrobromide. Lane 9: HMW-uPA and plasminogen. Lane 10: HMW-uPA, plasminogen and BC11 hydrobromide. Lane 11: Not in use. Lane 12: Standard containing human proMMP-9 and human proMMP-2. Arrow indicates the position of active plasmin.

Figure S8 Quantified gelatinolytic activity in tongue tumours. ZBF-fixed uPAR1 and EV1 tongue tumours were sectioned and analysed for the presence of gelatinolytic activity using DQ-gelatin *in situ* zymography. The quantification of fluorescence intensity (analysed using Volocity as described in materials and methods) for a minimum of 5 images per tumour is presented as mean values. A total of three tumours per cell line were analysed. Each bar represents the mean fluorescence values from each of the three individual tumours (no.1- no.3). The error bars show the standard deviation (+SD) between the five images analysed for each tumour. Mann-Whitney rank sum test; $^{***}p<0.001$, $^{**}p<0.01$, $^{*}p<0.05$.

File S1 Specificity of the anti-uPAR antibody (AF534).

File S2 Less efficient knock-down of *Plaur* in bulk transfected cells.

File S3 Quantification of leiomyoma invasion.

File S4 Inhibition of uPA hinders cleavage of uPAR expressed by AT84.

Acknowledgments

The authors are indebted to Professor Edward Shillitoe, Upstate Medical University, NY, USA for kindly providing the AT84 cell line. The authors thank Cristiane Cavalcanti Jacobsen, Eli Berg, Bente Mortensen and Marit Nilsen for excellent technical assistance, Peter McCourt for linguistic revision of the manuscript, Roy Lyså at the Imaging core facility (UiT – The Arctic University of Norway) for technical assistance with FACS analysis, Jack-Ansgar Bruun and Toril Anne Grønset at the Proteomic core facility (UiT – The Arctic University of Norway) for the mass spectrometry analysis, and Siri Knutsen at the Unit of Comparative Medicine for guidance and assistance with the animal experiments.

Author Contributions

Conceived and designed the experiments: SM EHO JOW LUH GS. Performed the experiments: SM EHO NL EP SES RH. Analyzed the data: SM EHO NL EP SES RH TS JOW LUH GS. Contributed reagents/materials/analysis tools: SM EHO NL EP SES RH TS JOW GS. Contributed to the writing of the manuscript: SM EHO NL EP SES RH TS JOW LUH GS.

References

1. Funk GF, Karnell LH, Robinson RA, Zhen WK, Trask DK, et al. (2002) Presentation, treatment, and outcome of oral cavity cancer: a National Cancer Data Base report. Head Neck 24: 165–180.
2. Rothenberg SM, Ellisen LW (2012) The molecular pathogenesis of head and neck squamous cell carcinoma. J Clin Invest 122: 1951–1957.
3. Jemal A, Bray F, Center MM, Ferlay J, Ward E, et al. (2011) Global cancer statistics. CA Cancer J Clin 61: 69–90.
4. Siegel R, Naishadham D, Jemal A (2012) Cancer statistics, 2012. CA Cancer J Clin 62: 10–29.
5. Andreasen PA, Egelund R, Petersen HH (2000) The plasminogen activation system in tumor growth, invasion, and metastasis. Cell Mol Life Sci 57: 25–40.
6. Duffy MJ (2004) The urokinase plasminogen activator system: role in malignancy. Curr Pharm Des 10: 39–49.
7. Blasi F, Sidenius N (2010) The urokinase receptor: focused cell surface proteolysis, cell adhesion and signaling. FEBS Lett 584: 1923–1930.
8. Zhang Z, Pan J, Li L, Wang Z, Xiao W, et al. (2011) Survey of risk factors contributed to lymphatic metastasis in patients with oral tongue cancer by immunohistochemistry. J Oral Pathol Med 40: 127–134.
9. Schmidt M, Hoppe F (1999) Increased levels of urokinase receptor in plasma of head and neck squamous cell carcinoma patients. Acta Otolaryngol 119: 949–953.
10. Magnussen S, Rikardsen O, Hadler-Olsen E, Uhlin-Hansen L, Steigen SE, et al. (2014) Urokinase plasminogen activator receptor (uPAR) and plasminogen activator inhibitor-1 (PAI-1) are potential predictive biomarkers in early stage oral squamous cell carcinomas (OSCC) PLoS One In Press.
11. Smith HW, Marshall CJ (2010) Regulation of cell signalling by uPAR. Nat Rev Mol Cell Biol 11: 23–36.
12. Svineng G, Magnussen S, Hadler-Olsen E (2012) Plasmin and the plasminogen activator system in health and disease. In: Karamanos NK, editor. Extracellular Matrix: Pathobiology and Signaling. Germany: Walter de Gruyter GmbH & Co. 261–290.
13. Blasi F, Carmeliet P (2002) uPAR: a versatile signalling orchestrator. Nat Rev Mol Cell Biol 3: 932–943.
14. Hoyer-Hansen G, Ronne E, Solberg H, Behrendt N, Ploug M, et al. (1992) Urokinase plasminogen activator cleaves its cell surface receptor releasing the ligand-binding domain. J Biol Chem 267: 18224–18229.
15. Andolfo A, English WR, Resnati M, Murphy G, Blasi F, et al. (2002) Metalloproteases cleave the urokinase-type plasminogen activator receptor in the D1–D2 linker region and expose epitopes not present in the intact soluble receptor. Thromb Haemost 88: 298–306.
16. Hoyer-Hansen G, Pessara U, Holm A, Pass J, Weidle U, et al. (2001) Urokinase-catalysed cleavage of the urokinase receptor requires an intact glycolipid anchor. Biochem J 358: 673–679.
17. Montuori N, Visconte V, Rossi G, Ragno P (2005) Soluble and cleaved forms of the urokinase-receptor: degradation products or active molecules? Thromb Haemost 93: 192–198.
18. Behrendt N, Ronne E, Dano K (1996) Domain interplay in the urokinase receptor. Requirement for the third domain in high affinity ligand binding and demonstration of ligand contact sites in distinct receptor domains. J Biol Chem 271: 22885–22894.
19. Hoyer-Hansen G, Ploug M, Behrendt N, Ronne E, Dano K (1997) Cell-surface acceleration of urokinase-catalyzed receptor cleavage. Eur J Biochem 243: 21–26.
20. Fazioli F, Resnati M, Sidenius N, Higashimoto Y, Appella E, et al. (1997) A urokinase-sensitive region of the human urokinase receptor is responsible for its chemotactic activity. EMBO J 16: 7279–7286.
21. Resnati M, Pallavicini I, Wang JM, Oppenheim J, Serhan CN, et al. (2002) The fibrinolytic receptor for urokinase activates the G protein-coupled chemotactic receptor FPRL1/LXA4R. Proc Natl Acad Sci U S A 99: 1359–1364.
22. Montuori N, Carriero MV, Salzano S, Rossi G, Ragno P (2002) The cleavage of the urokinase receptor regulates its multiple functions. J Biol Chem 277: 46932–46939.
23. de Paulis A, Montuori N, Prevete N, Fiorentino I, Rossi FW, et al. (2004) Urokinase induces basophil chemotaxis through a urokinase receptor epitope that is an endogenous ligand for formyl peptide receptor-like 1 and -like 2. J Immunol 173: 5739–5748.
24. Wilhelm OG, Wilhelm S, Escott GM, Lutz V, Magdolen V, et al. (1999) Cellular glycosylphosphatidylinositol-specific phospholipase D regulates urokinase receptor shedding and cell surface expression. J Cell Physiol 180: 225–235.
25. Beaufort N, Leduc D, Rousselle JC, Magdolen V, Luther T, et al. (2004) Proteolytic regulation of the urokinase receptor/CD87 on monocytic cells by neutrophil elastase and cathepsin G. J Immunol 172: 540–549.
26. Ploug M, Ronne E, Behrendt N, Jensen AL, Blasi F, et al. (1991) Cellular receptor for urokinase plasminogen activator. Carboxyl-terminal processing and membrane anchoring by glycosyl-phosphatidylinositol. J Biol Chem 266: 1926–1933.
27. Solberg H, Romer J, Brunner N, Holm A, Sidenius N, et al. (1994) A cleaved form of the receptor for urokinase-type plasminogen activator in invasive transplanted human and murine tumors. Int J Cancer 58: 877–881.
28. Sidenius N, Sier CF, Blasi F (2000) Shedding and cleavage of the urokinase receptor (uPAR): identification and characterisation of uPAR fragments in vitro and in vivo. FEBS Lett 475: 52–56.
29. Wahlberg K, Hoyer-Hansen G, Casslen B (1998) Soluble receptor for urokinase plasminogen activator in both full-length and a cleaved form is present in high concentration in cystic fluid from ovarian cancer. Cancer Res 58: 3294–3298.
30. Riisbro R, Christensen IJ, Piironen T, Greenall M, Larsen B, et al. (2002) Prognostic significance of soluble urokinase plasminogen activator receptor in serum and cytosol of tumor tissue from patients with primary breast cancer. Clin Cancer Res 8: 1132–1141.
31. Piironen T, Haese A, Huland H, Steuber T, Christensen IJ, et al. (2006) Enhanced discrimination of benign from malignant prostatic disease by selective measurements of cleaved forms of urokinase receptor in serum. Clin Chem 52: 838–844.
32. Almasi CE, Christensen IJ, Hoyer-Hansen G, Dano K, Pappot H, et al. (2011) Urokinase receptor forms in serum from non-small cell lung cancer patients: relation to prognosis. Lung Cancer 74: 510–515.
33. Almasi CE, Brasso K, Iversen P, Pappot H, Hoyer-Hansen G, et al. (2011) Prognostic and predictive value of intact and cleaved forms of the urokinase plasminogen activator receptor in metastatic prostate cancer. Prostate 71: 899–907.
34. Almasi CE, Drivsholm L, Pappot H, Hoyer-Hansen G, Christensen IJ (2013) The liberated domain I of urokinase plasminogen activator receptor a new tumour marker in small cell lung cancer. APMIS 121: 189–196.
35. Thurison T, Lomholt AF, Rasch MG, Lund IK, Nielsen HJ, et al. (2010) A new assay for measurement of the liberated domain I of the urokinase receptor in plasma improves the prediction of survival in colorectal cancer. Clin Chem 56: 1636–1640.
36. Stephens RW, Nielsen HJ, Christensen IJ, Thorlacius-Ussing O, Sorensen S, et al. (1999) Plasma urokinase receptor levels in patients with colorectal cancer: relationship to prognosis. J Natl Cancer Inst 91: 869–874.
37. Stephens RW, Pedersen AN, Nielsen HJ, Hamers MJ, Hoyer-Hansen G, et al. (1997) ELISA determination of soluble urokinase receptor in blood from healthy donors and cancer patients. Clin Chem 43: 1868–1876.
38. Taubert H, Wurl P, Greither T, Kappler M, Bache M, et al. (2010) Co-detection of members of the urokinase plasminogen activator system in tumour tissue and serum correlates with a poor prognosis for soft-tissue sarcoma patients. Br J Cancer 102: 731–737.
39. Nurmenniemi S, Sinikumpu T, Alahuhta I, Salo S, Sutinen M, et al. (2009) A novel organotypic model mimics the tumor microenvironment. Am J Pathol 175: 1281–1291.
40. Lindberg P, Larsson A, Nielsen BS (2006) Expression of plasminogen activator inhibitor-1, urokinase receptor and laminin gamma-2 chain is an early coordinated event in incipient oral squamous cell carcinoma. Int J Cancer 118: 2948–2956.
41. Schultz-Hector S, Haghayegh S (1993) Beta-fibroblast growth factor expression in human and murine squamous cell carcinomas and its relationship to regional endothelial cell proliferation. Cancer Res 53: 1444–1449.
42. Teppo S, Sundquist E, Vered M, Holappa H, Parkkisenniemi J, et al. (2013) The hypoxic tumor microenvironment regulates invasion of aggressive oral carcinoma cells. Exp Cell Res 319: 376–389.
43. Lund LR, Ellis V, Ronne E, Pyke C, Dano K (1995) Transcriptional and post-transcriptional regulation of the receptor for urokinase-type plasminogen activator by cytokines and tumour promoters in the human lung carcinoma cell line A549. Biochem J 310 (Pt 1): 345–352.
44. Laufs S, Schumacher J, Allgayer H (2006) Urokinase-receptor (u-PAR): an essential player in multiple games of cancer: a review on its role in tumor progression, invasion, metastasis, proliferation/dormancy, clinical outcome and minimal residual disease. Cell Cycle 5: 1760–1771.
45. Yoshida E, Tsuchiya K, Sugiki M, Sumi H, Mihara H, et al. (1996) Modulation of the receptor for urokinase-type plasminogen activator in macrophage-like U937 cells by inflammatory mediators. Inflammation 20: 319–326.
46. Lund LR, Dano K (1992) Okadaic acid strongly increases gene transcription, mRNA and protein level for the urokinase receptor in human A549 cells. FEBS Lett 298: 177–181.

47. Leef G, Thomas SM (2013) Molecular communication between tumor-associated fibroblasts and head and neck squamous cell carcinoma. Oral Oncol 49: 381–386.
48. Moserle L, Casanovas O (2013) Anti-angiogenesis and metastasis: a tumour and stromal cell alliance. J Intern Med 273: 128–137.
49. Smith HA, Kang Y (2013) The metastasis-promoting roles of tumor-associated immune cells. J Mol Med (Berl) 91: 411–429.
50. Siren V, Myohanen H, Vaheri A, Immonen I (1999) Transforming growth factor beta induces urokinase receptor expression in cultured retinal pigment epithelial cells. Ophthalmic Res 31: 184–191.
51. Henic E, Sixt M, Hansson S, Hoyer-Hansen G, Casslen B (2006) EGF-stimulated migration in ovarian cancer cells is associated with decreased internalization, increased surface expression, and increased shedding of the urokinase plasminogen activator receptor. Gynecol Oncol 101: 28–39.
52. Gonias SL, Gaultier A, Jo M (2011) Regulation of the urokinase receptor (uPAR) by LDL receptor-related protein-1 (LRP1). Curr Pharm Des 17: 1962–1969.
53. Engelholm LH, Ingvarsen S, Jurgensen HJ, Hillig T, Madsen DH, et al. (2009) The collagen receptor uPARAP/Endo180. Front Biosci 14: 2103–2114.
54. Lin L, Gardsvoll H, Huai Q, Huang M, Ploug M (2010) Structure-based engineering of species selectivity in the interaction between urokinase and its receptor: implication for preclinical cancer therapy. J Biol Chem 285: 10982–10992.
55. Ploug M, Rahbek-Nielsen H, Nielsen PF, Roepstorff P, Dano K (1998) Glycosylation profile of a recombinant urokinase-type plasminogen activator receptor expressed in Chinese hamster ovary cells. J Biol Chem 273: 13933–13943.
56. Moller LB, Pollanen J, Ronne E, Pedersen N, Blasi F (1993) N-linked glycosylation of the ligand-binding domain of the human urokinase receptor contributes to the affinity for its ligand. J Biol Chem 268: 11152–11159.
57. Ragno P, Montuori N, Covelli B, Hoyer-Hansen G, Rossi G (1998) Differential expression of a truncated form of the urokinase-type plasminogen-activator receptor in normal and tumor thyroid cells. Cancer Res 58: 1315–1319.
58. Behrendt N, Ronne E, Ploug M, Petri T, Lober D, et al. (1990) The human receptor for urokinase plasminogen activator. NH2-terminal amino acid sequence and glycosylation variants. J Biol Chem 265: 6453–6460.
59. Montuori N, Rossi G, Ragno P (1999) Cleavage of urokinase receptor regulates its interaction with integrins in thyroid cells. FEBS Lett 460: 32–36.
60. Nieves EC, Manchanda N (2010) A cleavage-resistant urokinase plasminogen activator receptor exhibits dysregulated cell-surface clearance. J Biol Chem 285: 12595–12603.
61. Dube DH, Bertozzi CR (2005) Glycans in cancer and inflammation–potential for therapeutics and diagnostics. Nat Rev Drug Discov 4: 477–488.
62. Jo M, Thomas KS, Wu L, Gonias SL (2003) Soluble urokinase-type plasminogen activator receptor inhibits cancer cell growth and invasion by direct urokinase-independent effects on cell signaling. J Biol Chem 278: 46692–46698.
63. Piccolella M, Festuccia C, Millimaggi D, Locatelli A, Bologna M, et al. (2008) suPAR, a soluble form of urokinase plasminogen activator receptor, inhibits human prostate cancer cell growth and invasion. Int J Oncol 32: 185–191.
64. Workman P, Aboagye EO, Balkwill F, Balmain A, Bruder G, et al. (2010) Guidelines for the welfare and use of animals in cancer research. Br J Cancer 102: 1555–1577.
65. Kilkenny C, Browne WJ, Cuthill IC, Emerson M, Altman DG (2012) Improving bioscience research reporting: the ARRIVE guidelines for reporting animal research. Osteoarthritis Cartilage 20: 256–260.
66. Bitu CC, Kauppila JH, Bufalino A, Nurmenniemi S, Teppo S, et al. (2013) Cathepsin K is present in invasive oral tongue squamous cell carcinoma in vivo and in vitro. PLoS One 8: e70925.
67. Lou E, Kellman RM, Hutchison R, Shillitoe EJ (2003) Clinical and pathological features of the murine AT-84 orthotopic model of oral cancer. Oral Dis 9: 305–312.
68. Yatohgo T, Izumi M, Kashiwagi H, Hayashi M (1988) Novel purification of vitronectin from human plasma by heparin affinity chromatography. Cell Struct Funct 13: 281–292.
69. Livak KJ, Schmittgen TD (2001) Analysis of relative gene expression data using real-time quantitative PCR and the 2(-Delta Delta C(T)) Method. Methods 25: 402–408.
70. Hadler-Olsen E, Kanapathippillai P, Berg E, Svineng G, Winberg JO, et al. (2010) Gelatin in situ zymography on fixed, paraffin-embedded tissue: zinc and ethanol fixation preserve enzyme activity. J Histochem Cytochem 58: 29–39.
71. Shevchenko A, Wilm M, Vorm O, Mann M (1996) Mass spectrometric sequencing of proteins silver-stained polyacrylamide gels. Anal Chem 68: 850–858.

12

Distinct Innate Immune Gene Expression Profiles in Non-Melanoma Skin Cancer of Immunocompetent and Immunosuppressed Patients

Beda Muehleisen[1,2], Shang Brian Jiang[1], Julie A. Gladsjo[1], Monika Gerber[1], Tissa Hata[1], Richard L. Gallo[1,3,4]*

1 Division of Dermatology, University of California San Diego, La Jolla, California, United States of America, 2 Department of Dermatology, Zurich University Hospital, Zurich, Switzerland, 3 Department of Medicine, University of California San Diego, La Jolla, California, United States of America, 4 Veterans Administration San Diego Healthcare System, San Diego, California, United States of America

Abstract

Squamous cell carcinoma (SCC) and basal cell carcinoma (BCC) are the most frequent skin cancers in humans. An intact immune system is critical for protection against SCC since organ transplant recipients (OTR) have a 60- to 100-fold higher risk for developing these tumors. The role of the innate immune system in tumor immunosurveillance is unclear. Our aim was to determine the expression of selected innate immune genes in BCC and SCC arising in immunocompetent and OTR patients. Lesional and peri-lesional skin from 28 SCC and 19 BCC were evaluated for mRNA expression of toll-like receptors (TLR) 1–9, downstream TLR signaling molecules, and antimicrobial peptides. 11 SCC occurring in OTR patients were included in the analysis. We found that SCC but not BCC showed significantly elevated expression of TLRs 1–3, 5–8, TRIF and TRAF1. TNF was increased in SCC compared to normal skin. BCC showed increased IFNγ. hBD1, hBD2 and psoriasin mRNA and protein expression were significantly higher in SCC than in normal skin and higher than in BCC. SCC from OTR showed only an increase in hBD2 but no increase in hBD1 or psoriasin. We conclude that innate immune gene expression in SCC is distinct from normal skin and BCC. BCC shows lesser induction of innate immune genes. SCC from OTR patients have depressed expression of hBD1 and psoriasin compared to SCC from immunocompetent patients.

Editor: Amanda Ewart Toland, Ohio State University Medical Center, United States of America

Funding: This work was supported by United States National Institutes of Health grants R01 AR052728, R01 AI052453, R01 AI0833358, and the Swiss National Science Foundation (PBZHP3-125571, PASMP3_140073) to B.M. The funding institutions had no role in study design, data collection and analysis, decision to publish, or preparation of the manuscript.

Competing Interests: The authors have declared that no competing interests exist.

* E-mail: rgallo@ucsd.edu

Introduction

Basal cell carcinoma (BCC) and squamous cell carcinoma (SCC) are the most frequent non-melanoma skin cancers (NMSC) in humans [1]. In the U.S.A. more than 3 million cases of BCC and SCC are estimated to occur annually [2–3]. However, although significant progress has been made in understanding the pathogenesis of NMSC, the host immune defense mechanisms that predict patient outcome are still largely unknown. The highly increased incidence of skin cancers in immunosuppressed patients such as organ transplant recipients (OTRs) [4] has clearly shown the importance of the immune system in controlling the development of NMSC. Furthermore, because ultraviolet (UV) radiation has important immunomodulatory properties [5–6], its contribution as a major risk factor for NMSC is amplified.

Currently, most research on tumor immunosurveillance in NMSC, including those within the framework of cancer immunoediting [7–8], have focused mainly on T-cell mediated, adaptive immune mechanisms. However, there is evidence that innate immune mechanisms are also important in NMSC. Early studies by William Coley demonstrated spontaneous tumor regression after developing postsurgical infections [9], and experimental administration of *Streptococcus pyogenes* has also resulted in tumor regression [10]. Today it is well known that infectious agents can be recognized by keratinocytes and other immune cells through various genes of the innate immune system such as toll-like receptors (TLRs). Recognition of microbes results in expression of antimicrobial peptides (AMPs), cytokines and chemokines [11–15].

The activation of an innate immune response has diverse consequences. AMPs can kill microbes and prevent infection [13,16–17]. Furthermore, AMPs can act in a manner similar to chemokines and have pro- and anti-inflammatory effects, stimulate angiogenesis and induce cell death [12,14,18] - effects that might be relevant also in carcinogenesis. Prior work in tumors such as oral squamous cell carcinoma showed enhanced expression of the AMPs human β-defensin 2 and psoriasin and this correlated with the clinicopathological features [19–20]. Furthermore, the expression of cathelicidin by NK cells has been directly shown to limit the growth rate of melanoma in mouse models [21]. More evidence for a role of the innate immune system in NMSC stems from treatment with TLR7 agonist imiquimod which is effective against superficial primary skin tumors and cutaneous metastases, including BCC, actinic keratosis and Bowen's disease [22].

Since very little data has been published on innate immune responses in NMSC we wished to provide an overview of innate immune gene expression in a population of patients with SCCs and BCCs, focusing on TLRs, TLR-signaling intermediates, cytokines and antimicrobial peptides. Since OTRs have a significantly higher risk for SCC [4], this study also included 11 SCCs from OTRs to characterize innate immune gene expression in that high risk population. We report that NMSCs have distinct expression patterns of several genes critical to innate immunity.

Results

Enhanced mRNA Expression of Epidermal Differentiation Genes in SCC

A total population of 37 patients was included in this study, comprising 28 patients with SCC and 19 with BCC. SCCs came from 17 immunocompetent patients and 11 that were OTR. Patient demographics in each group were similar with the exception of OTR who were generally younger (**Figure 1a,b**). Samples for analysis were taken from distant normal skin, peritumoral skin, at the tumor margin, and from central tumor tissue (See methods and **Figure 1c**).

Cutaneous SCC typically retains characteristics of squamous differentiation. To further characterize the specimens in our study, we measured mRNA expression of several epidermal differentiation genes. Samples within the central tumor tissue of SCC showed significantly elevated mRNA expression of filaggrin (13.60±4.52-fold (mean ± SEM), $p<0.05$) and keratin 10 (10.83±0.51-fold, $p<0.001$) compared to normal skin. Filaggrin and keratin 10 expression in the tumor center was also higher compared to the tumor margin (0.44±0.22, $p<0.001$; 1.56±0.51, $p<0.05$) and to peritumoral tissue (0.62±0.18, $p<0.001$; 1.19±0.34, $p<0.01$). Filaggrin and keratin 10 expression in the tumor center of SCC was also significantly higher than in the tumor center of BCC (5.50±2.98, $p<0.05$; 0.39±0.09, $p<0.001$). For loricrin, reduced mRNA expression in the tumor margin of SCC was observed compared to normal skin (0.073±0.021, $p<0.001$), the tumor center (8.29±5.29, $p<0.001$) and peritumoral tissue (0.33±0.08, $p<0.05$) (**Figure 2**).

Enhanced TLR Expression in SCC

TLR1 mRNA expression in the SCC tumor center was 5.49±1.21-fold higher ($p<0.01$) than in normal skin and also significantly higher than in the tumor center of BCCs (1.82±1.21, $p<0.001$). TLR2 mRNA expression in the SCC tumor center was 7.90±1.76-fold higher ($p<0.01$) than in normal skin and also higher than in the tumor center of BCCs (1.41±0.35, $p<0.001$). TLR3 mRNA expression in the SCC tumor center was 8.51±2.11-fold higher ($p<0.01$) than in normal skin and also higher than in peritumoral tissue (1.61±0.70, $p<0.05$). TLR5 mRNA expression in the SCC tumor center showed the largest magnitude difference and was 30.8±22.9-fold higher ($p<0.05$) than in normal skin and also significantly higher than in the tumor center of BCCs (0.92±0.46, $p<0.01$). TLR6 mRNA expression was significantly higher in the SCC tumor center (4.48±1.44) than in the tumor margin (0.96±0.48, $p<0.05$). TLR7 mRNA expression in the SCC tumor center was 15.6±3.70-fold higher than in normal skin ($p<0.001$) and also significantly higher than in peritumoral tissue (3.37±1.35, $p<0.01$) and than in the tumor center of BCCs (1.98±0.53, $p<0.001$).

Of note, TLR8 mRNA expression was significantly higher in the peritumoral tissue of SCC (13.93±0.57) as well as in the tumor center (7.46±4.99) compared to normal skin ($p<0.05$ for both) and significantly higher compared to BCC peritumoral (0.36±0.21) and BCC tumor center tissue (0.35±0.14) ($p<0.01$ for both) (**Figure 3**).

Enhanced TRIF, TRAF1 and TNF Expression in SCC. Enhanced TNF and IFNγ Expression in BCC

Consistent with the increased expression of TLRs in SCC, gene products that are either downstream of the TLR signaling cascade, or inducible by TLR activation, were also elevated in SCC. TRIF mRNA expression in the SCC tumor center was 17.11±5.14-fold higher than in normal skin ($p<0.01$), in peritumoral tissue (3.89±2.51, $p<0.05$) and also significantly higher than in the tumor center of BCCs (3.13±1.36, $p<0.001$). TRAF1 mRNA expression in the SCC tumor center was 9.62±2.18-fold higher than in normal skin ($p<0.01$) and also significantly higher than in the tumor center of BCCs (3.40±2.36, $p<0.05$). TNF mRNA expression in the SCC tumor center was 515±144-fold higher than in normal skin ($p<0.001$) and also significantly higher than in the tumor center of BCCs (55.5±29.3, $p<0.001$). In SCC, TNF mRNA expression was also significantly elevated in the tumor margin compared to normal skin (176.2±89.4, $p<0.05$). BCC showed also significantly higher TNF expression (55.5±29.3 vs. 1.02±0.55, $p<0.05$) and higher IFNγ expression (17.1±4.1 vs. 1.01±0.04, $p<0.05$) than in normal skin (**Figure 4**).

Enhanced Expression of hBD1 and 2 and Psoriasin in SCC. BCC Shows Less Expression of CAMP, hBD1-3, RNase7 and Psoriasin than SCC

hBD1 mRNA expression in the SCC tumor center was 50.36±28.90-fold higher than in normal skin ($p<0.05$), in the tumor margin (0.93±0.44, $p<0.05$) and also significantly higher than in the tumor center of BCCs (1.08±0.45, $p<0.001$). In BCC hBD1 mRNA expression was significantly lower in the tumor margin than in the tumor center (0.15±0.04 vs. 1.08±0.45, $p<0.05$). hBD2 mRNA expression in the SCC tumor center was 4748±3934-fold higher than in normal skin ($p<0.005$), in the tumor margin (5.02±2.11, $p<0.01$) and also significantly higher than in the tumor center of BCCs (58.36±40.56, $p<0.05$). In BCC hBD2.

mRNA expression was significantly higher in the tumor center (58.36±40.56) than in the tumor margin (0.61±0.26, $p<0.05$) or in the peritumoral tissue (0.30±0.11, $p<0.01$). Psoriasin(S100A7) is an abundant protein in the epidermis with much different antimicrobial activity than hBDs or cathelicidins. At protein concentrations exceeding 100 ug/ml psoriasin can partially inhibit the growth of Gram negative bacteria while hBDs and cathelicidins act at low micromolar concentrations against a broad range of bacteria, viruses and fungi [12,23–26]. mRNA expression for psoriasin in the SCC tumor center was 1334±690-fold higher than in normal skin ($p<0.05$) and also significantly higher than in the tumor center of BCCs (27.41±14.50, $p<0.001$). Cathelicidin and hBD3 mRNA expression were significantly lower in the tumor center of BCC compared to SCC (0.72±0.14 vs. 1.71±0.39, $p<0.05$; 9.59±5.15 vs. 2497±1447, $p<0.001$) (**Figure 5**). In line with elevated mRNA expression, immunofluorescence staining also revealed enhanced protein expression for hBD1, hBD2 and psoriasin in SCC compared to normal skin or BCC (**Figure 6**).

Lack of an Increase of hBD1 and psoriasin Expression in OTR

A direct comparison was made between the expression of all target genes in OTR and immunocompetent patients (ICP).

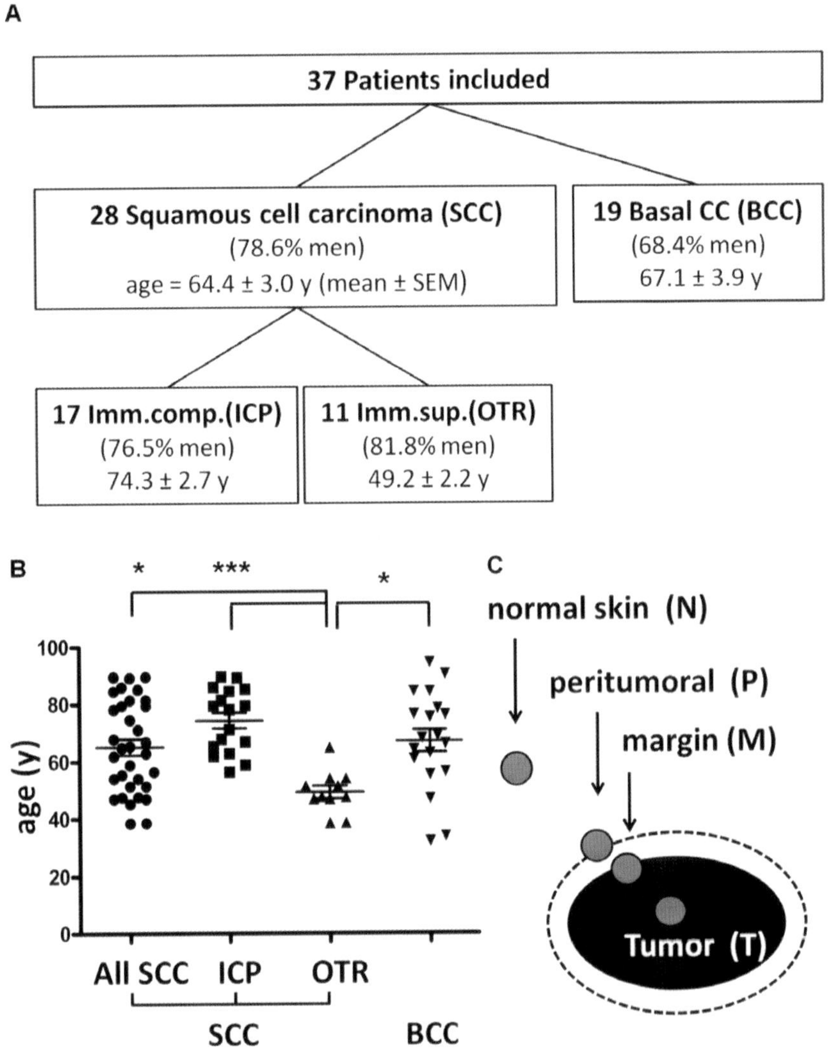

Figure 1. Patients enrolled and sample collection. 1A) Patients enrolled in the study, tumor diagnoses and immune status. SCC = squamous cell carcinoma. BCC = basal cell carcinoma. Imm'comp. (ICP) = immunocompetent patients. Imm.sup.(OTR) = organ transplant recipients (immunosuppressed patients). Gender (percentage male) and age (mean ± SEM) distribution in each group of patients is shown. 1 B) Age distribution in patient groups. Scatter plots including mean ± SEM are shown. *$p < 0.05$, ***$p < 0.005$ (one-way ANOVA with Bonferroni's post-test). 1 C) From each case, a specimen was collected from the center of the tumor (T), from the tumor margin (M) including tumor cells as well as non-tumor cells, from peritumoral tissue (P) that does not contain any tumor cells, and from normal control skin (N) in far distance from the tumor.

Differences in gene expression between OTR and ICP were only found for antimicrobial peptide genes and are displayed in **figure 7**. For all other genes in this study with similar expression between ICP and OTR, both patient categories were merged (n = 28 SCC) for statistical comparison to BCCs and for presentation in figures 2–4.

As in ICPs, SCC in OTRs showed enhanced hBD2 mRNA expression in the tumor center (233.5±149.2) compared to the tumor margin (3.11±2.16, $p<0.05$), peritumoral tissue (1.22±0.95, $p<0.01$) and normal skin (2.14±1.61, $p<0.05$). However, in contrast to ICPs, SCC in OTRs did not overexpress hBD1 or psoriasin. Psoriasin mRNA expression in the tumor center of SCC in OTRs was significantly lower than in ICPs (71.9±49.1 vs. 1334±690, $p<0.01$) (**Figure 7**). Further supporting these findings were our results from immunohistofluorescence staining showing also lower hBD1 and psoriasin protein expression in SCC from OTRs compared to ICPs (Figure 6).

Discussion

This study sought to provide an in depth analysis of innate immune gene expression in NMSC. The goal of this work was to further understand how our skin responds to the development of tumors and thus gain essential information that can help guide therapy. The candidate genes evaluated represented those such as TLRs that are involved in the innate immune recognition of danger, cytoplasmic molecules such as TRIF and TRAF that transmit information detected by these receptors, and molecules triggered by this process. These last groups of effector molecules are the AMPs and cytokines responsible for mediating the host response once danger is detected. Results show a dramatic difference in expression of many of these critical molecules in SCC, suggesting that this tumor type has enhanced many elements of innate immune response compared to normal skin. Since many of the effector molecules may play a role in the growth of the tumor or resistance to infection, and some are further altered in

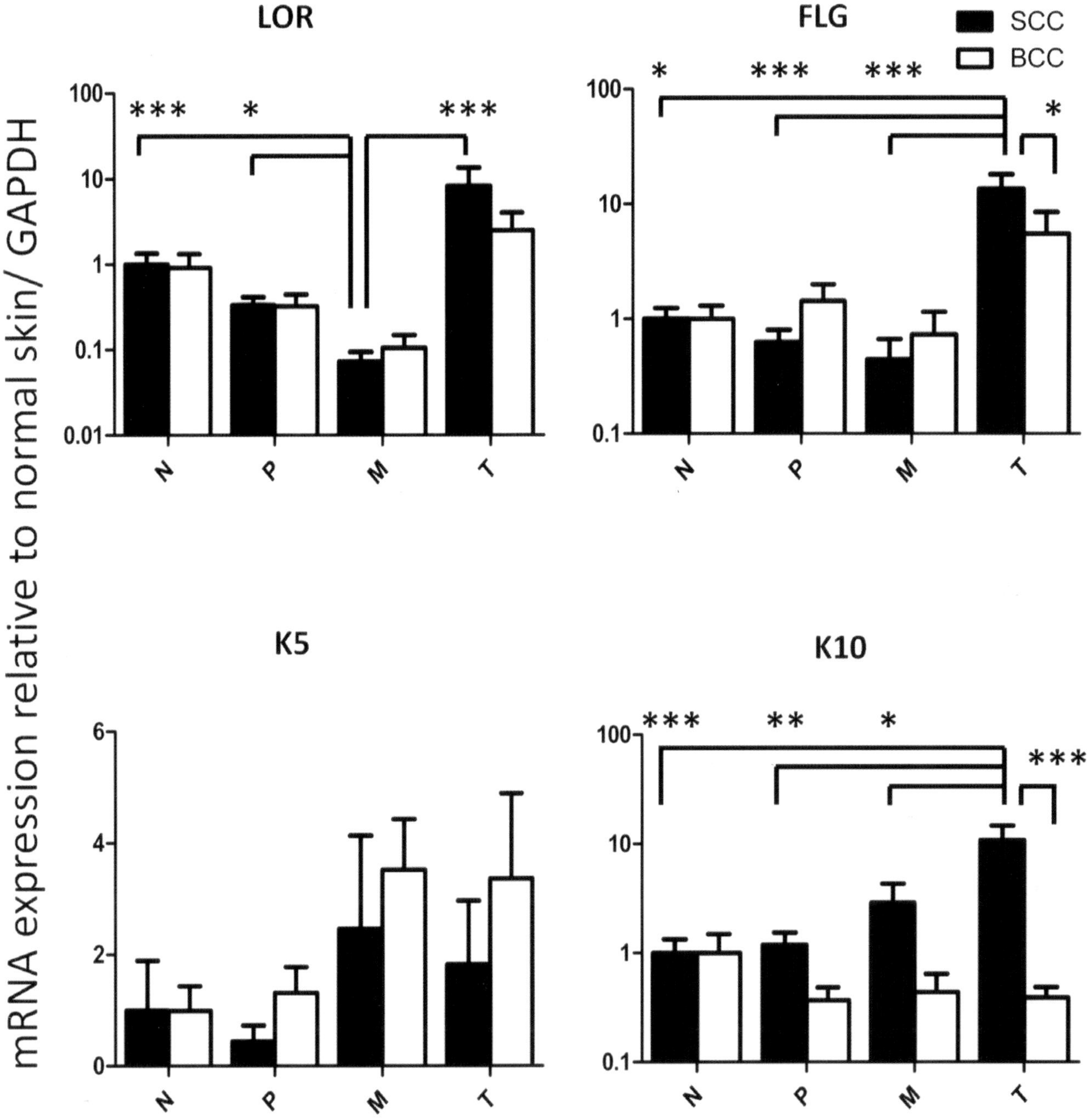

Figure 2. Distinct mRNA expression of differentiation genes in non-melanoma skin cancer. mRNA expression of differentiation gene loricrin (LOR), filaggrin (FLG), keratin 5 (K5) and keratin 10 (K10) in the tumor center (T), tumor margin (M), peritumoral tissue (P) and distant normal skin (N) in cutaneous squamous cell carcinoma (SCC, black bars) and basal cell carcinoma (BCC, white bars). Relative mRNA expression to glyceraldehyde 3-phosphate dehydrogenase (GAPDH) and normalized to normal skin is shown. Depicted are mean ± SEM values. *$p<0.05$, **$p<0.01$, ***$p<0.001$ by Kruskal-Wallis test with Dunn's post-test for comparison between N, P, M and T and by Mann Whitney U test for comparison between SCC and BCC in each group. N = 28 SCC and 19 BCC.

the immunocompromised host, these may partially explain the natural progression of NMSC.

Although full coverage of all molecules that participate in innate immunity would involve transcriptional profiling of several thousand gene products, and would be best approached by micro-array analysis [27] or RNASeq [28], the approach of real-time PCR analysis used here is the most quantitative and is commonly used for validation of high-throughput transcriptional profiling results. Sample selection from each patient involved the tumor itself, peritumoral tissue and normal skin. Since each tissue specimen represented a heterogenous collection of cell types, our evaluation is limited by the inability to attribute the mRNA measured to specific resident cells, the malignancy itself, or recruited cell types. However, the data obtained reflected expected expression patterns for the tumor. For example, cutaneous SCC typically retains characteristics of squamous differentiation [29],

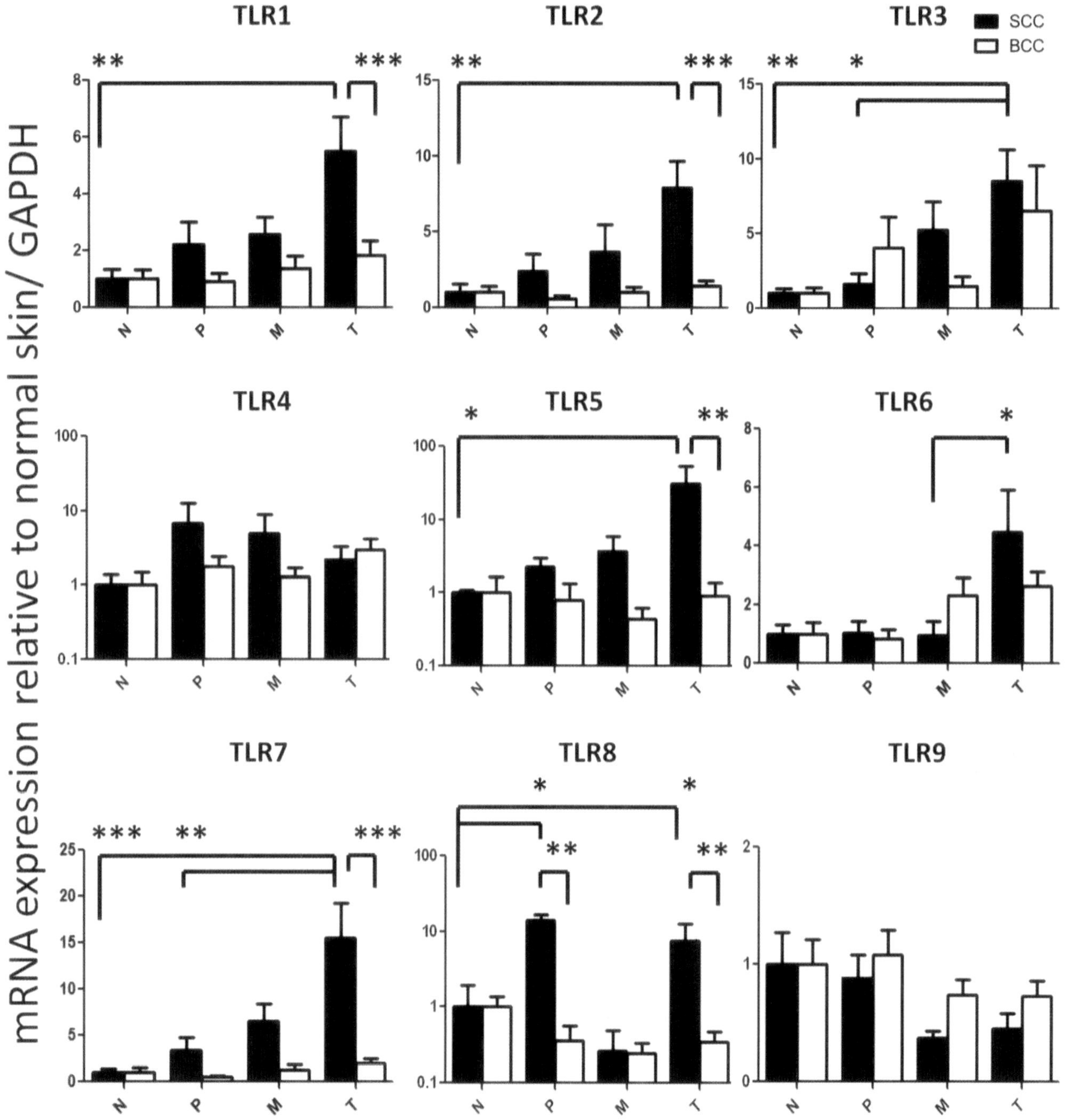

Figure 3. Distinct expression of toll like receptor genes in non-melanoma skin cancer. mRNA expression of toll like receptor genes 1–9 (TLR1-9) in the tumor center (T), tumor margin (M), peritumoral tissue (P) and distant normal skin (N) in cutaneous squamous cell carcinoma (SCC, black bars) and basal cell carcinoma (BCC, white bars). Relative mRNA expression to glyceraldehyde 3-phosphate dehydrogenase (GAPDH) and normalized to normal skin is shown. Depicted are mean ± SEM values. *$p<0.05$, **$p<0.01$, ***$p<0.001$ by Kruskal-Wallis test with Dunn's post-test for comparison between N, P, M and T and by Mann Whitney U test for comparison between SCC and BCC in each group. N = 28 SCC and 19 BCC.

and we found elevated filaggrin and keratin 10 gene expression in the SCC tissue of the tumor center. Expression was not only higher than in normal skin but also higher than in the tumor margin and in BCC. These results underline substantial differences in differentiation between SCC, BCC and normal skin, and served to validate the samples selected.

Activation of TLRs can result in a wide variety of responses that include apoptosis, inflammatory and non-inflammatory reactions (reviewed in [11]). TLRs are known to be expressed on a variety of murine and human cancer cells (reviewed in [30]). However, little information is available on TLR expression in SCC, and this has come mostly from cervical [31–32] or head and neck SCC [33–34], but not from cutaneous SCC. Our study showed significantly elevated expression of TLR1,2,3,5,6,7 and 8 in cutaneous SCC. For several TLRs a 5- to 10-fold induction was seen in SCC. Notable responses unique to SCC included TLR5 (responsible for

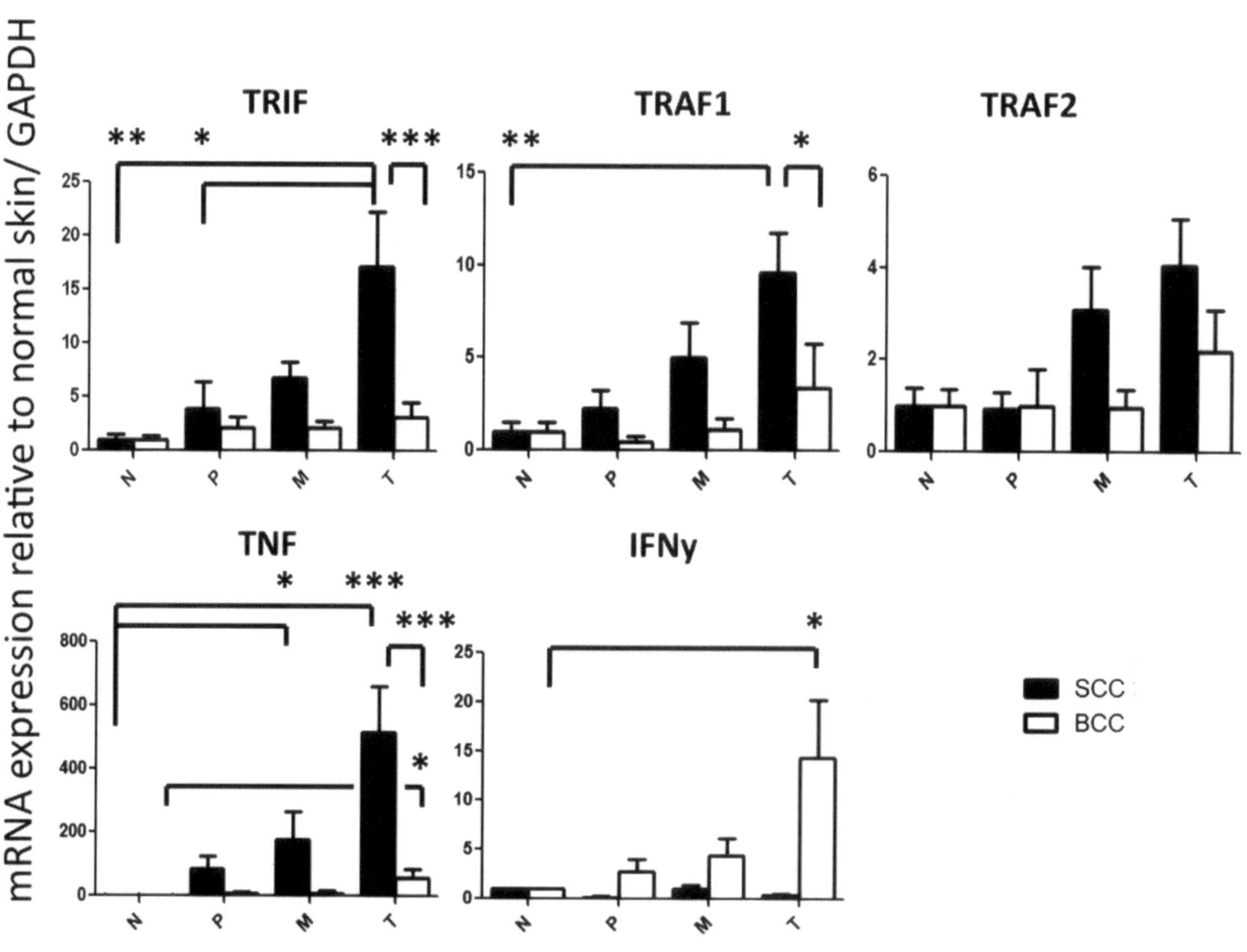

Figure 4. Distinct expression of innate immune receptor signaling molecules and cytokines in non-melanoma skin cancer. mRNA expression of TIR-domain-containing adaptor-inducing interferon-β (TRIF), TNF receptor-associated factors 1 and 2 (TRAF1 and 2), tumor necrosis factor (TNF) and interferon-γ (IFNγ) in the tumor center (T), tumor margin (M), peritumoral tissue (P) and distant normal skin (N) in cutaneous squamous cell carcinoma (SCC, black bars) and basal cell carcinoma (BCC, white bars). Relative mRNA expression to glyceraldehyde 3-phosphate dehydrogenase (GAPDH) and normalized to normal skin is shown. Depicted are mean ± SEM values. *$p<0.05$, **$p<0.01$, ***$p<0.001$ by Kruskal-Wallis test with Dunn's post-test for comparison between N, P, M and T and by Mann Whitney U test for comparison between SCC and BCC in each group. N = 28 SCC and 19 BCC.

recognition of flagellin), TLR7 (the target of imiquimod), and TLR8, which along with TLR7, can recognize RNA. The TLR8 response was particularly interesting as it also included an induction in the peri-tumoral region. We also observed high TLR2 expression in SCC which could be a characteristic of SCC or a result of a defective skin barrier in SCC. In this way the increase is comparable to the TLR2 upregulation seen in skin wounds [35]. Equally remarkable was the relatively little change in innate immune gene expression seen in BCC. This may be a pertinent negative response given that some TLR induction would be expected from damaged skin. To define a potential functional role of TLR overexpression in cutaneous SCC, further functional studies are needed.

TRIF and TRAF are downstream signaling molecules of TLR activation and their expression correlated with increased TLR expression in SCC. Similarly, the cytokine response was highest in SCC and correlated with increased TLR expression and signaling. However, in BCC TNF was significantly elevated compared to normal skin despite a lesser TLR response. Increased IFNγ was seen only in BCC. This underlines fundamental differences of innate immune receptor signaling and cytokine expression in BCC and SCC and likely reflects both the local expression of these molecules and expression in recruited inflammatory cells.

Because of the action of AMPs to alter cell growth and differentiation [36], their expression may be highly relevant in cancer. This association has been directly demonstrated for cathelicidin, where in mouse tumor models a lack of cathelicidin resulted in much more rapid tumor growth [21]. In the present study we found increased hBD1, hBD2, hBD3 and psoriasin in SCC compared to normal skin, but no increase in cathelicidin. Previously, enhanced hBD2 expression was also reported for oral SCC tumor cells and intratumoral vascular endothelia [29,37–38]. Furthermore, previous studies reported increased hBD3 in *in-situ* and invasive oral SCC, correlating with specific macrophage recruitment to the lesion site [20,39]. In contrast, the expression of AMPs in BCCs was much different than SCC. We found a significant decrease of hBD1 expression in the invading tumor margin of BCC but not in the tumor center. A decrease in hBD1 was previously reported in BCC [40]. The functional significance of altered hBD expression in cancer is unclear at present. However, treatment of head and neck SCC (HNSCC) cell lines

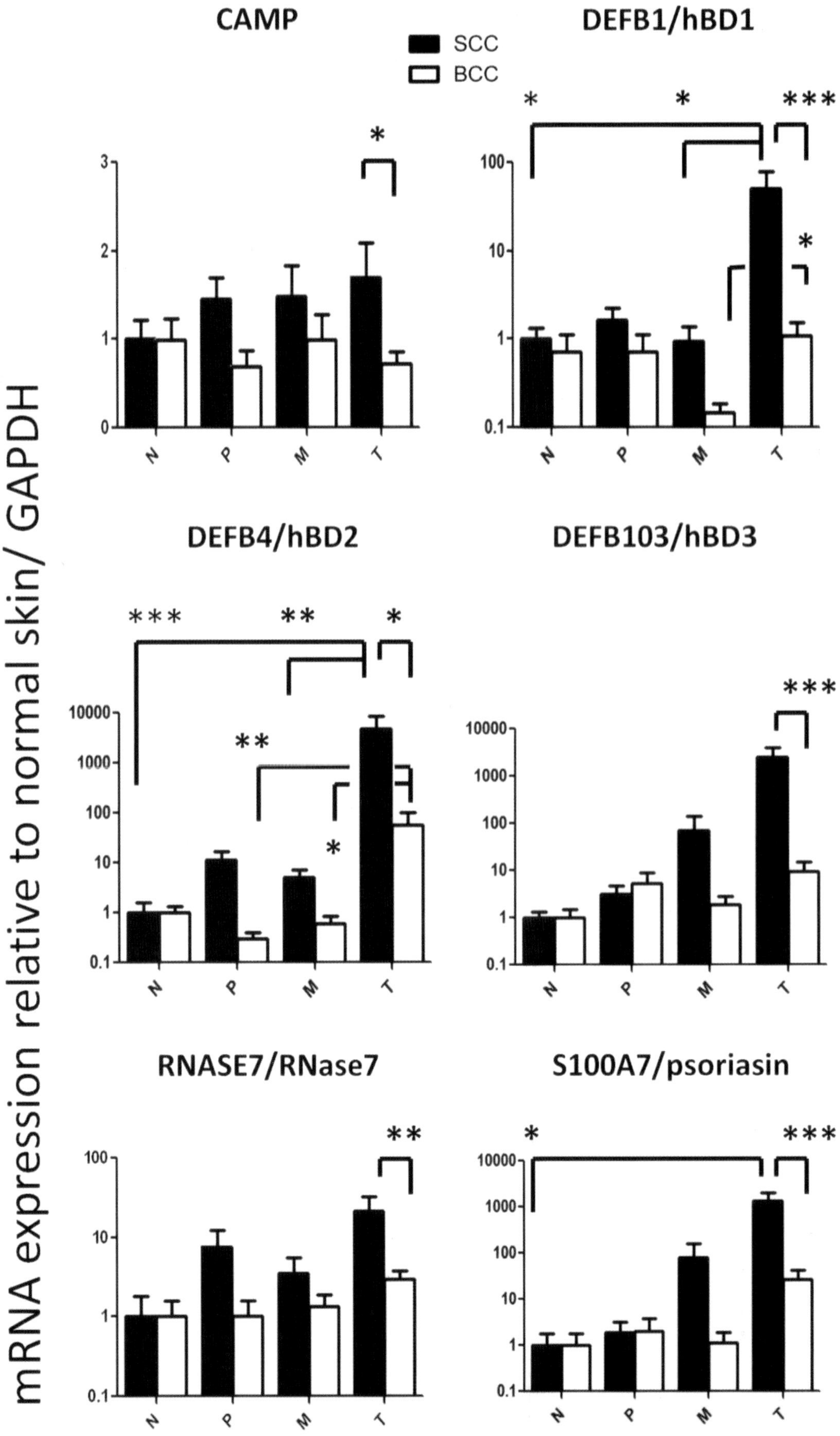
mRNA expression relative to normal skin/ GAPDH
CAMP
DEFB1/hBD1
SCC
BCC
DEFB4/hBD2
DEFB103/hBD3
RNASE7/RNase7
S100A7/psoriasin
N
P
M
T

Figure 5. Distinct expression of antimicrobial peptides in non-melanoma skin cancer. mRNA expression of cathelicidin antimicrobial peptide (*CAMP*), human β-defensins 1–3 (hBD1–3, genes *DEFB1*, *DEFB4* and *DEFB103*), RNase 7 (*RNASE7*) and psoriasisin (S100A7) in the tumor center (T), tumor margin (M), peritumoral tissue (P) and distant normal skin (N) in cutaneous squamous cell carcinoma (SCC, black bars) and basal cell carcinoma (BCC, white bars). Relative mRNA expression to glyceraldehyde 3-phosphate dehydrogenase (GAPDH) and normalized to normal skin is shown. Depicted are mean ± SEM values. *p<0.05, **p<0.01, ***p<0.001 by Kruskal-Wallis test with Dunn's post-test for comparison between N, P, M and T and by Mann Whitney U test for comparison between SCC and BCC in each group. N = 17 SCC from immunocompetent patients (ICP) and 19 BCC.

with hBD3 improved resistance against cis-platin, indicating that higher hBD expression may enhance tumor survival [41].

Psoriasin (S100A7) represents a much different type of molecule than the hBDs or cathelicidin and warrents separate discussion. Psoriasin is a much larger protein, is found in much greater abundance in skin, and has different antimicrobial activity (reviewed in [25]). It also does not appear to be expressed by bone marrow derived cells as is the case with many antimicrobial peptides. Rather, psoriasin is expressed primarily in a variety of epithelia. The functions of psoriasin in immunity are thus less clear although it has been associated with resistance to skin surface colonization by *E. coli* [24]. A previous study described elevated

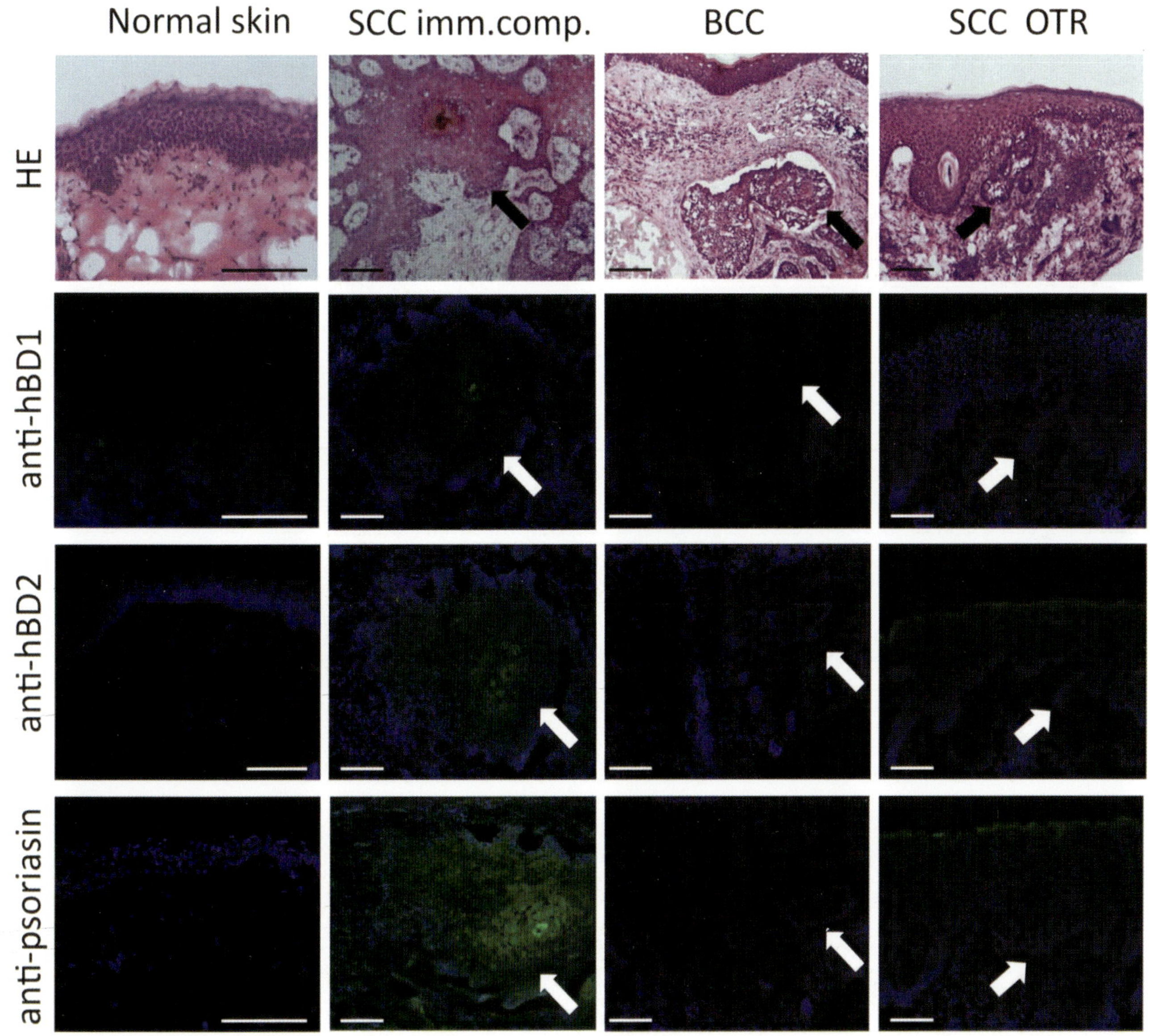

Figure 6. Distinct protein expression of the antimicrobial peptides hBD1, hBD2 and psoriasin in squamous cell carcinoma of immunocompetent patients and organ transplant recipients. Protein expression of the antimicrobial peptides hBD1, hBD2 and psoriasin as detected by immunofluorescence staining (green) in normal skin, basal cell carcinoma (BCC) and squamous cell carcinomas in immunocompetent patients (SCC imm.comp.) and organ transplant recipients (SCC OTR). Nuclei were visualized with 4′-6-diamidino-2-phenylindole (DAPI, blue). The top row shows hematoxylin and eosin (HE) staining of the same skin samples. Arrows point at groups of tumor cells. Bar = 100 µm. Data are representative of five samples each.

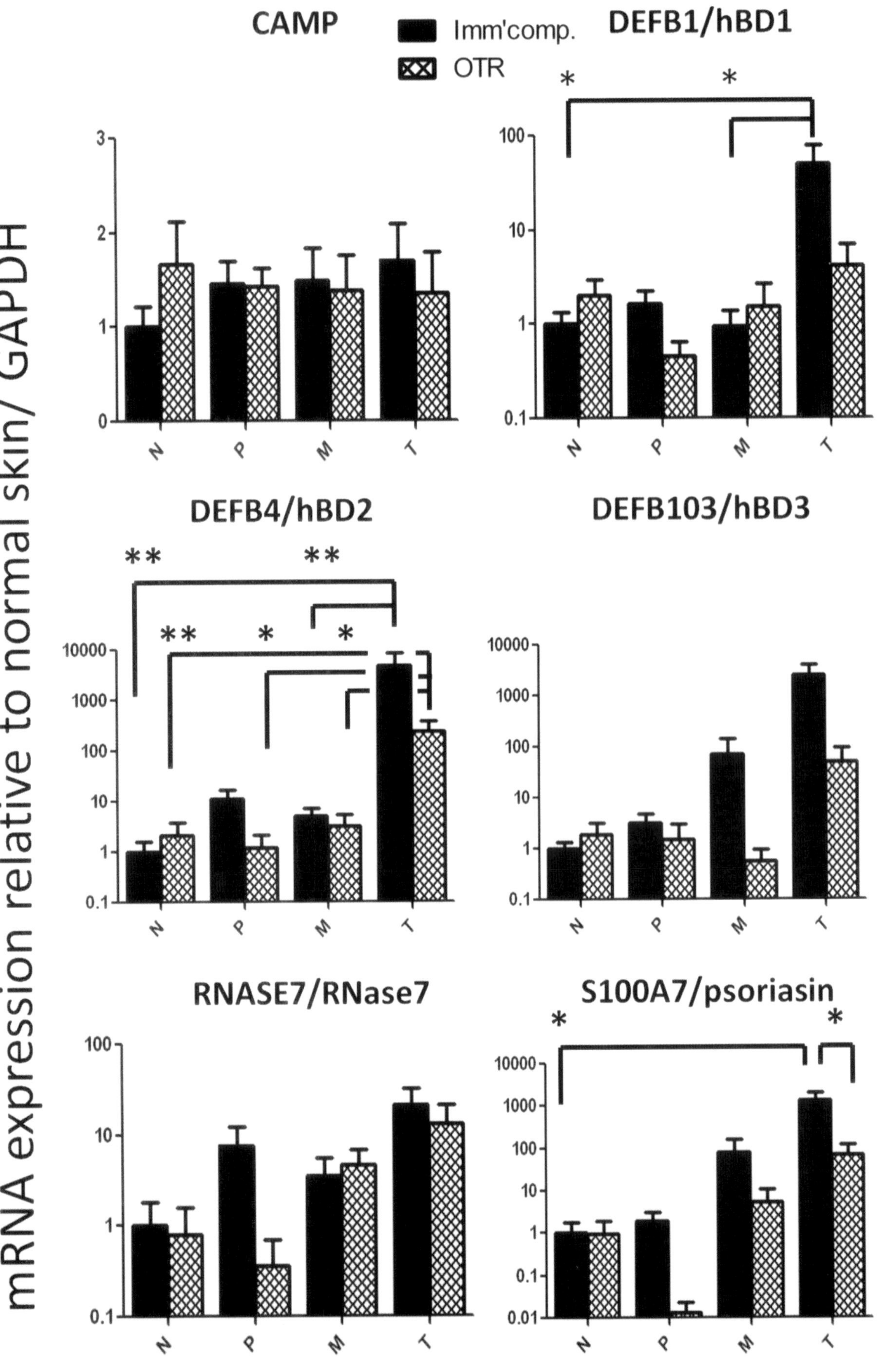
CAMP
Imm'comp.
OTR
DEFB1/hBD1
DEFB4/hBD2
DEFB103/hBD3
RNASE7/RNase7
S100A7/psoriasin
mRNA expression relative to normal skin/ GAPDH
N
P
M
T

Figure 7. Distinct expression of antimicrobial peptides in squamous cell carcinoma of organ transplant recipients. mRNA expression of cathelicidin antimicrobial peptide (*CAMP*), human β-defensins 1-3 (hBD1-3, genes *DEFB1, DEFB4* and *DEFB103*), RNase 7 (*RNASE7*) and psoriasisin (S100A7) in the tumor center (T), tumor margin (M), peritumoral tissue (P) and distant normal skin (N) in cutaneous squamous cell carcinoma (SCC) of immunocompetent (Imm'comp., black bars) and immunosuppressed patients (OTR = organ transplant recipients, cross-hatched bars). Relative mRNA expression to glyceraldehyde 3-phosphate dehydrogenase (GAPDH) and normalized to normal skin is shown. Depicted are mean ± SEM values. *$p<0.05$, **$p<0.01$, ***$p<0.001$ by Kruskal-Wallis test with Dunn's post-test for comparison between N, P, M and T and by Mann Whitney U test for comparison between immunocompetent and immunosuppressed patients in each group. N = 17 SCC from immunocompetent patients (ICP) and 11 SCC from organ transplant recipients (OTR).

psoriasin mRNA expression in *in-situ* and invasive SCC [42], and thus agreed with our results. Psoriasin overexpression has also been reported for other tumors such as breast cancer [43], where persistent expression in invasive tumor areas was associated with poorer prognosis [44–46]. Upregulation of psoriasin at transcriptional and protein level was recently also reported for early oral SCC [19]. Psoriasin can bind αvβ6-integrin to promote invasive behavior in oral SCC cells [47]. Therefore, as was discussed for TLRs and their signaling intermediates, the current findings validate the need for further study of the functional relevance of these antimicrobial peptides and proteins.

Immunocompromised patients such as organ transplant recipients (OTRs) have a 60- to 100-fold increased risk for SCC [4], however the exact mechanisms for how immunosuppressive drugs increase the risk for more frequent and more aggressive SCCs are still largely unknown. Long-term immunosuppressive drug treatment in OTR was recently shown to alter the composition of the SCC peritumoral inflammatory infiltrate. Reduced proportions of CD3+, CD8+, and CD14+ (monocytes), FOXP3+ (regulatory T cells) and 123+ (plasmacytoid dendritic cells) cells but more CD138+ plasma cells in SCC of OTR compared to immunocompetent patients have been reported [48–49]. Most OTRs are treated with several immunosuppressive drugs simultaneously, making it difficult to elucidate the exact mechanisms how an immunosuppressant contributes to the increased SCC risk.

To investigate if drug-induced immunosuppression altered innate immune gene expression, we included 11 SCC from OTRs for comparison with SCC from immunocompetent patients. All patients in our study were on a treatment regimen with corticosteroids and the mTOR inhibitor rapamycin for at least a year before tumor diagnosis and excision. In epidemiological studies, switching from an immunosuppressive therapy with calcineurin inhibitors to the mTOR-inhibitor sirolimus was effective to reduce skin carcinogenesis in renal transplant patients by 50% [50]. In our study, comparison of expression of all innate immune genes revealed that in contrast to immunocompetent patients, SCC in OTR had lower hBD1 and psoriasin expression, but the abundance of expression of other genes measured was similar to SCC from immunocompetent patients. It would be of interest to determine if the lower expression of hBD1 and psoriasin might be functionally relevant and related to the worse outcome in these patients.

In summary, this study clearly shows that the expression of several genes involved in the innate immune response is different in SCC than normal tissues. There are many possible reasons why skin tumors showed elevated expression of these innate immune genes. Tumor infiltrating immune cells such as $CD4^+$, $CD8^+$ and $FOXP3^+$ T-cells and macrophages secrete soluble effector molecules such as interferons, IL-6 and TNF, and some of these can directly influence innate immune gene expression in keratinocytes (reviewed in [12]). The higher degree of differentiation in SCC compared to BCC or normal basal keratinocytes might be another reason for overexpression of some innate immune genes, since highly differentiated keratinocytes showed enhanced expression of human β-defensins 2 and 3 [51]. A third driver of innate immune gene expression in SCC could be a defective skin barrier in these tumors. Skin SCCs often rupture and form wounds. Previous studies in non-malignant, sterile wounding experiments showed a strong induction of TLR2 and antimicrobial peptides in the wound edge [35]. Furthermore, uncontrolled growth of tumor cells and tissue necrosis lead to release of molecules such as cellular DNA, heat shock proteins and fibrinogen, all of which are danger signals that can activate TLRs and their downstream signaling and effector molecules [52–53]. However, even though these mechanisms might be responsible for part of the profile of innate immune gene expression which we found in our study, they provide only an incomplete explanation. Moreover, we believe that expression of some of these innate immune genes is tumor-intrinsic and independent from the tumor environment. Further studies are needed to better understand the exact mechanisms that lead to this distinct innate immune gene expression.

The approach of sampling tissue from the tumor margin and periphery distinguished expression of some genes of interest and provides an example of how basic research might be integrated in well established standardized clinical surgical procedures such as Mohs surgery. Furthermore, it would be a mistake to overlook the remarkably low response seen in BCC for some gene products. The expression (or lack of expression) of unique elements of the innate immune system provides clues to development of the next generation of targeted immune therapy for NMSC.

Materials and Methods

Patients

The study was designed to include 10 – 20 specimens each from SCC in immunocompetent patients, from SCC in organ transplant recipients and from basal cell carcinomas. Following approval by the Human Research Protection Program at the University of California, San Diego (IRB ref. # 071032), and upon receiving written informed consent prior to biopsy, skin specimens from subsequent patients undergoing Mohs surgery for non-melanoma skin cancer at the Division of Dermatology, University of California, San Diego, from December 2009 to June 2010 were collected. The only inclusion criterion was the tumor diagnosis. There were no exclusion criteria. None of the patients in this study was pregnant or had other underlying skin disorders in the areas from which skin samples were obtained. Storage and use of all tissues included in the work presented here was carried out in accordance with the Helsinki declaration. 37 patients were included. 19 patients had a basal cell carcinoma (BCC) and 28 squamous cell carcinoma (SCC). Because immunosuppressed patients such as organ transplant recipients (OTR) have a 60–100-fold greater risk for SCCs this study was designed to include 11 SCCs from OTRs for comparison with 17 SCC from immunocompetent patients (ICP). In the BCC patient group, 68.4% were men, and mean age was 67.1±3.9 years (± SEM). In the SCC ICP group, 76.5% were men and mean age was 74.3±2.7 years. In the SCC OTR group, 81.8% were men. As expected and published before [4,54], OTRs in this study developed SCC significantly earlier than ICPs (at 49.2±2.2 y, $p<0.001$) (**Figure 1A,B**). Transplanted organs were as follows: 8 kidneys, 1 liver and 2 hearts. Time since transplantation was ranging from 8 to 31 years. The current immunosuppressive regimens for at least one year before Mohs surgery were rapamycin & prednisone.

Collection of Human Skin Specimens

Mohs microscopically controlled surgery of these skin tumors was performed as described before [55]. During the course of Mohs surgery, 2x2x2 mm^3 specimens were collected from the center of the tumor (T), from the margin of the tumor (M) consisting of tumor cells and non-tumor cells, from the peritumoral region (P) in close proximity to the tumor but without any tumor cells, and from normal skin (N) in far distance from the tumor, used to reconstruct the skin defect after complete tumor excision (**Figure 1C**). This approach allowed comparison of not only tumor tissue with normal skin in the same patients but also with the peritumoral microenvironment and with the invading tumor edge.

Quantitative Real-time PCR (qPCR)

Total RNA was isolated using TRIzol reagent (Invitrogen, Carlsbad, CA) and 1 µg RNA was reverse transcribed using iScript (BioRad, Hercules, CA). Expression of the cathelicidin gene (*CAMP*) was evaluated using the FAM-CAGAGGATTGT-GACTTCA-MGB probe with primers 5′-CTTCAC-CAGCCCGTCCTTC-3′ and 5′-CCAGGACGACACAG-CAGTCA-3′. Taqman gene expression assays detecting human loricrin (Hs01894962_s1), filaggrin (Hs00856927_g1), keratin 5 (Hs00361185_m1), keratin 10 (Hs00196158_m1), TLR1-9 (Hs00413978_m1, Hs00610101_m1, Hs01551078_m1, Hs00152937_m1, Hs01019558_m1, Hs00271977_s1, Hs00607866_m1, Hs00370913_s1), TRIF (Hs00706140_s1), TRAF1 (Hs01090170_m1) TRAF2 (Hs00184186_m1), TNFα (Hs00174128_m1), IFNγ (Hs00989291_m1), human β-defensins 1-3 (Hs00608345_m1, Hs00823638_m1, Hs00218678_m1), RNAse7 (Hs00261482_m1) and S100A7 (Hs00161488_m1) were purchased from Applied Biosystems (ABI, Foster City, CA). Gene expression was normalized against GAPDH. For GAPDH expression a VIC CATCCATGACCACCCCTGGCCAAG-MGB probe with primers 5′-CTTAGCACCCCTGGCCAAG-3′ and 5′-TGGTCATGAGTCCTTCCACG-3′ was used. RT-qPCR was run on a 7300 Real Time PCR System (ABI). The ΔΔCt method was used to calculate relative expression normalized to normal skin.

Immunostaining

For immunohistofluorescence, frozen sections (6 µm) were fixed with 4% paraformaldehyde, blocked with 3% BSA in phosphate-buffered saline (PBS), and incubated with mouse monoclonal anti-psoriasin antibody (47C1068, sc-52948, Santa Cruz Biotechnology), rabbit anti-hBD1 (FL-68, sc-20797, Santa Cruz) or anti-hBD2 antibody (FL-64, sc-20798, Santa Cruz). Normal mouse IgG (sc-3877, Santa Cruz) and rabbit pre-immune serum were used as negative controls (**Figure S1**). After washing with PBS, FITC-conjugated goat anti-mouse IgG (Sigma-Aldrich) or FITC-conjugated goat anti-rabbit IgG (Jackson Immuno Research Laboratories, West Grove, PA) was used as second antibody. Sections were mounted in ProLong Gold Anti-Fade reagent with 4′-6-diamidino-2-phenylindole (Molecular Probes/Invitrogen, Eugene, OR). Images were obtained using an Olympus BX41 fluorescent microscope (Scientific Instrument Company, Temecula, CA).

Statistical Analysis

Statistical analysis was performed using GraphPad Prism software v5.0 (GraphPad Software Inc., La Jolla). The means and standard errors of the mean (SEM) were calculated for each data set. Data were analyzed by analysis of variance (ANOVA) or the Kruskal-Wallis test with post-tests when appropriate, Mann-Whitney U test and unpaired t test. P-values < 0.05 were considered significant.

Supporting Information

Figure S1 Negative control staining for hBD1, hBD2 and psoriasin. Squamous cell carcinomas from immunocompetent patients (SCC imm.comp.) and basal cell carcinomas (BCC) were stained with normal control antibodies. For hBD1 and hBD2 (top row) normal rabbit pre-immune serum was used. For psoriasin (bottom row) normal mouse IgG control antibody was used. FITC-conjugated goat anti-rabbit and goat anti-mouse IgG (green) were used as secondary antibodies. Nuclei were visualized with 4′-6-diamidino-2-phenylindole (DAPI, blue).

Acknowledgments

The authors thank Cuong Nguyen for assistance with experiments and Lars E. French for scientific advice.

Author Contributions

Performed the experiments: BM. Analyzed the data: BM RLG. Contributed reagents/materials/analysis tools: BM SJ MG JG TH. Wrote the paper: BM RLG.

References

1. Lomas A, Leonardi-Bee J, Bath-Hextall F (2012) A Systematic Review of worldwide incidence of Non-melanoma skin cancer. Br J Dermatol.
2. Jemal A, Siegel R, Ward E, Hao Y, Xu J, et al. (2009) Cancer statistics, 2009. CA Cancer J Clin 59: 225–249.
3. Rogers HW, Weinstock MA, Harris AR, Hinckley MR, Feldman SR, et al. (2010) Incidence estimate of nonmelanoma skin cancer in the United States, 2006. Arch Dermatol 146: 283–287.
4. Berg D, Otley CC (2002) Skin cancer in organ transplant recipients: Epidemiology, pathogenesis, and management. J Am Acad Dermatol 47: 1–17; quiz 18–20.
5. Norval M (2001) Effects of solar radiation on the human immune system. J Photochem Photobiol B 63: 28–40.
6. O'Dell BL, Jessen RT, Becker LE, Jackson RT, Smith EB (1980) Diminished immune response in sun-damaged skin. Arch Dermatol 116: 559–561.
7. Dunn GP, Bruce AT, Ikeda H, Old LJ, Schreiber RD (2002) Cancer immunoediting: from immunosurveillance to tumor escape. Nat Immunol 3: 991–998.
8. Schreiber RD, Old LJ, Smyth MJ (2011) Cancer immunoediting: integrating immunity's roles in cancer suppression and promotion. Science 331: 1565–1570.
9. Coley WB (1991) The treatment of malignant tumors by repeated inoculations of erysipelas. With a report of ten original cases. 1893. Clin Orthop Relat Res: 3–11.
10. Starnes CO (1992) Coley's toxins in perspective. Nature 357: 11–12.
11. Lai Y, Gallo RL (2008) Toll-like receptors in skin infections and inflammatory diseases. Infect Disord Drug Targets 8: 144–155.
12. Lai Y, Gallo RL (2009) AMPed up immunity: how antimicrobial peptides have multiple roles in immune defense. Trends Immunol 30: 131–141.
13. Ong PY, Ohtake T, Brandt C, Strickland I, Boguniewicz M, et al. (2002) Endogenous antimicrobial peptides and skin infections in atopic dermatitis. N Engl J Med 347: 1151–1160.
14. Schauber J, Gallo RL (2009) Antimicrobial peptides and the skin immune defense system. J Allergy Clin Immunol 124: R13–18.
15. Zanetti M (2005) The role of cathelicidins in the innate host defenses of mammals. Curr Issues Mol Biol 7: 179–196.

16. Dorschner RA, Pestonjamasp VK, Tamakuwala S, Ohtake T, Rudisill J, et al. (2001) Cutaneous injury induces the release of cathelicidin anti-microbial peptides active against group A Streptococcus. J Invest Dermatol 117: 91–97.
17. Nizet V, Ohtake T, Lauth X, Trowbridge J, Rudisill J, et al. (2001) Innate antimicrobial peptide protects the skin from invasive bacterial infection. Nature 414: 454–457.
18. Koczulla R, von Degenfeld G, Kupatt C, Krotz F, Zahler S, et al. (2003) An angiogenic role for the human peptide antibiotic LL-37/hCAP-18. J Clin Invest 111: 1665–1672.
19. Kesting MR, Sudhoff H, Hasler RJ, Nieberler M, Pautke C, et al. (2009) Psoriasin (S100A7) up-regulation in oral squamous cell carcinoma and its relation to clinicopathologic features. Oral Oncol 45: 731–736.
20. Yoshimoto T, Yamaai T, Mizukawa N, Sawaki K, Nakano M, et al. (2003) Different expression patterns of beta-defensins in human squamous cell carcinomas. Anticancer Res 23: 4629–4633.
21. Buchau AS, Morizane S, Trowbridge J, Schauber J, Kotol P, et al. (2010) The host defense peptide cathelicidin is required for NK cell-mediated suppression of tumor growth. J Immunol 184: 369–378.
22. Wagstaff AJ, Perry CM (2007) Topical imiquimod: a review of its use in the management of anogenital warts, actinic keratoses, basal cell carcinoma and other skin lesions. Drugs 67: 2187–2210.
23. Braff MH, Bardan A, Nizet V, Gallo RL (2005) Cutaneous defense mechanisms by antimicrobial peptides. J Invest Dermatol 125: 9–13.
24. Glaser R, Harder J, Lange H, Bartels J, Christophers E, et al. (2005) Antimicrobial psoriasin (S100A7) protects human skin from Escherichia coli infection. Nat Immunol 6: 57–64.
25. Glaser R, Koten B, Wittersheim M, Harder J (2011) Psoriasin: key molecule of the cutaneous barrier? J Dtsch Dermatol Ges 9: 897–902.
26. Kisich KO, Howell MD, Boguniewicz M, Heizer HR, Watson NU, et al. (2007) The constitutive capacity of human keratinocytes to kill Staphylococcus aureus is dependent on beta-defensin 3. J Invest Dermatol 127: 2368–2380.
27. Pollack JR, Perou CM, Alizadeh AA, Eisen MB, Pergamenschikov A, et al. (1999) Genome-wide analysis of DNA copy-number changes using cDNA microarrays. Nat Genet 23: 41–46.
28. Wang Z, Gerstein M, Snyder M (2009) RNA-Seq: a revolutionary tool for transcriptomics. Nat Rev Genet 10: 57–63.
29. Hudson LG, Gale JM, Padilla RS, Pickett G, Alexander BE, et al. (2010) Microarray analysis of cutaneous squamous cell carcinomas reveals enhanced expression of epidermal differentiation complex genes. Mol Carcinog 49: 619–629.
30. Huang B, Zhao J, Unkeless JC, Feng ZH, Xiong H (2008) TLR signaling by tumor and immune cells: a double-edged sword. Oncogene 27: 218–224.
31. Kelly MG, Alvero AB, Chen R, Silasi DA, Abrahams VM, et al. (2006) TLR-4 signaling promotes tumor growth and paclitaxel chemoresistance in ovarian cancer. Cancer Res 66: 3859–3868.
32. Lee JW, Choi JJ, Seo ES, Kim MJ, Kim WY, et al. (2007) Increased toll-like receptor 9 expression in cervical neoplasia. Mol Carcinog 46: 941–947.
33. Szczepanski M, Stelmachowska M, Stryczynski L, Golusinski W, Samara H, et al. (2007) Assessment of expression of toll-like receptors 2, 3 and 4 in laryngeal carcinoma. Eur Arch Otorhinolaryngol 264: 525–530.
34. Vahle AK, Kerem A, Ozturk E, Bankfalvi A, Lang S, et al. (2012) Optimization of an orthotopic murine model of head and neck squamous cell carcinoma in fully immunocompetent mice–role of toll-like-receptor 4 expressed on host cells. Cancer Lett 317: 199–206.
35. Schauber J, Dorschner RA, Coda AB, Buchau AS, Liu PT, et al. (2007) Injury enhances TLR2 function and antimicrobial peptide expression through a vitamin D-dependent mechanism. J Clin Invest 117: 803–811.
36. Frye M, Bargon J, Gropp R (2001) Expression of human beta-defensin-1 promotes differentiation of keratinocytes. J Mol Med (Berl) 79: 275–282.
37. Kawsar HI, Ghosh SK, Hirsch SA, Koon HB, Weinberg A, et al. (2010) Expression of human beta-defensin-2 in intratumoral vascular endothelium and in endothelial cells induced by transforming growth factor beta. Peptides 31: 195–201.
38. Sawaki K, Mizukawa N, Yamaai T, Yoshimoto T, Nakano M, et al. (2002) High concentration of beta-defensin-2 in oral squamous cell carcinoma. Anticancer Res 22: 2103–2107.
39. Jin G, Kawsar HI, Hirsch SA, Zeng C, Jia X, et al. (2010) An antimicrobial peptide regulates tumor-associated macrophage trafficking via the chemokine receptor CCR2, a model for tumorigenesis. PLoS One 5: e10993.
40. Gambichler T, Skrygan M, Huyn J, Bechara FG, Sand M, et al. (2006) Pattern of mRNA expression of beta-defensins in basal cell carcinoma. BMC Cancer 6: 163.
41. Mburu YK, Abe K, Ferris LK, Sarkar SN, Ferris RL (2011) Human beta-defensin 3 promotes NF-kappaB-mediated CCR7 expression and anti-apoptotic signals in squamous cell carcinoma of the head and neck. Carcinogenesis 32: 168–174.
42. Moubayed N, Weichenthal M, Harder J, Wandel E, Sticherling M, et al. (2007) Psoriasin (S100A7) is significantly up-regulated in human epithelial skin tumours. J Cancer Res Clin Oncol 133: 253–261.
43. Wolf R, Voscopoulos C, Winston J, Dharamsi A, Goldsmith P, et al. (2009) Highly homologous hS100A15 and hS100A7 proteins are distinctly expressed in normal breast tissue and breast cancer. Cancer Lett 277: 101–107.
44. Al-Haddad S, Zhang Z, Leygue E, Snell L, Huang A, et al. (1999) Psoriasin (S100A7) expression and invasive breast cancer. Am J Pathol 155: 2057–2066.
45. Emberley ED, Alowami S, Snell L, Murphy LC, Watson PH (2004) S100A7 (psoriasin) expression is associated with aggressive features and alteration of Jab1 in ductal carcinoma in situ of the breast. Breast Cancer Res 6: R308–315.
46. Leygue E, Snell L, Hiller T, Dotzlaw H, Hole K, et al. (1996) Differential expression of psoriasin messenger RNA between in situ and invasive human breast carcinoma. Cancer Res 56: 4606–4609.
47. Morgan MR, Jazayeri M, Ramsay AG, Thomas GJ, Boulanger MJ, et al. (2011) Psoriasin (S100A7) associates with integrin beta6 subunit and is required for alphavbeta6-dependent carcinoma cell invasion. Oncogene 30: 1422–1435.
48. Krynitz B, Lundh Rozell B, Lindelof B (2010) Differences in the peritumoural inflammatory skin infiltrate between squamous cell carcinomas in organ transplant recipients and immunocompetent patients. Acta Derm Venereol 90: 379–385.
49. Muhleisen B, Petrov I, Gachter T, Kurrer M, Scharer L, et al. (2009) Progression of cutaneous squamous cell carcinoma in immunosuppressed patients is associated with reduced CD123+ and FOXP3+ cells in the perineoplastic inflammatory infiltrate. Histopathology 55: 67–76.
50. Mathew T, Kreis H, Friend P (2004) Two-year incidence of malignancy in sirolimus-treated renal transplant recipients: results from five multicenter studies. Clin Transplant 18: 446–449.
51. Liu AY, Destoumieux D, Wong AV, Park CH, Valore EV, et al. (2002) Human beta-defensin-2 production in keratinocytes is regulated by interleukin-1, bacteria, and the state of differentiation. J Invest Dermatol 118: 275–281.
52. Asea A, Rehli M, Kabingu E, Boch JA, Bare O, et al. (2002) Novel signal transduction pathway utilized by extracellular HSP70: role of toll-like receptor (TLR) 2 and TLR4. J Biol Chem 277: 15028–15034.
53. Kuhns DB, Priel DA, Gallin JI (2007) Induction of human monocyte interleukin (IL)-8 by fibrinogen through the toll-like receptor pathway. Inflammation 30: 178–188.
54. Euvrard S, Kanitakis J, Claudy A (2003) Skin cancers after organ transplantation. N Engl J Med 348: 1681–1691.
55. Cumberland L, Dana A, Liegeois N (2009) Mohs micrographic surgery for the management of nonmelanoma skin cancers. Facial Plast Surg Clin North Am 17: 325–335.

13

Prognosis of Sentinel Node Staged Patients with Primary Cutaneous Melanoma

Otmar Elsaeßer[1]ᶺ, Ulrike Leiter[1*]ᶺ, Petra G. Buettner[2], Thomas K. Eigentler[1], Friedegund Meier[1], Benjamin Weide[1], Gisela Metzler[1], Helmut Breuninger[1], Claus Garbe[1,2]

1 Center for Dermatooncology, Department of Dermatology, and Central Malignant Melanoma Registry of the German Dermatological Society, Eberhard-Karls-University of Tuebingen, Tuebingen, Germany, 2 Skin Cancer Research Group, School of Public Health and Tropical Medicine, James Cook University, Townsville, Queensland, Australia

Abstract

Background: This study investigated survival probabilities and prognostic factors in sentinel lymph node biopsy (SLNB) staged patients with cutaneous melanoma (CM) with the aim of defining subgroups of patients who are at higher risk for recurrences and who should be considered for adjuvant clinical trials.

Methods: Patients with primary CM who underwent SLNB in the Department of Dermatology, University of Tuebingen, Germany, between 1996 and 2009 were included into this study. Survival probabilities and prognostic factors were evaluated by Kaplan-Meier and multivariate Cox proportional hazard models.

Results: 1909 SLNB staged patients were evaluated. Median follow-up time was 44 months. Median tumor thickness was 1.8 mm, ulceration was present in 31.8% of cases. The 5-year Overall Survival (OS) was 90.3% in SLNB negative patients (IB 96.2%, IIA 87.0%, IIB 78.1%, IIC 72.6%). Patients with micrometastases (stage IIIA/B) had a 5-year OS rate of 70.9% which was clearly less favorable than for stages I–II. Multivariate analysis revealed tumor thickness, ulceration, body site, histopathologic subtype and SLNB status as independent significant prognostic factors.

Conclusion: Survival rates of patients with primary CM in stages I–II were shown to be much more favorable than previously reported from non sentinel node staged collectives. For future clinical trials, sample size calculations should be adapted using survival probabilities based on sentinel node staging.

Editor: H. Peter Soyer, The University of Queensland, Australia

Funding: These authors have no support or funding to report.

Competing Interests: The authors have declared that no competing interests exist.

* E-mail: ulrike.leiter@med.uni-tuebingen.de

ᶺ These authors contributed equally to this work.

Introduction

Sentinel lymph node biopsy (SLNB) is a minimally invasive procedure with minor morbidity for patients with cutaneous melanoma (CM). SLNB allows to ascertain the status of the regional node field and assists with exact staging [1–3]. During the last decade SLNB has become a routinely performed procedure in most melanoma centers worldwide [4–6] There is international consent that SLNB should be discussed with and recommended to patients when at least one of the following indications is present [1]: (1) the risk of clinically occult nodal metastases is sufficient to justify the procedure (approximately 10%); (2) the prognostic information from SLNB would be of value to the patient and the treating physicians; (3), the tumor status of the SLN would be useful in guiding decisions regarding complete lymphadenectomy and adjuvant therapy; (4) nodal staging information is important for entry into clinical trials if the patient is interested; and/or (5) the risks of SLNB are acceptable to the physician and the patient [7]. SLNB is regarded to be a valuable procedure for CM patients allowing to stage regional lymph nodes with little morbidity [5,8].

The accuracy of SLNB staging has been shown through a long-term follow-up of SLNB negative patients. These patients have an improved survival compared to the SLNB positive group, and have less regional recurrences in the mapped node fields [3]. In SLNB staged patients nodal recurrences seem to occur less frequent but so far recurrence rates were reported in only a few case series, some of which had limited follow-up [4,9–14]. As the presence of nodal micrometastases is the single most important prognostic factor [5] patients want to get this information to be considered for new therapies under evaluation in clinical trials, and to make an informed decision about complete lymphadenectomy and adjuvant therapy. In addition, the information provided by a positive SN can be used to counsel patients regarding enrollment into clinical trials and can serve as the basis for discussing screening and follow-up regimen [15].

So far, few data on survival probabilities and prognostic factors in SLNB staged patients were reported. In order to validate the AJCC classification, Balch and Co-workers evaluated stage I/III CM patients who were considered as clinically node negative [16].

Table 1. Five-year **overall survival** (OS) and **disease-free** survival (DFS) probabilities based on Kaplan-Meier in sentinel node staged patients with CM (n = 1909).

Prognostic Factor	Number of Patients n (%)	Censored (%) at OS	P value 5-year OS [95% CI]	Censored (%) at DFS	P-value 5-year DFS [95% CI]
Thickness			P<0.0001		P<0.001
≤1.00 mm	188 (9.8%)	96.8	97.5 [94.6, 100]	94.1	96.9 [94.2, 99.6]
1.01–2.00 mm	934 (48.9%)	93.9	93.0 [90.7, 95.3]	86.6	84.2 [81.3, ,87.1]
2.01–4.00 mm	565 (29.6%)	86.2	82.8 [78.7, 86.9]	71.9	64.2 [59.7, 68.7]
>4 mm	222 (11.6%)	77.9	68.3 [60.1, 76.5]	61.7	55.3 [47.1, 63.5]
Ulceration			P<0.0001		P<0.001
absent	1094 (68.2%)	93.3	93.2 [91.3, 95.1]	87.3	86.2 [83.9, 88.5]
present	511 (31.8%)	83.0	75.8 [70.9, 80.7]	66.9	57.7 [52.5, 62.9]
Body site			P<0.0001		P<0.001
Head and Neck	231 (12.1%)	91.3	88.7 [83.0, 94.4]	79.1	75.5 [68.5, 82.6]
Trunk	729 (38.2%)	87.0	84.3 [81.0, 87.6]	78.1	74.1 [66.3, 78.0]
Upper limb	343 (18.0%)	97.1	95.6 [92.7, 98.5]	91.3	89.2 [85.1, 93.3]
Lower limb	606 (31.7%)	89.3	88.7 [85.6, 91.8]	76.4	72.6 [68.5, 76.7]
AJCC Stage			p<0.001		p<0.001
I A	90 (5.3%)	100.0	100.0	95.2	97.2 [95.2, 99.2]
I B	824 (43.2%)	96.0	96.2 [94.4, 98.0]	90.9	90.3 [89.0, 91.6]
II A	434 (22.7%)	90.6	87.0 [82.9, 91.1]	80.6	75.4 [72.9, 77.9]
II B	260 (13.6%)	83.8	78.1 [71.2, 85.0]	67.7	58.2 [54.2, 62.2]
II C	87 (4.6%)	80.5	72.6 [59.5, 83.9]	59.8	50.7 [43.0, 58.4]
III A	119 (6.2%)	73.1	72.6 [62.8, 82.4]	53.8	45.9 [40.4, 51.4]
III B	95 (5.0%)	73.7	65.6 [53.4, 77.8]	54.7	44.9 [38.7, 51.1]
Age			P = 0.035		P = 0.001
< = 45-year	531 (27.8%)	92.1	92.0 [89.3, 94.7]	84.0	82.6 [78.9, 86.3]
46–60 years	529 (27.7%)	87.7	86.3 [82.8, 89.8]	78.8	76.8 [72.7, 80.9]
61–70 years	454 (23.8%)	88.1	85.0 [80.7, 89.3]	78.0	73.7 [68.8, 78.6]
>70 years	395 (20.7%)	92.7	88.0 [83.1, 92.9]	79.0	70.2 [64.1, 76.3]
Gender			P = 0.068		P = 0.135
Male	1012 (53.0%)	88.8	86.2 [79.6, 93.0]	78.8	74.6 [74.5, 77.9]
Female	897(47.0%)	91.4	89.5 [87.0, 92.0]	81.6	78.0 [74.7, 81.3]
Clark-Level			P<0.0001		P<0.001
Level II	12 (0.7%)	100.0	100.0	91.7	85.7 [80.7, 88.2]
Level III	209 (12.6%)	95.7	93.1 [91.0, 95.1]	89.0	88.2 [83.3, 93.1]
Level IV	1350 (81.4%)	90.8	89.1 [88.0, 90.2]	80.6	76.9 [76.8, 79.6]
Level V	88 (5.3%)	75.0	82.3 [79.1, 85.5]	60.2	55.1 [43.0, 67.2]
Histological Subtype			P<0.001		P<0.001
SSM	993 (54.6%)	90.2	91.0 [89.9, 92.1]	82.6	80.6 [79.5, 81.7]
NM	437(24.0%)	86.2	82.9 [79.7, 82.3]	74.8	69.1 [66.4, 71.8]
LMM	81 (4.5%)	96.3	95.2 [69.5, 79.1]	88.9	86.2 [81.4, 91.0]
ALM	150 (8.2%)	81.3	74.3 [92.5, 97.9]	65.3	56.2 [51.2, 61.7]
Other	158 (8.7%)	95.6	93.2 [87.9, 98.5]	89.2	83.8 [76.2, 91.4]
SLNB status			P<0.001		P<0.001
negative	1697 (88.9%)	92.0	90.3 [88.5, 92.1]	83.3	80.6 [78.2, 83.0]
positive	212 (11.1%)	74.5	70.9 [63.3, 78.5]	54.2	46.0 [38.0, 54.1]

SD = Standard Deviation; IQR = Inter-Quartile Range; SSM = superficial spreading melanoma, NM = nodular melanoma, LMM = lentigious malignant melanoma, ALM = Acral lentigious melanoma; AJCC = American Joint Committee of Cancer.

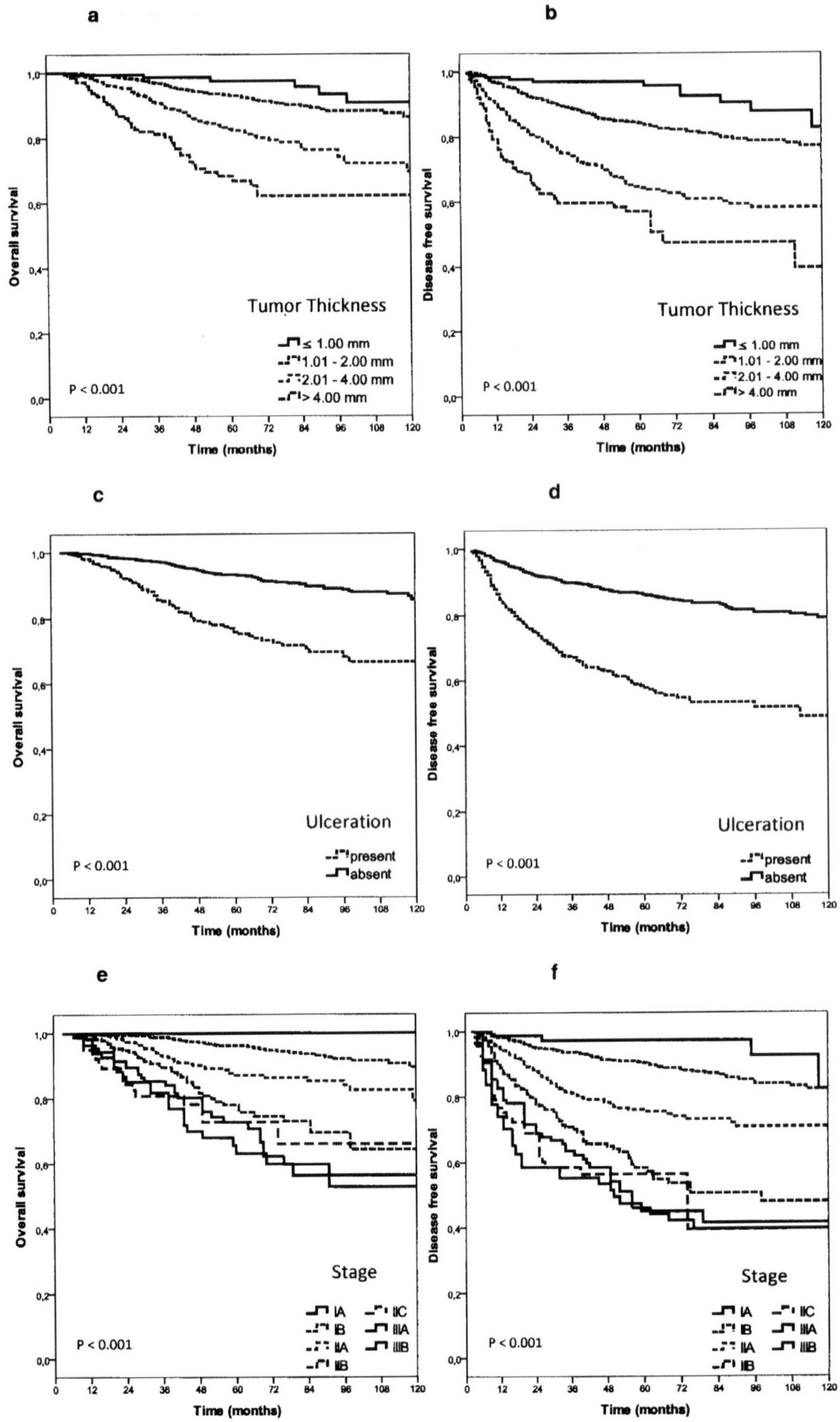
a
Overall survival
Tumor Thickness
≤ 1.00 mm
1.01 - 2.00 mm
2.01 - 4.00 mm
> 4.00 mm
P < 0.001
Time (months)
b
Disease free survival
Tumor Thickness
≤ 1.00 mm
1.01 - 2.00 mm
2.01 - 4.00 mm
> 4.00 mm
P < 0.001
Time (months)
c
Overall survival
Ulceration
present
absent
P < 0.001
Time (months)
d
Disease free survival
Ulceration
present
absent
P < 0.001
Time (months)
e
Overall survival
Stage
IA
IB
IIA
IIB
IIC
IIIA
IIIB
P < 0.001
Time (months)
f
Disease free survival
Stage
IA
IB
IIA
IIB
IIC
IIIA
IIIB
P < 0.001
Time (months)

Figure 1. Survival in sentinel node staged patients. a) Overall survival according to primary tumor thickness ($p<0.001$). b) Disease free survival according to primary tumor thickness ($p<0.001$). c) Overall survival in patients with and without ulcerated primary tumors ($p<0.001$). d) Disease-free survival in patients with and without ulcerated primary tumors ($p<0.001$). e) Overall survival according to AJCC stage of primary tumor ($p<0.001$). f) Disease-free survival according to AJCC stage of primary tumor ($p<0.001$).

SLNB staging had been performed for a part of these patients and there are only few cohorts of melanoma patients with a long-term follow-up after negative SLNB staging. The present study was performed to evaluate survival probabilities and prognostic factors of 1909 SLNB staged CM patients with the aim to define groups of patients who are at higher risk for recurrences and who should be considered for adjuvant clinical trials and undergo a closer follow-up.

Methods

The present analysis included patients with cutaneous melanoma (CM) diagnosed and treated by the Department of Dermatology, University Tuebingen, Germany. Patients included were diagnosed with incident invasive (Clark's level of invasion II or more) primary CM between January 1st 1996 and June 30th 2009. All patients had given their written informed consent (Supporting Information S1), the local Ethic committee statement had no concern (Supporting Information S2). At the University Department of Dermatology in Tuebingen, Germany, sentinel lymph node biopsy was introduced in January 1996 and has been routinely performed by four dermato-surgeons over the entire time period in all CM patients with a tumor thickness of 1.00 mm or more. SLNB was also performed in 101 patients with smaller tumors if additional unfavorable prognostic factors as a level of invasion IV–V, ulceration or tumor regression were present.

Follow-up examinations were performed according to the recommendations of the German Society of Dermatology comprising physical examinations every three months during years 1–5 after primary tumor diagnosis, twice yearly in years 6–10 and, twice respectively once yearly, lymph node ultrasound and blood tests [17]. Body site of the primary melanoma was classified into five anatomical sites: head with scalp and neck, anterior trunk, posterior trunk, upper and lower extremities. Histopathological analysis of sentinel lymph nodes was based on four serial sections performed at each of two levels. The sections from each level were stained with H&E and immunohistochemical stains for S-100 protein, HMB-45, and Melan-A. Reports of the responsible dermato-histopathologists were documented. SLNB containing isolated positive tumor cells or micrometastases of ≤0.1 mm were not judged as positive, in agreement with the 2002 AJCC melanoma classification [18].

Recurrences during follow-up were distinguished as loco-regional metastases (satellite/in-transit metastases), regional lymph node metastases and distant metastases. Loco-regional, nodal and distant recurrences were analyzed. Satellite metastasis was defined as recurrence in the first melanoma field 2 cm of the edge of the wide excision margin. In-transit metastasis was defined as subcutaneous metastases from 2 cm to the first nodal site. Only the first recurrence was considered for this analysis. False-negative SNBs were defined as procedures in which the initial histopathologic evaluation was negative, but the patients tumor recurred in the same node field. Patients whose tumor recurred as satellite or in-transit disease, followed by regional node field recurrence, were not considered to have a false-negative SNB on the assumption that the disease may not have been present in the regional nodes at the time of biopsy.

Statistical analysis

Statistical analyses were performed with the statistic software SPSS 19 (PASW, IBM SPSS, Chicago, IL, USA). Numerical variables were described by mean value and standard deviation (SD) if approximately normally distributed or median value and inter-quartile range (IQR) if skewed. Proportions were presented with 95% confidence intervals (95%-CI).

The time between primary excision of histological diagnosed CM and the date of the last follow-up visit or the date of death was used to calculate the follow-up time for melanoma-specific overall survival (OS), and the date of first recurrence for the disease-free survival (DFS), respectively. Only deaths due to CM (melanoma specific deaths) were considered "events". In case that mortality and cause of death was not directly reported, registration offices were systematically addressed. Survival probabilities with 95%-CI were calculated according to Kaplan-Meier and compared with log-rank test statistics. Multivariate Cox proportional hazard models were calculated to judge significant independent prognostic factors. Forward and backward stepwise procedures of the multivariate modeling process resulted in the same model. Results of Cox proportional hazard modeling were described as relative risks (hazard ratios) together with 95%-CI and p-values. Throughout the analysis, p-values less than 0.05 were considered as statistically significant.

Results

Selection of patients

From January 1996 to June 2009, a total of 6,028 patients with primary cutaneous melanoma were documented by the Department of Dermatology, Tuebingen, Germany. Patients with advanced disease, unknown primary or melanoma in extra-cutaneous localization ($n=660$), patients without SLNB ($n=3{,}330$) and patients with follow-up less than 3 months ($n=129$) were excluded. The present cohort consisted of 1,909 SLNB staged patients, of these 1,697 (88.9%) with negative and 212 (11.1%) with positive SLNB. Of 1,697 SLNB negative patients, 99 (5.8%) presented with a tumor thickness of less than 1.00 mm while there were two (0.9%) of 212 SLNB positive patients with a tumor thickness below 1 mm. Before SLNB was performed all patients underwent physical examinations and lymph node ultrasound. If these examinations suggested metastases these findings were judged as macrometastases as they were detected by clinical methods, and these patients were not included in the present analysis.

Description of sample

The collective of 1909 SLNB staged CM patients consisted of 53.0% males and 47.0% females. The mean age at diagnosis was 55.9 years (SD±16.1), the median tumor thickness was 1.80 mm (IQR = [1.2, 2.8]). Ulceration was present in 31.8% of the primary lesions (Table 1). The total rate of patients with recurrences was 20.2% ($N=385$), 35.1% of the first recurrences were satellite/intransit metastases ($N=135$), 30.9% were regional lymph node metastases ($N=119$) and 34.0% were distant metastases ($N=131$). If metastases on different sites occurred simultaneously, the metastasis with the worst prognosis counted as first metastasis. The rate of false negative SLN for the entire series was 13.1%.

a

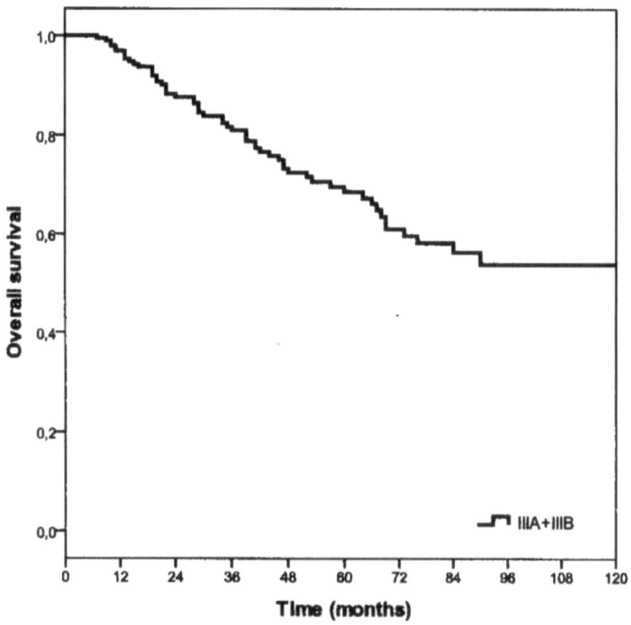

Survival probabilities and 95% CI				
Stage	1 year	3 years	5 years	10 years
IIIA+B	96.9%	81.1%	68.6%	53.9%
IIIA+B	[94.5; 99.3]	[75.2; 87.0]	[60.8; 76.4]	[43.5; 64.3]

b

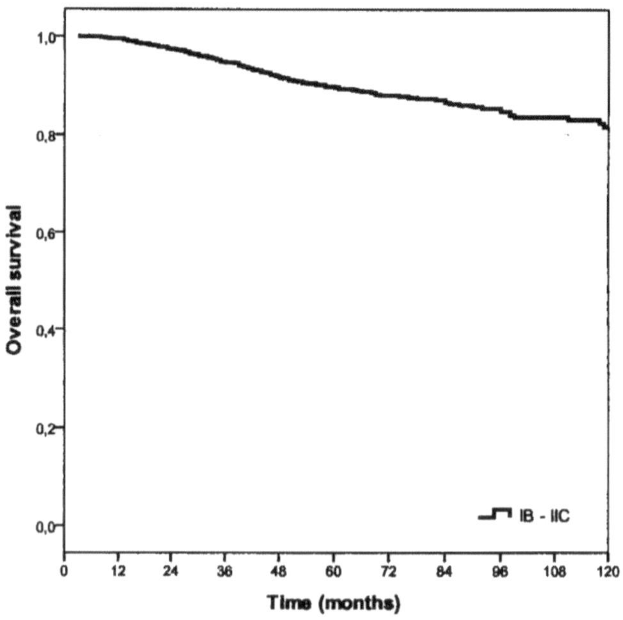

Survival probabilities and 95% CI				
Stage	1 year	3 years	5 years	10 years
IB-IIC	99.5%	94.7%	89.7%	81.7%
IB-IIC	[99.1; 99.9]	[93.3; 96.1]	[87.7; 91.7]	[78.0; 85.4]

c

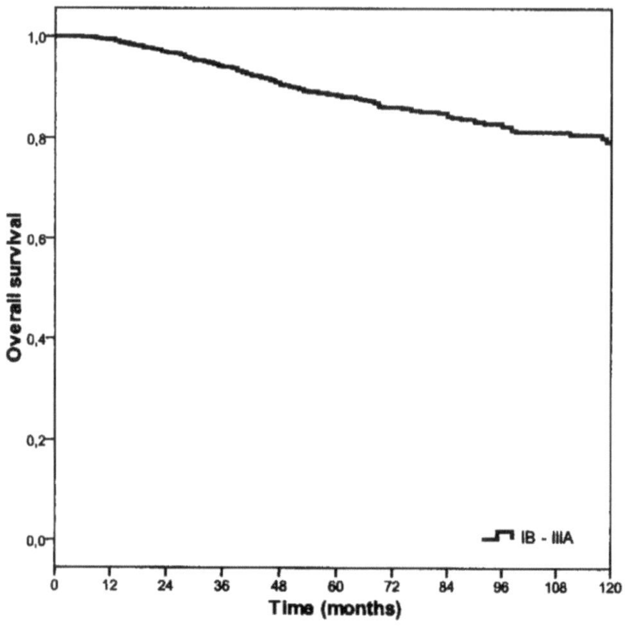

Survival probabilities and 95% CI				
Stages	1 year	3 years	5 years	10 years
IB-IIIA	99.4	93.9	88.4	79.4
IB-IIIA	[99.0; 99.8]	[92.5; 95.3]	[86.4; 90.4]	[75.7; 83.1]

d

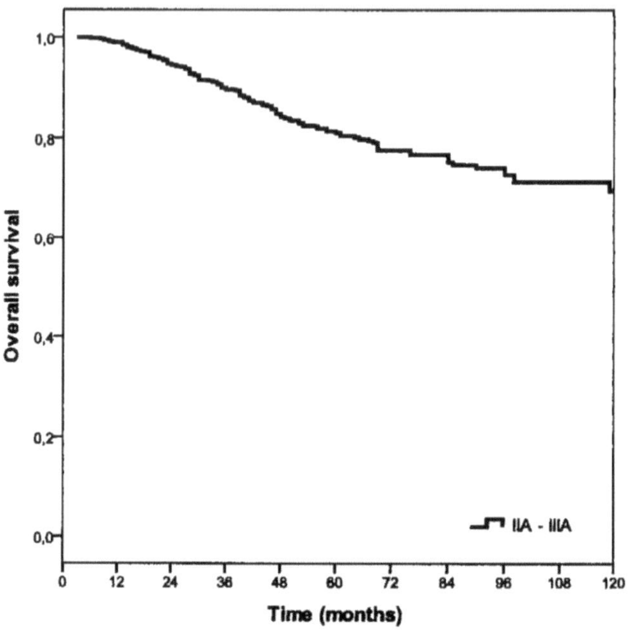

Survival probabilities and 95% CI				
Stages	1 year	3 years	5 years	10 years
IIA-IIIA	99.0	89.6	81.1	69.5
IIA-IIIA	[98.4; 99.6]	[87.2; 92.0]	[77.8; 84.4]	[63.4; 75.6]

Figure 2. Overall survival in different stages of primary tumors according to AJCC 2009. a) Overall survival in stage IIIA CM patients. b) Overall survival in stage IB- IIC CM patients. c) Overall survival in stage IB- IIIA CM patients. d) Overall survival in stage IIA-IIIA CM patients.

Disease related deaths occurred in 10% (n = 190; 95%CI = 8.7, 11.4). Follow up information for a period of 5-year or more was available for 35.3% of patients, 52% of all patients were diagnosed later than 2004 and did not yet reach a five-years follow-up at the timepoint of the analysis. The median OS time for the whole collective was 44 months (IQR = 21, 74); while the median DFS was 38 months (IQR = 15, 68).

Prognostic factors in SLNB staged patients

Kaplan-Meier analysis of OS identified age (p = 0.035), tumor thickness (p<0.001), body site (p<0.001), ulceration (p<0.001), Clark level of invasion (p<0.001), histological subtype (p<0.001) and SLNB status (p<0.001) as significant prognostic factors (see Table 1 and Figure 1a–f). Similar results were found for DFS for age (p = 0.001), tumor thickness (p<0.001), body site (p<0.001), ulceration (p<0.001), Clark level of invasion (p<0.001), histological subtype (p<0.001) and SLNB status (p<0.001) (see Table 1).

The 5-year melanoma-specific survival probabilities were 90.3% (95%CI: 88.5; 92.1) for node-negative patients compared to 70.9% (95%CI: 63.3, 78.5; p<0.001) for node-positive patients (see Table 1, Figure 2a–d). The 5-year DFS for SLNB negative patients was 80.6% (95%CI: 78.2, 83.0), vs 46.0% (95% CI: 38.0, 54.1) for SLNB positive patients.

Analyzing stages according to AJCC 2009, no significant differences could be found for OS in stages IB-IIC compared to IB-IIIA, the 5-year OS was 89.7% and. 88.4%, respectively, Figures 2b–c. Stage IIC patients showed a similar 5-year OS as stage IIIA patients (72.6%), the DFS was 50.7% and 45.9%, respectively, see Table 1. The results of the current study are listed and compared to those of Balch et al. [15] in Table 2.

Multivariate Cox proportional hazard analyses identified tumor thickness, ulceration, body site, histological subtype and SLNB status as independent significant prognostic factors for melanoma-specific and disease-free survival, Table 3. Tumors with a thickness of >4 mm had an increased relative risk to die of CM (5.2, 95%CI: 2.1, 12.7) compared to CM of ≤1.0 mm thickness (p<0.001, Table 3). Patients with positive SLNB status were 2.3 (95%CI: 1.6, 3.1) times more likely to die from melanoma compared to patients with negative SLNB (p<0.001). Age, gender and Clark's level of invasion failed to be independent significant prognostic factors for overall and disease-free survival.

Table 2. Five and 10-year melanoma-specific survival in sentinel node-staged cutaneous melanoma patients (n = 1909). compared to in 27,000 stage I/II and 2,587 stage IIIA/B patients reported by Balch et al. [15,18].

Stage	5-year OS		10-Years OS	
	Balch	Present Study	Balch	Present study
IB	n.g*	96%	n.g.	89.5%
T1b			85%	
T2			80%	
IIA	79–82%	87.0%	n.g.	79.2%
IIB	68–71%	78.1%	n.g.	64.3%
IIC	53%	72.6%	n.g.	66.0%
Micrometastases	67%	70.9%	n.g.	53.9%
IIIA	78%	72.6%	n.g.	56.4%
IIIB	59%	65.6%	n.g.	52.8%

*: n.g.: not given.

Discussion

In the last two decades, sentinel lymph node biopsy has become a standard procedure for nodal staging in patients with primary CM and clinically uninvolved lymph nodes. If SLNB was not part of the management of a CM patient, this patient might not be considered eligible for clinical trials [1]. This exclusion would not only slow the development of more effective therapies but could

Table 3. Prognostic factors of overall (OS) and disease-free (DFS) survival in sentinel node-staged CM patients (n = 1909). Results of multivariate Cox proportional hazard analysis.

	OS#			DFS##		
Prognostic factor	**RR**	**95% CI**	**p value**	**RR**	**95% CI**	**p value**
Tumor thickness			<0.001			<0.001
≤1.0 mm	1			1		
1.01–2.0 mm	1.6	0.69, 3.8		2.1	1.1, 3.8	
2.01–4.0 mm	3.1	1.3, 7.2		3.8	2.0, 7.2	
>4.0 mm	5.2	2.1, 12.7		5.7	3.0, 11.1	
Ulceration*			<0.001			<0.001
Absent	1			1		
Present	2.1	1.5, 3.0		2.2	1.7, 2.9	
Body site			<0.001			<0.001
Upper limb	1			1		
Head and Neck	3.8	1.7, 8.3		3.1	1.9, 5.0	
Lower limb	2.5	1.3, 4.9		2.4	1.6, 3.6	
Trunk	4.9	2.5, 9.6		2.9	1.9, 4.3	
SLNB status			<0.001			<0.001
Negative	1			1		
Positive	2.3	1.6, 3.1		2.3	1.8, 3.0	
Histological subtype**			= 0.034			= 0.014
SSM	1			1		
NM	1.1	0.73, 1.5		0.82	0.63, 1.1	
LMM	0.72	0.20, 2.5		0.56	0.26, 1.2	
ALM	2.2	1.3, 3.7		1.3	0.91, 1.9	
Other	0.64	0.29, 1.4		0.54	0.32, 0.91	
Gender			= 0.422			= 0.639
Age			= 0.166			= 0.133
Clark's level			= 0.823			= 0.747

RR = hazard ratio; 95% CI = 95% confidence interval.
*Adjusted for 304 missing values; Adjusted for 90 missing values;
#Model for melanoma-specific survival was adjusted for the confounding effects of age and gender;
##Model for disease-free survival was adjusted for the confounding effect of age.

also disadvantage patients by preventing them from receiving adequate therapy [1].

The current study was performed in order to evaluate survival probabilities and prognostic factors in 1909 SLNB staged CM patients. Only few cohorts of patients with primary CM and complete nodal staging with SLNB have been published so far [2,12,13,19]. In most published cohorts analyzing survival, nodal staging was either incomplete or not comparable to the present results [3,16,19]. We found more favorable survival probabilities compared to previously published cohorts which had incomplete nodal staging [18]. In addition, we calculated survival probabilities for groups of patients with different stages who were at elevated risk for recurrences and who might be eligible for adjuvant treatments. These stage-specific survival probabilities may be useful for sample size calculations for future melanoma trials.

In the 2009 AJCC staging classification Balch and co-workers investigated 27000 CM patients in stage I/II and 2313 in stage III with complete follow-up data in the AJCC melanoma staging database [15,18]. For the 27000 stage I/II patients with primary CM, tumor thickness, mitotic rate and ulceration were the most dominant prognostic factors.

Comparing the results of Balch et al. [18] to those of the present study, our patients showed an advanced 5-/10 year survival-probability, see Table 2. These discrepancies and improved survival for stage IB-IIC in our analysis may be caused by the fact that the data of 27000 patients in stages I/II published by Balch et al [18], may also include patients who had not undergone SLNB and were not truly negative for micro-metastases [18]. In particular, in stages IIB-IIC the discrepancies between our results and Balch's are greatest (Table 2). However, in these stages the 27000 patients were at the highest risk of unrecognized micro-metastases [18].

Several studies on prognostic factors in primary melanoma patients with negative SLNB have been published in the last years [3,18,19] confirming the impact of tumor thickness and ulceration. Yee et al reported a similar 5-year OS of 90% for all SLNB negative patients, ranging from 78% to 94% for patients with or without ulceration which is nearly identical to our results (Table 1a,b) [3]. In the present study SLNB containing isolated positive tumor cells or micrometastases of ≤ 0.1 mm were not judged as positive. This is in accordance to a recent publication from Eggermont's group [20]. In this study of 1,080 patients from van der Ploeg et al the 5 years OS of 91% in patients with micrometastases <0.1 mm in diameter was shown to be similar to those of SLNB negative patients. These results are in accordance to the five-years OS (90.6%) in SLNB negative patients in the current analysis [20]. Patients with micrometastases from 0.1 to 1.0 mm showed a similar 5-years OS of 74% [20] than stage IIIA patients in our study (72.6%).

Ulceration remains the second important prognostic factor associated with unfavorable survival [7,15,16,18]. Survival rates of patients with an ulcerated CM were previously found similar to those of patients with a non-ulcerated CM of the next higher tumor thickness category [15,18]. This is in concordance to our results, where ulceration proofed to be an independent significant prognostic factor in primary CM and in the total collective of SLNB staged patients (Tables 1, 3 and Figure 1c,d).

In our collective of positive and negative SLNB staged patients, SLNB status, tumor thickness, ulceration, histological subtype and body site were identified as independent significant prognostic factors for DFS and OS during multivariate analyses. In order to define subgroups for clinical trials, histological subtype and body site may provide additional prognostic information. The SLN status was shown to be a highly significant prognostic factor with a 5-year OS of about 90.3% in negative SLNB and 70.9% in positive SLNB. The impact of the SLN status, tumor thickness and ulceration on DFS and OS has been confirmed by various publications [3,4,12,13]. In addition, histological subtype was reported to be a further significant independent prognostic factor [21,22] for OS and DFS. Studies in SLNB negative patients did not show this effect [3]. In patients with stage III disease body site was shown to be a further prognostic factor [15].

One limitation of the present study is the missing information for mitotic rate. Until January 2010, the mitotic rate of primary melanoma was not determined in Germany. However we do not expect that this limitation would change our results markedly. A positive mitotic rate upstages patients with tumor thickness less than 1.0 mm which would then be classified as stage IB instead of IA. In our collective the number of patients with tumor thickness less than 1 mm was small (5.3%), and hence a marked change of the OS and DFS is unlikely.

Conclusion

The current study was performed to evaluate the survival probabilities and prognostic factors of 1909 SLNB staged CM patients. Five year survival rates for different subgroups eligible for adjuvant trials were found to be quite favourable (five years Overall Survival rates of 89.7% in stages IB – IIC, 88.4% in stages IB – IIIA, 81.1% in stages IIA – IIIA, 68.8% in stages IIIA/B). The prognosis for primary CM patients without micro-metastases in SLNB seems to be more favorable than previously reported. It is suggested that this is mainly due to the exclusion of sentinel-node positive patients from stages I–II. It is necessary to adapt sample size calculations for survival probabilities classified by the presently valid AJCC staging system.

Author Contributions

Conceived and designed the experiments: UL CG. Performed the experiments: OE UL PB CG. Analyzed the data: OE UL PB CG. Contributed reagents/materials/analysis tools: TE FM BW GM HB UL. Wrote the paper: OE UL PB CG.

References

1. Balch CM, Morton DL, Gershenwald JE, McMasters KM, Nieweg OE, et al. (2009) Sentinel node biopsy and standard of care for melanoma. J Am Acad Dermatol 60: 872–5.
2. Phan GQ, Messina JL, Sondak VK, Zager JS (2009) Sentinel lymph node biopsy for melanoma: indications and rationale. Cancer Control 16: 234–9.
3. Yee VS, Thompson JF, McKinnon JG, Scolyer RA, Li LX, et al. (2005) Outcome in 846 cutaneous melanoma patients from a single center after a negative sentinel node biopsy. Ann Surg Oncol 12: 429–39.
4. Essner R, Conforti A, Kelley MC, Wanek L, Stern S, et al. (1999) Efficacy of lymphatic mapping, sentinel lymphadenectomy, and selective complete lymph node dissection as a therapeutic procedure for early-stage melanoma. Ann Surg Oncol JID - 9420840 6: 442–9.
5. Morton DL, Thompson JF, Cochran AJ, Mozzillo N, Elashoff R, et al. (2006) Sentinel-node biopsy or nodal observation in melanoma. N Engl J Med 355: 1307–17.
6. Morton DL, Cochran AJ, Thompson JF (2008) The rationale for sentinel-node biopsy in primary melanoma. Nat Clin Pract Oncol 5: 510–1.

7. McMasters KM, Wong SL, Edwards MJ, Ross MI, Chao C, et al. (2001) Factors that predict the presence of sentinel lymph node metastasis in patients with melanoma. Surgery 130: 151–6.
8. Morton DL, Cochran AJ, Thompson JF, Elashoff R, Essner R, et al. (2005) Sentinel node biopsy for early-stage melanoma: accuracy and morbidity in MSLT-I, an international multicenter trial. Ann Surg 242: 302–11.
9. Cascinelli N, Belli F, Santinami M, Fait V, Testori A, et al. (2000) Sentinel lymph node biopsy in cutaneous melanoma: the WHO Melanoma Program experience. Ann Surg Oncol 7: 469–74.
10. Chao C, Wong SL, Ross MI, Reintgen DS, Noyes RD, et al. (2002) Patterns of early recurrence after sentinel lymph node biopsy for melanoma. Am J Surg 184: 520–4.
11. Gadd MA, Cosimi AB, Yu J, Duncan LM, Yu L, et al. (1999) Outcome of patients with melanoma and histologically negative sentinel lymph nodes. Arch Surg 134: 381–7.
12. Gershenwald JE, Colome MI, Lee JE, Mansfield PF, Tseng C, et al. (1998) Patterns of recurrence following a negative sentinel lymph node biopsy in 243 patients with stage I or II melanoma. J Clin Oncol JID - 8309333 16: 2253–60.
13. Nowecki ZI, Rutkowski P, Nasierowska-Guttmejer A, Ruka W (2003) Sentinel lymph node biopsy in melanoma patients with clinically negative regional lymph nodes–one institution's experience. Melanoma Res 13: 35–43.
14. Wagner JD, Gordon MS, Chuang TY, Coleman JJ, III (2000) Current therapy of cutaneous melanoma. Plast Reconstr Surg 105: 1774–99.
15. Balch CM, Gershenwald JE, Soong SJ, Thompson JF, Ding S, et al. (2010) Multivariate analysis of prognostic factors among 2,313 patients with stage III melanoma: comparison of nodal micrometastases versus macrometastases. J Clin Oncol 28: 2452–9.
16. Balch CM, Soong SJ, Gershenwald JE, Thompson JF, Reintgen DS, et al. (2001) Prognostic factors analysis of 17,600 melanoma patients: validation of the American Joint Committee on Cancer melanoma staging system. J Clin Oncol JID - 8309333 19: 3622–34.
17. Garbe C (2003) A rational approach to the follow-up of melanoma patients. Recent Results Cancer Res JID - 0044671 160: 205–15.
18. Balch CM, Gershenwald JE, Soong SJ, Thompson JF, Atkins MB, et al. (2009) Final version of 2009 AJCC melanoma staging and classification. J Clin Oncol 27: 6199–206.
19. Zogakis TG, Essner R, Wang HJ, Turner RR, Takasumi YT, et al. (2005) Melanoma recurrence patterns after negative sentinel lymphadenectomy. Arch Surg 140: 865–71.
20. van der Ploeg AP, van Akkooi AC, Rutkowski P, Nowecki ZI, Michej W, et al. (2011) Prognosis in patients with sentinel node-positive melanoma is accurately defined by the combined Rotterdam tumor load and Dewar topography criteria. J Clin Oncol 29: 2206–14.
21. Kunte C, Geimer T, Baumert J, Konz B, Volkenandt M, et al. (2010) Prognostic factors associated with sentinel lymph node positivity and effect of sentinel status on survival: an analysis of 1049 patients with cutaneous melanoma. Melanoma Res 20: 330–7.
22. Mandala M, Imberti GL, Piazzalunga D, Belfiglio M, Labianca R, et al. (2009) Clinical and histopathological risk factors to predict sentinel lymph node positivity, disease-free and overall survival in clinical stages I–II AJCC skin melanoma: outcome analysis from a single-institution prospectively collected database. Eur J Cancer 45: 2537–45.

14

Dysregulated ΔNp63α Inhibits Expression of Ink4a/arf, Blocks Senescence, and Promotes Malignant Conversion of Keratinocytes

Linan Ha[1], Roshini M. Ponnamperuma[1], Steven Jay[2], M. Stacey Ricci[1¤], Wendy C. Weinberg[1*]

1 Division of Monoclonal Antibodies, Center for Drug Evaluation and Research/Food and Drug Administration (CDER/FDA), Bethesda, Maryland, United States of America, **2** SAIC-Frederick, Inc., Frederick, Maryland, United States of America

Abstract

p63 is critical for squamous epithelial development, and elevated levels of the ΔNp63α isoform are seen in squamous cell cancers of various organ sites. However, significant controversy exists regarding the role of p63 isoforms as oncoproteins or tumor suppressors. Here, lentiviruses were developed to drive long-term overexpression of ΔNp63α in primary keratinocytes. Elevated levels of ΔNp63α *in vitro* promote long-term survival and block both replicative and oncogene-induced senescence in primary keratinocytes, as evidenced by the expression of SA-β-gal and the presence of nuclear foci of heterochromatin protein 1γ. The contribution of ΔNp63α to cancer development was assessed using an *in vivo* grafting model of experimental skin tumorigenesis that allows distinction between benign and malignant tumors. Grafted lenti-ΔNp63α keratinocytes do not form tumors, whereas lenti-GFP/v-ras^{Ha} keratinocytes develop well-differentiated papillomas. Lenti-ΔNp63α/v-ras^{Ha} keratinocytes form undifferentiated carcinomas. The average volume of lenti-ΔNp63α/v-ras^{Ha} tumors was significantly higher than those in the lenti-GFP/v-ras^{Ha} group, consistent with increased BrdU incorporation detected by immunohistochemistry. The block in oncogene-induced senescence corresponds to sustained levels of E2F1 and phosphorylated AKT, and is associated with loss of induction of p16^{ink4a}/p19^{arf}. The relevance of p16^{ink4a}/p19^{arf} loss was demonstrated in grafting studies of p19^{arf}-null keratinocytes, which develop malignant carcinomas in the presence of v-ras^{Ha} similar to those arising in wildtype keratinocytes that express lenti-ΔNp63α and v-ras^{Ha}. Our findings establish that ΔNp63α has oncogenic activity and its overexpression in human squamous cell carcinomas contributes to the malignant phenotype, and implicate its ability to regulate p16^{ink4a}/p19^{arf} in the process.

Editor: Mikhail V. Blagosklonny, Roswell Park Cancer Institute, United States of America

Funding: Supported by intramural funding to the Food and Drug Administration (FDA) and the National Cancer Institute (NCI). LH and MSR were fellows of the Interagency Oncology Task Force Fellowship Program. These funding providers had no role in study design, data collection and analysis, decision to publish, or preparation of the manuscript. Steven Jay is an employee of SAIC-Frederick Inc. and helped perform the experiments.

Competing Interests: Steven Jay is an employee of SAIC-Frederick Inc. There are no patents, products in development or marketed products to declare. This does not alter the authors' adherence to all the PLoS ONE policies on sharing data and materials.

* E-mail: wendy.weinberg@fda.hhs.gov

¤ Current address: Division of Biological Oncology Products, Center for Drug Evaluation and Research/Food and Drug Administration (CDER/FDA), Silver Spring, Maryland, United States of America

Introduction

p63 is a p53 homologue. The *p63* gene contains the three functional domains homologous to those of p53, which mediate transactivation (TA), DNA binding (DBD) and oligomerization (OD) [1]. However, in contrast to p53's well established role as a tumor suppressor [2], p63 has been primarily considered a critical developmental regulator of epithelium. It is well understood that temporal regulation of individual p63 isoforms is required for both normal development and maintenance of mature epidermis. This is evidenced by studies in p63 null mice, which are born with severe abnormalities, including the lack of epidermis and many ectodermal derivatives, truncated limbs and craniofacial malformations [3,4] and further supported by studies of postnatal keratinocytes in which p63 isoforms have been manipulated [5,6].

Despite similarities in their structures, p63 is also distinct from p53 in its role in tumorigenesis. While *p53* is one of the most commonly mutated genes recognized to date in human malignancies, *p63* is rarely mutated in human cancers [7], though *p63* gene amplification and/or overexpression has been reported in human squamous cell carcinomas (SCC) of the head and neck, lung, cervix and skin [1,8–12].

p63 is further distinct from p53 in its role in cell senescence. It is now well appreciated that senescence represents a potent anticancer mechanism to prevent tumor progression from premalignant to malignant lesions [13,14]. In contrast to p53's established role in promoting this tumor-suppressive machinery, it has been shown that p63 deficiency leads to the activation of cell senescence and accelerated aging in mice [15].

Significant controversy exists regarding the role of *p63* as an oncogene or as a tumor suppressor gene [7]. In a study by Flores *et al.* [16], $p63^{+/-}$ mice were found to have increased susceptibility to spontaneous tumorigenesis. A complex tumor phenotype was observed in the mutant mice, which included squamous cell carcinomas, histiocytic sarcomas and adenomas. Mice heterozygous for null mutations in both *p53* and *p63* developed higher tumor burdens and had higher rates of metastases compared to $p63^{+/+}/p53^{+/-}$ mice. These findings indicate that loss of p63 may cooperate in tumor formation with p53 loss-of-function. In contrast, an independent study by Keyes *et al.* [17] reported that $p63^{+/-}$ mice were less prone to either spontaneous or chemically induced tumors. The neoplasms that did develop in *p63+/−* mice included lymphomas, sarcomas and carcinomas. In the latter study, mice heterozygous for null mutations in both *p63* and *p53* were found to have fewer tumors than $p63^{+/+}/p53^{+/-}$ mice. These findings suggest that loss of p63 may prevent tumor formation mediated by p53 loss-of-function.

The complexity of *p63* contributes to the confusion surrounding the role of p63 in tumorigenesis [7]. p63 protein may refer to multiple variants arising from alternate promoter usage and/or alternative splicing. The *p63* gene is transcribed into two subclasses, TA and ΔN, which differ at the amino-terminus [1]. Additionally, alternative splicing gives rise to COOH-terminal variants p63α, -β and -γ within both TA- and ΔN-subclasses. TAp63 isoforms contain a p53-like N-terminal transactivation (TA) domain and are capable of transactivating known p53-responsive genes. ΔNp63 isoforms are transcribed from an alternate promoter and lack this transactivation domain, while still retaining transactivation activity [1,18–20]. ΔN isoforms have also been shown to be capable of acting in a dominant-negative manner to block transactivation mediated by TAp63 isoforms as well as by p53 [1].

Accumulating evidence implies that the TA and ΔN isoforms have distinct or even opposing functions in neoplasia. Although it has been suggested that the tumor suppressor phenotype of p63 might come from TAp63 but not ΔNp63 isoforms [18], significant controversy still exists regarding the role of individual p63 isoforms in tumorigenesis. Decreased TAp63 levels have been linked to poor clinical outcomes in buccal and laryngeal squamous cell carcinomas [21,22]. TAp63 functions as a robust mediator of cell senescence and inhibits tumorigenesis *in vivo* [23]. TAp63 isoforms have been found to promote cell apoptosis through death receptors and activating proapoptotic Bcl-2 family members [24]. A role of TAp63 in DNA damage-induced cell cycle arrest and cell death has also been demonstrated [25]. Conversely, Koster *et al.* reported, using an inducible transgenic mouse model, that embryonic induction of TAp63α causes keratinocyte hyperproliferation, and inhibits terminal differentiation [26], and that post-natal induction of TAp63α accelerates tumor development and progression [27].

ΔNp63 has been reported to be over-expressed in several different human cancers [8,12]. ΔNp63α is the predominant isoform in basal keratinocytes, and its expression correlates with proliferation in human cancers [28]. ΔNp63α has been shown to promote survival in squamous epithelial malignancy by repressing a p73-dependent proapoptotic transcriptional program [29]. However, it has also been reported that ΔNp63α promotes basal keratinocyte withdrawal from the cell cycle and commitment to terminal differentiation or apoptosis [30,31].

We have previously reported that transient overexpression of ΔNp63α causes enhanced cell proliferation and inhibition of morphological and biochemical differentiation in primary mouse keratinocytes [20,32]. The long-term biological effects of ΔNp63α and the consequences of it's overexpression, as seen in human squamous cell carcinomas, remain unknown. In this study we apply a well-established model of squamous cancer to elucidate the role of elevated levels of p63 in distinct stages of tumorigenesis. We report that sustained elevated levels of ΔNp63α in normal cells block the $p16^{ink4a}/p19^{arf}$ pathways and promote keratinocyte survival. However, elevated levels of ΔNp63α alone are insufficient to confer a tumor phenotype *in vivo*. In addition to its effect on replicative senescence, elevated ΔNp63α blocks oncogene-induced senescence and associated induction of $p16^{ink4a}/p19^{arf}$, and cooperates with v-ras^{Ha} to enhance malignant conversion *in vivo*. These findings indicate an oncogenic role for the elevated levels of ΔNp63α that have been observed in human squamous cell cancers.

Results

Lentivirus infection drives long term and stable gene expression in primary keratinocytes

To mimic the sustained high level expression of ΔNp63 that has been observed in human SCC, lentiviruses encoding green fluorescent protein (lenti-GFP) or ΔNp63α (lenti-ΔNp63α) were developed and their ability to drive long-term gene expression was assessed in cultures of primary epidermal keratinocytes. Under optimized conditions, the infection efficiency as assessed with lenti-GFP was 92.05% in primary keratinocytes five days following lentiviral infection (Figure 1A). Lenti-ΔNp63α expression was monitored over time by western blotting (Figure 1B). At five days following infection, lenti-ΔNp63α levels resembled those at the peak of adenoviral-driven gene expression (days 2–3, left panel), and remained stable for at least 14 days (right panel). Consistent with the FACS analysis shown for lenti-GFP in figure 1A, lenti-ΔNp63α expression observed by immunohistochemistry was distributed uniformly across the cell population (Figure 1C).

Long-term ΔNp63α overexpression promotes survival and blocks replicative senescence of primary keratinocytes

The effect of elevated levels of ΔNp63α on long-term *in vitro* survival of primary keratinocyte cultures was assessed by microscopic evaluation over 14 days following introduction of lenti-GFP or lenti-ΔNp63α. As shown in Figure 2A, lenti-ΔNp63α cultures remain confluent and appeared healthier at 14 days compared to lenti-GFP control cultures. Proliferation status was assessed by BrdU uptake followed by FACS analysis (Figure 2B). The S-phase population was initially similar across the two cell populations, as seen 5 days following introduction of the lentiviruses (18.18% *vs.* 17.58% in lenti-ΔNp63α- *vs.* lenti-GFP-expressing keratinocytes, respectively). While the S-phase population declined in both cell populations over 2 weeks in culture, it was maintained at higher levels in lenti-ΔNp63α cultures *vs.* the parallel lenti-GFP control cultures (11.12% *vs.* 4.12% BrdU-positive cells, respectively, at 10 days; 5.12% *vs.* 1.59% BrdU-positive cells, respectively, at day 14).

The continually decreasing BrdU uptake levels in both lenti-ΔNp63α and control cultures indicate that other mechanisms, in addition to cell proliferation, are involved in the prolonged maintenance of ΔNp63α overexpressing cells. Therefore, we tested the notion that overexpression of ΔNp63α facilitates the capacity of the cell to overcome replicative senescence, as originally described by Hayflick in cultured cells [33]. A previous study by Keyes *et al.*, showed that inactivation of all p63 isoforms in mice lead to cellular senescence and accelerated aging [15]. However, the role of individual p63 isoforms in cellular senescence has remained unclear. Here, keratinocytes were infected with lenti-GFP or lenti-ΔNp63α, and the cell senescence status at day 14 was determined by the nuclear presence of prominent HP1γ-positive senescence-associated heterochromatin foci [34]. As shown in Figure 2C, distinct HP-1γ nuclear foci were observed in control keratinocytes that express lenti-GFP, but not in keratinocytes that express lenti-ΔNp63α. Double staining with both HP-1γ and p63

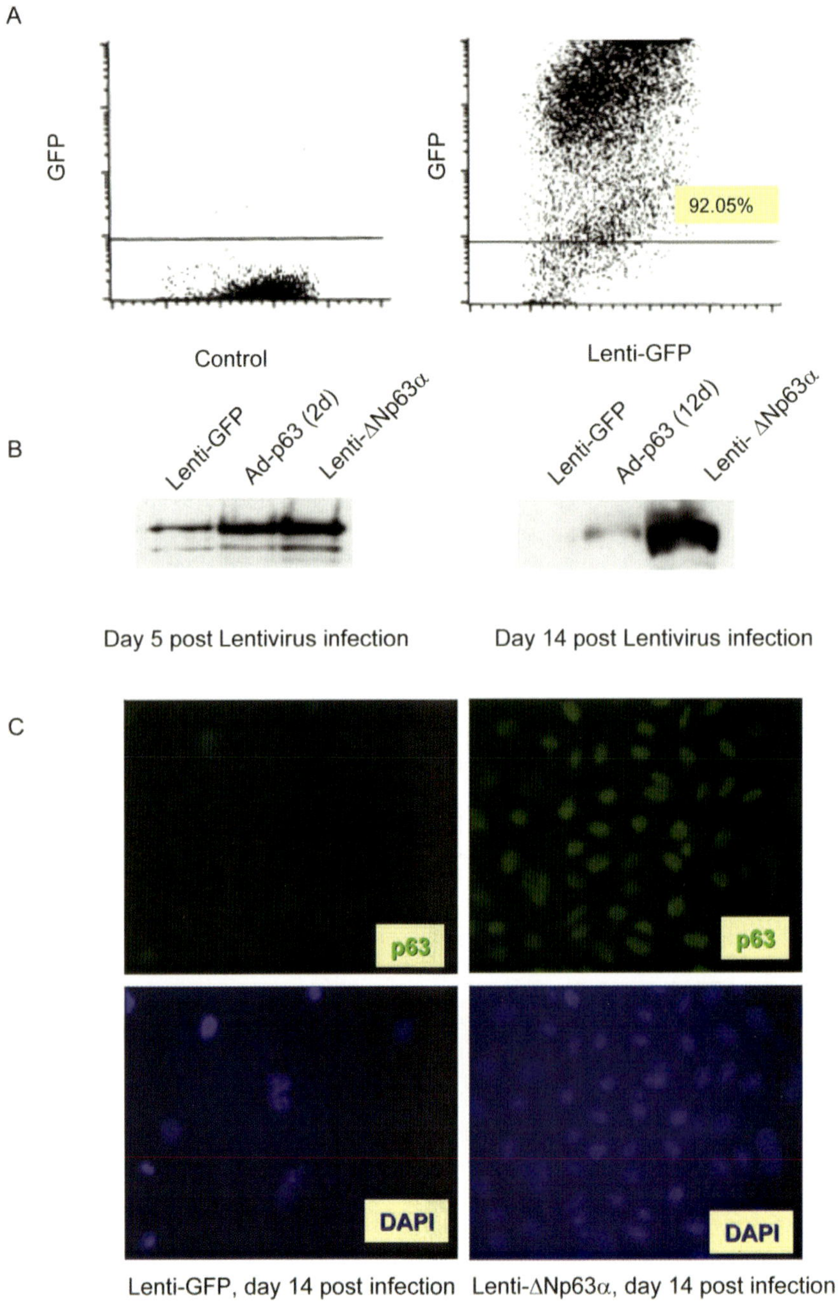

Figure 1. Lentivirus infection drives long term and stable gene expression in primary keratinocytes. A, Primary mouse keratinocytes were infected with lentivirus encoding GFP, and infection efficiency was assessed by FACS analysis at day 5 post-infection. Y-axis indicates the intensity of GFP, X-axis represents forward angle light scatter. B, Primary keratinocytes were infected with lentivirus encoding GFP or ΔNp63α and whole cell protein was collected at day 5 and 14 and analyzed for p63 expression by western blot. C, Primary keratinocyte cultures expressing lenti-GFP or lenti-ΔNp63α were fixed at 14 days post-lentiviral transduction and incubated with anti-p63 antibody, followed by a secondary antibody conjugated with Alexa-488. The cells were then stained with DAPI to visualize the cell nuclei.

antibodies demonstrated that the formation of HP-1γ foci is associated with lower p63 expression (Figure 2C, arrows).

Senescence in most cells is regulated through some combination of activities within the RB and p53 pathways, but frequently operates in a context-dependent and complex manner [13]. We examined the status of the RB and p53 pathways in keratinocytes that differ in their senescence status due to expression of either lenti-GFP or lenti-ΔNp63α. The induction of p53, p21, $p16^{ink4a}$, $p19^{arf}$ and E2F1 were examined by western blot. No induction of p53 or p21 was observed during the timepoints studied (data not shown). In contrast, up-regulation of $p19^{arf}$ followed by $p16^{ink4a}$ was observed beginning by day 3 in control lenti-GFP keratinocytes cultures (Figure 3A). This expression of $p16^{ink4a}$ and $p19^{arf}$ increased over time in lenti-GFP cultures, but was attenuated and delayed in lenti-ΔNp63α-expressing keratinocytes (Figure 3A). As expected, the upregulation of $p16^{ink4a}$ and $p19^{arf}$ correlates with decreased levels of E2F1. The down-regulation of E2F1 was delayed and attenuated in cells over-expressing ΔNp63α

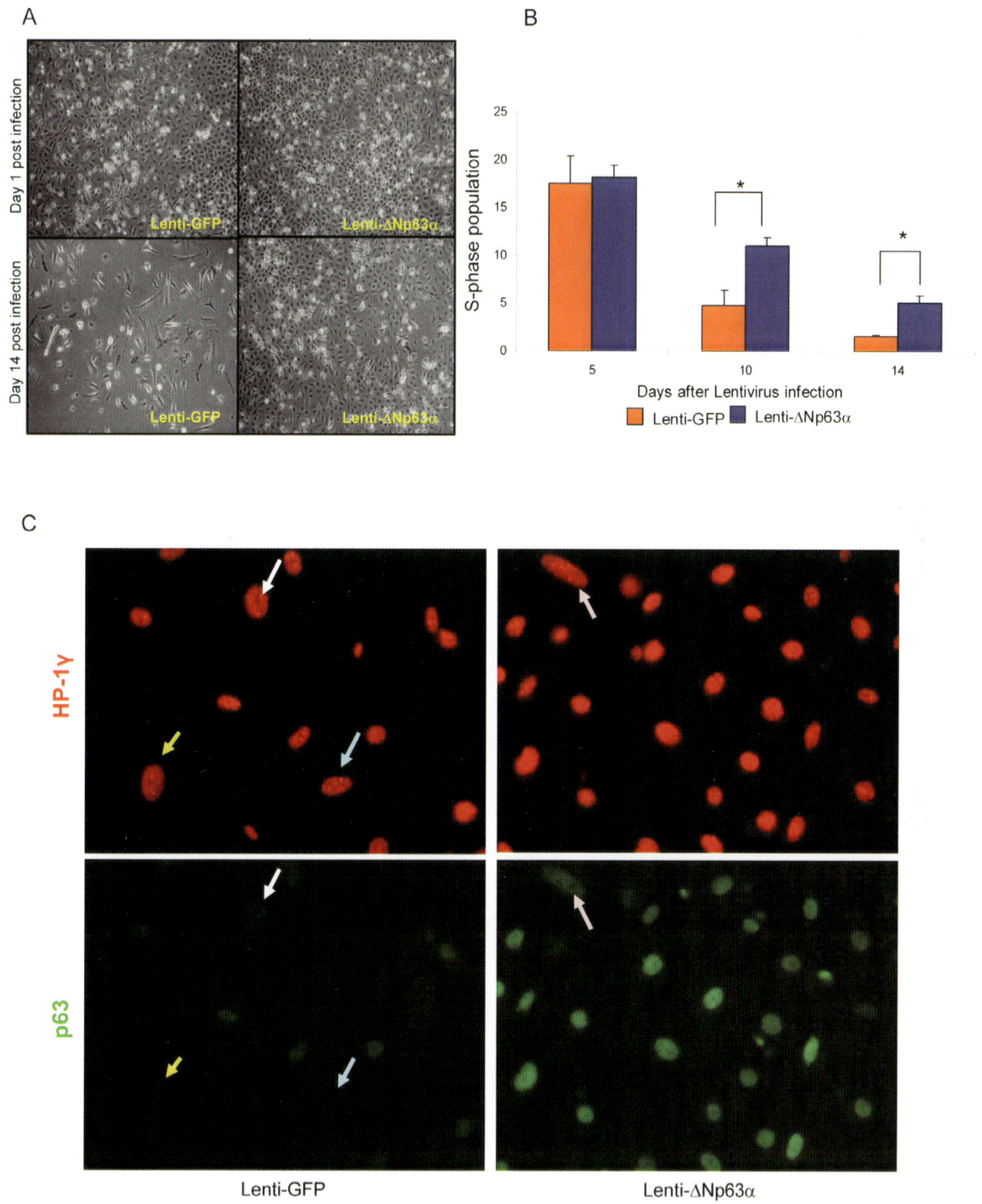

Figure 2. Dysregulated expression of ΔNp63α promotes survival and blocks replicative senescence of primary keratinocytes. A, Phase morphology of lenti-GFP- and lenti-ΔNp63α expressing keratinocytes cultured for 1 and 14 days post-infection. Results shown are representative of three independent experiments. B, Quantification of BrdU positive cells in lenti-GFP or lenti-ΔNp63α cultures at timepoints noted following lentiviral gene transduction. Data shown represent the means ± S.E. of three independent experiments. * indicates a statistically significant difference between lenti-GFP and lenti-ΔNp63α infected cells at $p<0.05$. C, Primary keratinocytes expressing lenti-GFP (left panel) or lenti-ΔNp63α (right panel) were fixed at 14 days post-lentiviral transduction. The cell senescence status was assessed by the presence of HP-1γ nuclear foci (red). The cells were double stained with p63 antibodies (green). Matched arrows indicate the same cell stained with both different antibodies. The image presented is representative of three independent experiments.

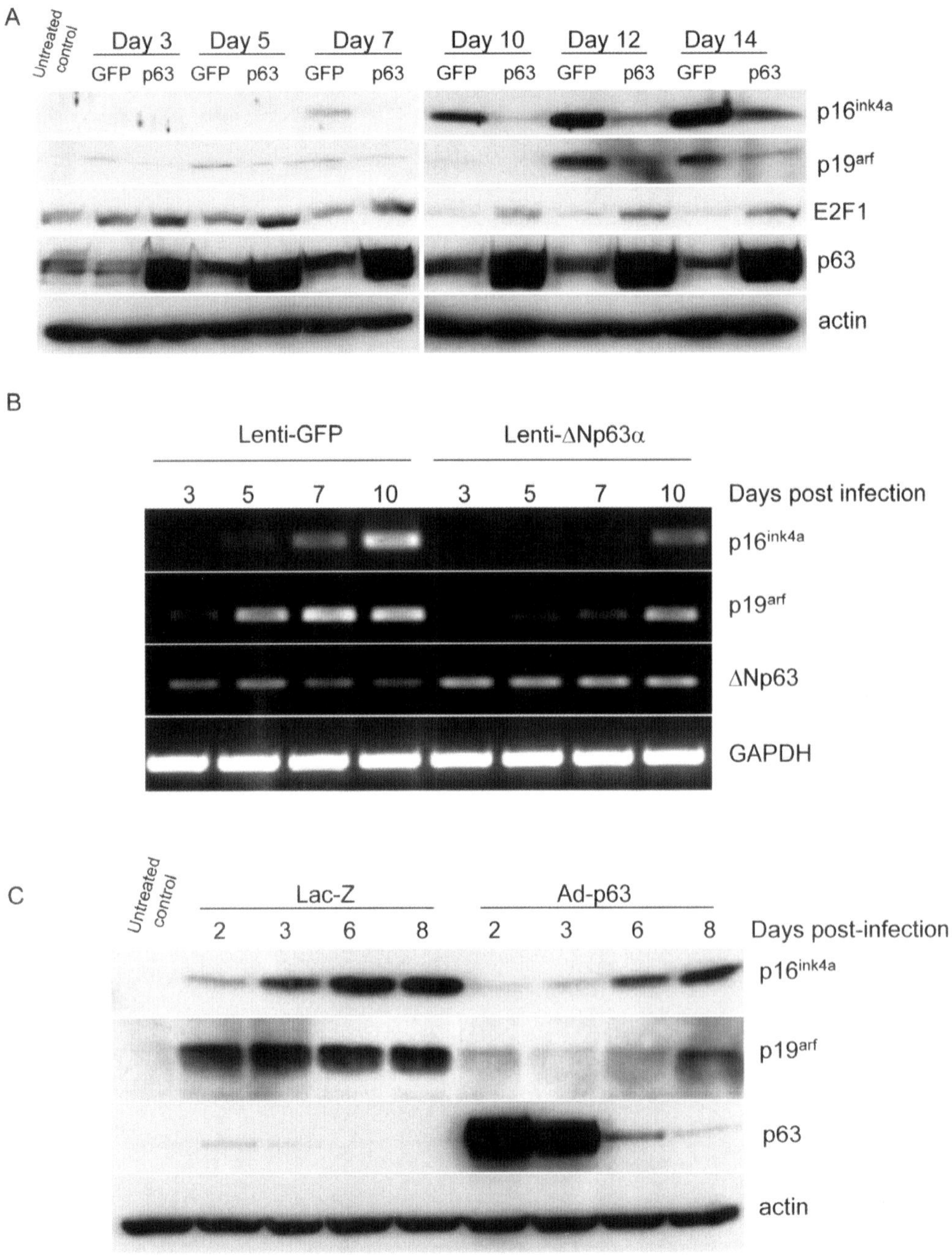

Figure 3. Overexpression of ΔNp63α inhibits the up-regulation of p16^{ink4a} and p19^{arf} associated with cell senescence. A, Whole cell protein was collected from primary keratinocytes expressing lenti-GFP or lenti-ΔNp63α at timepoints indicated following lentiviral gene transduction. Expression levels of p16^{ink4a}, p19^{arf}, E2F1 and p63 were detected by western blot. Equal protein loading was confirmed by immunoblotting for β-actin. B, Primary keratinocytes were infected with lentivirus encoding ΔNp63α or GFP at day 3 after plating. Total RNA was harvested at day 3, 5, 7 and 10 post-infection and reverse transcribed. Expression of p16^{ink4a} and p19^{arf} was determined by PCR amplification. PCR amplification of GAPDH was used as a loading control. C, Primary keratinocytes were cultured for 7 days after plating and then infected with adenovirus encoding ΔNp63α or LacZ. Whole cell lysates were collected at day 2, 3, 6 and 8 post-adenovirus infection (equivalent to day 9, 10, 13 and 15 post-plating). The expression levels of p16^{ink4a}, p19^{arf} and p63 were detected by western blot. Equivalent protein loading was confirmed by immunoblotting for actin.

(Figure 3A). We further used RT-PCR to confirm that the regulation of p16^{ink4a} and p19^{arf} by ΔNp63α occurs at the transcriptional level. RT-PCR analysis on p16^{ink4a} and p19^{arf} transcription was carried out on primary keratinocytes at day 3, 5, 7 and 10 post-lenti-GFP or lenti-ΔNp63α infection. As shown in figure 3B, p16^{ink4a} and p19^{arf} mRNA began to increase in lenti-GFP cells at day 5 post-infection. This induction was delayed in lenti-ΔNp63α overexpressing cells. These findings are consistent with a previous report, using cells null for all p63 isoforms, demonstrating that p63 directly represses p16^{Ink4a} and p19^{Arf} expression [35]. To further challenge the relationship between ΔNp63α and p16^{ink4a}/p19^{arf}, a transient induction of ΔNp63α was achieved using adenoviral-mediated gene transduction and used to assess its impact on temporal expression of p16^{ink4a}/p19^{arf}.

Primary keratinocytes were infected with adenoviral constructs encoding Lac-Z or ΔNp63α at day 7 after plating, when $p16^{ink4a}$ and $p19^{arf}$ levels normally begin to increase. The expression levels of $p16^{ink4a}$, $p19^{arf}$ and p63 were evaluated at days 2, 3, 6 and 8 after adenoviral infection (equivalent to days 9, 10, 13 and 15 after plating, and to the time point of day 6, 7, 10 and 12 following introduction of lentivirus in Figure 3A). As shown in Figure 3C, adenoviral-driven gene expression of ΔNp63α peaked at day 2 post-infection and then rapidly declined. In control Ad-lacZ cultures, both $p16^{ink4a}$ and $p19^{arf}$ levels were seen to increase 2 to 3 days following adenovirus infection, in association with the onset of senescence typically seen in these cultures 10 days after plating. This upregulation was abrogated in parallel cultures in which Ad-ΔNp63α had been introduced. As Ad-ΔNp63α levels declined, levels of both $p16^{ink4a}$ and $p19^{arf}$ were once again up-regulated.

Elevated ΔNp63α levels enhance malignant conversion in v-ras^{Ha}-expressing keratinocytes

The role of ΔNp63α in promoting cell proliferation and blocking the $p16^{ink4a}$/$p19^{arf}$ pathways of cell senescence, as shown in Figures 2 and 3, indicate that ΔNp63α might function as an oncogene in carcinogenesis. To determine the contribution of ΔNp63α to cancer pathogenesis, we applied a well established *in vivo* grafting model of experimental skin cancer that allows distinctions between benign and malignant tumor phenotypes. We introduced lenti-GFP or lenti-ΔNp63α into primary murine keratinocytes, either alone or in combination with retrovirus encoding a v-ras^{Ha} oncogene, and cultures were grafted onto the dorsal surface of nude mice in combination with cultured dermal fibroblasts as previously described [36]. No tumors were observed in grafts of lenti-GFP or lenti-ΔNp63α keratinocytes following grafting (Figure 4A and Table 1). Graft sites on 4 of the 15 animals that received lenti-GFP/v-ras^{Ha}-expressing keratinocytes developed benign, well-differentiated papillomas with an average tumor volume of 25 mm^3. In contrast, when v-ras^{Ha} was expressed in combination with lenti-ΔNp63α, all grafts (20 mice) gave rise to undifferentiated carcinomas with an average tumor volume of 831.9 mm^3 (figure 4A, B and Table 1). The increased tumor size corresponded to increased BrdU incorporation, as detected by immunohistochemistry (Figure 4B and C), reflecting a higher proliferation status in these tumors.

Long term ΔNp63α overexpression blocks oncogene-induced senescence and supports long term survival of v-ras^{Ha}-expressing primary keratinocytes

It has been well documented that normal keratinocytes undergo a transient hyperproliferation response followed by senescence after oncogenic v-ras^{Ha} activation [37]. Oncogene-induced senescence is now well appreciated to be a crucial barrier to malignant conversion [13]. The above results (Figure 4) demonstrate that elevated ΔNp63α levels enhance malignant conversion in v-ras^{Ha}-expressing keratinocytes and suggest that ΔNp63α may play a role in blocking oncogene-induced senescence as well as replicative senescence. Primary keratinocytes were transduced with retrovirus encoding oncogenic v-ras^{Ha} followed by lentivirus encoding either lenti-GFP (Figure 5A, left) or lenti-ΔNp63α (Figure 5A, right). Oncogene-induced senescence was demonstrated at day 14 with the presence of nuclear foci of HP-1γ (Figure 5A, upper panels) or SA-β-Gal staining (Figure 5A, lower panels). While both of these well-defined markers of senescence were observed in lenti-GFP/v-ras^{Ha} cultures, they were diminished in lenti-ΔNp63α/v-ras^{Ha} keratinocytes.

p53 has been shown to direct cell fate between quiescence *vs.* senescence, and this has been linked to the status of the mTOR pathway [38,39]. We evaluated levels of phospho-S6 as a marker of mTOR activity in v-ras^{Ha}-expressing primary keratinocytes that had been transduced with either lenti-GFP or lenti-ΔNp63α. No change was observed in phospho-S6 levels due to the ΔNp63α status at days 5, 7 and 14 post-lentiviral infection, the timeframe during which control cultures are transitioning through senescence. These findings indicate that suppression of senescence in this system is not mediated *via* inhibition of mTOR (data not shown).

Similar to results seen with keratinocytes undergoing replicative senescence (Figure 3A), western blotting revealed up-regulation of both $p16^{ink4a}$ and $p19^{arf}$ in the presence of v-ras^{Ha} (lenti-GFP/v-ras^{Ha}) that was attenuated and delayed in the additional presence of elevated ΔNp63α (Figure 5B). Furthermore, consistent with the increased proliferation status observed in tumors generated from lenti-ΔNp63α/v-ras^{Ha} keratinocytes (Figure 4B and C), the levels of E2F1 and phosphorylated AKT (serine 473) remain stable in lenti-ΔNp63α/v-ras^{Ha} keratinocytes, but start to decrease at day 7 in lenti-GFP/v-ras^{Ha} keratinocytes (Figure 5B).

We have shown that sustained dysregulation of ΔNp63α in keratinocytes supports cell proliferation and facilitates an escape from oncogene-induced senescence (Figure 5A and B). We tested whether co-expression of ΔNp63α and v-ras^{Ha} would cooperate to immortalize cells and allow multiple passaging of primary mouse keratinocytes. Primary cultures of v-ras^{Ha}-expressing keratinocytes were transduced with lentiviruses encoding lenti-GFP or lenti-ΔNp63α. The cells were trypsinized 14 days following lentivirus introduction and reseeded. As shown in Figure 6A, lenti-GFP/v-ras^{Ha} keratinocytes display a senescence-like morphology 3 days after replating that is not observed in lenti-ΔNp63α/v-ras^{Ha} keratinocytes. Furthermore, lenti-ΔNp63α/v-ras^{Ha} keratinocytes re-attached and expanded for at least two passages, whereas lenti-GFP/v-ras^{Ha} keratinocytes stopped proliferation after the initial reseeding (Figure 6B).

Loss of $p19^{arf}$ cooperates with v-ras^{Ha} in malignant conversion, similar to lenti-ΔNp63α-expressing keratinocytes

To determine whether ΔNp63α-mediated downregulation of $p16^{ink4a}$ or $p19^{arf}$ could enhance malignant conversion, $p19^{arf}$-null primary keratinocytes were transduced with v-ras^{Ha}-encoding retrovirus, followed by lenti-GFP or lenti-ΔNp63α and grafted onto the dorsal surface of nude mice as previously described [36]. Wildtype primary keratinocytes expressing lenti-GFP or lenti-ΔNp63α in combination with v-ras^{Ha} were used as negative and positive controls. Out of 10 animals grafted with $p19^{arf}$-null keratinocytes expressing lenti-GFP and v-ras^{Ha}, 9 animals gave rise to undifferentiated carcinomas, which appeared similar to the tumor phenotype derived from keratinocytes overexpressing ΔNp63α. The remaining animal developed a well differentiated papilloma (Figure 7A and B, Table 2). A significantly larger tumor volume was observed in tumors derived from lenti-ΔNp63α/v-ras^{Ha}-expressing $p19^{arf}$-null keratinocytes when compared to tumors derived from $p19^{arf}$-null cells that express v-ras^{Ha} alone (Figure 7B).

Discussion

Expression of ΔNp63α is associated with proliferation of both normal and neoplastic epithelium, with elevated levels observed in human squamous cancer tissues [1,8–12]. Here, we provide a mechanistic link between the elevated levels of ΔNp63α and development of squamous cell cancers. The grafting model applied

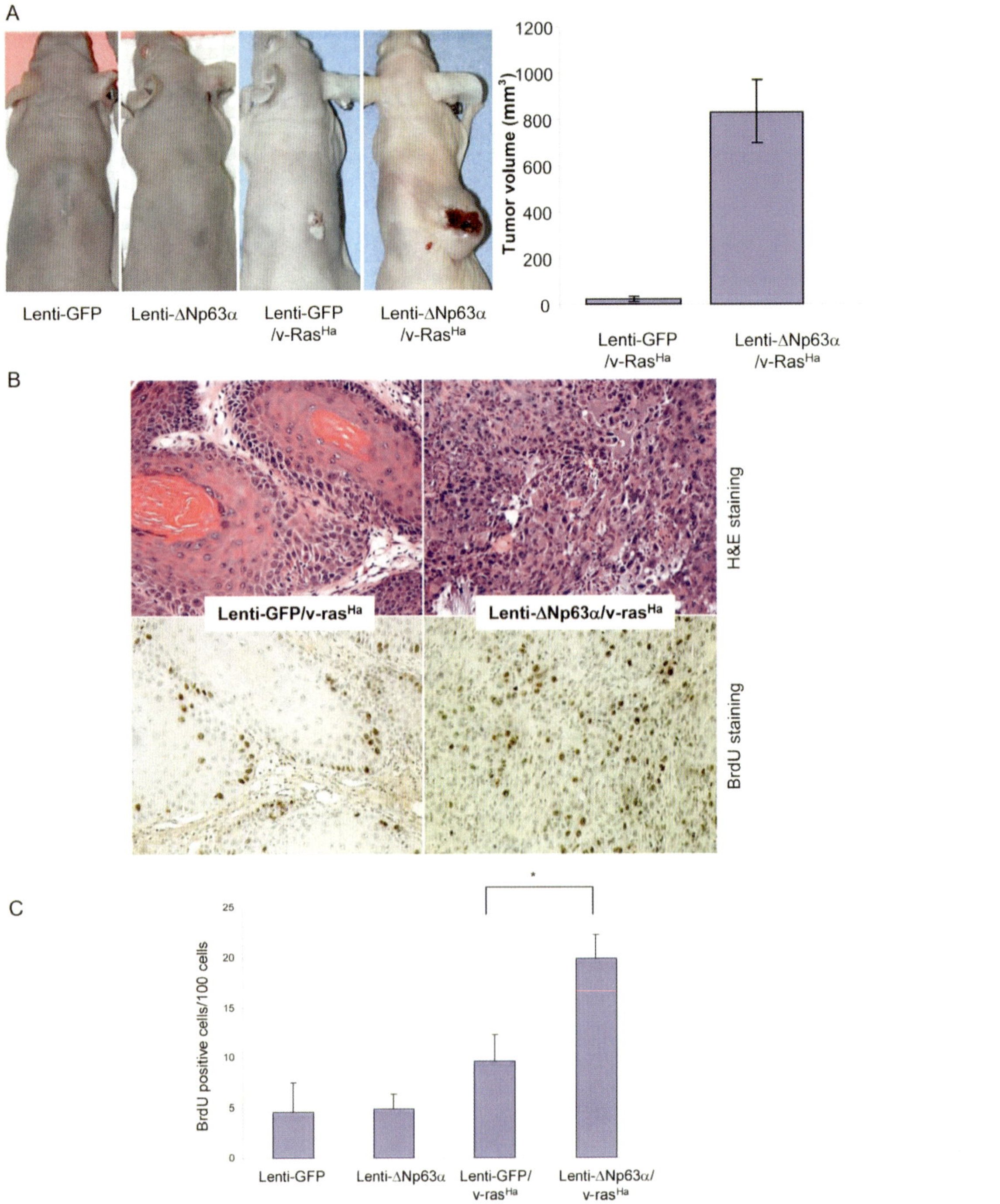

Figure 4. Elevated expression of ΔNp63α enhances malignant conversion in v-ras^{Ha}-expressing keratinocytes. A, *In vivo* phenotype of ΔNp63α-overexpressing keratinocytes in the presence and absence of oncogenic ras. Primary mouse keratinocytes were infected with lentivirus encoding lenti-GFP or lenti-ΔNp63α or sequentially with retrovirus encoding v-ras^{Ha} followed by lenti-GFP or lenti-ΔNp63α. The final tumor phenotype was assessed at 5 weeks following grafting. Final tumor volumes at 4 weeks are presented as the mean tumor volume ± S.E. B, Upper panel, representative H&E sections of tumor tissues obtained from grafting sites. Lower panel, BrdU incorporation in grafted tissue samples. C, Quantification of BrdU incorporation levels. Data are presented as the mean % of BrdU positive cells ± S.E. * indicates a statistically significant difference between lenti-GFP/v-ras^{Ha} and lenti-ΔNp63α/v-ras^{Ha} groups at $p<0.05$.

in this study is relevant to the normal tissue distribution of p63, and allows the discrimination of genetic alterations that contribute to distinct stages of cancer development. We demonstrate that ΔNp63α overexpression alone does not confer a neoplastic phenotype upon normal primary keratinocytes under the conditions used, but enhances malignant conversion of benign tumors arising from primary murine keratinocytes that express oncogenic ras. This phenotypic change appears to be due, at least in part, to the ability of ΔNp63α to enhance cell survival through suppression of $p16^{ink4a}/p19^{arf}$, key mediators of cell senescence.

Table 1. Elevated ΔNp63α levels enhance malignant conversion in v-ras^{Ha}-expressing keratinocytes.

	Normal Skin	Papilloma	Carcinoma	Total	Conversion rate
Lenti-GFP	10	0	0	10	0%
Lenti-ΔNp63α	10	0	0	10	0%
Lenti-GFP/v-ras^{Ha}	11 (73.3%)	4 (26.7%)	0	15	0%
Lenti-ΔNp63α/v-ras^{Ha}	0	0	20 (100%)	20	100%

Tumor incidence and conversion rate of grafted keratinocytes are presented at 5 weeks post-grafting. Tumor phenotypes were confirmed histologically.

Cell senescence was initially described as a form of irreversible growth arrest in cultured human cells [33]. It is now understood that it can be prematurely induced by multiple stimuli including DNA damage, oxidative stress, and excessive mitogenic stimuli [40], [41], and represents a potent anticancer mechanism to prevent malignant conversion [14]. The complexities of the signaling pathways mediating the senescence response, and the dependence of this response on p53, are underscored by the contrasting results observed *in vitro* and *in vivo* in keratinocytes undergoing senescence induced by p63 ablation [15].

The inhibition of cell senescence by ΔNp63α is linked to its ability to repress the expression of p16^{ink4a} and p19^{arf} (Figure 5). While p16^{ink4a} and p19^{arf} play well-defined roles in controlling cell cycle and senescence, their regulation remains poorly understood. Our finding that ΔNp63α negatively regulates p16^{ink4a} and p19^{arf} in primary mouse keratinocytes is consistent with recent studies linking p63 to cellular senescence and organismal aging, in which keratinocytes of p63-deficient mice display increased levels of p16^{ink4a}/p19^{arf} [15]. The ability of p63 to bind putative p53/p63 consensus sites on the p16^{ink4a}/p19^{arf} promoters, as demonstrated by ChIP analysis using cells null for all isoforms of p63, raises the possibility that p63 acts as a direct repressor of the p16^{ink4a}/p19^{arf} locus. A function for p16^{ink4a} downstream of p63 is also supported by the observation that germline disruption of both p16^{ink4a} and p19^{arf} was found to significantly alleviate the phenotypic consequences of p63 ablation during embryonic epidermal development [35]. Despite the above studies, the relationship between ΔNp63α and p16^{ink4a} in cancer remains unclear. Consistent with the findings reported here, a recent study by Keyes *et al.* [2] demonstrated that overexpression of ΔNp63α bypasses oncogenic ras-induced senescence and drives tumorigeneisis *in vivo*. However, in contrast to our results, Keyes *et al.* reported that the level of p16^{ink4a} remains stable in oncogenic ras and ΔNp63α expressing cells, and concluded that the inhibition of senescence by ΔNp63α occurs *via* an additional pathway, but not through modulating p16^{ink4a}. This indicates the complexity of the pathways interacting with p63 family members, and underscores the need for additional studies to understand the role of p63 and its downstream effectors in tumorigenesis and senescence.

p63 is recognized as a regulator of epidermal cell fate and lineage commitment [42,43]. The pathways involved in regulating epidermal development as well as homeostasis and differentiation of postnatal keratinocytes continue to be targets of active investigation [6,28,44]. Much effort has focused on the identification of downstream pathways of ΔNp63α contributing to neoplasia, including NFκB/c-Rel, EGF-R and COX-2 [45–47]. Furthermore, the ability of ΔNp63α to inhibit transcriptional regulatory activity of other p53 family members may contribute to a loss of genomic stability that could enhance progression to malignancy [1]. Our laboratory has previously demonstrated that NFκB/c-Rel mediates the aberrant growth regulation observed in ΔNp63α-overexpressing keratinocytes [43]. Here, we establish that the ability of ΔNp63α to overcome senescence and drive malignancy is linked to its downregulation of the p16^{ink4a}/p19^{arf} pathways. As proof of principle that the loss of p16^{ink4a}/p19^{arf} can contribute to ΔNp63α-induced malignant conversion, an *in vivo* grafting study showed that, similar to lenti-ΔNp63α-expressing keratinocytes, p19^{arf} null keratinocytes formed malignant carcinomas in the presence of v-ras^{Ha} (Figure 7). However, a significantly larger tumor volume was observed in tumors derived from lenti-ΔNp63α/v-ras^{Ha}-expressing p19^{arf} null keratinocytes when compared to tumors derived from p19^{arf} null cells expressing v-ras^{Ha} alone (Figure 7B). Our results suggest that additional mechanisms, *e.g.* p16^{ink4a} or c-Rel, contribute to ΔNp63α -induced malignant tumor formation [45]. Future studies are required to dissect the relative roles of each individual downstream pathway influenced by p63 and their cooperative contribution to discrete steps of cancer pathogenesis.

Materials and Methods

Ethics Statement

All animal work was performed in accordance with NIH (National Institutes of Health) established guidelines, in accordance with accepted standards of humane animal care under protocols approved by the Animal Care and Use Committee of the Center for Biologics Evaluation and Research of the Food and Drug Administration.

Cell Culture

Primary keratinocytes and dermal fibroblasts were isolated from the skin of 1–2 day-old C57Bl/6NCr mice, cultured and plated as described [20]. Keratinocytes were maintained at a final concentration of 0.05 mM Ca^{2+}. Fibroblasts were cultured for 9 days in DMEM prior to use in grafting studies.

Adenovirus encoding ΔNp63α has been previously described [20]. The replication-defective Psi-2 retroviral vector encoding v-ras^{Ha} was used to introduce a v-ras^{Ha} oncogene at day-2 post-plating as previously described [36]. The infection of adenovirus encoding Lac-Z or ΔNp63α was performed as previously described [20].

Lentivirus construction and infection

Lentivirus encoding human ΔNp63α was generated by ligating the complete coding region of ΔNp63α cDNA excised from pBMNiGFP–human ΔNp63α plasmid into lentiviral expression vector 960-X5-685 (pSICO-FerH-eGFP). The constructed pSICO-hFerH-human ΔNp63α was verified *via* restriction enzyme mapping and sequencing analysis. A similarly constructed lentiviral vector encoding GFP was used as a matched control. Lentiviruses were produced in HEK293T cells (Open Biosystems, Huntsville, AL). The producer cells were washed and incubated with standard keratinocyte medium 24 hours before harvesting (SAIC, Inc., Frederick, MD).

Keratinocytes, 3 days post-plating, were incubated for 3 hours in lentivirus-containing supernatant and 4 µg/mL polybrene (500 µl/60 mm^2 dish). Fresh medium was added at the end of the incubation. The induction of lenti-ΔNp63α was evaluated by western blot and immunofluorescent staining.

In vivo grafting and tumor sample collection

Keratinocyte cultures were infected with retrovirus encoding v-ras^{Ha} one day prior to infection with lentivirus encoding either

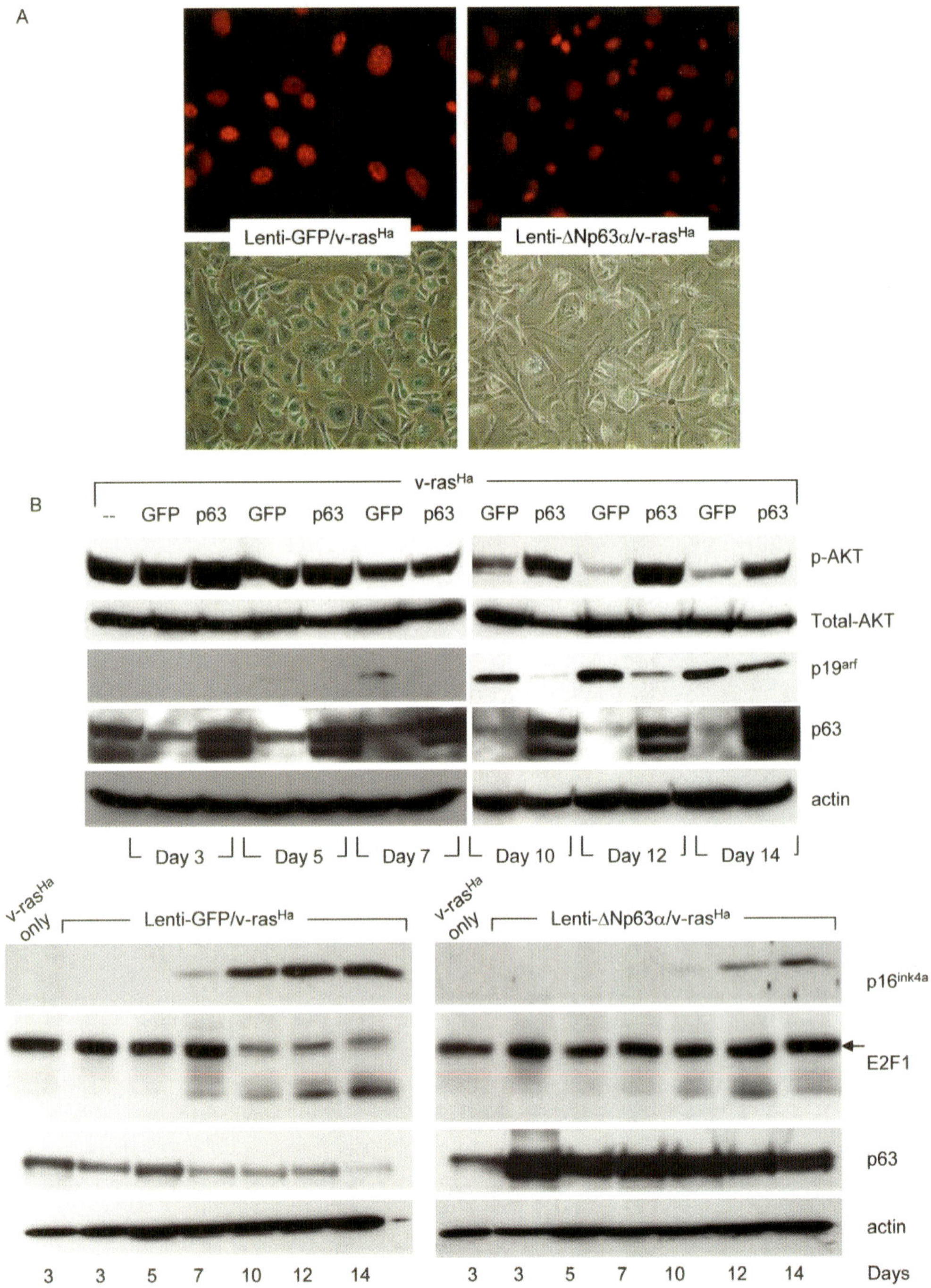

Figure 5. Long term ΔNp63α overexpression blocks oncogene-induced senescence. A, Primary keratinocytes were infected sequentially with retrovirus encoding oncogenic v-ras^{Ha}, followed by lentivirus encoding GFP or ΔNp63α. Oncogene-induced senescence was assessed 14 days post-lentivirus infection by immunofluorescent analysis of nuclear foci of HP-1γ (upper panel), or enzymatic activity of SA-β-gal (lower panel). The images shown are representative of three independent experiments. B, Whole cell protein was collected from keratinocytes infected sequentially with retrovirus encoding oncogenic v-ras^{Ha} followed by lentivirus encoding GFP or ΔNp63α at timepoints indicated following lentiviral gene transduction. The levels of phosphorylated AKT, total AKT, p19^{arf} and p63 were detected by western blot (upper panels). p16^{ink4a} and E2F1 levels with corresponding p63 expression are presented in the lower panels. Equal protein loading was confirmed by immunoblotting for β-actin.

ΔNp63α or GFP. Cells were harvested six days following lentivirus infection and 4×10^6 keratinocytes were mixed with 8×10^6 cultured dermal cells and transferred to a grafting chamber freshly implanted onto the dorsum of a nude mouse [36,48]. The chamber was removed 1 week following grafting. Tumor volume was measured every 3 days following the initial appearance of a tumor. Mice were injected with 250 µl of 50 mM 5-bromo-2′-deoxyuridine (BrdU, Sigma Chemical, St. Louis, MO) 1 hour prior to euthanasia and tumor harvest to allow immunohistochemical analysis of DNA synthesis in the grafted cells. Tumor tissues were collected 4 weeks after removing the chambers and fixed in formalin-buffered saline.

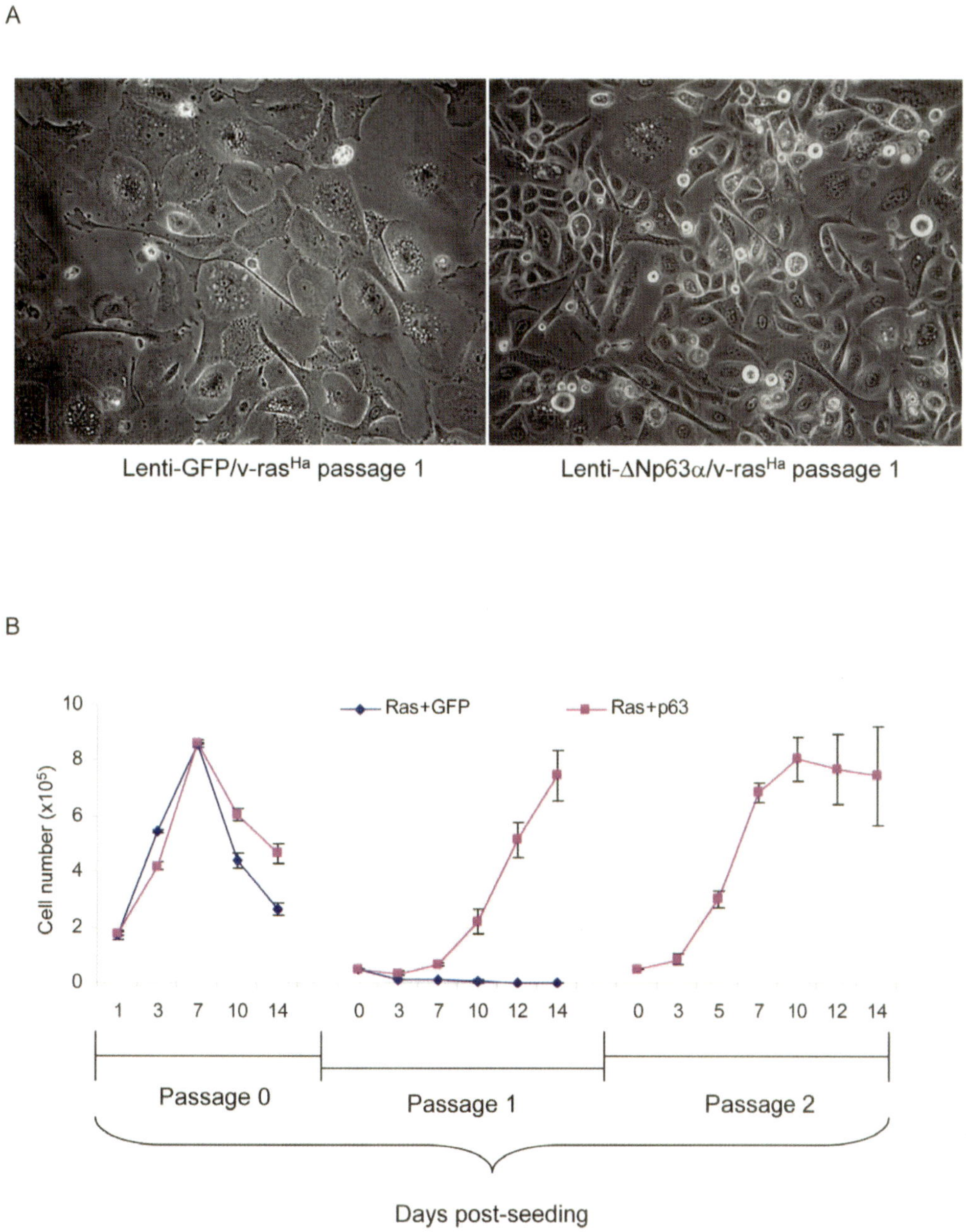

Figure 6. Overexpression of ΔNp63α supports long term survival of v-ras^{Ha}-expressing primary keratinocytes. Primary keratinocytes were infected sequentially with retrovirus encoding oncogenic v-ras^{Ha} and lentivirus encoding GFP or ΔNp63α, as noted. On post-infection day 14, the cells were trypsinized and reseeded. A, cell morphology was recorded at day 3 after the initial reseeding. B, growth curves of keratinocytes expressing v-ras^{Ha} in conjunction with lenti-GFP or lenti-ΔNp63α. Cell numbers were counted at days 1, 3, 7, 10 and 14 post-lentivirus infection (passage 0), or at the same timepoints following each reseeding. Data are expressed as cell number per well and represent the means ± S.D. of two independent experiments.

BrdU incorporation

BrdU incorporation in the grafted tissue sample was detected by immunohistochemical staining using an antibody against BrdU (B44, BD Biosciences, San Jose, CA) and tissues were counter-stained with Contrast Green (KPL, Inc., Gaithersburg, MD). At least 100 basal cells were scored for each sample; in the case of undifferentiated carcinomas 100 cells/field were counted. BrdU incorporation *in vitro* was detected by Fluorescent Activated Cell Sorting (FACS) analysis as previously described [32].

Senescence assays

For HP1γ detection, culture dishes were fixed with methanol at −20°C and incubated with antibody directed to HP1γ (MAB3450, Chemicon International, Billerica, MA), and p63 (4A4, Santa Cruz Biotechnology, Santa Cruz, CA). Cells were then incubated with a FITC- or rhodamine-labeled secondary antibody (Invitrogen) and viewed under a fluorescence microscope. Senescence-associated β-galactosidase (SA-β-gal) staining was performed as previously described [36].

A

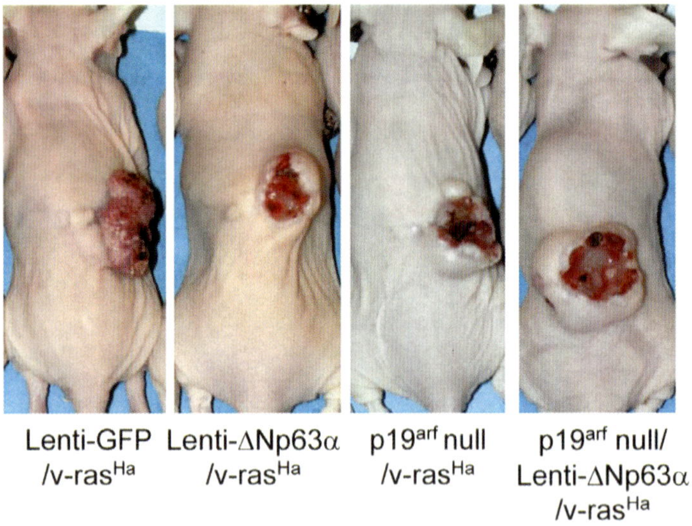

B

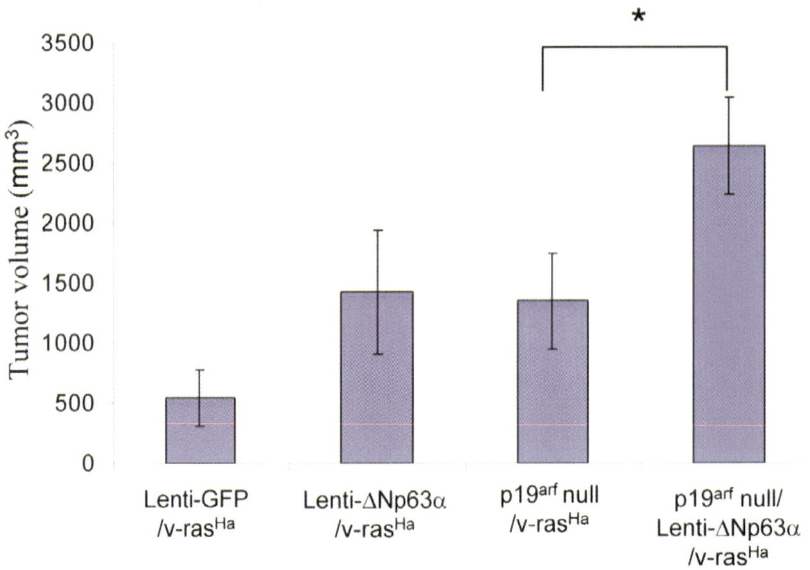

Figure 7. v-ras^{Ha}-expressing p19^{arf} null keratinocytes display a tumor phenotype similar to v-ras^{Ha}/ΔNp63α overexpressing keratinocytes. A, p19^{arf} null primary keratinocytes were infected with lenti-GFP or lenti-ΔNp63α in combination with v-ras^{Ha}, and grafted onto the dorsal side of nude mice as previously described [36]. Wild type primary keratinocytes expressing lenti-GFP or lenti-ΔNp63α in combination with v-ras^{Ha} were used as negative and positive controls. The final tumor phenotype was assessed at 5 weeks after grafting. B, Final tumor volumes at 5 weeks are presented as the mean tumor volume ± S.E. * indicates a statistically significant difference between p19^{arf} null/v-ras^{Ha} and p19^{arf} null/lenti-ΔNp63α/v-ras^{Ha} groups at $p<0.05$.

Keratinocyte growth curve

Keratinocytes were infected with retrovirus encoding v-ras^{Ha}, followed by lenti-ΔNp63α or lenti-GFP. Cells were collected by trypsinization and counted using a hemocytometer (Hausser Scientific, Horsham, PA) at timepoints noted. At 14 days post-infection, the cultures were trypsinized and reseeded at 0.5×10^5 cells per well, then counted as above at timepoints noted.

Immunoblot Analysis

Immunoblot analysis was performed using standard procedures. The following primary antibodies were used: p63 (4A4, Santa Cruz Biotechnology), E2F1 (C-20, Santa Cruz Biotechnology), p16 (M-156, Santa Cruz Biotechnology), p19 (5-C3-1, Santa Cruz Biotechnology), β-actin (Clone AC-15, Sigma Chemical), phospho-AKT (ser473) (D9E, Cell Signaling Technology, Boston, MA), AKT (pan) (C67E7, Cell Signaling Technology) and phospho-S6 (Ser235/236) (D27.2.2E) and S6 (5G10) (Cell signaling Technology).

RNA isolation and Reverse Transcription-PCR

Total RNA was harvested using TRIzol reagent (Invitrogen) and reverse transcribed (1 μg) using the SuperScript III first strand

Table 2. Loss of $p19^{arf}$ cooperates with $v\text{-}ras^{Ha}$ in malignant conversion.

	Normal Skin	Papilloma	Carcinoma	Total	Conversion rate
Lenti-GFP/$v\text{-}ras^{Ha}$	0	5	0	5	0%
Lenti-ΔNp63α/$v\text{-}ras^{Ha}$	0	0	5	5	100%
$p19^{arf}$ null/$v\text{-}ras^{Ha}$	0	1	9	10	90%
$p19^{arf}$ null/Lenti-ΔNp63α/$v\text{-}ras^{Ha}$	0	0	10	10	100%

Tumor incidence and conversion rate of grafted $p19^{arf}$ null keratinocytes are presented at 5 weeks post-grafting. Tumor phenotypes were confirmed histologically.

cDNA synthesis kit (Invitrogen) with an oligo(dT) primer. Expression of p16 and p19 mRNA was determined by PCR amplification using primers specific for the mouse p16/p19 gene (p16: sense 5′-GCTGCAGACAGACTGGCCA-3′; antisense 5′-GTCCTCGCAGTTCGAATCTG-3′) [49]. p19: sense 5′-GTCGCAGGTTCTTGGTCACT-3′; antisense 5′-ATGTT-CACGAAAGCCAGAGC-3′) [50]. PCR amplification of GAPDH was used as a loading control. The PCR reaction program was as follows: denaturation, 94°C, 30 s; annealing, 53°C, 30 s; elongation, 72°C, 30 s for 35 cycles.

Acknowledgments

We thank Drs. Stuart Yuspa, Glenn Merlino and Chi-ping Day for helpful discussions. We thank Dr. Glenn Merlino for providing $p19^{arf}$ null mice. We acknowledge Drs. Kathryn King and Milos Dokmanovic for critical reading of the manuscript.

Author Contributions

Conceived and designed the experiments: LH WCW. Performed the experiments: LH SJ RMP MSR. Analyzed the data: LH WCW. Wrote the paper: LH WCW.

References

1. Yang A, Kaghad M, Wang Y, Gillett E, Fleming MD, et al. (1998) p63, a p53 homolog at 3q27-29, encodes multiple products with transactivating, death-inducing, and dominant-negative activities. Mol Cell 2: 305–316.
2. Levine AJ, Oren M (2009) The first 30 years of p53: growing ever more complex. Nat Rev Cancer 9: 749–758.
3. Mills AA, Zheng B, Wang XJ, Vogel H, Roop DR, et al. (1999) p63 is a p53 homologue required for limb and epidermal morphogenesis. Nature 398: 708–713.
4. Yang A, Schweitzer R, Sun D, Kaghad M, Walker N, et al. (1999) p63 is essential for regenerative proliferation in limb, craniofacial and epithelial development. Nature 398: 714–718.
5. Candi E, Rufini A, Terrinoni A, Dinsdale D, Ranalli M, et al. (2006) Differential roles of p63 isoforms in epidermal development: selective genetic complementation in p63 null mice. Cell Death Differ 13: 1037–1047.
6. Truong AB, Kretz M, Ridky TW, Kimmel R, Khavari PA (2006) p63 regulates proliferation and differentiation of developmentally mature keratinocytes. Genes & Development 20: 3185–3197.
7. DeYoung MP, Ellisen LW (2007) p63 and p73 in human cancer: defining the network. Oncogene 26: 5169–5183.
8. Hibi K, Trink B, Patturajan M, Westra WH, Caballero OL, et al. (2000) AIS is an oncogene amplified in squamous cell carcinoma. Proc Natl Acad Sci U S A 97: 5462–5467.
9. Wrone DA, Yoo S, Chipps LK, Moy RL (2004) The expression of p63 in actinic keratoses, seborrheic keratosis, and cutaneous squamous cell carcinomas. Dermatol Surg 30: 1299–1302.
10. Lin Z, Nan Y, Zhang X, Zhao Y, Kim C, et al. (2006) Reverse transcription-polymerase chain reaction and western blotting analysis for detection of p63 isoforms in uterine cervical cancers. International Journal of Gynecological Cancer 16: 1643–1647.
11. Nylander K, Coates PJ, Hall PA (2000) Characterization of the expression pattern of p63 alpha and delta Np63 alpha in benign and malignant oral epithelial lesions. Int J Cancer 87: 368–372.
12. Nylander K, Vojtesek B, Nenutil R, Lindgren B, Roos G, et al. (2002) Differential expression of p63 isoforms in normal tissues and neoplastic cells. J Pathol 198: 417–427.
13. Mooi WJ, Peeper DS (2006) Oncogene-induced cell senescence - Halting on the road to cancer. New England Journal of Medicine 355: 1037–1046.
14. Michaloglou C, Vredeveld LCW, Soengas MS, Denoyelle C, Kuilman T, et al. (2005) BRAF(E600)-associated senescence-like cell cycle arrest of human naevi. Nature 436: 720–724.
15. Keyes WM, Wu Y, Vogel H, Guo XC, Lowe SW, et al. (2005) p63 deficiency activates a program of cellular senescence and leads to accelerated aging. Genes & Development 19: 1986–1999.
16. Flores ER, Sengupta S, Miller JB, Newman JJ, Bronson R, et al. (2005) Tumor predisposition in mice mutant for p63 and p73: evidence for broader tumor suppressor functions for the p53 family. Cancer Cell 7: 363–373.
17. Keyes WM, Vogel H, Koster MI, Guo X, Qi Y, et al. (2006) p63 heterozygous mutant mice are not prone to spontaneous or chemically induced tumors. Proc Natl Acad Sci U S A 103: 8435–8440.
18. Ghioni P, Bolognese F, Duijf PH, van Bokhoven H, Mantovani R, et al. (2002) Complex Transcriptional Effects of p63 Isoforms: Identification of Novel Activation and Repression Domains. Mol Cell Biol 22: 8659–8668.
19. Helton ES, Zhu JH, Chen XB (2006) The unique NH2-terminally deleted (Delta N) residues, the PXXP motif, and the PPXY motif are required for the transcriptional activity of the Delta N variant of p63. Journal of Biological Chemistry 281: 2533–2542.
20. King KE, Ponnamperuma RM, Yamashita T, Tokino T, Lee LA, et al. (2003) ΔNp63α functions as a positive and negative transcriptional regulator and blocks in vitro differentiation of murine keratinocytes. Oncogene 22: 3635–3644.
21. Chen YK, Hsue SS, Lin LM (2004) Expression of p63 (TA and deltaN isoforms) in human primary well differentiated buccal carcinomas. Int J Oral Maxillofac Surg 33: 493–497.
22. Pruneri G, Pignataro L, Manzotti M, Carboni N, Ronchetti D, et al. (2002) p63 in laryngeal squamous cell carcinoma: evidence for a role of TA-p63 down-regulation in tumorigenesis and lack of prognostic implications of p63 immunoreactivity. Lab Invest 82: 1327–1334.
23. Guo X, Keyes WM, Papazoglu C, Zuber J, Li W, et al. (2009) TAp63 induces senescence and suppresses tumorigenesis in vivo. Nat Cell Biol 11: 1451–1457.
24. Gressner O, Schilling T, Lorenz K, Schulze SE, Koch A, et al. (2005) TAp63alpha induces apoptosis by activating signaling via death receptors and mitochondria. EMBO J 24: 2458–2471.
25. Suh EK, Yang A, Kettenbach A, Bamberger C, Michaelis AH, et al. (2006) p63 protects the female germ line during meiotic arrest. Nature 444: 624–628.
26. Koster MI, Kim S, Mills AA, DeMayo FJ, Roop DR (2004) p63 is the molecular switch for initiation of an epithelial stratification program. Genes Dev 18: 126–131.
27. Koster MI, Lu SL, White LD, Wang XJ, Roop DR (2006) Reactivation of developmentally expressed p63 isoforms predisposes to tumor development and progression. Cancer Res 66: 3981–3986.
28. Candi E, Dinsdale D, Rufini A, Salomoni P, Knight RA, et al. (2007) TAp63 and Delta Np63 in cancer and epidermal development. Cell Cycle 6: 274–284.
29. Rocco JW, Leong CO, Kuperwasser N, DeYoung MP, Ellisen LW (2006) p63 mediates survival in squamous cell carcinoma by suppression of p73-dependent apoptosis. Cancer Cell 9: 45–56.
30. Koster MI, Dai D, Marinari B, Sano Y, Costanzo A, et al. (2007) p63 induces key target genes required for epidermal morphogenesis. Proc Natl Acad Sci U S A 104: 3255–3260.
31. Zhu L, Rorke EA, Eckert RL (2007) DeltaNp63alpha promotes apoptosis of human epidermal keratinocytes. J Invest Dermatol 127: 1980–1991.
32. King KE, Ponnamperuma RM, Gerdes MJ, Tokino T, Yamashita T, et al. (2006) Unique domain functions of p63 isotypes that differentially regulate distinct aspects of epidermal homeostasis. Carcinogenesis 27: 53–63.
33. Hayflick L (1965) The Limited in vitro lifetime of human diploid cell strains. Exp Cell Res 37: 614–636.
34. Narita M, Narita M, Krizhanovsky V, Nunez S, Chicas A, et al. (2006) A novel role for high-mobility group A proteins in cellular senescence and heterochromatin formation. Cell 126: 503–514.

35. Su XH, Cho MS, Gi YJ, Ayanga BA, Sherr CJ, et al. (2009) Rescue of key features of the p63-null epithelial phenotype by inactivation of Ink4a and Arf. Embo Journal 28: 1904–1915.
36. Ponnamperuma RM, King KE, Elsir T, Glick AB, Wahl GM, et al. (2009) The transcriptional regulatory function of p53 is essential for suppression of mouse skin carcinogenesis and can be dissociated from effects on TGF-beta-mediated growth regulation. Journal of Pathology 219: 263–274.
37. Tremain R, Marko M, Kinnimulki V, Ueno H, Bottinger E, et al. (2000) Defects in TGF-beta signaling overcome senescence of mouse keratinocytes expressing v-Ha-ras. Oncogene 19: 1698–1709.
38. Korotchkina LG, Leontieva OV, Bukreeva EI, Demidenko ZN, Gudkov AV, et al. (2010) The choice between p53-induced senescence and quiescence is determined in part by the mTOR pathway. Aging (Albany NY) 2: 344–352.
39. Leontieva OV, Blagosklonny MV (2010) DNA damaging agents and p53 do not cause senescence in quiescent cells, while consecutive re-activation of mTOR is associated with conversion to senescence. Aging (Albany NY) 2: 924–935.
40. Serrano M, Lin AW, McCurrach ME, Beach D, Lowe SW (1997) Oncogenic ras provokes premature cell senescence associated with accumulation of p53 and p16(INK4a). Cell 88: 593–602.
41. Campisi J (2001) Cellular senescence as a tumor-suppressor mechanism. Trends in Cell Biology 11: S27–S31.
42. Romano RA, Ortt K, Birkaya B, Smalley K, Sinha S (2009) An active role of the DeltaN isoform of p63 in regulating basal keratin genes K5 and K14 and directing epidermal cell fate. PLoS One 4: e5623.
43. Koster MI, Huntzinger KA, Roop DR (2002) Epidermal differentiation: transgenic/knockout mouse models reveal genes involved in stem cell fate decisions and commitment to differentiation. J Investig Dermatol Symp Proc 7: 41–45.
44. Pozzi S, Zambelli F, Merico D, Pavesi G, Robert A, et al. (2009) Transcriptional network of p63 in human keratinocytes. PLoS One 4: e5008.
45. King KE, Ponnamperuma RM, Allen C, Lu H, Duggal P, et al. (2008) The p53 homologue DeltaNp63alpha interacts with the nuclear factor-kappaB pathway to modulate epithelial cell growth. Cancer Res 68: 5122–5131.
46. Perez CA, Pietenpol JA (2007) Transcriptional programs regulated by p63 in normal epithelium and tumors. Cell Cycle 6: 246–254.
47. Boldrup L, Coates PJ, Gu X, Nylander K (2009) DeltaNp63 isoforms differentially regulate gene expression in squamous cell carcinoma: identification of Cox-2 as a novel p63 target. J Pathol 218: 428–436.
48. Weinberg WC, Montano NE, Deng C (1997) Loss of p21CIP1/WAF1 does not recapitulate accelerated malignant conversion caused by p53 loss in experimental skin carcinogenesis. Oncogene 15: 685–690.
49. Frost SJ, Simpson DJ, Clayton RN, Farrell WE (1999) Transfection of an inducible p16/CDKN2A construct mediates reversible growth inhibition and G(1) arrest in the AtT20 pituitary tumor cell line. Molecular Endocrinology 13: 1801–1810.
50. Ha L, Ichikawa T, Anver M, Dickins R, Lowe S, et al. (2007) ARF functions as a melanoma tumor suppressor by inducing p53-independent senescence. Proc Natl Acad Sci U S A 104: 10968–10973.

Miz1 Is a Critical Repressor of *cdkn1a* during Skin Tumorigenesis

Jan Hönnemann[1], Adrián Sanz-Moreno[1], Elmar Wolf[2], Martin Eilers[2], Hans-Peter Elsässer[1]*

1 Department of Cytobiology, Philipps-University Marburg, Germany, **2** Theodor-Boveri-Institute, Biocentre, University of Würzburg, Germany

Abstract

The transcription factor Miz1 forms repressive DNA-binding complexes with the Myc, Gfi-1 and Bcl-6 oncoproteins. Known target genes of these complexes encode the cyclin-dependent kinase inhibitors (CKIs) *cdkn2b* ($p15^{Ink4}$), *cdkn1a* ($p21^{Cip1}$), and *cdkn1c* ($p57^{Kip2}$). Whether Miz1-mediated repression is important for control of cell proliferation *in vivo* and for tumor formation is unknown. Here we show that deletion of the Miz1 POZ domain, which is critical for Miz1 function, restrains the development of skin tumors in a model of chemically-induced, Ras-dependent tumorigenesis. While the stem cell compartment appears unaffected, interfollicular keratinocytes lacking functional Miz1 exhibit a reduced proliferation and an accelerated differentiation of the epidermis in response to the tumor promoter 12-O-tetradecanoylphorbol-13-acetate (TPA). Tumorigenesis, proliferation and normal differentiation are restored in animals lacking *cdkn1a*, but not in those lacking *cdkn2b*. Our data demonstrate that Miz1-mediated attenuation of cell cycle arrest pathways via repression of *cdkn1a* has a critical role during tumorigenesis in the skin.

Editor: Klaus Roemer, University of Saarland Medical School, Germany

Funding: This work was supported by the Deutsche Forschungsgemeinschaft (Sonderforschungsbereich Transregio 17, Project B5, and International GRK 767). The funders had no role in study design, data collection and analysis, decision to publish, or preparation of the manuscript.

Competing Interests: The authors have declared that no competing interests exist.

* E-mail: elsaesse@mailer.uni-marburg.de

Introduction

Miz1 (*M*yc-*i*nteracting *z*inc finger protein 1; Zbtb17) is a zinc finger transcription factor that forms a complex with the Myc oncoprotein [1]. In addition to 13 zinc fingers that are clustered in the central and C-terminal part of the protein, Miz1 bears a POZ (*po*xvirus *z*inc finger protein) domain at the N-terminus [2]. POZ domains are found in a variety of different transcription factors and can confer hetero- or homodimerization as well as tetramerisation [3,4]. The POZ domain of Miz1 forms tetramers [3] and is required for a stable association of Miz1 with chromatin [5,6]. In addition, Miz1 lacking the POZ domain can also interact with other proteins. As a result, the POZ domain is required both for transcriptional activation and repression by Miz1.

Among the proteins which interact with Miz1 independent of the POZ domain is Myc, which binds to Miz1 between the zinc finger domains 12 and 13 [1]. This complex represses the transcription of genes including *cdkn2b* (encoding $p15^{Ink4b}$), *cdkn1a* (encoding $p21^{Cip1}$), *cdkn1c* (encoding $p57^{Kip2}$) and *mxd4* (encoding Mad4) [7–10]. In the absence of Myc, Miz1 activates transcription of a number of genes including Bcl-2 [11], clusterin, several integrins and other proteins involved in cell adhesion [12], in a concerted manner with other transcription factors. For example, Miz1 synergizes with the Smad complex during the TGF-ß mediated activation of *cdkn2b* expression [7,8]. Similarly, increased transcription of *cdkn1a* depends on Miz1 in response to DNA damage [9] as well as in models of cellular differentiation [13–15]. Miz1 also forms repressive complexes with the Bcl-6 and Gfi-1 oncoproteins. Both complexes are capable of repressing expression of *cdkn1a*, and, in the case of Gfi-1, also of *cdkn2b*. These observations suggest that Miz1 functions as a general mediator of repression in association with several transcription factors [13,16,17].

The constitutive knockout of Miz1 is lethal at embryonic day E7.5 [18]. We previously analysed the function of Miz1 in keratinocytes using a conditional Cre/lox knockout model, in which the Cre recombinase is targeted via the keratin 14 promoter to the basal layer of both intra- and interfollicular epidermis [19], where Miz1 is predominantly expressed [12]. In this model, loxP sites flank exons 3 and 4, which encode the POZ domain [2], and deletion of these exons results in expression of a truncated Miz1 protein lacking the POZ domain [20]. Consistent with the biochemical model described above, keratinocytes lacking the Miz1 POZ domain show an attenuated expression of Miz1 target genes in response to TGF-β [20]. Furthermore, animals homozygous for this deletion exhibit an impaired morphogenesis of hair follicles with irregular order and extended length of the follicle, formation of epidermal cysts, delayed catagen during the hair cycle, loss of zig-zag hairs, as well as the occurrence of pigment incontinence in older animals [20].

The model described above suggests that Miz1 has a repressive function in highly proliferative and tumor tissues that express high levels of Myc, which may not be revealed during normal development [21]. Recent work by Trumpp and colleagues demonstrated that endogenous Myc is required for the formation of skin papillomas. The critical function of endogenous Myc in this context is to repress expression of *cdkn1a*, since deletion of *c-myc* leads to a loss of tumor formation as well as elevated levels of $p21^{Cip1}$, and co-deletion of *cdkn1a* fully restores tumor formation [22]. We now used the conditional Miz1-POZ domain knockout model to test the role of Miz1 in proliferation, differentiation and tumorigenesis in keratinocytes. We report here that the deletion of the Miz1 POZ domain leads to increased differentiation and reduced proliferation of keratinocytes when skin is challenged by the tumor promoter agent 12-O-tetradecanoylphorbol-13-acetate (TPA) as well as strongly decreased papilloma formation. These alterations are dependent on an altered regulation of *cdkn1a expression*. Our findings show that Miz1 is part of a repressor complex that is critical for restraining p21^{Cip1} expression in response to stimuli that enhance proliferation and promote skin carcinogenesis.

Results

The number of label retaining cells and the distribution of stem cell markers are unaffected in Miz1ΔPOZ mice

The homozygous deletion of the Miz1 POZ domain in keratinocytes, using a mouse strain that expresses Cre recombinase under the control of the keratin 14 promoter (hereafter called *Miz1ΔPOZ* mice; corresponding control animals do not express Cre recombinase; see also Material and Methods), revealed a complex skin phenotype [20]. To assess whether a defect of the stem cell compartment, located at the bulge region of the hair follicle, can account for the observed phenotypes in *Miz1ΔPOZ* mice, we visualized label-retaining cells (LRCs; [23]) by injecting BrdU on day 10 post partum (P10) and analysed the number and location of LRCs on P24. No significant morphological difference in number and location of BrdU positive cells of the bulge region was detected comparing control and *Miz1ΔPOZ* animals (Figure 1 A and B and Figure S1). To test whether enhanced proliferation has an impact on LRCs, we applied 12-O-tetradecanoylphorbol-13-acetate (TPA), a known enhancer of keratinocyte proliferation [24], once per day over five days. Again, no significant difference in number and location of LRCs of the bulge region was observed between control and *Miz1ΔPOZ* animals (Figure 1 C and D and Figure S1).

In addition, immunohistochemical stainings for the stem cell markers K15 (Figure 1 E–H) and CD34 (Figure 1 I–L) [25,26] revealed no difference in the number and location of labelled cells between control and *Miz1ΔPOZ* animals, irrespective of TPA or control treatment. Our data indicate that the deletion of the *Miz1ΔPOZ* domain has little effect on the location, number and proliferation of stem cells in the bulge region of *Miz1ΔPOZ* mice.

Alterations of differentiation and proliferation after TPA treatment are dependent on p21^{cip1}

Since Miz1, together with Myc, regulates the expression of genes encoding cyclin dependent kinase inhibitors like *cdkn2b* (encoding p15^{Ink4b}) or *cdkn1a* (encoding p21^{Cip1}) we next asked whether proliferation, differentiation and apoptosis of interfollicular keratinocytes are affected when a functional Miz1 protein is missing. The epidermis of control and *Miz1ΔPOZ* mice showed no difference in the expression pattern of the differentiation markers keratin 1 (Figure 2 A and C), loricrin (Figure 2 E and G) or filaggrin (Figure S2F and H). Additionally, the number and location of cells positive for the proliferation marker Ki67 was unaltered (Figure 2 I, K and M). When mice were treated with TPA, the thickness of the epidermis increased as expected (Figure S2A–E), and the expression of the suprabasal differentiation markers keratin 1 and loricrin, but not filaggrin, was undetectable in large areas of the epidermis from control animals (Figure 2 B, F and Figure S2F and G). In contrast, thickening of the epidermis was slightly but significantly reduced in *Miz1ΔPOZ* mice under TPA treatment (Figure S2E) and all three markers of differentiation remained prominent throughout the epidermis of *Miz1ΔPOZ* mice (Fig. 2 D, H and Figure S2H and I). Furthermore, skin from *Miz1ΔPOZ* mice exhibited keratin 1 staining in lower suprabasal cell layers, relative to control animals, where keratin 1 expression was mostly restricted to superficial epidermal cell layers (Figure 2 B and D). We conclude that treatment with TPA delays the differentiation of keratinocytes in control, but not in *Miz1ΔPOZ* mice.

Consistent with these observations, application of TPA over five days significantly enhanced the number of Ki67 positive cells in the epidermis of control animals, but to a much lesser extent in the epidermis of *Miz1ΔPOZ* animals (Figure 2 J, L and M). In addition, while a considerable number of Ki67 positive cells were located in suprabasal cell layers in control mice, this was not observed in *Miz1ΔPOZ* mice (Figure 2 J, L), strongly indicating that the absence of the Miz1 POZ domain prevents cell cycle entry in response to TPA. Taken together, our findings show that a decrease of cell proliferation and an earlier onset of increased differentiation attenuate the effect of TPA in the epidermis of *Miz1ΔPOZ* mice.

To genetically test whether one of the Miz1 regulated cyclin dependent kinase inhibitors, p15^{Ink4b} or p21^{Cip1}, have a role in restricting proliferation and promoting differentiation of keratinocytes in *Miz1ΔPOZ* mice, we generated *Miz1ΔPOZ* mice that lack either *cdkn2b* or *cdkn1a*. TPA treatment of *Miz1ΔPOZ;cdkn2b*$^{-/-}$ mice revealed no difference to *Miz1ΔPOZ;cdkn2b*$^{+/+}$ *mice* in regard to differentiation and proliferation of interfollicular keratinocytes, indicating that p15^{Ink4b} is not required for restraining proliferation of *Miz1ΔPOZ* keratinocytes (Figure 3E, Figure S3A–D, E). In line with these findings we didn't observe changes in p15^{ink4b} expression by quantitative RT-PCR (data not shown). In contrast, keratinocyte proliferation was induced by TPA to the same extent in *Miz1ΔPOZ;cdkn1a*$^{-/-}$ animals as in control animals (Figure 3A–D and F, Figure S3F). In addition, the extended focal ablation of differentiation markers that was observed in control animals also occurred in *Miz1ΔPOZ;cdkn1a*$^{-/-}$ mice, in contrast to *Miz1ΔPOZ* mice (Figure S4). These genetic data show that the impact of Miz1 on keratinocyte proliferation and differentiation depends on p21^{Cip1}.

To determine the biochemical basis of these observations, we analysed p21^{cip1} expression by immunoblot analysis of skin from control and knockout animals with a *cdkn1a*$^{+/+}$ background (Fig. 3I). Without TPA treatment, expression of p21^{cip1} was below the limit of detection in the skin from control animals but gave a clear signal in skin from *Miz1ΔPOZ* animals. TPA treatment induced the expression of p21^{cip1} in control animals and led to a further increase in p21^{cip1} expression in *Miz1ΔPOZ* mice. Under both conditions p21^{cip1} expression was increased in *Miz1ΔPOZ* animals compared to control animals, demonstrating directly that the Miz1 POZ domain restrains expression of p21^{cip1} *in vivo*.

To rule out the possibility that the increased p21^{cip1} expression was an indirect effect of an altered signal transduction in *Miz1ΔPOZ* animals, we first analysed Myc levels and found by immunoblot analysis that addition of TPA elevated Myc levels to a similar extent in control and *Miz1ΔPOZ* animals (Figure S5A). Second, we evaluated the activity of the Ras-Raf-MEK pathway via detection of phosphorylated ERK (p-ERK) [22]. Immunoblot analysis revealed a similar phosphorylation of ERK after TPA treatment in control and *Miz1ΔPOZ* animals (Figure S5A). In addition, p-ERK was detected in the suprabasal cell layers of the epidermis independent of the genotype (Figure S5B–E). Third, analysis of expression of p53, a major regulator of *cdkn1a*, by immunoblot and immunohistochemistry revealed no evidence for a difference between *Miz1ΔPOZ* and control animals (Figure S5A, F and G).

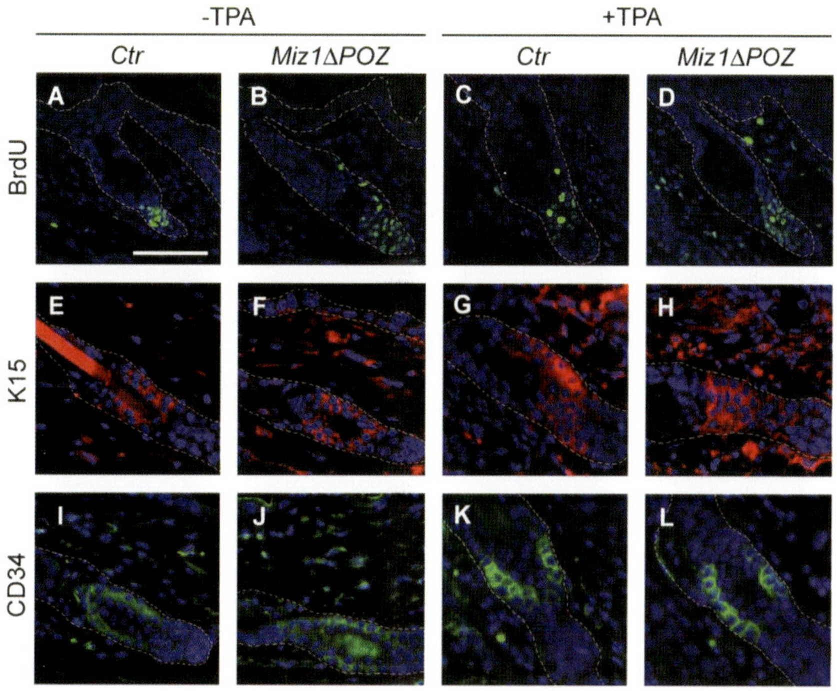

Figure 1. The skin stem cell compartment is unaltered in *Miz1ΔPOZ* mice. Animals, which were labelled on day P10 with BrdU, showed label-retaining cells two weeks later, predominantly located in the bulge region of the hair follicle. No difference was observed between control (*Ctr*) and *Miz1ΔPOZ* mice, neither without nor with TPA treatment (**A–D**). Skin stem cell markers Keratin 15 (K15; **E–H**) and CD34 (**I–L**) did not reveal differences between the different genotypes or treatments. Number of animals analysed: n = 3 for F–J and L; n = 4 for B, C and E; n = 5 for D and K; n = 6 for A. Bar: 50 μm.

To confirm that *cdkn1a* is a direct target gene of Miz1 and Myc in keratinocytes, we performed chromatin immunoprecipitation (ChIP) assays with antibodies directed against Miz1 and Myc, respectively. Since the isolation of primary keratinocytes takes several hours under harsh conditions and since it is almost impossible to obtain sufficient primary keratinocytes for efficient chromatin isolation, we used the murine keratinocyte cell line PAM212 [27], which responds to TPA similarly as primary keratinocytes [28]. Using chromatin isolated from these cells, ChIP assays revealed that both Miz1 and Myc were bound to the core promoter region of *cdkn1a*, but not to a control region located about 20 Mb downstream of *cdkn1a*. The binding of Miz1 to the *cdkn1a* promoter was not altered under TPA treatment (Figure 3G and H).

Taken together our data show that (a) *cdkn1a* is a direct target gene of Myc and Miz1 in murine keratinocytes,(b) that the POZ domain of Miz1 is critical for repressing $p21^{Cip1}$ expression *in vivo* and (c) that elevated levels of $p21^{Cip1}$ restrain TPA-stimulated keratinocyte proliferation in *Miz1ΔPOZ* mice.

Reduced skin tumorigenesis in Miz1ΔPOZ mice

The reduced proliferation response to TPA treatment in the skin of *Miz1ΔPOZ* animals led us to ask whether Miz1 plays a role in skin tumorigenesis. We applied the well-established two-stage skin carcinogenesis protocol using 7,2-dimethylbenz(a)anthracene (DMBA) as tumor initiator and 12-O-tetradecanoylphorbol-13-acetate (TPA) as tumor promoter [29]. Tumors initially emerged between weeks 8 and 9 of the TPA treatment both in control (see Materials and Methods) and in *Miz1ΔPOZ* animals, indicating that the principal time course of tumor development is similar in both mouse strains (Figure 4A). However, whereas 50% of the control animals developed tumors between weeks 10 and 11 of TPA treatment (n = 23), it took 15–16 weeks until 50% of the *Miz1ΔPOZ* animals exhibited tumors (Figure 4A; n = 26; $p<0.001$). To exclude that the tumors observed in *Miz1ΔPOZ* mice developed from keratinocytes that have escaped Cre recombination, we isolated DNA from tumor samples and genotyped them by PCR. In all 45 tumors tested we could confirm efficient Cre-mediated recombination (Figure S6I). Since skin papillomas in this animal model are usually monoclonal [29,30], a recombinant band indicates that the tumor has descended from a recombined keratinocyte. The non-recombined bands almost certainly come from cells of epidermal (melanocytes, dendritic cells) and/or dermal (fibroblasts, dendritic cells and many others) origin, in which the Cre recombinase is not active. This indicates that the tumors have not grown from escaper clones, but from cells lacking the Miz1 POZ domain. The gross morphology of tumors of comparable size from control and *Miz1ΔPOZ* animals was identical. No difference in the pattern of outfoldings was observed. In both genotypes, the thicknesses of the epidermis and of the cornified layer, and the amount of keratohyalin granules were increased compared to the interfollicular epidermis. Finally, no spread of epidermal cells into the dermal compartment occurred (Figure S6A–H).

The decreased tumorigenesis in *Miz1ΔPOZ* mice was further reflected by a reduced tumor burden per mouse, since the number of tumors was significantly lower in *Miz1ΔPOZ* compared to control animals (*Miz1ΔPOZ*: n = 3.38±4.30 tumors per mouse measured in 26 mice; control: n = 8.35±5.16 tumors per mouse measured in 23 mice; $p<0.001$; Figure 4B). Furthermore, tumors at the end of TPA treatment were significantly smaller in *Miz1ΔPOZ* mice than in control mice (1.94±1.64 mm vs 2.93±1.73 mm; Figure 4E and H). To exclude that the reduced tumor size is caused by increased apoptosis, we performed a

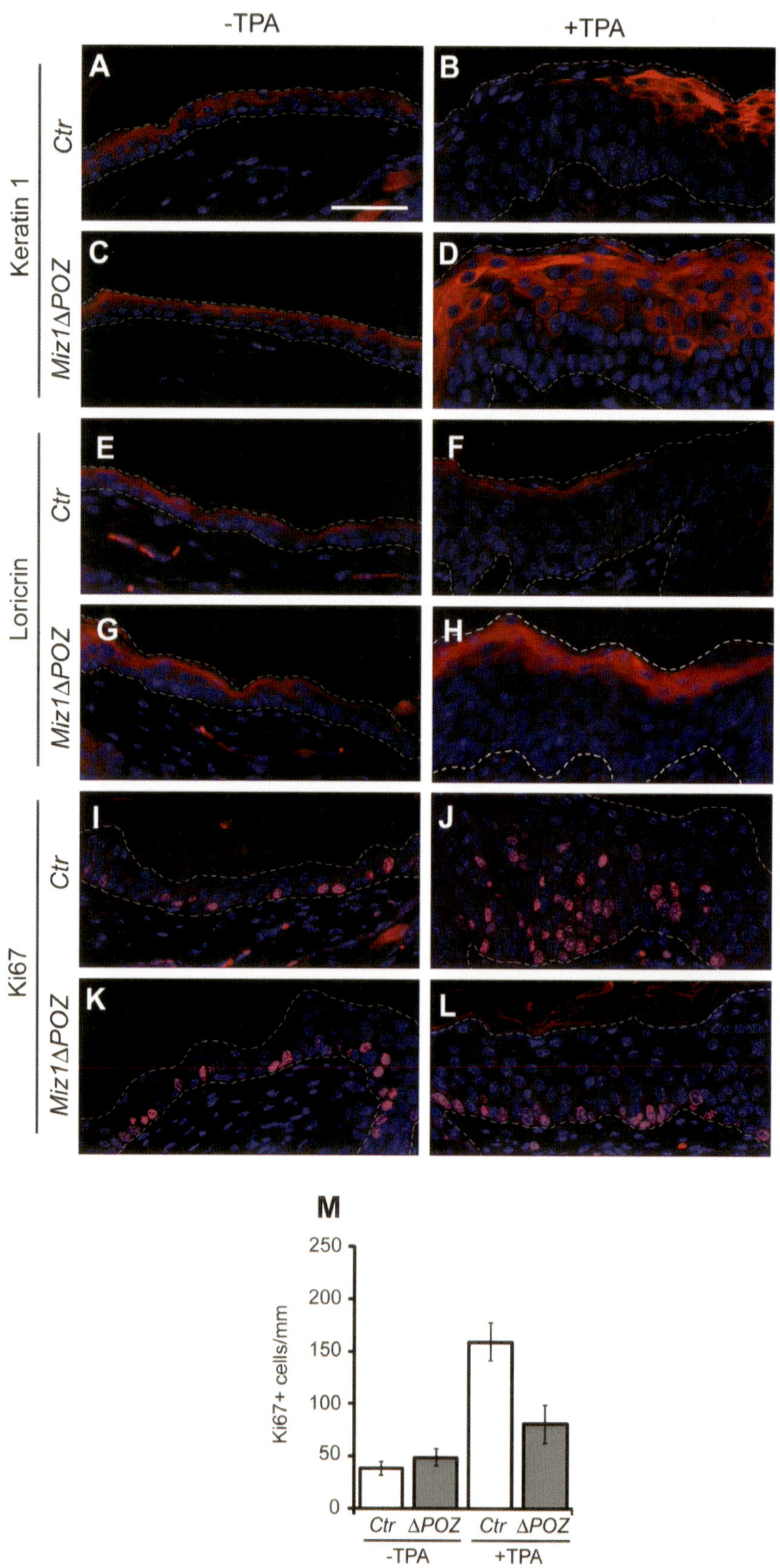

Figure 2. Epidermal differentiation and proliferation is altered upon TPA treatment. Immunohistochemical staining revealed no difference in the expression of the differentiation markers keratin 1 or loricrin (A, C and E, G) in the epidermis of untreated control (*Ctr*) or *Miz1ΔPOZ* mice. When *Ctr* animals were treated with TPA, focal areas were observed lacking these differentiation markers (B, F). In contrast, such foci did not

occur in the skin of *Miz1ΔPOZ* mice (D, H). Immunohistochemistry for the proliferation marker Ki67 revealed positive cells in the basal cell layer of untreated skin in both genotypes (I, K) and the labelling index was not significantly different (M, −TPA; n = 5 for each genotype). After TPA treatment, the Ki67 labelling index in *Ctr* animals was about twice as high as in *Miz1ΔPOZ* animals (M, +TPA; n = 5 for each genotype; *Ctr* vs *Miz1ΔPOZ* for ± TPA: $p<0.0001$). In addition, Ki67 positive cells were scattered through the suprabasal cell layers of the epidermis in *Ctr* but not in *Miz1ΔPOZ* animals (J, L). Bar: 50 μm.

TUNEL assay. TUNEL positive cells were rarely found in the tumors of both genotypes and were almost absent in the interfollicular epidermis (Figure S7A), indicating that the tumor size in *Miz1ΔPOZ* mice is not affected by increased programmed cell death. Finally, when TPA treatment was finished after 20 weeks and mice were subsequently observed for further 17 weeks, tumor diameter increased about threefold in control animals but remained constant in *Miz1ΔPOZ* mice (Figure S7B and C). We conclude that tumor development and growth is strongly reduced in *Miz1ΔPOZ* mice.

Strikingly, immunohistochemistry of papillomas revealed low levels of $p21^{cip1}$ in keratinocytes from 19 out of 21 tumors from control animals, but high $p21^{cip1}$ levels in keratinocytes from 14 out of 15 tumors of *Miz1ΔPOZ* mice (Figure 4F and G; Figure S8A). Additionally, increase of $p21^{cip1}$ in papillomas from *Miz1ΔPOZ* mice was observed by immunoblot analysis (Figure S8B). To test the impact of $p21^{cip1}$ genetically, we monitored tumor development in a cohort of *Miz1ΔPOZ;cdkn1a*$^{-/-}$ mice. In these experiments, we noted that the tumor burden per mouse in *cdkn1a*$^{-/-}$ control animals (Figure 4D) was lower than in *cdkn1a*$^{+/+}$ control animals (Figure 4B), most likely due to subtle differences in the overall genetic background of the animals used in the two experiments (see Materials and Methods) or possibly to a general lower tumor incidence in $p21^{cip1}$ deficient animals [31,32]. Importantly, *Miz1ΔPOZ;cdkn1a*$^{-/-}$ animals developed tumors with a time course that was indistinguishable from control *cdkn1a*$^{-/-}$ animals (Figure 4C; $p=0.6933$). Furthermore, the difference of tumor burden between *cdkn1a*$^{-/-}$*;Miz1ΔPOZ* and their corresponding control mice was smaller (5.04 ± 7.03 vs 6.27 ± 5.74 tumors per mouse, measured in 22 control and 26 *cdkn1a*$^{-/-}$*;Miz1ΔPOZ* mice; $p=0.5139$) than in an *cdkn1a*$^{+/+}$ background (8.35 vs 3.38 tumors per mouse, see above). Finally, there was no difference in the tumor size between control and *Miz1ΔPOZ* animals in a *cdkn1a*$^{-/-}$ background (Figure 4I), in contrast to control and *Miz1ΔPOZ* animals with a *cdkn1a*$^{+/+}$ background (Figure 4H). Taken together, we conclude that the reduced tumorigenicity observed in *Miz1ΔPOZ* mice depends on the upregulation of $p21^{Cip1}$ expression.

Discussion

One well characterized function of Miz1 is the regulation of the cyclin dependent kinase inhibitor genes *cdkn2b* (encoding $p15^{Ink4b}$), *cdkn1a* (encoding $p21^{Cip1}$) and *cdkn1c* (encoding $p57^{Kip2}$) [33], although a number of other genes are now known to be expressed in a Miz1-dependent manner [6,11,12]. The current model proposes that Miz1, complexed with nucleophosmin, binds to the core promoter of its target genes to enhance gene expression. Transactivation is blocked when the Myc/Max complex binds to Miz1, thereby releasing nucleophosmin [34,35]. In this model, Miz1 has a dual role in expression of its target genes. In the absence of Myc, Miz1 contributes to target gene activation. However, Miz1 also serves to recruit Myc leading to the formation of a repressive complex. This suggests that abrogation of Miz1 function will enhance target gene expression in conditions of high Myc expression. The allele of Miz1 used here lacks the POZ domain, which is necessary both for the transactivating properties of Miz1 [1,9] and for its stable association with chromatin [6,21].

We observed fewer and smaller tumors in *Miz1ΔPOZ* animals. A detailed analysis revealed that a reduced proliferation of keratinocytes in response to the tumor promoter, TPA, can account for the reduction of tumor growth in these animals, while changes in the stem cell compartment could not be uncovered. Interestingly, proliferation was completely restored in a *cdkn1a* null background, strongly suggesting that the increase in $p21^{Cip1}$ expression that is observed in *Miz1ΔPOZ* mice is responsible for the observed phenotype. This notion is further supported 1) by an immunoblot analysis revealing elevated $p21^{cip1}$ levels in the skin from *Miz1ΔPOZ* mice compared to their wildtype counterparts (Fig. 3I), 2) by immunohistochemical data showing that $p21^{Cip1}$ is consistently expressed in tumors of *Miz1ΔPOZ* mice, but is hardly detectable in control tumors (Fig. 4F, G) and 3) by the genetic experiment exhibiting a rescue of the reduced proliferation reflected by Ki67 positive cells (Figure 3A–D and F), a rescue of the tumor development (Figure 4C) and partial rescue of the tumor burden (Figure 4D) in *Miz1ΔPOZ* mice on a *cdkn1a* null background. In contrast, *Miz1ΔPOZ* mice with a *cdkn2b* null background exhibited only a small and statistically insignificant increase in Ki67 positive cells (Figure 3E; Figure S3A–E), suggesting that upregulation of $p15^{Ink4b}$ is not involved in restraining proliferation of *Miz1ΔPOZ* keratinocytes in response to TPA treatment.

While our data show that Miz1 has a critical role in repressing *cdkn1a* expression during skin carcinogenesis, they do not directly address the mechanism by which Miz1 acts in this system. For example, Miz1 has been suggested to associate with p53 [36]. While deletion of the POZ domain does not affect levels of p53 (Figure S5A), it is possible that it enhances p53 function in more subtle ways, leading to enhanced $p21^{cip1}$ expression. Furthermore, we do not know which of the several oncoproteins that can repress transcription via Miz1 (see Introduction) are functional during skin carcinogenesis. However, our data can account for the results obtained using tamoxifen inducible *c-myc*$^{-/-}$ mice [22]. In these mice, DMBA/TPA treatment led to elevated expression of $p21^{Cip1}$ and skin tumors could only be induced in the absence of $p21^{Cip1}$, demonstrating that endogenous Myc has a critical function in repressing *cdkn1a* during skin tumor development. It should be noted, that a related model in which *c-myc* is deleted during development by a constitutively active Cre recombinase expressed under the keratin 5 promoter shows more severe phenotypes, suggesting that Myc has functions in addition to repressing $p21^{cip1}$ during skin development [37].

Our data extend observations on Myc-induced lymphomagenesis in mice expressing a mutant allele of Myc that is selectively deficient in binding to Miz1 (MycV349D). Mice expressing this mutant display a reduced tumorigenesis, at least in part because binding of Myc to Miz1 is required to restrain expression of $p15^{Ink4b}$ and of $p57^{kip2}$ in the lymphomas [38]. Importantly, lymphomas arising in these mice showed an accumulation of senescent cells, suggesting that binding of Myc to Miz1 may be required to antagonize senescence during tumorigenesis.

$p21^{Cip1}$ is a key player during the induction of senescence of human fibroblasts [39], keratinocytes [40], melanocytes [41] and mammary epithelial cells [42]. While we did not detect senescent cells in tumors that arose in either wild type or *Miz1ΔPOZ*

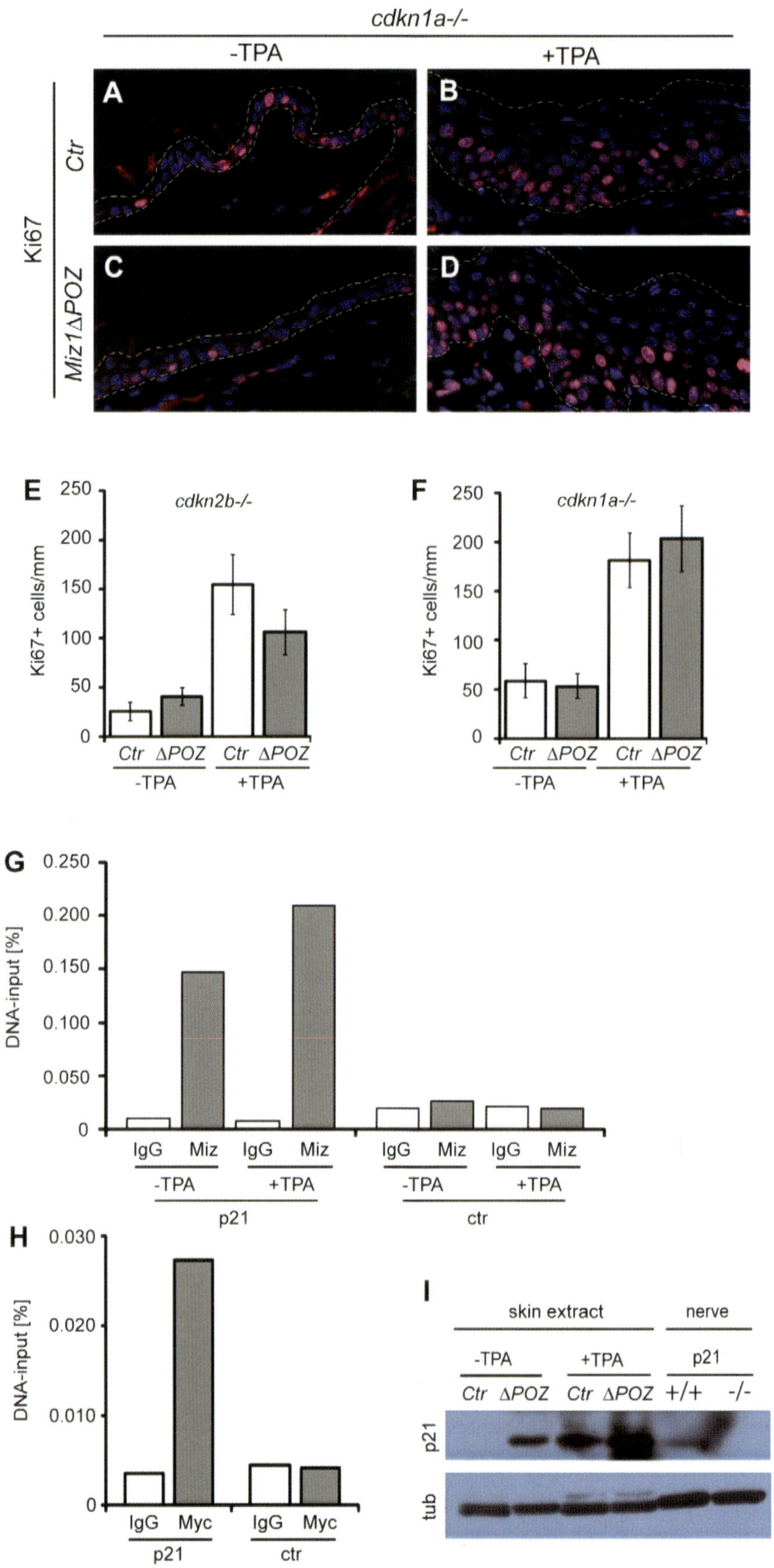
cdkn1a-/-
-TPA
+TPA
A
B
C
D
Ki67
Ctr
Miz1ΔPOZ
E
cdkn2b-/-
Ki67+ cells/mm
Ctr ΔPOZ Ctr ΔPOZ
-TPA +TPA
F
cdkn1a-/-
G
DNA-input [%]
IgG Miz IgG Miz IgG Miz IgG Miz
-TPA +TPA -TPA +TPA
p21
ctr
H
IgG Myc IgG Myc
I
skin extract
nerve
-TPA
+TPA
p21
Ctr ΔPOZ Ctr ΔPOZ +/+ -/-
p21
tub

Figure 3. Altered proliferation in the skin of *Miz1ΔPOZ* mice depends on $p21^{Cip1}$. TPA treatment of skin from control (*Ctr*) and *Miz1ΔPOZ* mice on a *cdkn1a* null background shows the same increase of the Ki67 labelling index and scattering of Ki67 positive cells in the suprabasal layers of the epidermis (**A–D** and **F**; n = 3 for each genotype and condition; *Ctr* vs *Miz1ΔPOZ* for −TPA: p = 0.4007; *Ctr* vs *Miz1ΔPOZ* for +TPA: p = 0.4494). In contrast, the equivalent experiment on a *cdkn2b* null background (**E**; n = 3 for each genotype and condition) exhibited the same result as in $cdkn2b^{+/+}$ animals (compare with Figure 2 M; *Ctr* vs *Miz1ΔPOZ* for ±TPA: $p<0.0001$). In $cdkn1a^{+/+}$ animals, $p21^{Cip1}$ is upregulated in protein extracts from *Miz1ΔPOZ*-mice (*ΔPOZ*) compared to extracts from control-mice (*Ctr*) either with or without TPA-treatment (**I**). Sciatic nerve extracts from $cdkn1a^{+/+}$ and $cdkn1a^{-/-}$ animals were used as positive and negative controls, respectively (see Materials and Methods). Chromatin immunoprecipitation assay using chromatin from murine PAM212 keratinocytes and antibodies against Miz1 and Myc (**G**; **H**; one representative experiment of three independent experiments each). The experiment demonstrates that both transcription factors bind to the *cdkn1a* promoter in this cell type. Miz1 binds to the *cdkn1a* promoter in PAM212 keratinocytes, without and with TPA treatment (100 nM for 4 hours). Primers used either amplified genomic DNA comprising part of the *cdkn1a* promoter (p21) or a *cdkna1a* unrelated sequence of chromosome 17 (ctr). For details see Materials and Methods. The graphs show the mean value of 2–3 technical replicas.

animals, a fraction of interfollicular and follicular keratinocytes and approximately 25% of the hair follicles stain positive for the senescence marker SA-ß-galactosidase in aged skin of *Miz1ΔPOZ* but not of control animals (Figure S9; [43]). We suggest, therefore, that repression via Miz1 may be more broadly involved in suppressing senescence and the reduced tumorigenesis in *Miz1Δ-POZ* mice may reflect the need to overcome $p21^{Cip1}$ mediated senescence during tumor formation [44,45]. While this remains to be formally demonstrated, the current data strongly support the view that the formation of a functional Miz1/Myc complex results in a context-dependent and cell type-specific attenuation, or even abrogation, of critical growth arrest pathways during tumorigenesis.

Materials and Methods

Transgenic mice

$Miz1^{lox/lox}$ mice [20] were crossed with K14Cre mice [19] to generate a conditional knockout of the POZ domain of Miz1 in murine basal epidermal cells as described elsewhere [20]. Mice were backcrossed 6 times on a 129S2/SvHsd background. Here, mice which are $K14cre^{+}$;$Miz1^{flox/flox}$ are designated *MizΔPOZ*-mice, while $K14Cre^{-}$;$Miz1^{flox/flox}$ mice were used as control animals designated *Ctr*. *MizΔPOZ* mice were crossed on a *cdkn2b* [46] and *cdkn1a* [47] deficient background, here designated *MizΔPOZ*;$cdkn2b^{-/-}$ and *MizΔPOZ*;$cdkn1a^{-/-}$ mice, respectively. $cdkn2b^{-/-}$ animals, with a FVB background, were a generous gift from A. Burns, Amsterdam. $cdkn1a^{-/-}$ animals, with a 129S4/SvJae genetic background, were purchased from Jackson laboratory (stock no. 008184).

49 d old mice were treated on 5 consecutive days with 5 nmol TPA (Sigma) in 100 µl acetone. TPA was locally applied on the dorsal skin, which was shaved 1 week before the first treatment. The mice were sacrificed 24 h after the last treatment.

In the 2-stage tumorigenesis experiment [29], 100 nmol DMBA (Sigma) in 100 µl acetone was once applied on the shaved dorsal skin of 49 d old mice. 1 week after the DMBA-application, the TPA treatment was started. Mice were then treated with 5 nmol TPA in 100 µl acetone for 20 weeks with two TPA applications per week.

Label-retaining cells (LCRs) were demonstrated in a bromodesoxyuridine (BrdU) pulse-chase experiment. On day 10 post partum (P10), 10 mg BrdU dissolved in 50 µl sterile PBS were injected intraperitoneally 5 times once every hour. On days P18 to P23 animals were treated with TPA as described above and the skin was prepared for histology. Immunocytochemical staining of BrdU was performed as described below.

Research involving mice have been conducted according to the German Animal Protection Law (Tierschutzgesetz). The application for the experiments was reviewed and approved by the responsible local authorities (Regierungspraesidium Giessen, reference numbers V 54 - 19 c 20/15 (1) MR20/10 Nr. 23/2005, V 54 - 19 c 20/15 (1) MR20/10 Nr. 95/2009 and V 54 - 19 c 20/15 (1) MR20/10 Nr. 66/2010)

Immunoblot analysis

Protein samples were extracted from dorsal skin and homogenized in RIPA buffer, containing 1% Triton X-100; 1% sodium deoxycholate; 0,1% SDS; 150 mM NaCl; 10 mM Na_2HPO_4; 2 mM EDTA; 1% Apronitin; 50 mM NaF; 200 mM Na_3VO_4; pH 7,4. As a positive control for $p21^{cip1}$, extracts from sciatic nerves were used [48]. Protein concentration was determined using the BCA-assay (Sigma). 20 µg per sample were separated on 10% polyacrylamide-SDS gels according to standard procedures. Proteins were blotted on nitrocellulose membranes and the blots were stained with antibodies against the following proteins: c-Myc (N-262, Santa Cruz; 1:400), p21 (C-19, Santa Cruz; 1:100), p-ERK (T202/Y204, Cell Signalling; 1:200), p53 (FL-393, Santa Cruz; 1:400), tubulin (YL1/2, Abcam; 1:2000) at 4°C overnight or for 72 hours in case of p53. Appropriate secondary peroxidase labelled antibodies (Biorad) were applied 1 hour at room temperature and antibody binding was visualized using the Lumi-Light Western blotting substrate from Roche.

Chromatin immunoprecipitation assay

Chromatin immunoprecipitation was carried out according to Boyd [49] using the mouse keratinocyte cell line PAM212 [27]. Briefly, the chromatin was sonicated at 4°C using a Bioruptor™ NextGen (Diagenode) for 15×30 sec at 20 Hz and 320 W with 30 sec breaks between each sonication step. The Immunoprecipitation Starter Pack (GE Healthcare) was used with antibodies directed against c-Myc (N-262; Santa Cruz) and Miz1 (10E2, Staller *et al.* 2001). For the isotype control, IgG from mouse and rabbit serum (Sigma) was used. After the crosslink reversion, the chromatin was purified with the QIAquick PCR Purification Kit (QIAGEN).

The promoter binding was detected by qPCR on a Mx3005p PCR machine (Stratagene/Agilent) with a QPCR SYBR Green Mix (Thermo Scientific), using CTCAGCTCTAACTG-TACTGTTGTTCA as forward and CTGGGCTATTCTC-TTGTCACG as reverse primer, to detect the *cdkn1a* promoter sequence by amplifying genomic DNA between basepairs 29.230.454–29.230.529 of chromosome 17. Control primers were TCATCCCACCCAGGAGTATT as forward primer and GAG-TACATTTAACCAACTATCAGAGCA as reverse primer, respectively, amplifying genomic DNA between basepairs 9.600.536–9.600.628 of chromosome 17 being unrelated to *cdkn1a*.

Histology

Skin samples were fixed in PBS buffered 3.7% formaldehyde and embedded in paraffin according to standard procedures. For immunohistochemistry, 3 µm sections were applied on silane-coated slides, preincubated with 10% goat serum (Sigma) and, if

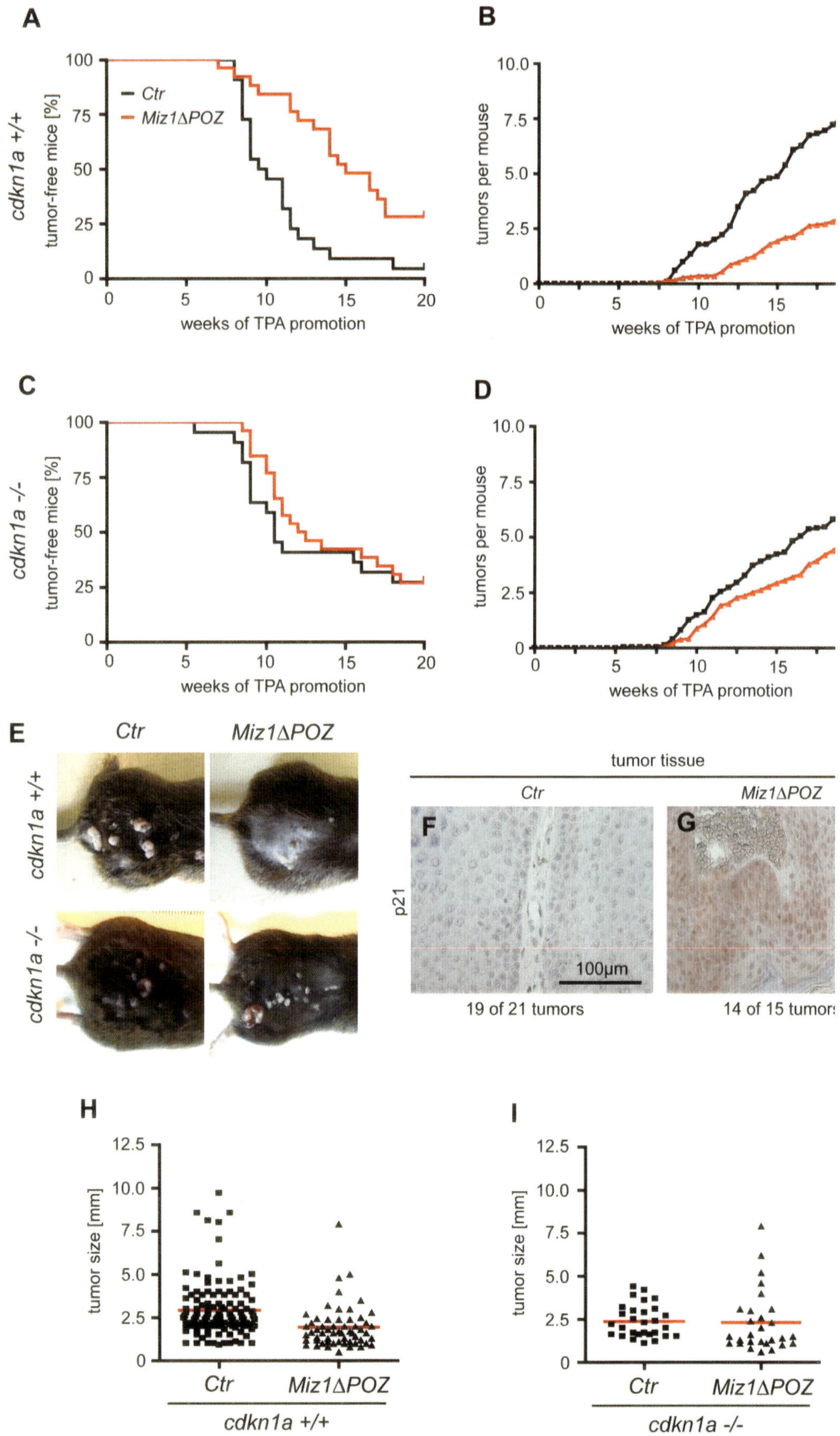
A
B
C
D
E
F
G
H
I
cdkn1a +/+
cdkn1a -/-
tumor-free mice [%]
Ctr
Miz1ΔPOZ
weeks of TPA promotion
tumors per mouse
tumor tissue
p21
100µm
19 of 21 tumors
14 of 15 tumors
tumor size [mm]

Figure 4. Formation of skin papillomas is decreased in *Miz1ΔPOZ* mice. (A) Animals with a conditional knockout of the *Miz1ΔPOZ* domain in keratinocytes (n = 26) showed a reduced development of skin papillomas relative to control (*Ctr*) mice (n = 23; $p<0.001$). In addition, the average number of tumors per mouse was significantly reduced in *Miz1ΔPOZ* animals compared to control animals (B). With a *cdkn1a* null background, tumor development (C) and average number of tumors per animal (D) in *Ctr* (n = 22) and *Miz1ΔPOZ* (n = 26) mice were not significantly different (tumor development: p = 0.9789; tumors per animal: p = 0.1585). In (E), representative tumors of all genotypes are shown documenting a smaller size of tumors in *Miz1ΔPOZ* mice with a *cdkn1a*$^{+/+}$ background. This is confirmed by the quantification of the tumor diameters (H; *Ctr* vs. *Miz1ΔPOZ*: $p<0.0001$). In contrast, tumor size on a *cdkn1a*$^{-/-}$ background was not significantly different between control and *Miz1ΔPOZ* animals (I; *Ctr* vs. *Miz1ΔPOZ*: p = 0.8788). When tumor tissue with a *cdkn1a*$^{+/+}$ background was stained with an antibody against p21^{Cip1}, 14 out of 15 tumors from 9 *Miz1ΔPOZ* mice exhibited a strong staining (G), while p21^{Cip1} expression was not detectable in 19 out of 21 tumors from 7 wild type mice (F) (see also Figure S8).

necessary, further treated as outlined below. For Ki67, p21^{Cip1} and p-ERK staining, slides were microwaved in 10 mM citrate buffer pH 6 for 3×5 min. For bromodesoxyuridine (BrdU) staining, slides were incubated for 30 min in 2 N HCl/0.5% Triton X-100, for 3 min in borax buffer (0.5 M sodium diborate/ 0,5 M boric acid, pH = 7.6) at RT and for 3 min in 0.025% trypsin in 0,05 M Tris/HCL, pH = 7.4. Primary antibodies were diluted in 10% goat serum (Dako) and incubated at 4°C overnight. Antibodies against the following antigens were used: Ki67 (Dako; 1:50), BrdU (Dianova; 1:100), p-ERK (T202/Y204, Cell Signalling; 1:100), CD34 (BD; 1:100), K15 (Abcam; 1:100), p21^{Cip1} (Abcam; 1:100), keratin 1 (Covance, 1:1000), loricrin (Covance; 1:1000). For visualization, appropriate secondary antibodies labelled either with FITC, TRITC (Molecular Probes) or with peroxidase were used. Slides were incubated 1 hour at room temperature and were subsequently covered with Mowiol. For documentation, a motorized BX61 microscope (Olympus) equipped with a F-View digital camera was used (Soft Imaging System, Münster, Germany).

The TUNEL assay was performed using the DeadEnd kit (Promega) according to manufacturer instructions. The staining for SA-ß-galactosidase was performed as described by Dimri et al. [43]. To ascertain the percentage of positive hair follicles, about 100 follicles per sample were counted.

Morphometric analysis

The number of Ki67 positive cells per mm of skin and the ratio of suprabasal Ki67 positive cells were measured using the program cell^{F} (Olympus). From 3 to 5 mice per condition (control, *MizΔPOZ*, *MizΔPOZ;cdkn2b*$^{-/-}$ and *MizΔPOZ;cdkn1a*$^{-/-}$; TPA-treated and untreated) 15–25 pictures were taken. In each picture, the length of the epidermis was measured and the related Ki67 positive basal and suprabasal cells were counted. The amount of all Ki67 positive cells per mm of skin was calculated. In addition, the ratio of basal to superbasal Ki67 positive cells was determined.

Statistical analysis

Mean values and standard deviations of the morphometric and ChIP data were calculated with Excel (Microsoft). The statistical significance of the morphometric data, the Kaplan-Meier estimator and the average number of tumors per mouse was calculated using the Student's *t*-test as implemented in the program GraphPad Prism (GraphPad Software).

Supporting Information

Figure S1 Label-retaining cells (LRCs) in the bulge region. (A) Documentation of LRC number variability in bulge regions from ctr and *Miz1ΔPOZ* animals, without and with TPA treatment. In (B), the percentage of LRCs (% BrdU positive cells) counted in the bulge region area are shown. 19 to 25 bulge regions per condition were evaluated for BrdU positive cells.

Figure S2 TPA treated control and *Miz1ΔPOZ* epidermis. HE-staining of control (A, B) and *Miz1ΔPOZ* epidermis (C, D) under TPA treatment (B, D) or in untreated skin (A, C). The size of scale bar in A is 50 µm. The average epidermal thickness of TPA treated and untreated control and *Miz1ΔPOZ* epidermis is shown in E. 100 single measurements per animal were done with 3 animals per condition. Fluorescence staining of filaggrin in control (F, G) and *Miz1ΔPOZ* (H, I) skin with and without TPA treatment (+/−TPA). Filaggrin is equally expressed in *Ctr* and *Miz1ΔPOZ* suprabasal epidermis, either with or without TPA treatment. Percentage of suprabasal Ki67 positive keratinocytes in untreated and TPA treated *Ctr* and *Miz1ΔPOZ* skin (J).

Figure S3 TPA treated control and *Miz1ΔPOZ* epidermis with a *cdkn2b*$^{-/-}$ background. Fluorescence staining of Ki67 in *Ctr* (A, B) and *Miz1ΔPOZ* (C, D) skin with a *cdkn2b* (encoding p15^{INK4b}) deficient background with and without TPA treatment (+/−TPA). The additional deletion of *cdkn2b* does not rescue the reduced proliferation in TPA treated *Miz1ΔPOZ* skin compared to TPA treated *Ctr* skin. Quantification of suprabasal Ki67 positive keratinocytes in untreated and TPA treated *Ctr* and *Miz1ΔPOZ* skin with either a p15^{INK4b} (E) or a p21^{cip1} (F) deficient background. Under TPA treatment, suprabasal Ki67 positive cells are significantly reduced in *Miz1ΔPOZ* skin compared to *Ctr* skin in mice with a *cdkn2b*$^{-/-}$ background (E; $p<0.0001$), as observed in *cdkna2b*$^{+/+}$ animals (compare with Figure S2 J). In contrast, a complete rescue was achieved in *cdkn1a*$^{-/-}$ animals where no difference of Ki67 suprabasal cells was observed between control and *Miz1ΔPOZ* mice (F; p = 0.9316).

Figure S4 Differentiation in *cdkn2b* or *cdkn1a* deficient *Miz1ΔPOZ* epidermis. Fluorescence staining of keratin 1 (A–H) and loricrin (I–P) in control and *Miz1ΔPOZ* skin with and without TPA treatment (+/−TPA) either with a *cdkn2b* (A–D and I–L) or *cdkn1a* (E–H and M–P) deficient background. In *cdkn2b*$^{-/-}$ mice and upon TPA treatment, keratin 1 expression is focally interrupted in *Ctr* skin while *Miz1ΔPOZ* skin shows continuous keratin 1 expression (B, D). With a *cdkn1a* deficient background, *Ctr* and *Miz1ΔPOZ* skin both show a focal interruption of keratin 1 expression after TPA (F, H). Also, with a *cdkn2b*$^{-/-}$ background, loricrin expression is focally reduced in *Ctr* skin (J) but not in *Miz1ΔPOZ* skin (L), while in *cdkn1a*$^{-/-}$ skin, focal reduction of loricrin expression can be observed in both *Ctr* (N) and *Miz1ΔPOZ* skin (P). The described expression patterns of keratin 1 and loricrin only occurred in TPA treated skin, whereas untreated skin did not show differences between *Ctr* and *Miz1ΔPOZ* animals in regard to keratin 1 and loricrin expression, neither with a *cdkn2b* (A, C, I, K), nor with a *cdkn1a* deficient background (E, G, M, O).

Figure S5 ERK-phosphorylation, c-Myc and p53 expression in *Miz1ΔPOZ* epidermis. Immunoblot of phosphorylated

ERK (p-ERK), c-Myc and p53 in extracts of murine Control (*Ctr*) and *Miz1ΔPOZ* skin (A), untreated or treated with TPA (−/+TPA). α-tubulin was used as a loading control. The expression of p-ERK was also visualized in murine epidermis via immunohistochemistry in control (B, C) and *Miz1ΔPOZ* samples (D, E) both untreated (B, D) or TPA treated (C, E). Furthermore, p53 stained by immunohistochemistry in tumors did not reveal a difference between control (*Ctr*) and *Miz1ΔPOZ* papillomas (F, G), in contrast to $p21^{cip1}$ expression (see Figure 4F, G and Figure S8).

Figure S6 Histology and genotyping of *Miz1ΔPOZ* papillomas. HE-staining of control (A, C, D, G) and *Miz1ΔPOZ* papillomas (B, E, F, H). The length of the scale bars is 600 µm in A and B, 100 µm in C–F and 50 µm in G and H. (I) Miz1 genotyping of murine tail skin (S) and tumor tissue (T). A control (*Ctr*) animal and one tumor with a floxed *Miz1* allele and no Cre recombinase expression was genotyped as a negative control. Animals 1–11 are *Miz1ΔPOZ* animals with a floxed *Miz1* allele which express Cre recombinase. The lower band at 180 bp indicates the recombinant allele, while the upper band at 311 bp indicates the floxed allele. A floxed allele can also be detected in tumors from *Miz1ΔPOZ* animals due to the presence in the samples of other (non-keratinocyte) epidermal and dermal cell types that do not express Cre recombinase.

Figure S7 Apoptosis and tumor growth in tissue from control (ctr) and *Miz1ΔPOZ* animals. (A) While there were essentially no TUNEL positive cells in the interfollicular skin, we occasionally observed TUNEL positive cells in tumors independent of the genotype, although most tumors from both genotypes lacked TUNEL positive cells. As a positive control for the assay we used either skin fixed in Carnoy's solution, where most nuclei should be positive because of an acidic hydrolysis of the DNA (due to the acetic acid which is a component of this fixative) or thymus which usually exhibits a large number of apoptotic T-cells, predominately in the cortex. (B) Tumor development during 17 weeks after the last TPA treatment. Representative pictures of control (*Ctr*) and *Miz1ΔPOZ* papillomas 17 weeks after the last TPA treatment (B). Measurement of the tumor diameter (C) revealed an increased tumor-size in *Ctr* animals but not in *Miz1ΔPOZ mice* (compare with Figure 4H).

Figure S8 p21-expression in *Miz1ΔPOZ* papillomas. Immunohistochemistry of control (*Ctr*) and *Miz1ΔPOZ* papillomas showing the expression of $p21^{cip1}$ (A). Each slide indicates a representative region of an individual tumor. In the majority of *Miz1ΔPOZ* papillomas, $p21^{cip1}$ was upregulated, whereas in most *Ctr* tumors $p21^{cip1}$ expression was not detectable. Expression of p21 protein in papillomas was also analyzed by immunoblot (B) in each of three (1–3) *Ctr* and *Miz1ΔPOZ* papillomas with $p21^{+/+}$. *Ctr* and *Miz1ΔPOZ* tumor samples with a $p21^{-/-}$ background are negative controls. All *Miz1ΔPOZ*-tumors have an increased p21 expression compared to *Ctr* tumors, while in $p21^{-/-}$ tumors, no p21 expression was detectable.
(TIF)

Figure S9 Tumors of *Miz1ΔPOZ* mice are not positive for SA-ß-galactosidase. Tumors from control (*Ctr*) (A) and *Miz1ΔPOZ* (B) animals after 20 weeks of TPA treatment were histochemically stained for SA-ß-galactosidase, but were not positive independent of the genotype. In contrast, skin from one year old *Miz1ΔPOZ mice* displayed a focal staining which was absent in *Ctr* animals (C, D). In addition, about 25% of hair follicles stained positive for SA-ß-galactosidase in *Miz1ΔPOZ* but not in *Ctr* animals (E). Arrowheads indicate sebaceous glands, which stain always positive for SA-ß-galactosidase.

Acknowledgments

The expert technical assistance of Waltraud Ackermann and Ursula Lehr is greatly acknowledged. We thank Salvador Aznar-Benitah, Centre for Genomic Regulation, for technical support with the BrdU staining, Karin Müller-Decker from the Deutsche Krebsforschungszentrum (DKFZ) for her introduction of the DMBA/TPA model and Thorsten Stiewe from the Institute of Molecular and Tumor Biology, Marburg for helpful discussions about p53. PAM212 cells were a generous gift from Stuart H. Yuspa from the Laboratory of Cancer Biology and Genetics, Center for Cancer Research, National Cancer Institute, Bethesda.

Author Contributions

Conceived and designed the experiments: JH ME HPE. Performed the experiments: JH ASM EW. Analyzed the data: JH ME HPE ASM EW. Contributed reagents/materials/analysis tools: ME HPE. Wrote the paper: HPE ME.

References

1. Peukert K, Staller P, Schneider A, Carmichael G, Hänel F, et al. (1997) An alternative pathway for gene regulation by Myc. EMBO J 16: 5672–5686. doi:10.1093/emboj/16.18.5672.
2. Bardwell VJ, Treisman R (1994) The POZ domain: a conserved protein-protein interaction motif. Genes Dev 8: 1664–1677.
3. Stead MA, Trinh CH, Garnett JA, Carr SB, Baron AJ, et al. (2007) A beta-sheet interaction interface directs the tetramerisation of the Miz-1 POZ domain. J Mol Biol 373: 820–826. doi:10.1016/j.jmb.2007.08.026.
4. Stogios PJ, Downs GS, Jauhal JJS, Nandra SK, Privé GG (2005) Sequence and structural analysis of BTB domain proteins. Genome Biol 6: R82. doi:10.1186/gb-2005-6-10-r82.
5. Möröy T, Saba I, Kosan C (2011) The role of the transcription factor Miz-1 in lymphocyte development and lymphomagenesis-Binding Myc makes the difference. Semin Immunol 23: 379–387. doi:10.1016/j.smim.2011.09.001.
6. Kosan C, Saba I, Godmann M, Herold S, Herkert B, et al. (2010) Transcription factor miz-1 is required to regulate interleukin-7 receptor signaling at early commitment stages of B cell differentiation. Immunity 33: 917–928. doi:10.1016/j.immuni.2010.11.028.
7. Seoane J, Pouponnot C, Staller P, Schader M, Eilers M, et al. (2001) TGFbeta influences Myc, Miz-1 and Smad to control the CDK inhibitor p15INK4b. Nat Cell Biol 3: 400–408. doi:10.1038/35070086.
8. Staller P, Peukert K, Kiermaier A, Seoane J, Lukas J, et al. (2001) Repression of p15INK4b expression by Myc through association with Miz-1. Nat Cell Biol 3: 392–399. doi:10.1038/35070076.
9. Herold S, Wanzel M, Beuger V, Frohme C, Beul D, et al. (2002) Negative regulation of the mammalian UV response by Myc through association with Miz-1. Mol Cell 10: 509–521.
10. Kime L, Wright SC (2003) Mad4 is regulated by a transcriptional repressor complex that contains Miz-1 and c-Myc. Biochem J 370: 291–298. doi:10.1042/BJ20021679.
11. Patel JH, McMahon SB (2007) BCL2 is a downstream effector of MIZ-1 essential for blocking c-MYC-induced apoptosis. J Biol Chem 282: 5–13. doi:10.1074/jbc.M609138200.
12. Gebhardt A, Frye M, Herold S, Benitah SA, Braun K, et al. (2006) Myc regulates keratinocyte adhesion and differentiation via complex formation with Miz1. J Cell Biol 172: 139–149. doi:10.1083/jcb.200506057.
13. Phan RT, Saito M, Basso K, Niu H, Dalla-Favera R (2005) BCL6 interacts with the transcription factor Miz-1 to suppress the cyclin-dependent kinase inhibitor p21 and cell cycle arrest in germinal center B cells. Nat Immunol 6: 1054–1060. doi:10.1038/ni1245.
14. Wu S, Cetinkaya C, Munoz-Alonso MJ, von der Lehr N, Bahram F, et al. (2003) Myc represses differentiation-induced p21CIP1 expression via Miz-1-dependent interaction with the p21 core promoter. Oncogene 22: 351–360. doi:10.1038/sj.onc.1206145.
15. van de Wetering M, Sancho E, Verweij C, de Lau W, Oving I, et al. (2002) The beta-catenin/TCF-4 complex imposes a crypt progenitor phenotype on colorectal cancer cells. Cell 111: 241–250.

16. Basu S, Liu Q, Qiu Y, Dong F (2009) Gfi-1 represses CDKN2B encoding p15INK4B through interaction with Miz-1. Proc Natl Acad Sci USA 106: 1433–1438. doi:10.1073/pnas.0804863106.
17. Liu J, Zhao Y, Eilers M, Lin A (2009) Miz1 is a signal- and pathway-specific modulator or regulator (SMOR) that suppresses TNF-alpha-induced JNK1 activation. Proc Natl Acad Sci USA 106: 18279–18284. doi:10.1073/pnas.0906328106.
18. Adhikary S, Peukert K, Karsunky H, Beuger V, Lutz W, et al. (2003) Miz1 is required for early embryonic development during gastrulation. Mol Cell Biol 23: 7648–7657.
19. Huelsken J, Vogel R, Erdmann B, Cotsarelis G, Birchmeier W (2001) beta-Catenin controls hair follicle morphogenesis and stem cell differentiation in the skin. Cell 105: 533–545.
20. Gebhardt A, Kosan C, Herkert B, Möröy T, Lutz W, et al. (2007) Miz1 is required for hair follicle structure and hair morphogenesis. J Cell Sci 120: 2586–2593. doi:10.1242/jcs.007104.
21. Möröy T, Saba I, Kosan C (2011) The role of the transcription factor Miz-1 in lymphocyte development and lymphomagenesis-Binding Myc makes the difference. Semin Immunol. Available:http://www.ncbi.nlm.nih.gov/pubmed/22000024. Accessed 3 November 2011.
22. Oskarsson T, Essers MAG, Dubois N, Offner S, Dubey C, et al. (2006) Skin epidermis lacking the c-Myc gene is resistant to Ras-driven tumorigenesis but can reacquire sensitivity upon additional loss of the p21Cip1 gene. Genes Dev 20: 2024–2029. doi:10.1101/gad.381206.
23. Bickenbach JR (1981) Identification and behavior of label-retaining cells in oral mucosa and skin. J Dent Res 60 Spec No C: 1611–1620.
24. Yuspa SH, Hennings H, Lichti U (1981) Initiator and promoter induced specific changes in epidermal function and biological potential. J Supramol Struct Cell Biochem 17: 245–257. doi:10.1002/jsscb.380170306.
25. Blanpain C, Lowry WE, Geoghegan A, Polak L, Fuchs E (2004) Self-renewal, multipotency, and the existence of two cell populations within an epithelial stem cell niche. Cell 118: 635–648. doi:10.1016/j.cell.2004.08.012.
26. Morris RJ, Liu Y, Marles L, Yang Z, Trempus C, et al. (2004) Capturing and profiling adult hair follicle stem cells. Nat Biotechnol 22: 411–417. doi:10.1038/nbt950.
27. Yuspa SH, Hawley-Nelson P, Koehler B, Stanley JR (1980) A Survey of Transformation Markers in Differentiating Epidermal Cell Lines in Culture. Cancer Research 40: 4694–4703.
28. Ridd K, Dhir S, Smith AG, Gant TW (2010) Defective TPA signalling compromises HaCat cells as a human in vitro skin carcinogenesis model. Toxicol In Vitro 24: 910–915. doi:10.1016/j.tiv.2009.11.017.
29. Kemp CJ (2005) Multistep skin cancer in mice as a model to study the evolution of cancer cells. Semin Cancer Biol 15: 460–473. doi:10.1016/j.semcancer.2005.06.003.
30. Nagase H, Mao J-H, Balmain A (2003) Allele-specific Hras mutations and genetic alterations at tumor susceptibility loci in skin carcinomas from interspecific hybrid mice. Cancer Res 63: 4849–4853.
31. Topley GI, Okuyama R, Gonzales JG, Conti C, Dotto GP (1999) p21(WAF1/Cip1) functions as a suppressor of malignant skin tumor formation and a determinant of keratinocyte stem-cell potential. Proc Natl Acad Sci USA 96: 9089–9094.
32. Weinberg WC, Denning MF (2002) p21WAF1 Control of Epithelial Cell Cycle and Cell Fate. Critical Reviews in Oral Biology & Medicine 13: 453–464. doi:10.1177/154411130201300603.
33. Wanzel M, Herold S, Eilers M (2003) Transcriptional repression by Myc. Trends Cell Biol 13: 146–150.
34. Wanzel M, Russ AC, Kleine-Kohlbrecher D, Colombo E, Pelicci P-G, et al. (2008) A ribosomal protein L23-nucleophosmin circuit coordinates Mizl function with cell growth. Nat Cell Biol 10: 1051–1061.
35. Herkert B, Dwertmann A, Herold S, Abed M, Naud J-F, et al. (2010) The Arf tumor suppressor protein inhibits Miz1 to suppress cell adhesion and induce apoptosis. J Cell Biol 188: 905–918. doi:10.1083/jcb.200908103.
36. Miao L, Song Z, Jin L, Zhu YM, Wen LP, et al. (2010) ARF antagonizes the ability of Miz-1 to inhibit p53-mediated transactivation. Oncogene 29: 711–722. doi:10.1038/onc.2009.372.
37. Zanet J, Pibre S, Jacquet C, Ramirez A, de Alborán IM, et al. (2005) Endogenous Myc controls mammalian epidermal cell size, hyperproliferation, endoreplication and stem cell amplification. J Cell Sci 118: 1693–1704. doi:10.1242/jcs.02298.
38. van Riggelen J, Müller J, Otto T, Beuger V, Yetil A, et al. (2010) The interaction between Myc and Miz1 is required to antagonize TGFbeta-dependent autocrine signaling during lymphoma formation and maintenance. Genes Dev 24: 1281–1294. doi:10.1101/gad.585710.
39. Brown JP, Wei W, Sedivy JM (1997) Bypass of senescence after disruption of p21CIP1/WAF1 gene in normal diploid human fibroblasts. Science 277: 831–834.
40. Sayama K, Shirakata Y, Midorikawa K, Hanakawa Y, Hashimoto K (1999) Possible involvement of p21 but not of p16 or p53 in keratinocyte senescence. J Cell Physiol 179: 40–44. doi:10.1002/(SICI)1097-4652(199904)179:1<40::AID-JCP5>3.0.CO;2-Z.
41. de Keizer PLJ, Packer LM, Szypowska AA, Riedl-Polderman PE, van den Broek NJF, et al. (2010) Activation of Forkhead Box O Transcription Factors by Oncogenic BRAF Promotes p21cip1-Dependent Senescence. Cancer ResAvailable: http://www.ncbi.nlm.nih.gov/pubmed/20959475. Accessed 1 November 2010.
42. Borgdorff V, Lleonart ME, Bishop CL, Fessart D, Bergin AH, et al. (2010) Multiple microRNAs rescue from Ras-induced senescence by inhibiting p21Waf1/Cip1. Oncogene 29: 2262–2271.
43. Dimri GP, Lee X, Basile G, Acosta M, Scott G, et al. (1995) A biomarker that identifies senescent human cells in culture and in aging skin in vivo. Proc Natl Acad Sci U S A 92: 9363–9367.
44. Campisi J (2010) Cellular senescence: putting the paradoxes in perspective. Curr Opin Genet Dev. Available: http://www.ncbi.nlm.nih.gov/pubmed/21093253. Accessed 5 January 2011.
45. Collado M, Serrano M (2010) Senescence in tumours: evidence from mice and humans. Nat Rev Cancer 10: 51–57. doi:10.1038/nrc2772.
46. Krimpenfort P, Ijpenberg A, Song J-Y, van der Valk M, Nawijn M, et al. (2007) p15Ink4b is a critical tumour suppressor in the absence of p16Ink4a. Nature 448: 943–946. doi:10.1038/nature06084.
47. Brugarolas J, Chandrasekaran C, Gordon JI, Beach D, Jacks T, et al. (1995) Radiation-induced cell cycle arrest compromised by p21 deficiency. Nature 377: 552–557. doi:10.1038/377552a0.
48. Atanasoski S, Boller D, De Ventura L, Koegel H, Boentert M, et al. (2006) Cell cycle inhibitors p21 and p16 are required for the regulation of Schwann cell proliferation. Glia 53: 147–157. doi:10.1002/glia.20263.
49. Boyd KE, Wells J, Gutman J, Bartley SM, Farnham PJ (1998) c-Myc target gene specificity is determined by a post-DNAbinding mechanism. Proc Natl Acad Sci USA 95: 13887–13892.

Increased IKKα Expression in the Basal Layer of the Epidermis of Transgenic Mice Enhances the Malignant Potential of Skin Tumors

Josefa P. Alameda[1]¶, Rodolfo Moreno-Maldonado[1]¶, M. Jesús Fernández-Aceñero[2], Manuel Navarro[1], Angustias Page[1], José L. Jorcano[1], Ana Bravo[3], Ángel Ramírez[1], M. Llanos Casanova[1]*

1 Division of Epithelial Biomedicine, CIEMAT, Madrid, Spain, **2** Department of Pathology, Fundación Jiménez Díaz, Madrid, Spain, **3** Department of Veterinary Clinical Sciences, Veterinary Faculty, University of Santiago de Compostela, Lugo, Spain

Abstract

Non-melanoma skin cancer is the most frequent type of cancer in humans. In this study we demonstrate that elevated IKKα expression in murine epidermis increases the malignancy potential of skin tumors. We describe the generation of transgenic mice overexpressing IKKα in the basal, proliferative layer of the epidermis and in the outer root sheath of hair follicles. The epidermis of K5-IKKα transgenic animals shows several alterations such as hyperproliferation, mislocalized expression of integrin-α6 and downregulation of the tumor suppressor maspin. Treatment of the back skin of mice with the mitogenic agent 12-*O*-tetradecanoylphorbol-13-acetate causes in transgenic mice the appearance of different preneoplastic changes such as epidermal atypia with loss of cell polarity and altered epidermal tissue architecture, while in wild type littermates this treatment only leads to the development of benign epidermal hyperplasia. Moreover, in skin carcinogenesis assays, transgenic mice carrying active Ha-*ras* (K5-IKKα-Tg.AC mice) develop invasive tumors, instead of the benign papillomas arising in wild type-Tg-AC mice also bearing an active Ha-*ras*. Therefore we provide evidence for a tumor promoter role of IKKα in skin cancer, similarly to what occurs in other neoplasias, including hepatocarcinomas and breast, prostate and colorectal cancer. The altered expression of cyclin D1, maspin and integrin-α6 in skin of transgenic mice provides, at least in part, the molecular bases for the increased malignant potential found in the K5-IKKα skin tumors.

Editor: Christophe Egles, Université de Technologie de Compiègne, France

Funding: This work was funded by grants from the Ministerio de Ciencia e Innovación (PI10/01480, SAF2010-22156) to MLC and AR respectively. The funders had no roles in study design, data collection and analysis, decision to publish, or preparation of the manuscript.

Competing Interests: The authors have declared that no competing interests exist.

* E-mail: llanos.casanova@ciemat.es

¶ These authors contributed equally to this work.

Introduction

Keratinocytes of the basal layer of the epidermis are mitotic, providing new cells to replace those that are shed. After moving to the suprabasal layers, the cells gradually differentiate and give rise to the cornified layer at the surface of the skin that protects the internal organs. Therefore, a balance between keratinocyte proliferation and differentiation is required to maintain epidermal homeostasis. IKKα (IκB kinase α) is a fundamental component of the IKK complex that regulates the NF-κB signalling pathway [1–3]. IKKα has a fundamental role in regulating keratinocyte proliferation and differentiation [4–8]. The epidermis of IKKα−/− newborn mice lacks a terminally differentiated cornified layer and exhibits marked thickening [6–8]. Reintroduction of IKKα or a kinase-inactive mutant IKKα induces terminal differentiation of keratinocyte and represses hyperproliferation [9,10]. This demonstrates that IKKα is necessary for epidermal differentiation independently of its kinase activity [9]. We have described that IKKα increases the differentiation of human keratinocytes by a mechanism dependent on E-cadherin [5]. Other adhesion molecules such as claudin-23, occludin and desmoglein 3 have also been found to be regulated by IKKα and to play a role in epidermal terminal differentiation and skin barrier function [11].

Non melanoma skin cancer (NMSC) is the most common malignancy in humans: BCCs (basal cell carcinomas) and SCCs (squamous cell carcinomas) represent the vast majority of the tumors diagnosed. The incidence of both benign and malignant NMSC has been rising at an alarming rate for the past several years. The role of IKKα in cancer development remains controversial: while it has been suggested that it functions as a tumor suppressor in skin cancer [4,12,13], there are also evidences that support a role of IKKα as promoter of cancer progression and metastasis in different types of neoplasias such as breast cancer [14], hepatocarcinomas [15], prostate cancer [16,17] and colorectal cancer [18,19]. Indeed, we have found, in xenograft assays, an increase in malignancy of skin tumors over-expressing IKKα [5].

In the last years it has been found that IKKα regulates the expression of molecules implicated in cancer development such as the tumor suppressor maspin (mammary serine protease inhibitor), twist, and adhesion proteins. It inhibits cellular motility, invasiveness and angiogenesis, and provides sensitivity to apoptosis in tumor cells [20,21]. Maspin expression predicts a better prognosis in different types of cancers: breast [22,23], prostate [24,25], colon [26], oral squamous cell carcinoma [27], lung [28], larynx [29], malignant melanoma [30] and ovarian cancer [31], although recently it has been reported that it might act as tumor promoter in colorectal or pancreatic cancers [32,33]. Maspin also acts as a suppressor of metastasis in different types of cancer such as prostate, liver and breast [17,34]. Interestingly, IKKα inhibits maspin expression and promotes cell metastasis in prostate cancer and hepatocarcinomas [15,17,35]. Twist is a basic-helix-loop-helix (bHLH) protein known to be essential during the embryogenesis which also plays an important role as mediator of EMT (epidermal mesenchymal transition) during tumor progression [36]. Twist is overexpressed in a large set of human and murine tumors including sarcomas, melanomas, gliomas and neuroblastomas [37,38] being the reactivation of Twist indicative of poor prognosis. Interestingly, it has been reported that IKKα null embryos express reduced levels of Twist [7] which suggest a positive regulation of Twist expression by IKKα. The altered expression of adhesion molecules has been related to tumor development, included skin cancer, i.e., overexpression of the adhesion protein integrin-α6 in the basal layer of epidermis and hair follicles has been reported to cause malignization of skin tumors in transgenic mice [39]. Moreover, α6β4 integrin expression in suprabasal strata serves as an early predictive marker to identify benign squamous tumors at high risk of malignant progression [40].

In this work we have analyzed the effect of increased levels of IKKα expression in the basal layer of the epidermis of transgenic (Tg) mice (K5-IKKα mice), and its repercussion in *in vivo* skin carcinogenesis. We have found that K5-IKKα mice exhibit in epidermis several alterations, such as increased proliferation, suprabasal integrin-α6 expression and downregulation of the tumor suppressor maspin. In line with these alterations, the application of a mitogenic agent, i.e. TPA in the back skin of mice leads in transgenic K5-IKKα mice to the appearance of preneoplastic features such as epidermal atypia with loss of cell polarity and altered epidermal tissue architecture, while in wild type (WT) littermates this treatment only leads to the development of benign epidermal hyperplasia. Moreover, in carcinogenesis experiments, tumors developed in transgenic mice carrying active Ha-*ras* (Tg.AC mice) are invasive tumors, in sharp contrast with the benign tumors originated in WT animals (also bearing an active Ha-*ras*). In addition to integrin-α6 suprabasal overexpression, tumors developed in the K5-IKKα mice show reactivation of the expression of Twist.

Materials and Methods

Ethics Statement

All experimental procedures were performed according to European and Spanish laws and regulations (European Convention ETS 123 on the use and protection of vertebrate mammals used in experimentation and other scientific purposes; Spanish R.D 1201/2005 of the Ministry of Agricultural, Food and Fisheries on the protection and use of animals in scientific research) and approved by the our institution's ethics committee. Approval ID: BME 3/06; BME 1/09 and BME 2–10 by the CIEMAT Institution's ethics commitee.

Generation of Tg mice

HA-tagged murine IKKα [5] was placed under the control of a 5.2 kb 5′-upstream fragment of bovine K5 promoter and a rabbit β-globin intron (Figure 1A). Tg mice were generated by microinjection of this construct into B6D2F2 embryos using standard techniques and Tg lines were maintained by crossing with B6D2F1 mice. Mice were genotyped by PCR analysis of tail genomic DNA using primers specific for the rabbit β-globin intron. Wild type non-transgenic littermates were used as control animals.

Western Blotting

Total or nuclear and cytoplasmic protein extracts (40 μg) were subjected to SDS/PAGE. The separated proteins were transferred to nitrocellulose membranes (Amersham, Arlington Heights, IL) and probed with antibodies against IKKα, IKKβ, IKKγ (IMGENEX, San Diego, CA, USA); HA epitope (Covance, California, USA); IκBα, p105/p50, p65, maspin, actin, fibrillarin, EGFR (Santa Cruz Biotechnology, Inc. Europe); p100/p52 (Abcam, Cambridge, UK); P-p65, P-IκBα (Cell Signaling Technology, Danvers, MA, USA); Cyclin D1 (NeoMarkers, Fremont, CA, USA); P-tyrosine (4G10; Upstate, NY, USA), and tubulin (Sigma, Saint-Louis, Missouri, USA). In all cases samples were subjected to luminography with the Supersignal West Pico Chemiluminescent Substrate (Pierce Biotechnology, Inc., Illinois, USA). Densitometric analysis of the blots was performed using the Molecular Analyst software package (Bio-Rad Laboratories Inc., Hercules, California, USA).

Histology and Immunohistochemistry

Skin and tumors were fixed in 10% buffered formalin or in 70% ethanol and embedded in paraffin. Sections were stained with H&E for histopathological evaluation or used for immunostaining using primary antibodies raised against IKKα (sc-7182, Santa Cruz Biotechnology, Inc. Europe; IMG-90454, IMGENEX), keratin K1, K5, K10, involucrin, loricrin, filaggrin (Covance); keratin K13, Twist (Abcam); integrin-α6 (CD49f; BD Pharmingen), BrdU (Roche, Mannheim, Germany) and Cleaved Caspase-3 (Cell Signaling Technology, Danvers, MA, USA). Sections were incubated with a biotinylated anti-mouse, anti-rat or anti-rabbit antibody, and then with streptavidin conjugated to horseradish peroxidase (DAKO A/S, Glostrp, Denmark). Antibody localization was determined using 3,3-diaminobenzidine (DAB) in PBS (Vector Laboratories; Burlingame, CA, USA).

BrdU treatment

Mice received an intraperitoneal injection of BrdU 120 mg/kg body weight 1 h before sample harvesting.

TNF-α *in vivo* treatment

3 days-old mice were subcutaneously injected with 20 μg/Kg of human TNF-α (Sigma) or with PBS (control). After the indicated times mice were sacrificed, skin samples removed and proteins extracted.

NF-κB activity assay

NF-κB DNA binding assays was determined by the NF-κB p50/p65 EZ-TFA Transcription Factor Assay (Millipore, Massachusetts, USA) following manufacturer's instructions [41]. Briefly, protein extracts from WT and Tg skins (12.5 μg) were mixed with a double stranded biotinylated oligonucleotide containing the consensus sequence for NF-κB binding. In this way, activated NF-κB (active p65) contained in the extracts binds to its consensus sequence. This mixture is transferred to a streptavidin coated plate and the bound NF-κB subunit, p65, is detected with a specific primary antibody. An HRP-conjugated secondary antibody is then used for detection and provides sensitive colorimetric detection that can be read in a spectrophotometric plate reader (Genios Pro, TECAN, Madrid, Spain; XFluor4Version V4.50).

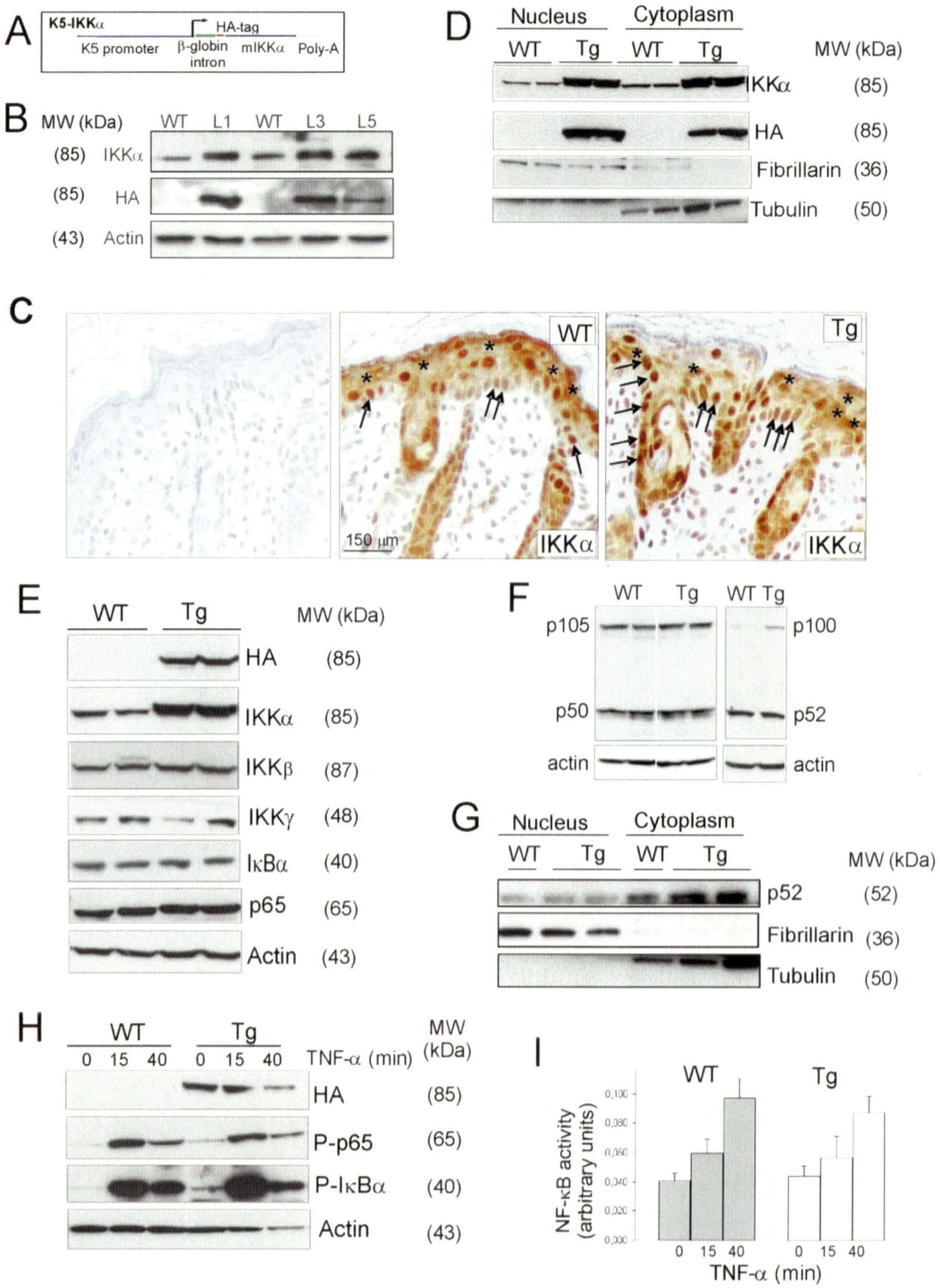

Figure 1. Characterization of K5-IKKα transgenic mice. (**A**) Recombinant DNA construct employed to generate transgenic mice. (**B**) Western blots showing IKKα and HA expression in WT and 3 different transgenic lines (L1, L3 and L5). Actin was used as a loading control. (**C**) Expression of the IKKα protein in back skin of 3-day-old mice. Immunostaining with the Sc-7182 antibody is showed (middle and right panels); similar results where obtained with the IMG-90454 anti IKKα antibody (not shown). Control without primary antibody (only with secondary biotinylated anti-rabbit antibody) is shown as control of specificity of the immunostaining against IKKα (left panel). Arrows show the expression of IKKα in basal epidermal keratinocytes and hair follicles. Asterisks indicate cytoplasmic expression of IKKα. (**D**) IKKα and HA detection in nuclear and cytoplasmic protein extracts from 5 day-old WT and Tg mice. Samples from two different mice of the line L1 and two different control littermates were loaded. Fibrillarin and tubulin show loading control and purity of the extracts. (**E**) Western blots analysis of the expression of different members of the NF-κB pathway in skin of WT and K5-IKKα transgenic mice. Total proteins from backskin of two different mice of the line L1 and two different control littermates were loaded. No differences were found between mice of both genotypes. (**F**) Western blot showing p100 and p105 processing in skin of WT and Tg mice. No differences were found. (**G**) Western blot showing the nuclear localization of p52 in skin of WT and Tg mice. No differences were found. (**H**) p65 and IκBα phosphorylation kinetics; actin: loading control. Newborn WT and Tg mice were injected with TNF-α and analyzed at the indicated times. (**I**) NF-κB activity in skin of non-stimulated and TNF-α injected mice for the indicated times. Experiments were repeated 3 times with similar results.

TPA treatment

To induce epidermal hyperplasia, six K5-IKKα 8-week-old mice and six WT mice of the same age (8 weeks) were used. Shaved dorsal skins were treated twice a week with 5 μg of 12-*O*-tetradecanoylphorbol-13-acetate (TPA; Sigma) for 3 weeks. Mice were sacrificed 24 hours after the last application.

Carcinogenesis assays

In the DMBA/TPA protocol, both, K5-IKKα and WT 9-week-old mice (9 animals respectively) were initiated with a single dose of 200 nmol of 7,12-dimethyl-benz[a]anthracene (DMBA) (Sigma) on shaved dorsal skin. Two weeks later, tumor growth was promoted by treating with 5 μg of TPA twice a week per 20 weeks. In the carcinogenesis experiments in Tg.AC background, female homozygous v-Ha-*ras* transgenic Tg.AC mice [42] were mated with K5-IKKα males. Double transgenic K5-IKKα-TgAC and WT-TgAC 9-week-old mice (11 animals respectively) were treated twice weekly with topical applications of 5 μg of TPA in 200 μl acetone for 7 weeks according to standard protocols. Experimental procedures were performed according to European and Spanish laws on experimental animal protection.

Statistics

Statistical significance of data was assessed using the t-test and the Mann-Whitney (Wilcoxon) W test.

Results

Increased expression of IKKα in basal keratinocytes of K5-IKKα transgenic mice

We generated the K5-IKKα transgenic mice overexpressing a mouse IKKα cDNA tagged with an epitope from hemagglutinin A (HA) (Figure 1A). The keratin 5 (K5)-derived sequences included in this construct drive transgene expression to the basal cells of the epidermis and outer root sheath (ORS) of hair follicles, as well as to internal stratified epithelia [43,44]. K5-IKKα transgenic mice developed normally and showed no obvious alterations. Immunoblotting analysis using specific antibodies against IKKα revealed increased expression of IKKα in the skin of different K5-IKKα Tg lines (Figure 1B). HA epitope was detected in skin of K5-IKKα-Tg mice but not in skin of WT mice (Figure 1B). L1 and L3 were the highest IKKα expressing lines and similar results were obtained in the analysis of both of them, therefore we performed most of the following experiments in line L1. The immunohistochemical staining of IKKα in back skin of WT and Tg mice showed higher IKKα staining in the basal layer of the epidermis and the ORS of hair follicles of K5-IKKα-Tg mice than in WT littermates (Figure 1C). IKKα immunostaining was performed with two different antibodies (see Mat and Met section) and repetitively IKKα expression was detected both in the cytoplasm and in the nucleus of suprabasal and basal keratinocytes in WT and Tg animals (Figure 1C). WB analysis confirmed this nuclear and cytoplasmic localization of IKKα and also its overexpression in K5-IKKα-Tg skin (Figure 1D). HA immunostaining gave similar results (data not shown).

Classical and non-canonical NF-κB activation pathways are not affected in the K5-IKKα-Tg mice

The state of the NF-κB pathway in WT and K5-IKKα mice was analyzed. In agreement with other studies [8], we found that changes in IKKα expression do not alter the expression of other members of the NF-κB pathway such as IKKβ, IKKγ, IκBα and p65 (Figure 1E). In addition no differences were found in p100 or p105 processing, nor in nuclear p52 localization in WT and Tg mice skin (Figure 1F, G), indicating that the non-canonical pathway of NF-κB does not seem altered by IKKα overexpression. Treatment of newborn mice with tumor necrosis factor α (TNF-α) led to similar kinetics and extension of p65 and IκBα phosphorylation in WT and Tg mice (Figure 1H). In addition, we analyzed the NF-κB pathway by measuring NF-κB binding activity in protein extracts from skins of mice of each genotype and found no differences in non-stimulated skin as well as after TNF-α subcutaneous injection of WT and K5-IKKα mice (Figure 1I). Together, these results indicate that the classical IKK/NF-κB pathway is not modified in K5-IKKα Tg mice, and are in accordance with our previous data in human HaCaT keratinocytes [5] where the overexpression of IKKα did not alter this signalling pathway.

Delocalized integrin-α6 suprabasal expression, increased proliferation and maspin inhibition in epidermis of K5-IKKα-Tg mice

As IKKα has an essential role in epidermal morphogenesis and differentiation, we analyzed early and late differentiation markers of the epidermis such as K1, involucrin, loricrin, and filaggrin (Figure 2A). No appreciable differences were found between WT and K5-IKKα-Tg mice, suggesting that no alterations of the normal epidermal differentiation program occur in these animals. The expression of K5 and K6 also was unaltered (data not shown). We also analyzed the proliferative capability of WT and K5-IKKα-Tg mice skin by measuring BrdU incorporation. We observed increased BrdU-positive cells in the basal layer of the epidermis of K5-IKKα mice (11.4±2.7% in Tg mice *versus* 7.6±1.7% in WT mice; $n=6$; $P<0.05$) (Figure 2B). Cyclin D1, another marker of proliferation was also increased in the skin of Tg mice (Figure 2C). In an attempt to discover a possible cause for the increased proliferation observed in skin of transgenic mice, we measured EGFR expression, as this is an important factor for keratinocyte proliferation [45]; however, we found no differences in EGFR levels nor in EGFR phosphorylation in skin of WT and K5-IKKα Tg mice (Figure 2D). Another reason for the increase in the number of proliferating cells in the skin of Tg mice could be the altered expression of adhesion molecules; in particular, the suprabasal expression of integrin-α6 has been found to be associated with hyperproliferative conditions in dermal equivalent cultures of keratinocytes [46]. We therefore analyzed the expression of integrin-α6 in the back skin of WT and Tg newborn mice and found that while WT mice skin exhibit integrin-α6 expression restricted to the basal layer of the epidermis, K5-IKKα-Tg mice showed increased and delocalized integrin-α6 expression in basal as well as suprabasal keratinocytes (Figure 2B). As these parameters (i.e. increased proliferation and altered expression of integrin-α6 in epidermis) are signals that may precede a malignization process [39], we checked the expression of maspin, a tumor suppressor known to be negatively regulated by IKKα. We found by Western blotting of total skin extracts that maspin was downregulated in the skin of K5-IKKα-Tg mice (Figure 2C), in agreement with other studies where IKKα overexpression leads to the inhibition of maspin expression [15,17].

Epidermal atypia of the epidermis in K5-IKKα transgenic mice treated with TPA

To analyze whether the alterations found in the skin of transgenic K5-IKKα mice could predispose these mice to the development of more severe lesions when subjected to skin insult, we applied multiple doses of the mitogenic agent, TPA, to the back

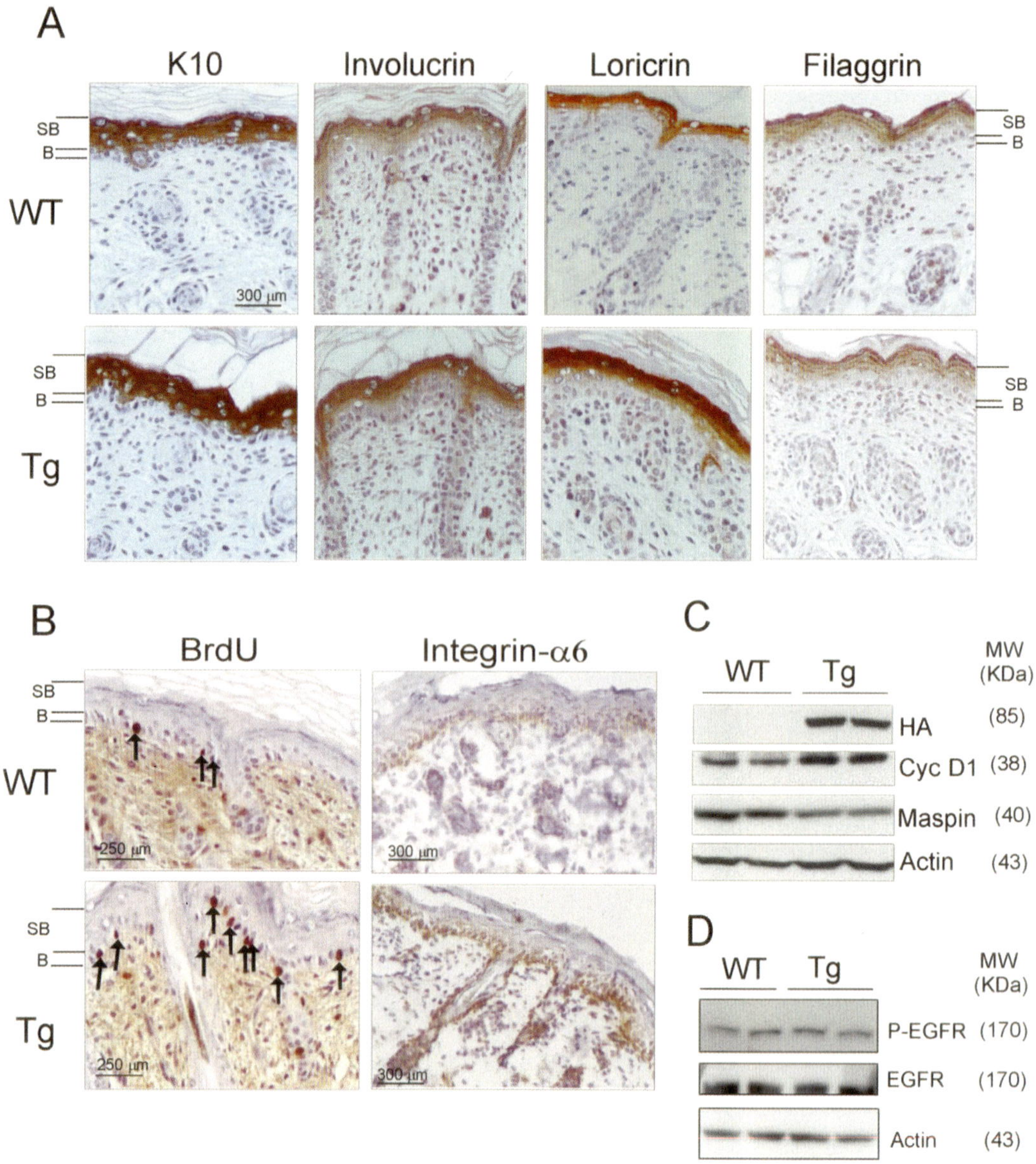

Figure 2. Alterations found in back skin of K5-IKKα-Tg mice. (**A**) Immunohistochemical analysis of epidermal differentiation markers in back skin of 3-day-old WT and K5-IKKα mice. No differences were found between mice of both genotypes. B, SB, basal and suprabasal keratinocyte layers respectively. (**B**) Images show the increased number of basal keratinocytes that incorporate BrdU in epidermis of Tg mice. Integrin α6 is expressed in basal as well as suprabasal keratinocytes in skin of Tg mice. (**C; D**) Analysis of cyclin D1 (Cyc D1), maspin and EGFR protein levels as well as EGFR phosphorylation (P-EGFR) in total protein extracts of skin of WT and K5-IKKα-Tg mice. Total proteins from backskin of two different mice of the line L1 and two different control littermates were loaded.

skin of WT and Tg mice in the second telogen phase of the hair follicles. As expected, 3 weeks of treatment provoked in WT animals the entry of hair follicles into the anagen phase as well as the development of epidermal hyperplasia (7 to 10 layers of epidermal keratinocytes *versus* 2 to 4 layers observed in non-treated epidermis of adult mice; Figure 3 compare A and B). We observed that the hyperplasia was due to an increase both in the *stratum spinosum* and *granulosum* (see inset in B). This hyperplasia exhibit the typical increase in epidermal thickness, with keratinocytes of the *stratum basale* containing nuclei perpendicular to the basal membrane; keratinocytes of the *stratum spinosum* with round, central nuclei; and keratinocytes of the *stratum granulosum* showing progressive flattening of the cells, in parallel to the basal membrane, with smaller nucleus and scarce cytoplasm filled with keratohyaline granules. In Tg mice, TPA application also induces hair follicle anagen phase and epidermal hyperplasia (Figure 3 compare C and D). However, in these mice the hyperplasia was associated with epidermal atypia, characterized by a disorganized architecture of the different keratinocyte layers where cells lose their polarity and normal differentiation; it was not possible to distinguish the *stratum basale*, *spinosum* and *granulosum* because most keratinocytes appeared as round cells with central nucleus and there was no sign of terminal differentiation (i.e. lack of keratohyaline granules in the upper suprabasal layers) (see inset in Figure 3D and compare with inset in B). There was also a great heterogeneity in the nuclear staining of keratinocytes from Tg-TPA-treated mice showing many condensed, highly basophilic pyknotic nuclei. Elevated rates of keratinocyte proliferation (measured as BrdU incorporation) were observed in the epidermis of both WT and Tg mice treated with TPA (Figure 3 E, F), being significantly higher the number of proliferating cells in the K5-IKKα mice (Figure 3F) compared with WT siblings (Figure 3E) (labelling index, Tg = 29.1±3.7; WT = 18.8±4.0; n = 6; $P<0.05$). The treatment with TPA in addition to a mitogenic effect also provokes an inflammatory response. We have analyzed this effect in skin of WT and transgenic mice and have found a similar response in both cases i.e. a mild lichenoid inflammation with diffuse infiltrates of mononuclear cells in the superficial dermis (Figure 3B and D asterisks).

Enhanced malignant potential of tumors developed in K5-IKKα transgenic mice

We performed two different approaches to investigate the susceptibility of K5-IKKα mice to develop skin cancer. We initiated WT and K5-IKKα mice with a single dose of DMBA followed by TPA application in a conventional two-stage (DMBA/TPA) tumorigenesis protocol. DMBA activates Ha-*ras* to initiate skin tumors [47]. During the course of the experiment we did not observe significant differences in the number of tumors between WT and Tg mice (Figure S1A). Tumors were traced until week 27, when they were collected. The average tumor size was also similar in both groups (data not shown). In the other approach we performed TPA treatments in F1 crosses of K5-IKKα mice with the Tg.AC mice strain, carrying an activated Ha-*ras* transgene that triggers the classic initiation event [42,44,48]. Both groups of mice (WT-TgAC and K5-IKKα-TgAC) developed papillomas with a similar latency period (5–7 weeks, Figure S1B). The percentage of animals that developed tumors, as well as the tumor multiplicity, was similar in both genotypes. From week 17 on, the number of tumors in WT mice in both approaches was reduced, due probably to a higher regression rate (Figure S1A, B).

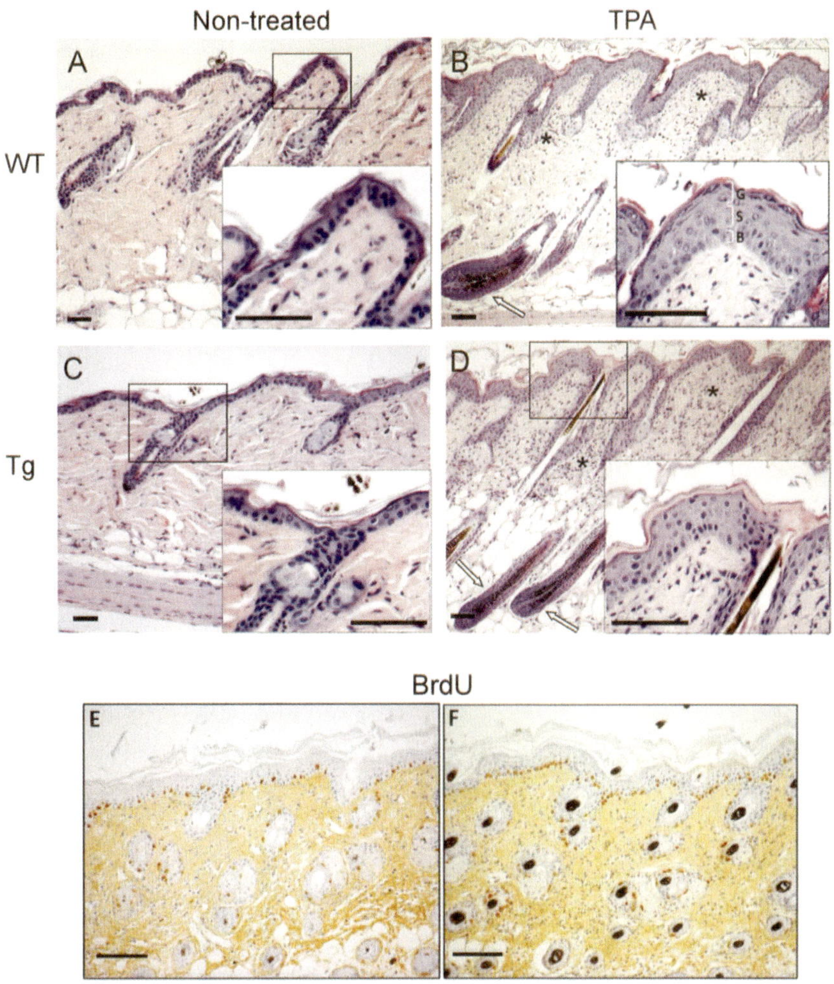

Figure 3. Atypical epidermal hyperplasia in skin of K5-IKKα-Tg mice subjected to TPA treatment. (**A–D**) Representative paraffin-sections of skin from WT (**A–B**) and K5-IKKα-Tg mice (**C–D**) were stained with hematoxilin/eosin. (**A, C**) Non-treated skins; (**B, D**) TPA treated skins. (**B**) Hyperplastic epidermis induced by topical application of TPA in WT mice. White arrow indicates a hair follicle in the anagen phase. (Inset in B) B: *stratum basale*, S: *stratum spinosum*, G: *stratum granulosum*. Conservation of squamous differentiation is clear in WT epidermis where marked hyperplasia of *stratum spinosum* (acantosis) and *stratum granulosum* (hipergranulosis) are observed as common facts of typical epidermal hyperplasia. (**D**) Hyperplasia and epidermal atypia with loss of cellular architecture in TPA-treated Tg skin. White arrows indicate hair follicles in the anagen phase. (Inset in D) Epidermal hyperplasia in K5-IKKα-Tg mice shows an atypical proliferating epithelium with all strata conformed by keratinocytes with round, central nuclei highly basophilic (pyknosis). The *stratum granulosum* of flattened cells with cytoplasm filled with keratohyaline granules were not formed. Asterisks in B, D points to regions of the lichenoid inflammation with diffuse infiltrates of mononuclear cells found in skin of both WT and Tg mice after TPA treatment. (**E, F**) BrdU incorporation in skins from WT (**E**) and Tg (**F**) mice treated with TPA. (**A–F**): scale bars = 50 μm.

We checked by Western blot analysis that the tumors developed in Tg mice in both carcinogenesis protocols express higher levels of IKKα than WT tumors and also express the HA-tag (Figure 4A, F). The histological study showed important differences between tumors developed in WT and K5-IKKα mice in the two approaches. Thus, while tumors arising in WT mice in the DMBA/TPA tumorigenesis were benign papillomas with a well conserved differentiation pattern of the epidermis (Figure 4B, C), those developed by K5-IKKα mice exhibited extended areas of epithelial atypia (Figure 4D, E), indicating a higher malignant potential. These lesions resemble those found in the epidermis of Tg mice treated with TPA (Figure 3D) although of higher aggressive potential. The tumorigenesis assays in Tg.AC mice showed that tumors from WT-TgAC animals were benign papillomas (Figure 4G, H), while tumors from K5-IKKα-TgAC mice showed areas of focal invasion, i.e., microinvasive infiltration, indicating a higher degree of malignant progression (Figure 4I, J). The immunohistochemical analysis of tumors developed in WT mice in both types of carcinogenesis protocols showed a diffuse expression of IKKα in the suprabasal cells (Figure 5A). By contrast, a higher staining for IKKα was detected in the K5-IKKα tumors obtained by both approaches (Figure 5A'), in accordance with the results of the Western blot analysis of IKKα in tumors (Figures 4A and F). IKKα was mainly located in the basal cells, where the K5 promoter directs the transgene expression although it was also detected in the suprabasal layers (Figure 5A' inset). Differentiation markers such as the keratins K1/K10 are expressed at higher levels in WT tumors than in Tg tumors in both protocols of skin carcinogenesis (Figure 5B, B' and data not shown). K13, a keratin characteristic of internal stratified squamous epithelia which is aberrantly expressed in skin tumors (Figure 5C), indicating malignancy [49], was rarely expressed in WT tumors while it was extensively expressed in the K5-IKKα tumors (Figure 5C'). Low expression of keratins K1/K10 and elevated expression of K13 indicate a worse prognosis of tumors that express elevated levels of IKKα. Maspin expression was analyzed and found that it was lower in the K5-IKKα tumors (Figure 5D, D'). Panels A–D' in Figure 5 show staining of DMBA/TPA tumors although similar results were found in the Tg.AC tumors staining (data not shown).

Induction of twist and delocalized integrin-α6 expression in tumors developed in K5-IKKα Tg mice. We analyzed other markers of tumor progression, such as the expression of integrin-α6. In benign tumors, integrin-α6 is expressed by basal keratinocytes; however in malignant tumors it is also expressed in suprabasal layers [40,48]. We found that tumors developed in WT mice in both carcinogenesis protocols have a basal staining of integrin-α6 (Figure 5E); by contrast, tumors from K5-IKKα mice exhibit basal as well as delocalized suprabasal expression of integrin-α6 (Figure 5E').

Another marker of tumor malignancy is Twist, which is expressed in embryonic development and silenced in the adulthood. However, it is induced in malignant tumors and is associated with metastasis [36]. We found that while WT tumors do not express Twist (Figure 5F), it is highly induced in K5-IKKα tumors obtained by both protocols of carcinogenesis (Figure 5F'). It is detected in the basal layer of the epidermis, where the K5 promoter directs the expression of the IKKα transgene (Figure 5F').

As increased integrin-α6 expression is usually accompanied by increased proliferation [46], we next analyzed tumor cell proliferation, measured as BrdU incorporation, and found higher number of proliferating cells in the K5-IKKα tumors (Figure 5G, G'). However, the size of IKKα and WT tumors showed no significant differences; therefore, we examined the apoptosis in both types of tumors and found that WT papillomas exhibited low number of apoptotic cells (measured by cleaved-Caspase 3 immunostaining; Figure 5H). By contrast, the number of apoptotic cells in IKKα tumors was markedly higher (Figure 5H'). Nevertheless, the rate of proliferation is greater than that of apoptosis in transgenic tumors and these differences alone would not fully explain the similar size reached by both types of tumors. Panels E–H' in Figure 5 show staining of DMBA/TPA tumors although similar results were found in the Tg.AC tumors staining (data not shown). Altogether these results suggest that skin tumors overexpressing IKKα in the basal layer of the epidermis have a malignant potential due at least in part to the induction of Twist expression and the suprabasal expression of integrin-α6.

Discussion

We have found that the overexpression of IKKα in the epidermis of K5-IKKα mice causes several molecular alterations, such as increased cyclin D1 expression, delocalized suprabasal integrin-α6 expression and downregulation of the tumor suppressor maspin. These proteins are important for cancer development and progression, suggesting that the skin of these Tg mice could develop more aggressive lesions when subjected to skin injuries than WT skin. We have proved that in fact, after applying proliferative stimuli (such as TPA) in back skin, K5-IKKα mice develop epidermal atypia with loss of tissue architecture, being these pathological changes considered as preneoplastic signals. TPA also induces inflammation; the inflammatory response found both in WT and Tg mice following TPA treatment was similar, indicating that the alterations found in skin of Tg mice after TPA application are unlikely due to the proinflammatory activity of this agent. We have also found that in carcinogenesis assays Tg mice develop invasive tumors with higher malignant potential than the benign tumors developed in WT mice.

The first anomaly detected in the epidermis of the Tg K5-IKKα mice was an enhanced proliferation of basal keratinocytes that seems to be the consequence of both enhanced cyclin D1 expression and increased (and delocalized) integrin-α6 expression. Epidermal suprabasal integrin-α6 expression has been correlated with high proliferative activity in the basal layer of the epidermis, without occurrence of abnormal terminal differentiation or inflammation [46]. Our results are in line with these observations, since we find in K5-IKKα Tg mice increased proliferation of keratinocytes without inflammation or appreciable alterations in early or terminal differentiation. While our data are the first description of regulation of integrin-α6 by IKKα, the regulation of the expression of other adhesion proteins by IKKα has been previously reported: Changes in E-cadherin, desmoglein 3, claudin and occludin expression levels as a consequence of changes in IKKα expression have been described [5,11,50]. The induction of cyclin D1 expression by IKKα has also been previously reported [51]; in addition, we have also found increased cyclin D1 expression in human keratinocytes overexpressing IKKα (Alameda et al, unpublished data).

The suprabasal integrin-α6 expression found both in epidermis and skin tumors of Tg mice could also cause the increased skin malignancy of K5-IKKα tumors, as inappropriate suprabasal integrin-α6β4 expression in epidermis correlates with high risk of cancer progression [39]. In this regard, it is interesting to note that the delocalized integrin-α6 expression in papillomas is an early predictive marker for the identification of benign squamous tumors at high risk of malignant progression [40].

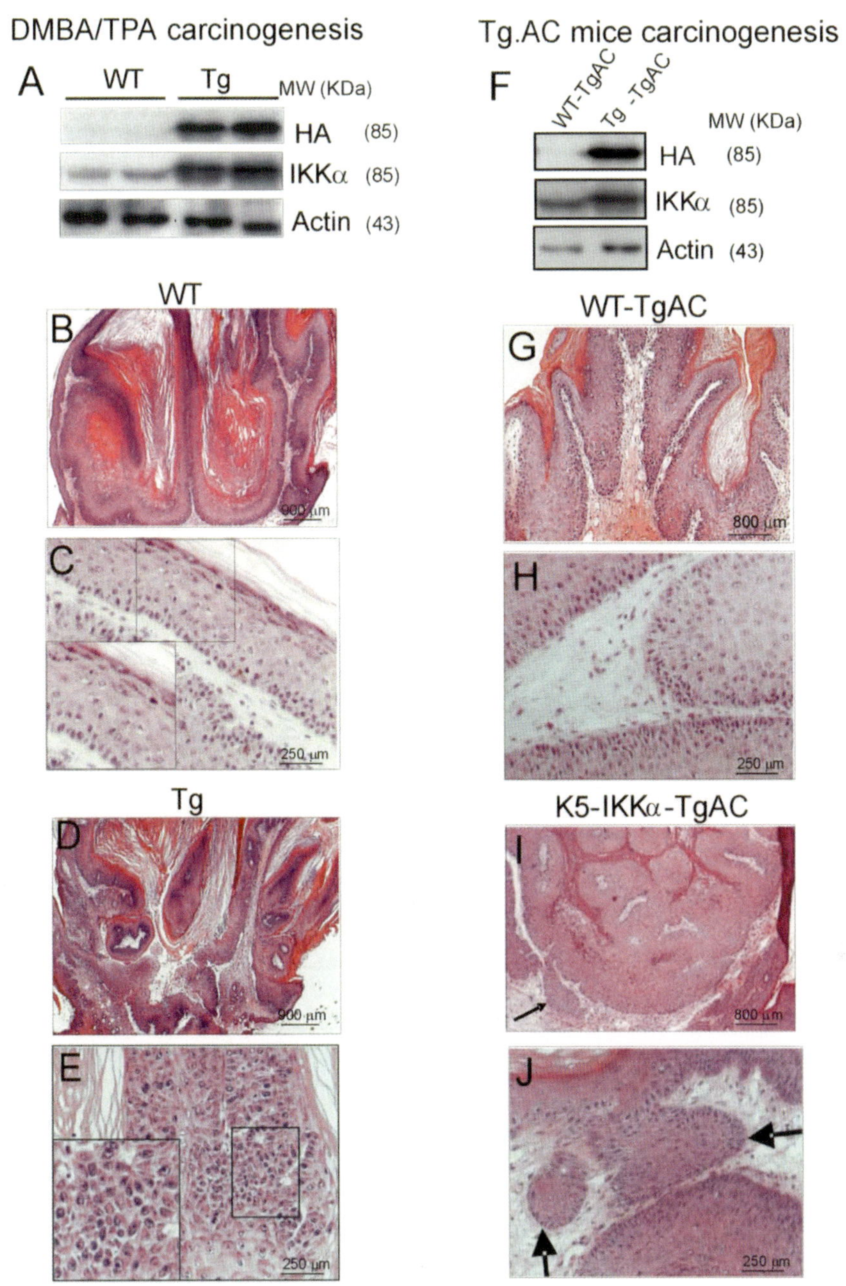

Figure 4. Tumors from K5-IKKα transgenic mice show increased malignancy. (**A, E**) Tumors developed in WT and Tg mice in the DMBA/TPA skin carcinogenesis assays. (**A**) Western blot showing the expression of the transgene in the tumors. Total protein extratcs from two different tumors developed in transgenic mice of the line L1 and proteins from two different control mice were loaded. (**B–E**) Histology of tumors arising in mice subjected to the DMBA/TPA approach. Note the epithelial atypia areas in Tg tumors (inbox in **E**) versus the well conserved tissue architecture in WT tumors (**C**). (**F–J**) Tumorigenesis in Tg.AC mice. (F) Western blot showing the expression of the transgene in the tumors. Total protein extratcs were loaded. (**G, H**) Development of benign tumors in WT-TgAC mice versus invasive tumors K5-IKKα-TgAC mice (**I, J**). (**J**) High magnification showing the rupture of the basement membrane and invasion of tumor epidermal cells into the stroma of transgenic tumors. Arrows in (**I, J**): focal invasion areas.

An interesting finding of this study has been the discovery of IKKα as negative regulator of the tumor suppressor maspin in the skin, since downregulation of this protein has been related to tumor progression and metastasis [17,20,21]. The downregulation of maspin by IKKα in epidermis has not been described before and we have confirmed this result in other different transgenic mice expressing distinct IKKα constructs (Alameda et al, unpublished results). Additionally, we have found that Twist expression which is silenced in adult tissues is induced in K5-IKKα tumors. In our experience searching in mouse skin cancer we have analyzed by immunohistochemistry more than 80 skin tumors obtained by both protocols of chemical carcinogenesis, and wee have never found before the induction of Twist expression in keratinocytes. Twist induction could be another plausible reason for the increased aggressiveness of the K5-IKKα tumors (developed in Tg.AC and DMBA-treated mice, carrying an activated Ha-*ras*), since recent findings show that in the presence of aberrant mitogenic signalling, such as Ha-*ras* activation, reactiva-

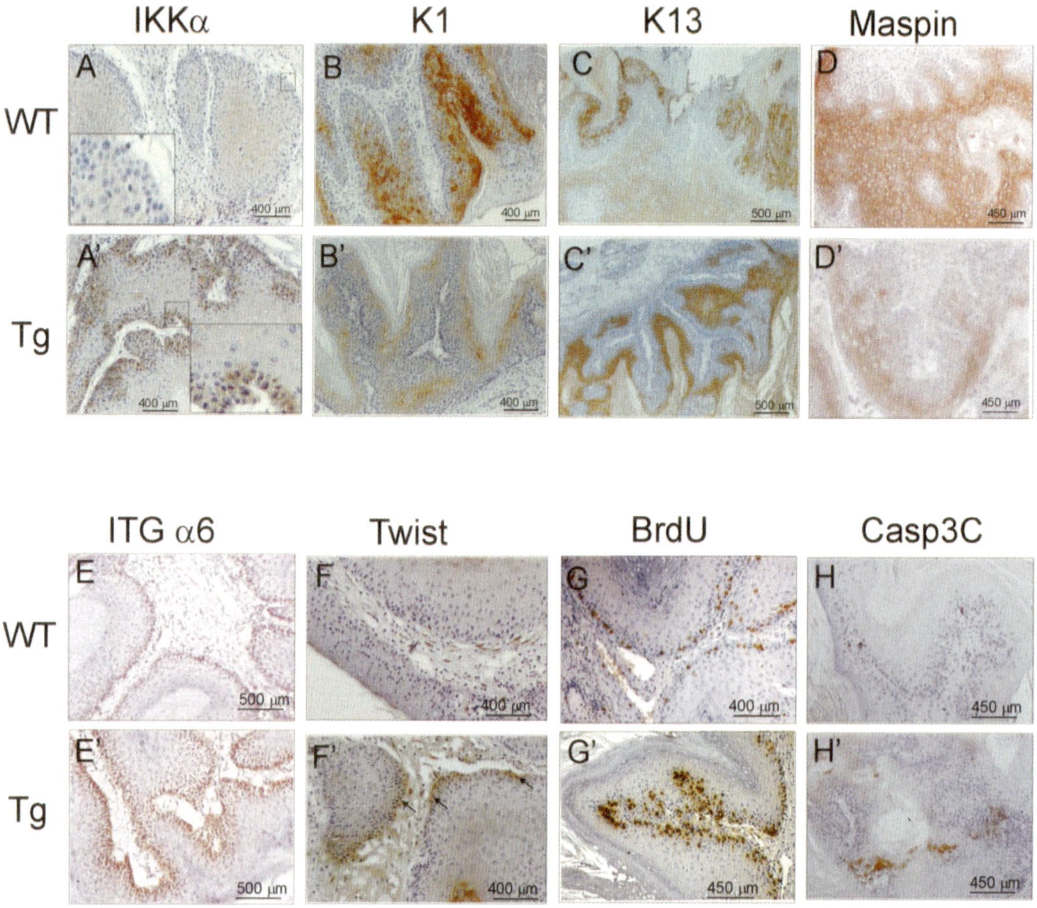

Figure 5. Immunohistochemical analysis of tumor markers in WT and K5-IKKα DMBA/TPA tumors. (**A, A'**) IKKα is scarcely and diffusely expressed in the suprabasal cells of WT tumors while it is strongly expressed in K5-IKKα tumors, mainly in the basal cells, although it is also detected in the suprabasal cells. (**B, B'**) Elevated expression of K1 is detected in WT tumors while Tg tumors exhibit scarce K1 staining. (**C, C'**) K13 immunostaining shows that it is weakly expressed in WT tumors versus the strong expression detected in Tg tumors. (**D, D'**) Lower staining of Maspin in K5-IKKα tumors. (**E, E'**) Strong and delocalized integrin α6 staining is detected in K5-IKKα tumors while WT tumors show integrin α6 basal expression. (**F, F'**) Twist is expressed in Tg tumors while it is not detected in WT tumors. (**G, G'**) Higher proliferation rate (measured as BrdU incorporation) is detected in Tg tumors (both in the basal and suprabasal layers) compared to the lower proliferating cells found in the basal layer of WT tumors. (**H, H'**) Increased Caspase 3 cleaved (Casp3C) staining in K5-IKKα tumors compared to that in WT tumors.

tion of Twist promotes the transition from a premalignant to a malignant stage by inactivation of innate failsafe programs [38]. It is well known that Twist is reactivated in different types of tumors and it is considered to play a key role in the development and progression of human cancer, being associated with advanced tumor stage and poor prognosis in rhabdomyosarcoma, gastric carcinoma, melanoma, glioma, liver carcinoma and breast, prostate, bladder and pancreatic cancer [37;52,53;36,54]. The regulation of Twist expression by IKKα has been previously noted, in other context, by Takeda et al., who described the downregulation of *twist* in IKKα−/− embryos [7].

During the last years several evidences have been reported indicating that IKKα functions as an oncogenic molecule. For instance, IKKα phosphorylates important molecules of signalling cascades (β-catenin, estrogen receptor-α transcriptional factor) which through induction of cyclin D1 and/or c-Myc expression enhances tumor proliferation [51,55,56,57]. Recently, a nuclear function of IKKα has been implicated in tumor progression: [58,59,19,60]. In this regard and in agreement with the data obtained in this study, it is interesting to mention the role of nuclear IKKα in promoting cancer through inhibition of maspin expression in pancreatic cancer [17,35]. Other evidences of the implication of IKKα in tumor promotion are that IKKα is induced by different proangiogenic agents such as TPA, UV radiation and Ets1 and that IKKα itself promotes angiogenesis and stimulates tumoral growth [61]. In this context, it is worth to note that IKKα KO mice have impaired angiogenesis [8]. In agreement with all these data, there is an increasing number of studies reporting the relationship of IKKα signaling to the development of different types of neoplasias: breast cancer [14]; hepatocarcinomas [15]; prostate cancer [17], and colorectal cancer [18]. Our group has also found an increase in the malignancy of skin tumors arising after injection of tumor epidermal cells overexpressing IKKα into nude mice [5].

On the other hand, other studies indicate a role for IKKα as a tumor suppressor in skin cancer. Therefore, Loricrin-IKKα transgenic mice that overexpress IKKα in the suprabasal terminally differentiated cells, which are mitotically inactive and committed to shed, develop less tumors in skin carcinogenesis experiments than WT mice [4]. However, this approach is not comparable to ours because we have targeted IKKα to basal keratinocytes, which are mitotically active cells. This is an important difference, because the tumorigenic properties of skin tumors strongly depend on the cell type targeted being the expression of a potential tumoral promoter more harmful in basal cells than in terminally differentiated cells [62]. Other studies on the role of IKKα in skin tumorigenesis have been performed in IKKα+/− mice and show that these animals develop more carcinomas with a lower latency period [13]. However, these mice are defective in IKK expression in both epidermis and dermis, and increasing evidences support the contribution of the tumor stroma to some of the most malignant characteristics of epithelial tumors [63]; therefore through this approach it is not possible to discern the role that the expression of IKKα specifically in keratinocytes plays for skin carcinogenesis. A different approach to this study would be the use of conditional knockout mice lacking IKKα specifically in keratinocytes. These mice have been generated by two different groups and the skin phenotypes obtained are completely different: while one model exhibits an hyperplastic skin with absence of terminal differentiation [12], the other shows a nearly normal skin with terminal differentiation and no signs of hyperplasia [11] being the reasons for this discrepancy not understood. Therefore, although skin carcinogenesis assays showing increased tumorigenesis in the IKKα conditional mice exhibiting a skin phenotype have been reported [12], the absence of the same experiments in the other IKKα conditional mice model casts doubts on the conclusiveness of the results.

Taking into account the different results published, it seems that the role that IKKα plays in carcinogenesis could depend on the type of tumor, the cell targeted in each tumor and the strain of mice employed in the studies. Our present study supposes a different approach for study the role of IKKα in skin carcinogenesis, targeting IKKα to the basal keratinocytes of the epidermis. Our results showing the increase in the malignant potential of skin tumors developed *in vivo*, in transgenic mice overexpressing IKKα in keratinocytes, are in line and strengthen our previous findings showing the enhanced aggressiveness of skin tumors arising after injection of tumor epidermal cells overexpressing IKKα into nude mice [5]. We have found that increased IKKα expression levels in the basal layer of the epidermis and ORS of the hair follicles of transgenic mice leads to alterations that originate lesions of higher malignant potential than those developed in WT mice when subjected to aberrant mitogenic stimuli. We have found that the altered expression of cyclin D1, maspin and integrin-α6 in skin of transgenic mice provide, at least in part, the molecular bases of the increase in the malignant potential of carcinomas originated in skin of K5-IKKα Tg mice.

Supporting Information

Figure S1 Graphical representation of the number of tumors developed in WT and Tg-K5-IKKα mice in the two skin carcinogenesis approaches. (**A**) K5-IKKα and WT 9-week-old mice (9 animals respectively) were subjected to DMBA/TPA carcinogenesis assay. Tumors were traced until week 26, when they were collected. (**B**) Double transgenic K5-IKKα-TgAC and WT-TgAC 9-week-old mice (11 animals respectively) were treated twice weekly with topical applications of TPA. Tumors were traced until week 30, when they were collected. No differences were found between number of tumors developed in WT and Tg animals in both approaches.
(TIF)

Acknowledgments

We thank M. Isabel de los Santos and Federico Sánchez-Sierra for histological assistance; Juan Manuel Luque for technical assistance and personnel of the Animal Unit for care of the mice.

Author Contributions

Conceived and designed the experiments: MLC AR. Performed the experiments: JPA RM-M MLC AP. Analyzed the data: MLC AB MJF-A AR MN. Contributed reagents/materials/analysis tools: MN JLJ AR. Wrote the paper: MLC.

References

1. Ghosh S, Karin M (2002) Missing pieces in the NF-kappaB puzzle. Cell 109: S81–S96.
2. Hayden MS, Ghosh S (2004) Signaling to NF-kappaB. Genes Dev 18: 2195–2224.
3. Shih VF, Tsui R, Caldwell A, Hoffmann A (2011) A single NFkappaB system for both canonical and non-canonical signaling. Cell Res 21: 86–102.
4. Liu B, Park E, Zhu F, Bustos T, Liu, J, et al. (2006) A critical role for I kappaB kinase alpha in the development of human and mouse squamous cell carcinomas. Proc Natl Acad Sci U S A 103: 17202–17207.
5. Moreno-Maldonado R, Ramirez A, Navarro M, Fernandez-Acenero MJ, Villanueva C, et al. (2008) IKKalpha enhances human keratinocyte differentiation and determines the histological variant of epidermal squamous cell carcinomas. Cell Cycle 7: 2021–2029.
6. Li Q, Lu Q, Hwang JY, et al. (1999) IKK1-deficient mice exhibit abnormal development of skin and skeleton. Genes Dev 13: 1322–1328.
7. Takeda K, Takeuchi O, Tsujimura T, Itami S, Adachi O, et al. (1999) Limb and skin abnormalities in mice lacking IKKalpha. Science 284: 313–316.
8. Hu Y, Baud V, Delhase M, Zhang P, Deerinck T, et al. (1999) Abnormal morphogenesis but intact IKK activation in mice lacking the IKKalpha subunit of IkappaB kinase. Science 284: 316–320.
9. Hu Y, Baud V, Oga T, Kim KI, Yoshida K, et al. (2001) IKKalpha controls formation of the epidermis independently of NF-kappaB. Nature 410: 710–714.
10. Sil AK, Maeda S, Sano Y, Roop DR, Karin M (2004) IkappaB kinase-alpha acts in the epidermis to control skeletal and craniofacial morphogenesis. Nature 428: 660–664.
11. Gareus R, Huth M, Breiden B, Nenci A, Rosch N, et al. (2007) Normal epidermal differentiation but impaired skin-barrier formation upon keratinocyte-restricted IKK1 ablation. Nat Cell Biol 9: 461–469.
12. Liu B, Xia X, Zhu F, Park E, Carbajal S, et al. (2008) IKKalpha is required to maintain skin homeostasis and prevent skin cancer. Cancer Cell 14: 212–225.
13. Park E, Zhu F, Liu B, Xia X, Shen J, et al. (2007) Reduction in IkappaB kinase alpha expression promotes the development of skin papillomas and carcinomas. Cancer Res 67: 9158–9168.
14. Merkhofer EC, Cogswell P, Baldwin AS (2010) Her2 activates NF-kappaB and induces invasion through the canonical pathway involving IKKalpha. Oncogene 29: 1238–1248.
15. Jiang R, Xia Y, Li J, Deng L, Zhao L, et al. (2010) High expression levels of IKKalpha and IKKbeta are necessary for the malignant properties of liver cancer. Int J Cancer 126: 1263–1274.
16. Mahato R, Qin B, Cheng K (2010) Blocking IKKalpha Expression Inhibits Prostate Cancer Invasiveness. Pharm Res; Epub ahead of print.
17. Luo JL, Tan W, Ricono JM, Korchynskyi O, Zhang M, et al. (2007) Nuclear cytokine-activated IKKalpha controls prostate cancer metastasis by repressing Maspin. Nature 446: 690–694.
18. Charalambous MP, Lightfoot T, Speirs V, Horgan K, Gooderham NJ (2009) Expression of COX-2, NF-kappaB-p65, NF-kappaB-p50 and IKKalpha in malignant and adjacent normal human colorectal tissue. Br J Cancer 101: 106–115.
19. Fernandez-Majada V, Aguilera C, Villanueva A, Vilardell F, Robert-Moreno A, et al. (2007) Nuclear IKK activity leads to dysregulated notch-dependent gene expression in colorectal cancer. Proc Natl Acad Sci U S A 104: 276–281.
20. Bailey CM, Khalkhali-Ellis Z, Seftor EA, Hendrix MJ (2006) Biological functions of maspin. J Cell Physiol 209: 617–624.
21. Khalkhali-Ellis Z (2006) Maspin: the new frontier. Clin Cancer Res 12: 7279–7283.
22. Shi HY, Zhang W, Liang R, Abraham S, Kittrell FS, et al. (2001) Blocking tumor growth, invasion, and metastasis by maspin in a syngeneic breast cancer model. Cancer Res 61: 6945–6951.
23. Futscher BW, O'Meara MM, Kim CJ, Rennels MA, Lu D, et al. (2004) Aberrant methylation of the maspin promoter is an early event in human breast cancer. Neoplasia 6: 380–389.
24. Abraham S, Zhang W, Greenberg N, Zhang M (2003) Maspin functions as tumor suppressor by increasing cell adhesion to extracellular matrix in prostate tumor cells. J Urol 69: 1157–1161.
25. Zhang M, Volpert O, Shi YH, Bouck N (2000) Maspin is an angiogenesis inhibitor. Nat Med 6: 196–199.

26. Boltze C (2005) Loss of maspin is a helpful prognosticator in colorectal cancer: a tissue microarray analysis. Pathol Res Pract 200: 783–790.
27. Yoshizawa K, Nozaki S, Okamune A, Rennels MA, Lu D, et al. (2009) Loss of maspin is a negative prognostic factor for invasion and metastasis in oral squamous cell carcinoma. J Oral Pathol Med 38: 535–539.
28. Zheng HC, Saito H, Masuda S, Wang ZG, Takano Y (2008) Cytoplasmic and nuclear maspin expression in lung carcinomas: an immunohistochemical study using tissue microarrays. Appl Immunohistochem Mol Morphol 16: 459–465.
29. Marioni G, Blandamura S, Giacomelli L, Calgaro N, Segato P, et al. (2005) Nuclear expression of maspin is associated with a lower recurrence rate and a longer disease-free interval after surgery for squamous cell carcinoma of the larynx. Histopathology 46: 576–582.
30. Chua R, Setzer S, Govindarajan B, Sexton D, Cohen C, et al. (2009) Maspin expression, angiogenesis, prognostic parameters, and outcome in malignant melanoma. J Am Acad Dermatol 60: 758–766.
31. O'Donnell JD, Linger RJ, Kruk PA (2010) BRCA1 185delAG mutant protein, BRAt, up-regulates maspin in ovarian epithelial cells. Gynecol Oncol 116: 262–268.
32. Cao D, Zhang Q, Wu LS, Salaria SN, Winter JW, et al. (2007) Prognostic significance of maspin in pancreatic ductal adenocarcinoma: tissue microarray analysis of 223 surgically resected cases. Mod Pathol 20: 570–578.
33. Dietmaier W, Bettstetter M, Wild PJ, Woenckhaus M, Rummele P, et al. (2006) Nuclear Maspin expression is associated with response to adjuvant 5-fluorouracil based chemotherapy in patients with stage III colon cancer. Int J Cancer 118: 2247–2254.
34. Stark AM, Schem C, Maass N, Hugo HH, Jonat W, et al. (2010) Expression of metastasis suppressor gene maspin is reduced in breast cancer brain metastases and correlates with the estrogen receptor status. Neurol Res 32: 303–308.
35. Karin M (2008) The IkappaB kinase - a bridge between inflammation and cancer. Cell Res 18: 334–342.
36. Yang J, Mani SA, Donaher JL, Ramaswamy S, Itzykson RA, et al. (2004) Twist, a master regulator of morphogenesis, plays an essential role in tumor metastasis. Cell 117: 927–939.
37. Puisieux A, Valsesia-Wittmann S, Ansieau S (2006) A twist for survival and cancer progression. Br J Cancer 94: 13–17.
38. Ansieau S, Bastid J, Doreau A, Morel AP, Bouchet BP, et al. (2008) Induction of EMT by twist proteins as a collateral effect of tumor-promoting inactivation of premature senescence. Cancer Cell 14: 79–89.
39. Owens DM, Romero MR, Gardner C, Watt FM (2003) Suprabasal alpha6beta4 integrin expression in epidermis results in enhanced tumourigenesis and disruption of TGFbeta signalling. J Cell Sci 116: 3783–3791.
40. Tennenbaum T, Weiner AK, Belanger AJ, Glick AB, Hennings H, et al. (1993) The suprabasal expression of alpha 6 beta 4 integrin is associated with a high risk for malignant progression in mouse skin carcinogenesis. Cancer Res 53: 4803–4810.
41. Alameda JP, Moreno-Maldonado R, Navarro M, Bravo A, Ramirez A, et al. (2010) An inactivating CYLD mutation promotes skin tumor progression by conferring enhanced proliferative, survival and angiogenic properties to epidermal cancer cells. Oncogene 29: 6522–6532.
42. Leder A, Kuo A, Cardiff RD, Sinn E, Leder P (1990) v-Ha-ras transgene abrogates the initiation step in mouse skin tumorigenesis: effects of phorbol esters and retinoic acid. Proc Natl Acad Sci U S A 87: 9178–9182.
43. Ramirez A, Bravo A, Jorcano JL, Vidal M (1994) Sequences 5′ of the bovine keratin 5 gene direct tissue- and cell-type-specific expression of a lacZ gene in the adult and during development. Differentiation 58: 53–64.
44. Casanova ML, Larcher F, Casanova B, Murillas R, Fernandez-Acenero MJ, et al. (2002) A critical role for ras-mediated, epidermal growth factor receptor-dependent angiogenesis in mouse skin carcinogenesis. Cancer Res 62: 3402–3407.
45. Jost M, Kari C, Rodeck U (2000) The EGF receptor - an essential regulator of multiple epidermal functions. Eur J Dermatol 10: 505–510.
46. Rikimaru K, Moles JP, Watt FM (1997) Correlation between hyperproliferation and suprabasal integrin expression in human epidermis reconstituted in culture. Exp Dermatol 6: 214–221.
47. Balmain A, Pragnell IB (1983) Mouse skin carcinomas induced in vivo by chemical carcinogens have a transforming Harvey-ras oncogene. Nature 303: 72–74.
48. Casanova ML, Bravo A, Martinez-Palacio J, Fernandez-Acenero MJ, Villanueva C, et al. (2004) Epidermal abnormalities and increased malignancy of skin tumors in human epidermal keratin 8-expressing transgenic mice. Faseb J 18: 1556–1558.
49. Winter H, Rentrop M, Nischt R, Schweizer J (1990) Tissue-specific expression of murine keratin K13 in internal stratified squamous epithelia and its aberrant expression during two-stage mouse skin carcinogenesis is associated with the methylation state of a distinct CpG site in the remote 5′-flanking region of the gene. Differentiation 43: 105–114.
50. Marinari B, Moretti F, Botti E, Giustizieri ML, Descargues P, et al. (2008) The tumor suppressor activity of IKKalpha in stratified epithelia is exerted in part via the TGF-beta antiproliferative pathway. Proc Natl Acad Sci U S A 105: 17091–17096.
51. Albanese C, Wu K, D'Amico M, Jarrett C, Joyce D, et al. (2003) IKKalpha regulates mitogenic signaling through transcriptional induction of cyclin D1 via Tcf. Mol Biol Cell 14: 585–599.
52. Ohuchida K, Mizumoto K, Ohhashi S, Yamaguchi H, Konomi H, et al. (2007) Twist, a novel oncogene, is upregulated in pancreatic cancer: clinical implication of Twist expression in pancreatic juice. Int J Cancer 120: 1634–1640.
53. Lee TK, Poon RT, Yuen AP, Ling MT, Kwok WK, et al. (2006) Twist overexpression correlates with hepatocellular carcinoma metastasis through induction of epithelial-mesenchymal transition. Clin Cancer Res 12: 5369–5376.
54. Zhang Z, Xie D, Li X, Wong YC, Xin D, et al. (2007) Significance of TWIST expression and its association with E-cadherin in bladder cancer. Hum Pathol 38: 598–606.
55. Lamberti C, Lin KM, Yamamoto Y, Verma U, Verma IM, et al. (2001) Regulation of beta-catenin function by the IkappaB kinases. J Biol Chem 276: 42276–42286.
56. Park KJ, Krishnan V, O'Malley BW, Yamamoto Y, Gaynor RB (2005) Formation of an IKKalpha-dependent transcription complex is required for estrogen receptor-mediated gene activation. Mol Cell 18: 71–82.
57. Wu RC, Qin J, Hashimoto Y, Wong J, Xu J, et al. (2002) Regulation of SRC-3 (pCIP/ACTR/AIB-1/RAC-3/TRAM-1) Coactivator activity by I kappa B kinase. Mol Cell Biol 22: 3549–3561.
58. Yamamoto Y, Verma UN, Prajapati S, Kwak YT, Gaynor RB (2003) Histone H3 phosphorylation by IKK-alpha is critical for cytokine-induced gene expression. Nature 423: 655–659.
59. Anest V, Hanson JL, Cogswell PC, Steinbrecher KA, Strahl BD, et al. (2003) A nucleosomal function for IkappaB kinase-alpha in NF-kappaB-dependent gene expression. Nature 423: 659–663.
60. Huang WC, Ju TK, Hung MC, Chen CC (2007) Phosphorylation of CBP by IKKalpha promotes cell growth by switching the binding preference of CBP from p53 to NF-kappaB. Mol Cell 26: 75–87.
61. DeBusk LM, Massion PP, Lin PC (2008) IkappaB kinase-alpha regulates endothelial cell motility and tumor angiogenesis. Cancer Res 68: 10223–10228.
62. Brown K, Strathdee D, Bryson S, Lambie W, Balmain A (1998) The malignant capacity of skin tumours induced by expression of a mutant H-ras transgene depends on the cell type targeted. Curr Biol 8: 516–524.
63. Trimboli AJ, Cantemir-Stone CZ, Li F, Wallace JA, Merchant A, et al. (2009) Pten in stromal fibroblasts suppresses mammary epithelial tumours. Nature 461: 1084–1091.

17

Occludin Is Involved in Adhesion, Apoptosis, Differentiation and Ca^{2+}-Homeostasis of Human Keratinocytes: Implications for Tumorigenesis

Susanne Rachow[1,2]¶, Michaela Zorn-Kruppa[1]¶, Ulrich Ohnemus[1], Nina Kirschner[1], Sabine Vidal-y-Sy[1], Peter von den Driesch[3], Christian Börnchen[1], Jürgen Eberle[4], Michael Mildner[5], Eik Vettorazzi[6], Rita Rosenthal[7], Ingrid Moll[1], Johanna M. Brandner[1]*

1 Department of Dermatology and Venerology, University Hospital Hamburg-Eppendorf, Hamburg, Germany, **2** Tabea Clinics GmbH, Hamburg, Germany, **3** Dermatological Center, Klinikum Stuttgart, Stuttgart, Germany, **4** Department of Dermatology, Venerology and Allergology, Skin Cancer Center, Charité, Berlin, Germany, **5** Department of Dermatology, Medical University of Vienna, Vienna, Austria, **6** Department of Medical Biometry and Epidemiology, University Hospital Hamburg-Eppendorf, Hamburg, Germany, **7** Institute of Clinical Physiology, Charité-Universitätsmedizin Berlin, Berlin, Germany

Abstract

Tight junction (TJ) proteins are involved in a number of cellular functions, including paracellular barrier formation, cell polarization, differentiation, and proliferation. Altered expression of TJ proteins was reported in various epithelial tumors. Here, we used tissue samples of human cutaneous squamous cell carcinoma (SCC), its precursor tumors, as well as sun-exposed and non-sun-exposed skin as a model system to investigate TJ protein alteration at various stages of tumorigenesis. We identified that a broader localization of zonula occludens protein (ZO)-1 and claudin-4 (Cldn-4) as well as downregulation of Cldn-1 in deeper epidermal layers is a frequent event in all the tumor entities as well as in sun-exposed skin, suggesting that these changes result from chronic UV irradiation. In contrast, SCC could be distinguished from the precursor tumors and sun-exposed skin by a frequent complete loss of occludin (Ocln). To elucidate the impact of downregulation of Ocln, we performed Ocln siRNA experiments in human keratinocytes and uncovered that Ocln downregulation results in decreased epithelial cell-cell adhesion and reduced susceptibility to apoptosis induction by UVB or TNF-related apoptosis-inducing ligand (TRAIL), cellular characteristics for tumorigenesis. Furthermore, an influence on epidermal differentiation was observed, while there was no change of E-cadherin and vimentin, markers for epithelial-mesenchymal transition. Ocln knock-down altered Ca^{2+}-homeostasis which may contribute to alterations of cell-cell adhesion and differentiation. As downregulation of Ocln is also seen in SCC derived from other tissues, as well as in other carcinomas, we suggest this as a common principle in tumor pathogenesis, which may be used as a target for therapeutic intervention.

Editor: Michel Simon, CNRS-University of Toulouse, France

Funding: Deutsche Forschungsgemeinschaft, Forschergruppe 721/2, TP9, Johann und Anny Thomas Stiftung, COST Action BM 0903 SkinBAD STSM. The funders had no role in study design, data collection and analysis, decision to publish, or preparation of the manuscript.

Competing Interests: The authors have declared that no competing interests exist.

* E-mail: brandner@uke.de

¶ These authors contributed equally to this work.

Introduction

Tight Junctions (TJs) are multiprotein complexes formed by transmembrane proteins, e.g. occludin (Ocln), claudins (Cldns), and junctional adhesion molecules (JAMs), which are associated with intracellular plaque proteins, e.g. ZO-1, 2 and 3 and MUPP-1. From simple epithelia it is known that TJs seal neighbouring cells and control the paracellular pathway for solutes, water, and cells (barrier function). In addition, they restrict the diffusion of apical and basolateral membrane components (fence function), coordinate signalling molecules and play a role in cell differentiation and proliferation [1,2,3,4,5,6]. A role of TJs in paracellular barrier function was also shown in the multi-layered epithelium of the skin [7,8], and an involvement of Cldn-1 in proliferation and differentiation of keratinocytes was suggested [9,10,11].

There are frequent changes in TJ protein localization and/or expression in the course of carcinogenesis. For Cldns, up- or downregulation, as well as altered localization were described, dependent on the tumor entity. For instance, in breast cancer Cldn-1, -2, and -7 are downregulated, while Cldn-4 is upregulated and in colorectal- and pancreatic-cancer Cldn-1, -2, and -7 are upregulated [12,13,14,15,16]. For Ocln, mainly a downregulation was observed in various tumors [17,18,19,20]. Downregulation of Ocln is a common feature of epithelial-mesenchymal-transition (EMT) in tumors derived from simple epithelial cells, and regulation of Ocln was described by the oncogenic Raf1 pathway as well as by the transcription factors slug, and snail [21,22,23,24,25]. Furthermore, an involvement of Ocln in apoptosis has been suggested, but there is conflicting evidence whether apoptosis is enhanced or suppressed (see also discussion) [26,27,28,29,30]. For ZO-1 down- or upregulation was observed in different tumor entities [17,31,32], and its redistribution from cell-cell-borders to the cytoplasm and nucleus was described in EMT [e.g. 33]. Decreased expression of TJ proteins suggests that tumorigenesis is accompanied by TJ disruption and loss of cell-cell adhesion followed by loss of differentiation, uncontrolled proliferation, and invasiveness as well as increased supply with nutrition. However, up-regulation of TJ proteins may also be an initial step which disturbs the balance of TJs and therefore cell homeostasis [12,15,34].

Squamous cell carcinoma (SCC) is the second most common skin malignancy accounting for the majority of non-melanoma skin cancer-related metastatic disease and death [35]. It can be categorized in well, moderately and poorly differentiated SCCs [36,37]. Epidermal differentiation marker involucrin was described to be present in lower malignant, well differentiated SCCs but to be decreased in higher malignant, poorly differentiated ones [38,39,40], Transglutaminase 1 (TG1) was described to be increased in the epidermal part of the SCCs but is absent in invasive parts [41]. Actinic keratoses (AK) and Bowen's disease (BD) are suggested to be precursors (*carcinomata in situ*) of SCC and their presence is a marker for increased risk for the occurrence of SCC [42]. Keratoacanthoma (KA) represents a closely related epithelial tumor and can transform to SCC especially in elderly persons [37]. SCC and its precursors mainly develop as the result of UV damage on chronically sun-exposed skin. Due to their good accessibility, SCC and its precursors are a good model system to investigate tumor progression from normal (non-sun-exposed skin) via stressed (sun-exposed skin) multi-layered epithelia to in-situ (AK, BD), low malignant (KA) and high malignant (SCC) carcinoma.

There is limited data about TJ protein alterations in human cutaneous SCC. Langbein et al. [43] investigated three cases and found punctate or extended cell-cell border structures positive for Ocln, Cldn-1, Cldn-4, cingulin, and ZO-1 in higher as well as in lower differentiated areas. On the other hand, Morita et al. [44] described a restriction of strong expression of Cldn-1, Cldn-4, Ocln, and ZO-1 to keratinized areas in 5 SCC. In unkeratinized tumor cells, Cldn-1 was heterogeneously expressed, ZO-1 was weak, whereas Ocln and Cldn-4 were absent. In 5 cases of BD, no loss of Ocln and Cldn-4 but an aberrant localization were seen [44].

These interesting but somewhat discrepant findings in only a limited number of SCC and BD cases and the putative impact of TJ protein alterations on tumor progression prompted us to investigate larger numbers of cutaneous SCC and their precursors including (chronically) sun-exposed skin, as well as healthy, non-sun-exposed skin with the aim to identify similarities and differences for TJ proteins. Because we observed a striking loss of Ocln in many malignant SCC in contrast to its precursors we hypothesized that this molecule might promote tumorigenic features in keratinocytes which was addressed by investigating the involvement of Ocln in cell-cell adhesion, apoptosis, proliferation, differentiation and Ca^{2+}-homeostasis in knock-down studies.

Materials and Methods

Ethics Statement

The samples for this study were obtained from our clinical department. They were used after diagnostic procedures had been completed. The local medical ethics committee (Aerztekammer Hamburg) approved this study (060900 and OB-008/04). All patients gave their written informed consent.

Tissues, Cells, Antibodies, qPCR Primers and siRNAs

Samples of human SCC (n = 46; 31 male, 15 female; age 19–93 y, mean: 73 y), BD (n = 26; 15 male, 11 female; age 33–94 y, mean 74 y), KA (n = 24; 15 male, 9 female; age 21–89 y; mean 59 y), AK (n = 25, 12 male, 13 female, age 61–92 y, mean 72 y) sun-exposed skin (n = 11, 4 male, 7 female; age 16–89 y, mean: 67 y) and non-sun-exposed skin (n = 17, 9 male, 8 female; age 20–78 y; mean 42 y) were obtained from our clinical department. Grading of the SCC was performed according to the world health organisation classification [37]. Human foreskin keratinocytes were isolated and cultured as described [45]. Antibodies used are summarized in Table 1. FAM™ dye-labeled real-time PCR (qRT-PCR) TaqMan® MGB probes for Ocln (Hs00170162_m1), involucrin (Hs0084307_s1), TG1 (Hs01070310_m1), Cldn-2 (Hs00252666_s1), Cldn-12 (Hs00221623_m1) and GAPDH (Hs03929097_g1) were purchased from Applied Biosystems (Carlsbad, CA, USA). Ready-to-use siRNAs for human Ocln (Hs_OCLN_7: SI03225999, Hs_OCLN_9: SI04360034), ZO-1 (SI02655149), and control siRNA (1027280) were purchased from QIAGEN (Hilden, Germany). Stealth siRNAs for gene silencing of Ocln in human organotypic skin models [46] were purchased from Life Technologies (Darmstadt, Germany; siRNA1: HSS107401; siRNA3: HSS181629; control: 12935–300). Due to technical reasons different siRNAs had to be used for cell culture and skin model experiments.

Immunofluorescence Microscopy

Immunofluorescence microscopy was performed as previously described [45]. For details see Table 1. An Axiophot-II microscope (Carl Zeiss; Jena/Oberkochen, Germany), a CCD-Camera (Hamamatsu Photonics; Hamamatsu City, Japan), and Openlab 2.0.9 software (Improvision; Coventry, UK) were utilized to visualize and evaluate the stained sections. ZO-1 and especially Ocln are very sensitive antigens influenced by slight deviations of fixation. Therefore samples were only evaluated when positive staining in the "uninvolved epidermis" (Figure 1) and/or internal positive controls (e.g. sweat glands) confirmed the success of staining procedure and stainings were repeated at least twice. The stainings were analyzed by two independent investigators (SR and JMB). The number of evaluated samples was as follows: SCC (Ocln: n = 35, ZO-1: n = 32, Cldn-1, JAM-A: n = 46; Cldn-4: n = 30, Inv: n = 41, TG1: n = 11; E-cadherin: n = 12; vimentin: n = 10), BD (Ocln: n = 19, ZO-1: n = 25, Cldn-1: n = 25, JAM-A: n = 26; Cldn-4: not tested), KA (Ocln: n = 18, ZO-1: n = 23, Cldn-1, JAM-A: n = 24; Cldn-4: not tested), AK (Ocln: n = 19, ZO-1: n = 22; Cldn-1: n = 24; JAM-1: n = 25; Cldn-4: n = 9), sun-exposed skin (Ocln: n = 9, ZO-1: n = 9; Cldn-1: n = 10; JAM-A: n = 9; Cldn-4: n = 11), non-sun-exposed healthy skin (Ocln: n = 11, ZO-1: n = 15; Cldn-1: n = 16; JAM-A: n = 15; Cldn-4: n = 15).

Human Organotypic Skin Models (3D Models)

Pre-confluent human primary keratinocytes were transfected with the respective siRNA using Lipofectamine 2000 (Invitrogen) according to the manufacturer's instructions. Keratinocytes were then incubated for 24 h before seeding onto a fibroblast collagen gel as described below.

Organotypic skin models were prepared as described previously [47]. Briefly, a 2.5 ml suspension of collagen type I (Advanced Biomatrix, San Diego, CA, USA) containing 2.5×10^5 fibroblasts was poured into cell-culture inserts (3 µm pore size; BD Bioscience, Bedford, MA, USA) and allowed to gel for 2 h at 37°C without CO_2. The gels were then equilibrated with KGM medium (Lonza, Basel, Switzerland) at 37°C in a CO_2 incubator for 2 h, and 1.5×10^6 keratinocytes, transfected with the respective siRNAs, were seeded onto each collagen gel. After overnight incubation at 37°C the medium was removed from both the inserts and external wells, and

Table 1. Antibodies and nuclear dyes.

Target	Clone/lot	Company	Dilution IF	Dilution Western-blot
Cldn-1	2H10D10	Zymed Laboratories	1:150	
Cldn-4	3E2CI	Zymed Laboratories	1:50	
Zo-1	1A12	Zymed Laboratories	1:80	
Ocln	OC-3F10 71–1500	Zymed Laboratories	1:80	1:2000
JAM-A	Rm-JAM-1	R&D systems	1:30	
TG1	BC1	Antibody online	1:20	1:500
Involucrin	SY5	Novo Castra	1:200	1:2000, pH 8.0
Ki67	MIB-1	DAKO	1:50	
E-Cadherin	NCH-38	DAKO	1:50	1:100
Vimentin	GP53	Progen	1:1000	1:500
Actin	AC-15	Sigma		1:10000
Tubulin	DM-1A	Calbiochem		1:2000
Nuclei	DAPI	Boehringer Mannheim	1:5000	

Abbreviations: Cldn, claudin; JAM, junctional adhesion molecule; IF, immuno-fluorescence; Ocln, occludin; TG1, transglutaminase 1; ZO, zonula occludens.
IF treatment for TG1: Citrate buffer, 2×10 min microwave, 0.001% trypsin, DAKO Block overnight. IF treatment for all others: TEC buffer, 2×10 min microwave, 0.001% trypsin, DAKO block.

10 ml serum-free keratinocyte defined medium (SKDM), consisting of KGM without bovine pituitary extract and supplemented with 1.3 mM calcium (Sigma, Vienna, Austria), 10 µg/ml transferrin (Sigma), 50 µg/ml ascorbic acid (Sigma), and 0.1% bovine serum albumin (Sigma), was added to each external well. The organotypic skin models were cultured for 7 days and medium was changed every second day.

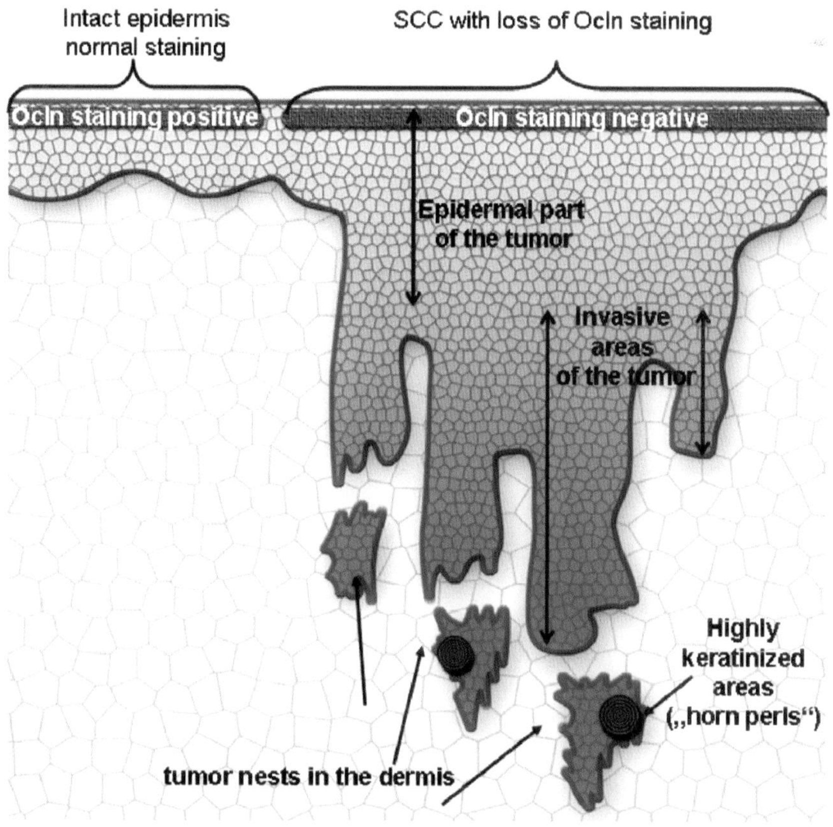

Figure 1. Schematic drawing of a squamous cell carcinoma denoting the different areas of the tumor.

siRNA Experiments

Primary human keratinocytes were transfected under low Ca^{2+} conditions by using HiPerFect Transfection reagent (Qiagen, Hilden, Germany) according to the manufacturer's instructions. Briefly, cells were transfected by a fast forward protocol. 100000 cells/ml were transfected with a 1:1 mixture of HiPerFect reagent (1:200) and 100 nM of Ocln-siRNA or control-siRNA, respectively. Efficiency of knock-down was controlled by Western-blot and qRT-PCR analysis after 2, 3 or 5 days (depending on the experiment). Silencing of Ocln in a human organotypic skin model was performed as described [46,47]. Briefly, transfection was performed using Lipofectamine 2000 (Invitrogen) according to the manufacturer's instructions with slight modifications. Third passage keratinocytes were grown to 70–80% confluency. Lipofectamine 2000 (50 µl) was mixed with 100 µl of a 20 µM siRNA solution and 5 ml OPTI-MEM medium (Gibco). After 30 min at room temperature, KGM (20 ml) was added and the solution was poured onto the keratinocytes monolayer (25 ml) for 24 h. After transfection keratinocytes were trypsinized and seeded onto a fibroblast collagen gel. Efficiency of knock-down was controlled by Western-blot and qRT-PCR analysis.

BrdU-assay

Proliferation experiments under low Ca^{2+} conditions were performed 48 h after seeding of 8000 cells/well and siRNA-treatment. Subsequently, Ca^{2+} levels were elevated to 2 mM to induce differentiation and 48 h later proliferation experiments were performed under high Ca^{2+} conditions. The BrdU-ELISA kit from Roche (Mannheim, Germany) was used following manufacturer's instructions.

Evaluation of Proliferative Cells in 3D Models

Proliferative (Ki67-positive) cells were stained by MIB-1 and at least 5 visual fields (0.25 mm^2) were evaluated per model (n = 4). In each visual field the number of Ki67 positive cells was normalized to the total number of basal cells which were evaluated by DAPI staining.

Cell Adhesion Assays

Intercellular adhesion under high Ca^{2+} conditions was tested using a hanging drop assay which was modified from [48]. Briefly, following 48 h of siRNA silencing cell suspensions of 550000 single cells per ml were prepared. 35 µl drops of the suspensions were placed under the lids of 60×15 mm tissue culture dishes. To limit evaporation 2 ml of PBS was added to the bottoms of the dishes. After indicated time points the drops were pipetted and placed in an improved Neubauer hemocytometer chamber. Pictures of 4×12 Neubauer-squares of 0.0625 mm^2 each were taken using a Leica DM LS microscope with 10× objective magnification and a Leica EC3 digital camera (*Leica* Biosystems *Nussloch* GmbH, *Nussloch*, Germany). The numbers of particles in the squares were determined automatically by utilizing FIJI software [49] and the particles analyzer tool. The relative cell adhesion activity was evaluated according to [50] by calculating the cell aggregation index $Nt/N0 \times 100$, where Nt is the number of particles at different time points and N0 the initial particle number. Lower numbers of particles reflect increased cell-cell adhesion.

TRAIL Treatment and UVB-irradiation

For TRAIL treatment and UVB-irradiation, keratinocytes were plated in 96-well plates (8000 cells/well) under low Ca^{2+} conditions and transfected for 48 h with the indicated siRNAs. Then cells were transferred to siRNA-free medium for another 24 h and subsequently exposed to TRAIL (25 ng/ml; Axxorra/Alexis Gruenberg, Germany) or irradiated with 150 mJ/cm^2 to induce apoptosis. Irradiation was performed in PBS, and then the solution was replaced by fresh medium.

Apoptosis and LDH Assay

Apoptosis was evaluated at 3 h and 20 h of TRAIL treatment and at 16 h after UVB-irradiation by using the Cell Death Detection ELISA^{PLUS} kit (Roche) according to the manufacturer's instructions. This assay is defined as release of mono- and oligonucleosomes due to DNA fragmentation in the cytoplasm of apoptotic cells. Cytotoxicity was determined after 3 h and 20 h of TRAIL treatment as well as 4 h and 16 h after UVB irradiation by a lactate dehydrogenase (LDH) release assay (Cytotoxicity Detection kit^{PLUS} - LDH; Roche). Relative apoptosis was calculated by dividing the absorbance of treated cells by the absorbance of non-transfected non TRAIL-or UV-treated control cells. The percentages of cytotoxicity were calculated according to a control with completely lysed cells due to lysis buffer treatment.

Analysis of Ca^{2+} Permeability

Determination of Ca^{2+} permeability was performed in Ussing chambers specially designed for the investigation of cell monolayers grown on culture plate inserts [51]. Keratinocytes were seeded on culture plate inserts (Millicell-PCF, pore size 0.4 µm, area 0.6 cm^2; Millipore), cultured under high Ca^{2+}-conditions for 48 h, and investigated in the Ussing chambers. Ca^{2+} permeability was determined from biionic potentials and the Goldman–Hodgkin–Katz equation as reported in detail previously [52].

Statistical Analysis

Statistical significance of proliferation, adhesion, Ca^{2+}-barrier-formation and apoptosis was determined by Student's t-test. TJ protein expressions were cross-tabulated with tumor grading, differentiation markers, and sun-exposure and the significance of associations were tested using Fisher's Exact Test. P-values <0.05 were considered as statistically significant (* $p<0.05$, ** $p<0.01$, *** $p<0.001$).

Results

Aberrant Localization Patterns of TJ Proteins in Cutaneous SCC

In normal, non-sun-exposed skin Cldn-1 and JAM-A were predominantly found at the cell-cell borders of all living epidermal layers, while localization of Cldn-4, Ocln and ZO-1 was mainly restricted to cell-cell borders of the stratum granulosum (Figure 2, 3). In addition, cytoplasmic staining was observed (Figure 2, 3).

In contrast, in SCC samples there was a complete loss of staining for ZO-1 in 25% of the tumors, for Ocln in 80% (Figure 3), for Cldn-1 in 9%, and for Cldn-4 in 17% (Table 2). Also in samples positive for these proteins there were some negative spots (data not shown). No cases were completely negative for JAM-A.

In 81% of the positive cases for Cldn-1, there was a downregulation of the protein in the lowermost and in 60% in the uppermost layers of epidermal tumor parts (Figure 1, 2, Table 2). JAM-A was downregulated in the upper layers in 85% of the samples (Figure 2, Table 2). Cldn-4 showed a broader localization in 91% of the samples (Figure 2), ZO-1 in 67%, and Ocln in 29% (Figure 3, Table 2).

In the invasive parts of the tumors (Figure 1), Ocln and Cldn-4 were absent, Cldn-1 was observed in one and ZO-1 in two cases. JAM-A was present in all cases (data not shown).

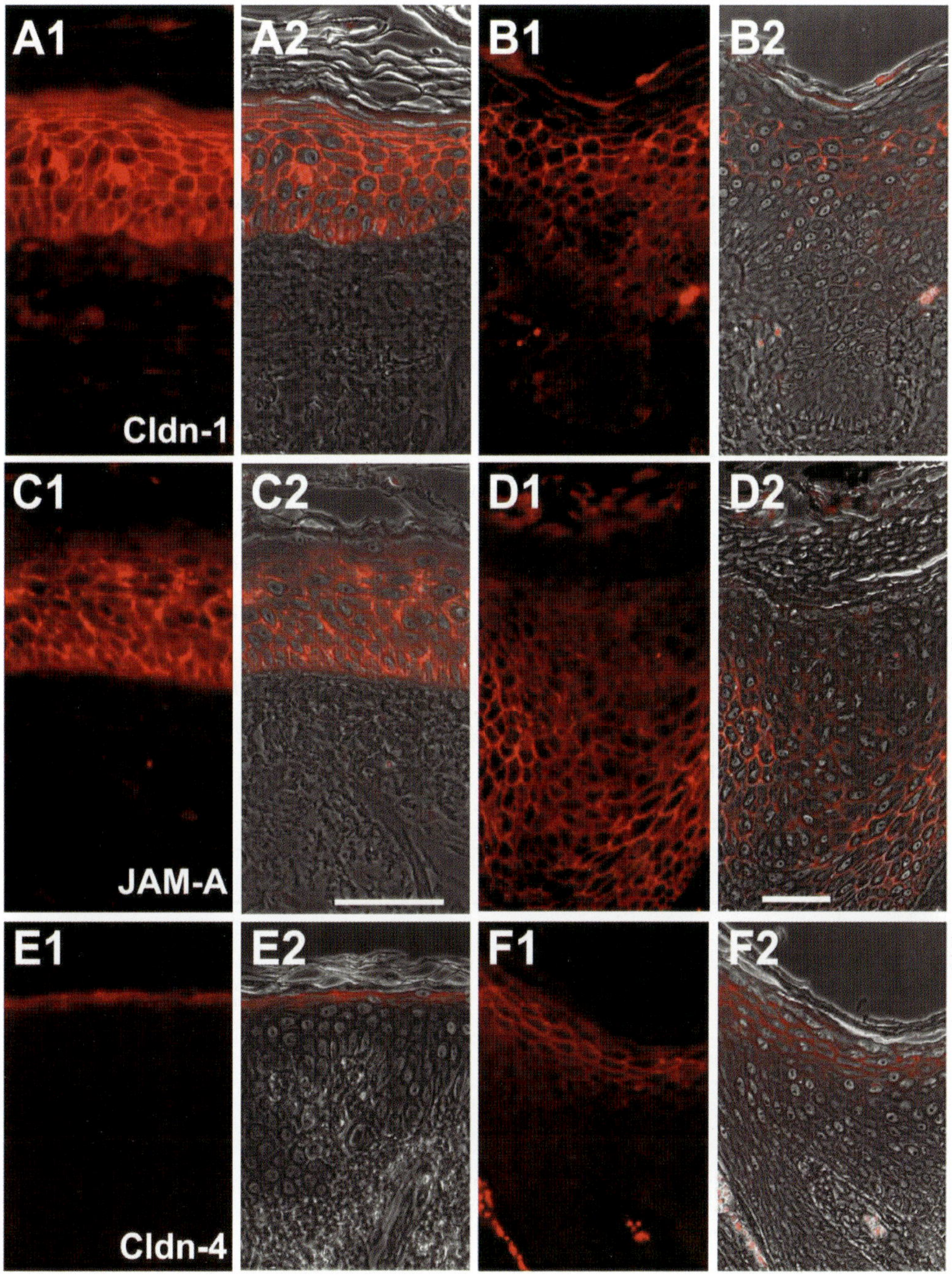

Figure 2. Immunolocalization of Cldn-1, JAM-A, and Cldn-4 in healthy, non-sun- exposed skin and SCC. Immunolocalization of Cldn-1 (A1, A2, B1, B2), JAM-A (C1, C2, D1, D2), and Cldn-4 (E1, E2, F1, F2) in healthy, non-sun-exposed skin (A1, A2, C1, C2, E1, E2) and SCC (B1, B2, D1, D2, F1, F2). (A1, B1, C1, D1, E1, F1: epifluorescence pictures; A2, B2, C2, D2, E2, F2: overlay of epifluorescence and phase contrast pictures). Note that Cldn-1 is downregulated in the uppermost and lowermost layers whereas JAM-A is primarily downregulated in the uppermost layers of SCC. Furthermore Cldn-4 demonstrates broader localization in SCC compared to healthy skin. Bars: 50 μm.

This indicates that complete loss of Ocln and downregulation of Cldn-1 in the lowermost and JAM-A and Cldn-1 in the uppermost layers is a frequent feature in SCC. This also applies for the broader localization of Cldn-4 and ZO-1.

Localization Patterns of TJ Proteins in AK, BD, and KA

We wondered whether the alterations found in SCC may also be seen in in-situ carcinomas (AK, BD) or in tumors of lower malignancy (KA).

Complete loss of Ocln was found in only 5% of AK, 11% of BD, and 29% of KA, demonstrating that its absence is much more characteristic for SCC (80%). Contrariwise, broader localization of Ocln was found more frequently in the precursor tumors (42–71%, as compared to 29%; Table 2).

For ZO-1, complete loss was observed in 9% of AK, 12% of BD but not in KA (25% in SCC). Frequency of broader localization was similar between the tumor entities. Furthermore, there was no clear-cut difference between SCC and the other tumors as

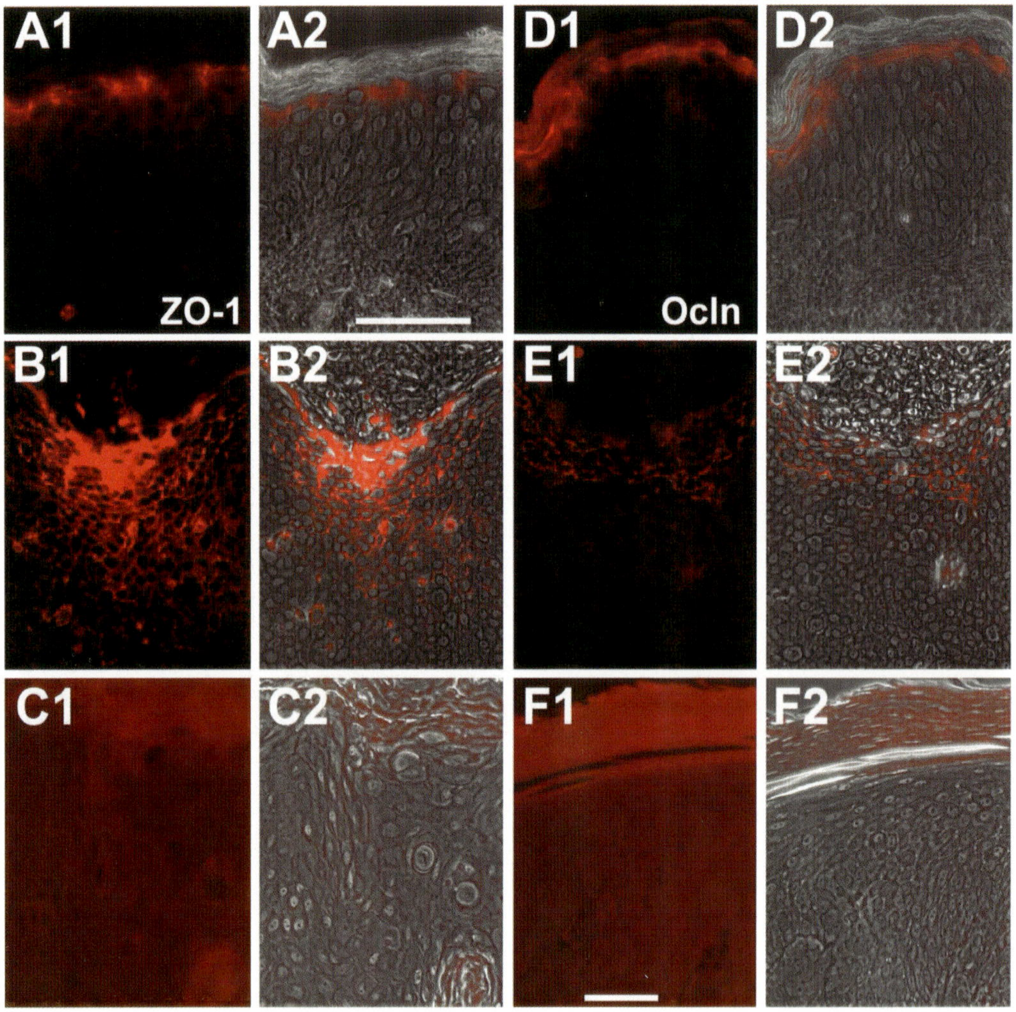

Figure 3. Immunolocalization of ZO-1 and Ocln in healthy, non-sun-exposed skin and SCC. Immunolocalization of ZO-1 (A1, A2, B1, B2, C1, C2), and Ocln (D1, D2, E1, E2, F1, F2), in healthy, non-sun-exposed skin (A1, A2, D1, D2) and SCC (B1, B2, C1, C2, E1, E2, F1, F2). (A1, B1, C1, D1, E1, F1: epifluorescence pictures; A2, B2, C2, D2, E2, F2: overlay of epifluorescence and phase contrast pictures). For both molecules an example of broader localization (B1, B2, E1, E2) and loss of the protein (C1, C2, F1, F2) are shown. Note that exposure time in C1, C2, F1, F2 was substantially higher than in the other figures in order to show that also with very high exposure time no Ocln or ZO-1 staining was seen in these samples. Bars: 50 μm.

Table 2. Protein expression and localization of TJ proteins in the various skin tumors.

	Squamous cell carcinoma		Kerato-acanthoma		Bowens Disease		Actinic keratoses	
	Loss	**Altered**	**Loss**	**Altered**	**Loss**	**Altered**	**Loss**	**Altered**
Cldn-1	9%	60%[1]/81%[2]	0%	68%[1]/80%[2]	4%	55%[1]/86%[2]	4%	83%[1]/83%[2]
Cldn-4	17%	91%[3]	Not tested	Not tested	Not tested	Not tested	0%	91%[3]
JAM-A	0%	85%[1]	0%	88%[1]	0%	78%[1]	4%	73%[1]
Ocln	80%	29%[3]	29%	71%[3]	11%	42%[3]	5%	54%[3]
ZO-1	25%	67%[3]	0%	88%[3]	12%	65%[3]	9%	75%[3]

Loss: complete loss of expression, altered: altered localization. % in "loss of expression" denotes the percentage of all tumors, % in "altered localization" denotes the percentage of positive tumors.

[1]downregulation in the uppermost layers.

[2]downregulation in the lowermost layers.

[3]broader expression.

Abbreviations see table 1.

concerning Cldn-1, Cldn-4, and JAM-A (Table 2). Similar to SCC samples, we observed also in the SCC precursor samples spots with lacking expression of TJ proteins.

The data indicate that alterations found for Cldn-1, Cldn-4, ZO-1, and JAM-A are common for UV-induced skin tumors while the frequent loss of Ocln appears as specific for SCC.

Localization Patterns of TJ Proteins in Sun-exposed Versus Non-sun-exposed Skin

Because the alterations for Cldn-1, Cldn-4, and ZO-1 were observed in all UV- promoted skin tumors and a broader localization of Ocln was frequent in all tumor entities except for SCC, we wondered whether these alterations could also be identified in chronically sun-exposed skin. Indeed, a broader localization of Ocln, ZO-1, and Cldn-4 was seen more frequent in the epidermis of sun-exposed as compared to non-sun-exposed skin with high statistical significance (Ocln: $p = 0.001$, ZO-1: $p = 0.001$, Cldn-4: $p = 0.001$) (Figure 4). We found no significant influence of age and sex on TJ protein localization. However, a complete loss of Ocln, as in SCC, was not observed in sun-exposed skin. Also spots with loss of staining were less frequent than in the tumors (data not shown). For Cldn-1, we observed a downregulation in the lowermost epidermal layers in sun-exposed skin which was less frequent in non-sun-exposed skin ($p<0.001$) (Figure 4). Downregulation in the uppermost layers - as frequently seen in the tumors - was not observed. From this data we conclude that most TJ protein alterations observed in skin tumors are likely to be induced by UV-irradiation, but loss of Ocln and downregulation of Cldn-1 in the uppermost layers may not be related to UV.

Knock-down of Occludin Alters Epidermal Differentiation Markers but not Markers for EMT

Altered differentiation is a common feature in tumor progression. Accordingly, irregularity of epidermal differentiation markers involucrin and TG1 was described in SCC [38,39,40]. Therefore we investigated whether downregulation of Ocln may influence epidermal differentiation. When using two different siRNAs in a 3D skin model, we could strongly downregulate Ocln protein expression (Figure 5A). This was associated with downregulation of the differentiation marker involucrin and an upregulation of TG1 (Figure 5A). The same effect was seen for involucrin when investigating 2D cell cultures (data not shown). On mRNA-level, a slight and partly significant upregulation for involucrin and TG1 was observed (Involucrin: Ocln siRNA1:1.4±0.4, n.s., Ocln siRNA3:2.2±0.5, $p<0.01$; TG1: Ocln siRNA1:1.4±0.1, $p<0.001$; Ocln siRNA3:1.7±0.6, n.s.; Ocln: Ocln siRNA1:0.4±0.2, $p<0.01$; Ocln siRNA3:0.4±0.2, $p<0.01$; $n = 3$).

Because Ocln was also described to be involved in epithelial-mesenchymal transition [21,22,25], we investigated E-cadherin as an epithelial marker as well as vimentin as a mesenchymal marker for EMT in the Ocln knock-down models. However, we did not find any changes of these markers (Figure 5A).

Further, we looked for correlations between involucrin, and TG1, on one hand and Ocln expression on the other hand in the SCC samples as well as for correlations of Ocln with the SCC grade. We found that Ocln-positive tumors were to a higher percentage differentiated tumors (Grade I; 57.1%) than Ocln-negative tumors (25.9%) (Table 3). Characteristically, all Ocln-positive tumors were also positive for involucrin (Table 4). However, also 84% of Ocln-negative tumors were still positive for involucrin (see Table 3, 4). For TG1, 71% of the Ocln-negative tumors showed an upregulation in the epidermal parts, however, this was also the case in 100% of Ocln-positive tumors (Table 4).

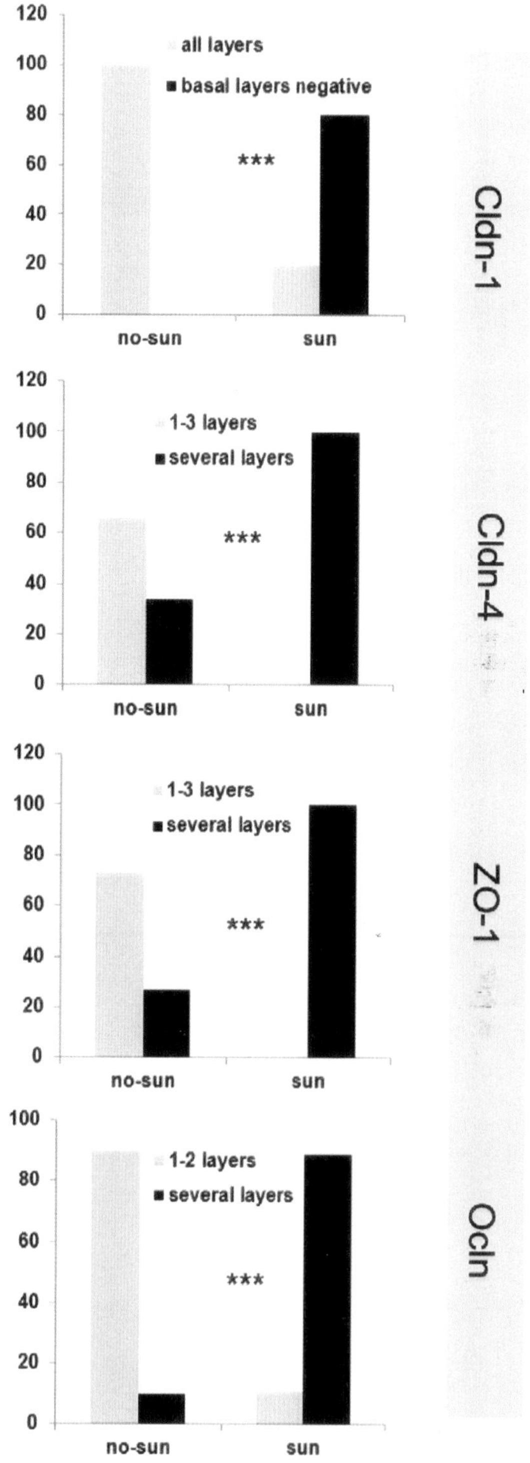

Figure 4. Distribution patterns of TJ proteins in normal skin from sun-exposed and non-sun-exposed areas. Percentages denote distribution patterns of the various TJ proteins in sun-exposed (sun; e. g. face, lower arms) and non-sun-exposed areas (no-sun; e. g. abdomen, bottom). ***: $p<0.001$ between sun-exposed and non-sun-exposed skin.

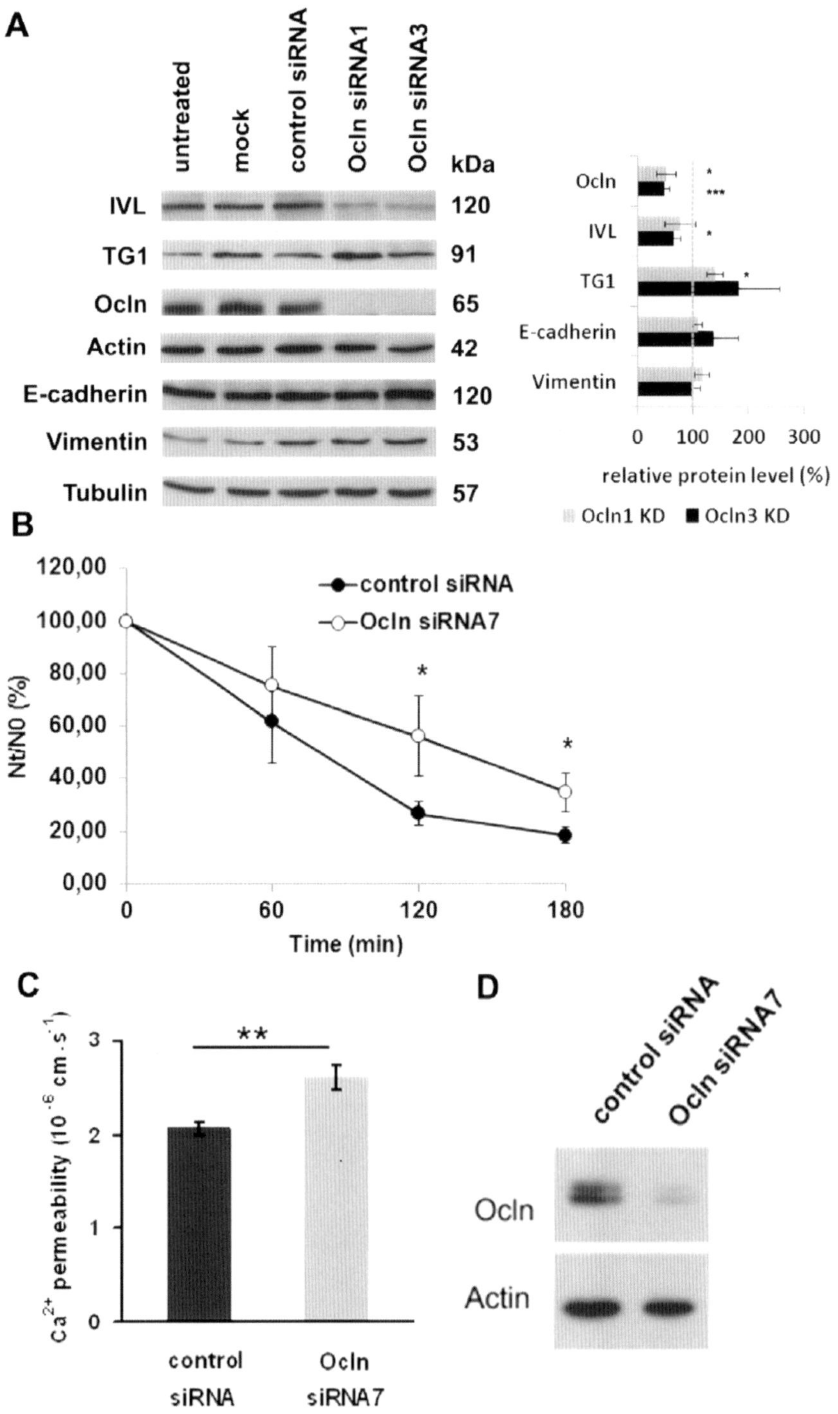

Figure 5. Influence of Ocln on epidermal differentiation and EMT markers, cell-cell adhesion and paracellular Ca^{2+} permeability. (A) (left side) Western Blot analysis of 3D skin models after silencing of Ocln with 2 different siRNAs shows downregulation of Ocln and of the epidermal differentiation marker involucrin and an upregulation of TG1. There is no alteration for the EMT markers E-cadherin and vimentin. Same amounts of protein were loaded and actin or tubulin were used as gel loading controls. A representative experiment is shown (n = 3). (right side) Semiquantitative analysis of Ocln, involucrin, TG1, E-cadherin and vimentin. Band intensities were normalized to actin (Inv, TG1) or tubulin (E-cad, vim). Subsequently, the values were normalized to control siRNA treated cells (n = 3; mean ± SEM; *p < 0.05, ***p < 0.001 compared to control siRNA). (B) Calcium induced cell-cell adhesion was investigated with a hanging drop assay at the indicated time points. Significantly greater numbers of particles (indicating less cell-cell adhesion) were found in the suspensions of Ocln knock-down cells compared to the controls (*: $p < 0.05$ $n = 3$), (C) Electrophysiological studies of paracellular Ca^{2+}-permeability in Ocln siRNA-treated cultured keratinocytes revealed an increase in paracellular permeability for Ca^{2+} in Ocln knock-down cells compared to cells treated with control siRNA (n = 6, mean ± SEM). (D) Example for the knock-down of Ocln in siRNA treated submerged cells. Mean knock-down of Ocln in the cells used for experiments in Figure 5 B, C and 6 was 76% +/−9%.

Table 3. Correlation of presence of TJ proteins and tumor grading of SCC.

	Ocln		ZO-1		Cldn-1		Cldn-4	
	Pos	Neg	Pos	Neg	Pos	Neg	Pos	Neg
Tumor grading								
I	57.1%	25.9%	27.3%	25.0%	32.5%	50%	20.8%	40%
II	28.6%	40.7%	45.4%	37.5%	42.5%	25%	50%	20%
III	14.3%	33.4%	27.3%	37.5%	25%	25%	29.2%	40%

Pos, positive; neg, negative. Further abbreviations see table 1.

Knock-down of Occludin Reduces Cell-cell Adhesion

We asked whether the alteration of Ocln might also influence keratinocyte adhesion, because loss of adhesion is also a prerequisite for tumor invasion and metastasis. Indeed, significantly reduced keratinocyte-keratinocyte adhesion was seen in response to Ocln knock-down, as shown by a cell adhesion assay in a time kinetic analysis (Figure 5B, D).

Knock-down of Occludin Increases Paracellular Permeability for Ca^{2+}

Cell-cell adhesion as well as cell-differentiation is dependent on Ca^{2+}-homeostasis. Therefore, we investigated whether decreased Ocln levels may also alter Ca^{2+} permeability of keratinocyte-sheets. Indeed, increased paracellular Ca^{2+} permeability (126% ±5%) was observed in Ocln knock-down cells as compared to control-siRNA-treated cells (Figure 5C, D). Consequently, knock-down of Ocln also reduced transepithelial resistance (data not shown). Because Cldn-2 and Cldn-12 are known to be key-players in Ca^{2+}-permeability in intestinal cells [53] we investigated the influence of Ocln knock-down on mRNA expression of these claudins. While there was no influence on Cldn-12, we observed a significant downregulation of Cldn-2 to 0.56+/−0.05 of the level of control cells (n = 3).

Knock-down of Occludin Reduces the Susceptibility of Keratinocytes for Induction of Apoptosis

A tumor-promoting effect may also result from inhibition of apoptosis. We therefore addressed the question whether down-regulation of Ocln may also result in a reduced sensitivity of keratinocytes for proapoptotic stimuli. We tested here TRAIL, which plays a particular role in keratinocyte regulation of apoptosis [54], and UVB-irradiation, a typical apoptosis inducing stimulus in the skin.

Indeed, significantly decreased apoptosis was evident after 3 h (data not shown) and 20 h (Figure 6A, B) of TRAIL-treatment in Ocln knock-down keratinocytes compared to control siRNA-treated cells as seen by using two different siRNAs (Figure 6A, B). In addition, a clear decrease of UVB-induced apoptosis was seen in Ocln knock-down cells (Figure 6C).

Thus, Ocln knock-down selectively prevented apoptosis induction by TRAIL and UVB, which may suggest a role of Ocln loss in tumor progression of SCC, based on apoptosis resistance to different stimuli.

Of note, the effects of Ocln knock-down were not seen in all keratinocyte cultures. The effects on TRAIL-induced apoptosis were seen in 50% of the primary keratinocyte cultures (n = 14) that originated from different donors, and the suppressive effects on UVB-induced apoptosis were seen in 40% of cultures (n = 10). This was independent from the level of Ocln knock-down. All primary cultures that showed an effect of Ocln knock-down on UVB-induced apoptosis showed a similar effect when using TRAIL.

No primary cytotoxicity (necrotic cell death) was seen in response to TRAIL at early time points (3 h). It was only enhanced in the TRAIL-treated keratinocyte cultures after 20 h, interestingly both in the Ocln-siRNA treated cells and in control cells (Figure 6D), arguing for a secondary cytotoxic effect due to absence of removal of apoptotic cells from cell culture.

Knock-down of Occludin Shows Only Minor Effects on Keratinocyte Proliferation

Increased proliferation represents a characteristic feature of in-situ and malignant tumors. Therefore, we asked whether Ocln

Table 4. Correlation of the presence of TJ proteins and differentiation markers involucrin and TG1 as well as EMT markers E-cadherin and vimentin in SCC.

	Involucrin		TG1		E-Cadherin		Vimentin	
	Pos	Neg	Normal	Up-regulated	Normal or slightly down-regulated	Strongly down-regulated	Pos	Neg
Ocln- pos	100% 7/7	0% 0/7	0% 0/4	100% 4/4	67% 4/6	23% 2/6	20% 1/5	80% 4/5
Ocln-neg	84% 21/25	16% 4/25	29% 2/7	71% 5/7	86% 6/7	14% 1/7	0% 0/5	100% 5/5

Abbreviations see table 1 and 3. n/m denotes the positive/negative or normal/upregulated cases compared to the total amount of cases of a specific category.

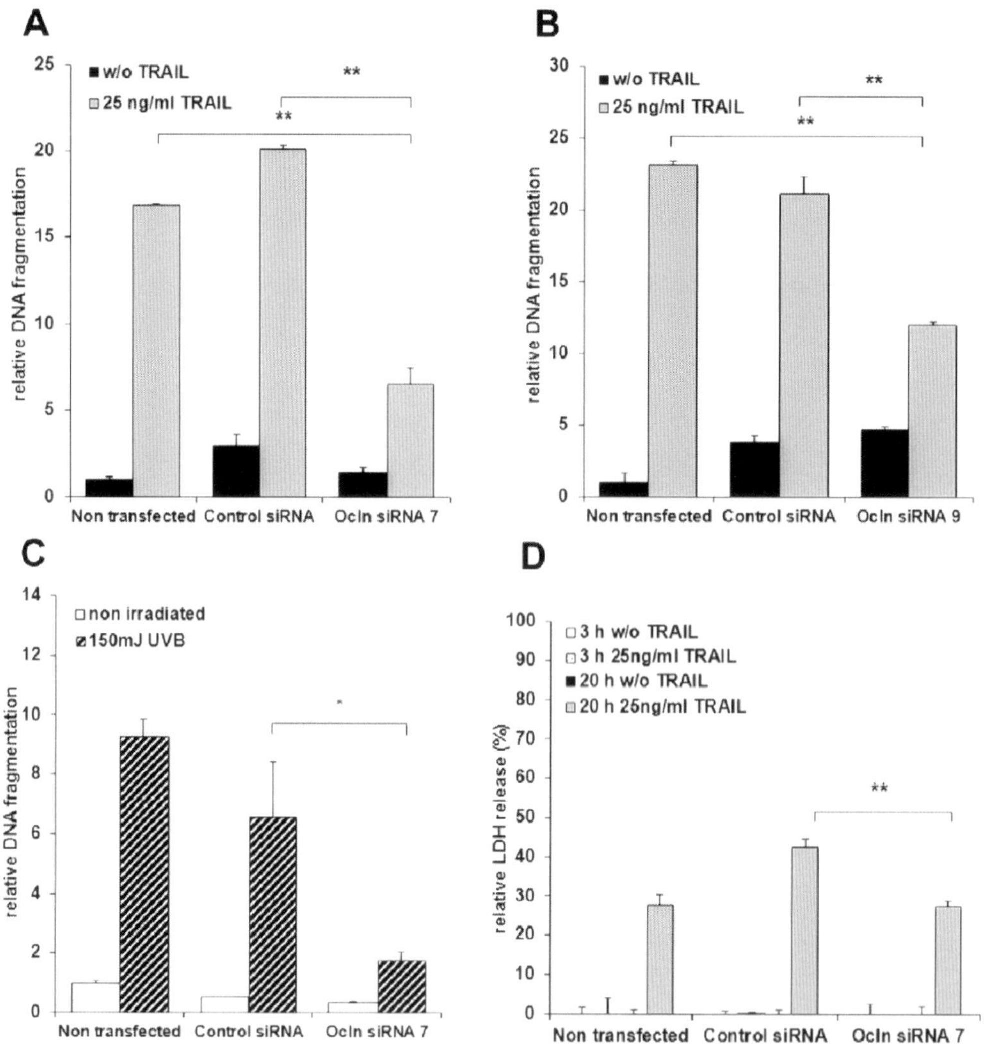

Figure 6. Influence of Ocln on DNA fragmentation after induction of apoptosis by TRAIL and UVB. Apoptotic response at 20 h of TRAIL treatment (25 ng/ml) (A+B) or 16 h after UVB-irradiation (C) in human keratinocyte cultures with or without Ocln knock-down due to Ocln siRNA7 (A+C+D) or Ocln siRNA9 treatment (B). A significant decrease of apoptotic DNA fragmentation induced by TRAIL and UV light was observed after downregulation of Ocln. (D) Cytotoxicity measured by LDH assay at 3 h and 20 h of TRAIL treatment (100% corresponds to complete lysis of the cells). Note that 3 h after TRAIL treatment (when apoptotic fragmentation was already detectable) cytotoxicity was not primarily influenced indicating an apoptotic rather than necrotic mechanism. Mean +/− SEM. *: $p<0.05$; ** $p<0.01$. Example of one out of at least 10 independent cell lines. All experiments were performed in triplicates.

might also contribute to the regulation of keratinocyte proliferation. We did, however, not observe increased proliferation of human keratinocytes in 2D cultures at low Ca^{2+} conditions when treated with Ocln-siRNA, whereas at high Ca^{2+} conditions cell proliferation was slightly reduced. Also in 3D skin models no significant influence of Ocln knock-down on keratinocyte proliferation was evident (data not shown).

Discussion

Here, we demonstrate that downregulation of Ocln in keratinocytes results in decreased cell-cell adhesion, reduced susceptibility to induction of apoptosis, altered epidermal differentiation, and altered Ca^{2+} homeostasis. This hints for a significance of the Ocln loss proven here in a large panel of cutaneous SCC as compared to SCC precursors and to normal skin. In addition, we demonstrate that changes of Cldn-1, Cldn-4, JAM-A, and ZO-1 can not only be found in SCC but also in precursor lesions and sun-exposed skin.

We identified a frequent loss of Ocln in cutaneous SCC which was not found in its precursors or sun-exposed and non-sun-exposed skin. In line with our results loss or downregulation of Ocln has also been described in most samples of lingual and bronchial SCC [55,56] suggesting Ocln downregulation as a common characteristic of SCC, irrespective from its origin. In addition, Ocln downregulation was also observed in other cancer entities, e.g. gastric cancer, hepatocellular carcinoma, and breast cancer [17,18,19], hinting for a general role in tumorigenesis. In breast cancer cell lines it was shown that overexpression of Ocln can decrease invasiveness and cell motility in vitro and inhibits tumor development and metastasis in mouse experiments in vivo [30]. On the other hand, knock-down of Ocln in breast cancer cell lines resulted in increased invasiveness [18].

Previous reports of cutaneous SCC could not identify such an Ocln loss though the protein was partly found to be restricted to cells with keratinization such as cancer pearls [43,44]. As we also observed Ocln staining in some of our SCC, this discrepancy might be due to the limited number of cases investigated before. Any staining procedure problems could be largely excluded because we exclusively evaluated tumors with internal positive controls (see materials and methods).

Addressing the question of consequences of reduced Ocln levels in keratinocytes, we investigated epidermal differentiation, markers for EMT, cell-cell adhesion, Ca^{2+}-permeability, apoptosis, and proliferation.

We demonstrate that downregulation of Ocln results in downregulation of involucrin and increase of TG1 protein levels in 3D skin models, indicating an influence of Ocln on epidermal differentiation. Several studies described a downregulation of involucrin in poorly differentiated SCC, while it was strongly expressed in highly differentiated SCC [38,39,40,44]. For TG1 increased staining intensity was described in the epidermal part of cutaneous SCC, [41], a frequent (69%) upregulation was also observed in SCC of the lung [57]. However, we do not see a clear correlation of downregulation of Ocln and changes of involucrin and TG1 in our SCC tissues. This reflects that tumor progression is influenced by various internal and external factors that, depending on the tumor-microenvironment, might overrule the effect of downregulation of Ocln and which we cannot mimic in our cell culture system. In addition, we cannot rule out that in SCC alteration of Ocln might not only be a cause but also a consequence of altered differentiation, because the chicken-egg question "TJs – differentiation" has not been solved yet [58]. Therefore the final contribution of Ocln downregulation to altered epidermal differentiation in SCC still has to be clarified.

As a putative underlying mechanism of altered epidermal differentiation we identified an increased paracellular Ca^{2+} permeability in keratinocytes and therefore altered Ca^{2+}-homeostasis. Increased permeability might result in an altered tissue Ca^{2+}-gradient which is known to influence keratinocyte differentiation [59,60,61]. Altered Ca^{2+}-homeostasis is also likely to be involved in reduced cell-cell adhesion observed in our Ocln knock-down keratinocytes, because Ca^{2+} is known to be essential for the formation of functional adherence junctions and desmosomes [62,63,64]. Reduced cell-cell interaction is a typical hallmark in tumor progression. Involvement of Ocln in cell-cell adhesion was described before for fibroblasts ectopically overexpressing Ocln [50]. Because increased Ca^{2+}-permeability in Ocln knock-down cells could also be a secondary effect due to the alteration of other TJ proteins, namely Cldn-2 and 12 which are critical for Ca^{2+}-permeability in the intestine [65] we also investigated the mRNA levels of these TJ proteins. There was no change of Cldn-12, but there was a significant decrease of Cldn-2. However, because Cldn-2 normally mediates Ca^{2+}-permeability, its downregulation counteracts the increased permeability and might be a compensation mechanism.

Downregulation of Ocln has been described to be involved in EMT. Especially in the context of TGFβ induced EMT recent studies in simple epithelial cells indicate high significance of Ocln as a key regulatory component mediating complex formation of PAR6 together with type I TGFβ receptors. Upon exposure to TGFβ, Par6 is phosphorylated and binds to Smurf1, an E3 ubiquitin ligase, which in turn mediates ubiquitination of RhoA. Loss of Rho is important for the dissolution of TJs and for EMT [66,67,68]. However, we did not observe an influence of Ocln knock-down on E-cadherin and vimentin, typical markers for EMT, in our 3D cultures. We also did not observe a correlation of presence/absence of Ocln and the downregulation of E-cadherin or the upregulation of vimentin in our SCC (Table 4). Therefore it is unlikely that Ocln plays a major role in EMT in cutaneous SCC. This might reflect a difference between tumors derived from simple and multilayered epithelia.

We observed a role of Ocln in apoptosis sensitivity of keratinocytes. Thus, reduced apoptotic responses of keratinocytes were seen in response to TRAIL and UVB after Ocln knock-down. TRAIL activates the extrinsic apoptotic pathway, while UVB may induce both, extrinsic and intrinsic apoptotic pathways [69,70]. In line with our results, a relation of Ocln with extrinsic apoptotic pathways has also been shown in mammary gland cells: Following disruption of TJs by an Ocln-specific peptide, Ocln became associated with the death-inducing signalling complexes (DISC) of death receptors and the extrinsic apoptotic pathway was activated. In mammary gland cells from Ocln knock-out mice this peptide did not induce apoptosis [27]. However, because TRAIL is less effective in differentiated keratinocytes [71,72], we investigated its effect under low Ca^{2+} conditions. Under these conditions only a low proportion of Ocln is present at the cell-cell borders [73,74]. Therefore the observed effect of Ocln knock-down in keratinocytes is likely to include an Ocln cell membrane localization-independent effect, while data presented for mammary gland cells suggest that Ocln moves through the plasma membrane to activate the death receptor [27]. In general, the role of Ocln in apoptosis is ambiguous and might depend on the cell type. In HeLa cells over-expression of Ocln enhanced the sensitivity to H_2O_2-induced cell death [30], suggesting, in line with our results and the results in mammary gland cells [27], a supportive role of Ocln for the induction of apoptosis. In contrast, in primary hepatocytes from Ocln-deficient mice increased numbers of apoptotic cells were observed and in immortalized cells from this origin apoptosis induced by serum-free conditions was more pronounced than in wild-type cells [28]. Yu et al [29] observed an increase of apoptotic cells in MDCKII cultures after siRNA-mediated Ocln knock-down but this increase was primarily due to the retention of apoptotic cells in the monolayers while overall apoptosis ratio was not affected compared to control cells. We do not observe a significant increase in the number of apoptotic cells in Ocln knock-down cells without treatment with UV or TRAIL compared to control cells. Therefore we conclude that the mechanism in MDCK II cells is different to keratinocytes. We also excluded by our experimental design that the reduced amount of apoptosis observed here in Ocln knock-down cells after induction of apoptosis with TRAIL and UV was due to decreased retention of the apoptotic cells in the monolayers. Interestingly, in our experiments only 40–50% of primary keratinocyte cultures from different donors revealed decreased response to proapoptotic stimuli after Ocln knock-down. Further clarification of the role of Ocln in keratinocyte apoptosis regulation will be a challenging task for future projects.

For Cldn-1, we found downregulation in uppermost and lowermost layers of cutaneous SCC and predominantly absence in the invasive parts, but a complete loss was only found in 9%. This is in agreement with Ouban et al [75] who found Cldn-1 in 91.7% of SCC from different origins. Concerning the downregulation in the uppermost and lowermost layers there was no difference for Cldn-1 between SCC and its precursors, hinting for an early event in skin hyperplasia. This is supported by findings in neoplasia induced by 7,12-dimethylbenz(a)anthracene and 12-O-tetradecanoyl-phorbol-13-acetate treatment of mouse models, which also exhibit downregulation of Cldn-1 in the basal cell layer [76].

Looking for explanations for the common alterations of Cldn-1, Cldn-4 and ZO-1 identified in the various skin tumors, we hypothesized that chronic UV exposure might induce some of these changes. Therefore, we investigated sun-exposed versus non-sun-exposed skin. Indeed, we observed a significant downregulation of Cldn-1 in lower layers and broader localization of Ocln, ZO-1, and Cldn-4 in a high proportion of chronically sun-exposed skin. Our data fit nicely to results reported in an UVB-irradiated murine skin model [77] describing a broader ZO-1 localization throughout the upper epidermis. A broader localization of ZO-1 was also shown in irradiated human skin xenografts and of Ocln in irradiated skin equivalents [78]. Downregulation of Cldn-1 in upper layers which was found in SCC and its precursors, was not observed in sun-exposed skin. Also, opposed to skin tumors, spots of loss for the various proteins were rarely seen in sun-exposed skin. Therefore these events seem to be independent from chronic UV-irradiation.

Conclusion

In conclusion, we demonstrate a frequent loss of Ocln in cutaneous SCC but not in its precursors. We confirm our hypothesis that Ocln knock-down in keratinocytes is involved in the promotion of tumorigenic features and show reduced susceptibility to TRAIL- and UV-induced apoptosis as well as reduced cell-cell adhesion. This may play a role in SCC tumorigenesis, as well as in other carcinomas, as loss of Ocln is a common feature in tumors. Other changes of TJ proteins were identified in cutaneous SCC as well as in precursor lesions and sun-exposed skin, and may therefore characterize initial steps in tumorigenesis induced by UV-irradiation.

Acknowledgments

We thank Nikolas K. Haass, Sydney, and Claudia Bohner, Hamburg for helpful discussions and Ewa Wladykowski for skilful technical assistance.

Author Contributions

Conceived and designed the experiments: SR MZK UO JE JMB. Performed the experiments: SR MZK UO NK SV MM RR CB. Analyzed the data: SR MZK UO NK PVDD EV RR IM JMB. Wrote the paper: SR MZK UO NK SV PVDD JE MM EV CB RR IM JMB.

References

1. Aijaz S, Balda MS, Matter K (2006) Tight junctions: molecular architecture and function. Int Rev Cytol 248: 261–298.
2. Balda MS, Matter K (2009) Tight junctions and the regulation of gene expression. Biochim Biophys Acta 1788: 761–767.
3. Ebnet K, Suzuki A, Ohno S, Vestweber D (2004) Junctional adhesion molecules (JAMs): more molecules with dual functions? J Cell Sci 117: 19–29.
4. Furuse M, Tsukita S (2006) Claudins in occluding junctions of humans and flies. Trends Cell Biol 16: 181–188.
5. Shen L, Weber CR, Raleigh DR, Yu D, Turner JR (2011) Tight junction pore and leak pathways: a dynamic duo. Annu Rev Physiol 73: 283–309.
6. Schneeberger EE, Lynch RD (2004) The tight junction: a multifunctional complex. Am J Physiol Cell Physiol 286: C1213–1228.
7. Furuse M, Hata M, Furuse K, Yoshida Y, Haratake A, et al. (2002) Claudin-based tight junctions are crucial for the mammalian epidermal barrier: a lesson from claudin-1-deficient mice. J Cell Biol 156: 1099–1111.
8. Kirschner N, Houdek P, Fromm M, Moll I, Brandner JM (2010) Tight junctions form a barrier in human epidermis. Eur J Cell Biol 89: 839–842.
9. De Benedetto A, Rafaels NM, McGirt LY, Ivanov AI, Georas SN, et al. (2011) Tight junction defects in patients with atopic dermatitis. J Allergy Clin Immunol 127: 773–786 e771–777.
10. Kirschner N, Haftek M, Niessen CM, Behne MJ, Furuse M, et al. (2011) CD44 regulates tight-junction assembly and barrier function. J Invest Dermatol 131: 932–943.
11. Kirschner N, Rosenthal R, Furuse M, Moll I, Fromm M, et al. (in revision) Contribution of tight junction proteins to ion, macromolecule, and water barrier in keratinocytes: no direct effect of claudin-1 on water barrier. J Invest Dermatol.
12. Oliveira SS, Morgado-Diaz JA (2007) Claudins: multifunctional players in epithelial tight junctions and their role in cancer. Cell Mol Life Sci 64: 17–28.
13. Swisshelm K, Macek R, Kubbies M (2005) Role of claudins in tumorigenesis. Adv Drug Deliv Rev 57: 919–928.
14. Tsukita S, Yamazaki Y, Katsuno T, Tamura A, Tsukita S (2008) Tight junction-based epithelial microenvironment and cell proliferation. Oncogene 27: 6930–6938.
15. Turksen K, Troy TC (2011) Junctions gone bad: Claudins and loss of the barrier in cancer. Biochim Biophys Acta 1816: 73–79.
16. Lanigan F, McKiernan E, Brennan DJ, Hegarty S, Millikan RC, et al. (2009) Increased claudin-4 expression is associated with poor prognosis and high tumour grade in breast cancer. Int J Cancer 124: 2088–2097.
17. Orban E, Szabo E, Lotz G, Kupcsulik P, Paska C, et al. (2008) Different expression of occludin and ZO-1 in primary and metastatic liver tumors. Pathol Oncol Res 14: 299–306.
18. Martin TA, Mansel RE, Jiang WG (2010) Loss of occludin leads to the progression of human breast cancer. Int J Mol Med 26: 723–734.
19. Tobioka H, Isomura H, Kokai Y, Tokunaga Y, Yamaguchi J, et al. (2004) Occludin expression decreases with the progression of human endometrial carcinoma. Hum Pathol 35: 159–164.
20. Tobioka H, Tokunaga Y, Isomura H, Kokai Y, Yamaguchi J, et al. (2004) Expression of occludin, a tight-junction-associated protein, in human lung carcinomas. Virchows Arch 445: 472–476.
21. Iseri OD, Kars MD, Arpaci F, Atalay C, Pak I, et al. (2011) Drug resistant MCF-7 cells exhibit epithelial-mesenchymal transition gene expression pattern. Biomed Pharmacother 65: 40–45.
22. Lemieux E, Bergeron S, Durand V, Asselin C, Saucier C, et al. (2009) Constitutively active MEK1 is sufficient to induce epithelial-to-mesenchymal transition in intestinal epithelial cells and to promote tumor invasion and metastasis. Int J Cancer 125: 1575–1586.
23. Sehrawat A, Singh SV (2011) Benzyl isothiocyanate inhibits epithelial-mesenchymal transition in cultured and xenografted human breast cancer cells. Cancer Prev Res (Phila) 4: 1107–1117.
24. Yang Z, Rayala S, Nguyen D, Vadlamudi RK, Chen S, et al. (2005) Pak1 phosphorylation of snail, a master regulator of epithelial-to-mesenchyme transition, modulates snail's subcellular localization and functions. Cancer Res 65: 3179–3184.
25. Vincent T, Neve EP, Johnson JR, Kukalev A, Rojo F, et al. (2009) A SNAIL1-SMAD3/4 transcriptional repressor complex promotes TGF-beta mediated epithelial-mesenchymal transition. Nat Cell Biol 11: 943–950.
26. Beeman N, Webb PG, Baumgartner HK (2012) Occludin is required for apoptosis when claudin-claudin interactions are disrupted. Cell Death Dis 3: e273.
27. Beeman NE, Baumgartner HK, Webb PG, Schaack JB, Neville MC (2009) Disruption of occludin function in polarized epithelial cells activates the extrinsic pathway of apoptosis leading to cell extrusion without loss of transepithelial resistance. BMC Cell Biol 10: 85.
28. Murata M, Kojima T, Yamamoto T, Go M, Takano K, et al. (2005) Down-regulation of survival signaling through MAPK and Akt in occludin-deficient mouse hepatocytes in vitro. Exp Cell Res 310: 140–151.
29. Yu AS, McCarthy KM, Francis SA, McCormack JM, Lai J, et al. (2005) Knockdown of occludin expression leads to diverse phenotypic alterations in epithelial cells. Am J Physiol Cell Physiol 288: C1231–1241.
30. Osanai M, Murata M, Nishikiori N, Chiba H, Kojima T, et al. (2006) Epigenetic silencing of occludin promotes tumorigenic and metastatic properties of cancer cells via modulations of unique sets of apoptosis-associated genes. Cancer Res 66: 9125–9133.
31. Nemeth Z, Szasz AM, Somoracz A, Tatrai P, Nemeth J, et al. (2009) Zonula occludens-1, occludin, and E-cadherin protein expression in biliary tract cancers. Pathol Oncol Res 15: 533–539.
32. Smalley KS, Brafford P, Haass NK, Brandner JM, Brown E, et al. (2005) Up-regulated expression of zonula occludens protein-1 in human melanoma associates with N-cadherin and contributes to invasion and adhesion. Am J Pathol 166: 1541–1554.
33. Polette M, Mestdagt M, Bindels S, Nawrocki-Raby B, Hunziker W, et al. (2007) Beta-catenin and ZO-1: shuttle molecules involved in tumor invasion-associated epithelial-mesenchymal transition processes. Cells Tissues Organs 185: 61–65.
34. Martin TA, Mason MD, Jiang WG (2011) Tight junctions in cancer metastasis. Frontiers in Bioscience 16: 898–936.
35. Alam M, Ratner D (2001) Cutaneous squamous-cell carcinoma. N Engl J Med 344: 975–983.
36. Bryne M, Koppang HS, Lilleng R, Stene T, Bang G, et al. (1989) New malignancy grading is a better prognostic indicator than Broders' grading in oral squamous cell carcinomas. J Oral Pathol Med 18: 432–437.
37. Weedon D, Morgan MB, Gross C, Nagore E, Yu LL (2006) Squamous cell carcinoma. In: LeBoit PE, Burg G, Weedon D, Sarasin A, editors. World Health Organisation Classification of Tumors Pathology and Genetics: Skin Tumours. Lyon: IARC press. 20–23.

38. Caldwell CJ, Hobbs C, McKee PH (1997) The relationship of Ki67 and involucrin expression in proliferative, pre-neoplastic and neoplastic skin. Clin Exp Dermatol 22: 11–16.
39. Sumitomo S, Kumasa S, Iwai Y, Mori M (1986) Involucrin expression in epithelial tumors of oral and pharyngeal mucosa and skin. Oral Surg Oral Med Oral Pathol 62: 155–163.
40. Watanabe S, Ichikawa E, Takahashi H, Otsuka F (1995) Changes of cytokeratin and involucrin expression in squamous cell carcinomas of the skin during progression to malignancy. Br J Dermatol 132: 730–739.
41. Duvic M, Nelson DC, Annarella M, Cho M, Esgleyes-Ribot T, et al. (1994) Keratinocyte transglutaminase expression varies in squamous cell carcinomas. J Invest Dermatol 102: 462–469.
42. Sober AJ, Burstein JM (1995) Precursors to skin cancer. Cancer 75: 645–650.
43. Langbein L, Pape U-F, Grund C, Kuhn C, Praetzel S, et al. (2003) Tight junction-related structures in the absence of a lumen: Occludin, claudins and tight junction plaque proteins in densely packed cell formations of stratified epithelia and squamous cell carcinomas. Eur J Cell Biol 82: 385–400.
44. Morita K, Tsukita S, Miyachi Y (2004) Tight junction-associated proteins (occludin, ZO-1, claudin-1, claudin-4) in squamous cell carcinoma and Bowen's disease. Br J Dermatol 151: 328–334.
45. Kirschner N, Poetzl C, von den Driesch P, Wladykowski E, Moll I, et al. (2009) Alteration of tight junction proteins is an early event in psoriasis: putative involvement of proinflammatory cytokines. Am J Pathol 175: 1095–1106.
46. Mildner M, Ballaun C, Stichenwirth M, Bauer R, Gmeiner R, et al. (2006) Gene silencing in a human organotypic skin model. Biochem Biophys Res Commun 348: 76–82.
47. Mildner M, Jin J, Eckhart L, Kezic S, Gruber F, et al. (2010) Knockdown of filaggrin impairs diffusion barrier function and increases UV sensitivity in a human skin model. J Invest Dermatol 130: 2286–2294.
48. Elbert M, Cohen D, Musch A (2006) PAR1b promotes cell-cell adhesion and inhibits dishevelled-mediated transformation of Madin-Darby canine kidney cells. Mol Biol Cell 17: 3345–3355.
49. Schindelin J, Arganda-Carreras I, Frise E, Kaynig V, Longair M, et al. (2012) Fiji: an open-source platform for biological-image analysis. Nat Methods 9: 676–682.
50. Van Itallie CM, Anderson JM (1997) Occludin confers adhesiveness when expressed in fibroblasts. J Cell Sci 110 (Pt 9): 1113–1121.
51. Kreusel KM, Fromm M, Schulzke JD, Hegel U (1991) Cl- secretion in epithelial monolayers of mucus-forming human colon cells (HT-29/B6). Am J Physiol Cell Physiol 261: C574–C582.
52. Gunzel D, Stuiver M, Kausalya PJ, Haisch L, Krug SM, et al. (2009) Claudin-10 exists in six alternatively spliced isoforms that exhibit distinct localization and function. J Cell Sci 122: 1507–1517.
53. Fujita H, Sugimoto K, Inatomi S, Maeda T, Osanai M, et al. (2008) Tight junction proteins claudin-2 and -12 are critical for vitamin D-dependent Ca2+ absorption between enterocytes. Mol Biol Cell 19: 1912–1921.
54. Rodust PM, Stockfleth E, Ulrich C, Leverkus M, Eberle J (2009) UV-induced squamous cell carcinoma–a role for antiapoptotic signalling pathways. Br J Dermatol 161 Suppl 3: 107–115.
55. Brusselbach S, Mohle-Steinlein U, Wang ZQ, Schreiber M, Lucibello FC, et al. (1995) Cell proliferation and cell cycle progression are not impaired in fibroblasts and ES cells lacking c-Fos. Oncogene 10: 79–86.
56. Paschoud S, Bongiovanni M, Pache JC, Citi S (2007) Claudin-1 and claudin-5 expression patterns differentiate lung squamous cell carcinomas from adeno-carcinomas. Mod Pathol 20: 947–954.
57. Martinet N, Bonnard L, Regnault V, Picard E, Burke L, et al. (2003) In vivo transglutaminase type 1 expression in normal lung, preinvasive bronchial lesions, and lung cancer. Am J Respir Cell Mol Biol 28: 428–435.
58. Kirschner N, Rosenthal R, Gunzel D, Moll I, Brandner JM (2012) Tight junctions and differentiation–a chicken or the egg question? Exp Dermatol 21: 171–175.
59. Proksch E, Brandner JM, Jensen JM (2008) The skin: an indispensable barrier. Exp Dermatol 17: 1063–1072.
60. Behne MJ, Jensen JM (2012) Calcium in epidermis. Adv Exp Med Biol 740: 945–953.
61. Vicanova J, Boelsma E, Mommaas AM, Kempenaar JA, Forslind B, et al. (1998) Normalization of epidermal calcium distribution profile in reconstructed human epidermis is related to improvement of terminal differentiation and stratum corneum barrier formation. J Invest Dermatol 111: 97–106.
62. Aberle H, Schwartz H, Kemler R (1996) Cadherin-catenin complex: protein interactions and their implications for cadherin function. J Cell Biochem 61: 514–523.
63. Troyanovsky SM (1999) Mechanism of cell-cell adhesion complex assembly. Curr Opin Cell Biol 11: 561–566.
64. Vasioukhin V, Fuchs E (2001) Actin dynamics and cell-cell adhesion in epithelia. Curr Opin Cell Biol 13: 76–84.
65. Gao Y, He L, Katsumi H, Sakane T, Fujita T, et al. (2008) Improvement of intestinal absorption of insulin and water-soluble macromolecular compounds by chitosan oligomers in rats. Int J Pharm 359: 70–78.
66. Barrios-Rodiles M, Brown KR, Ozdamar B, Bose R, Liu Z, et al. (2005) High-throughput mapping of a dynamic signaling network in mammalian cells. Science 307: 1621–1625.
67. Ozdamar B, Bose R, Barrios-Rodiles M, Wang HR, Zhang Y, et al. (2005) Regulation of the polarity protein Par6 by TGFbeta receptors controls epithelial cell plasticity. Science 307: 1603–1609.
68. Viloria-Petit AM, Wrana JL (2010) The TGFbeta-Par6 polarity pathway: linking the Par complex to EMT and breast cancer progression. Cell Cycle 9: 623–624.
69. Pustisek N, Situm M (2011) UV-radiation, apoptosis and skin. Coll Antropol 35 Suppl 2: 339–341.
70. Sayers TJ (2011) Targeting the extrinsic apoptosis signaling pathway for cancer therapy. Cancer Immunol Immunother 60: 1173–1180.
71. Jansen BJ, van Ruissen F, Cerneus S, Cloin W, Bergers M, et al. (2003) Tumor necrosis factor related apoptosis inducing ligand triggers apoptosis in dividing but not in differentiating human epidermal keratinocytes. J Invest Dermatol 121: 1433–1439.
72. Chaturvedi V, Qin JZ, Denning MF, Choubey D, Diaz MO, et al. (1999) Apoptosis in proliferating, senescent, and immortalized keratinocytes. J Biol Chem 274: 23358–23367.
73. Brandner JM, Kief S, Grund C, Rendl M, Houdek P, et al. (2002) Organization and formation of the tight junction system in human epidermis and cultured keratinocytes. Eur J Cell Biol 81: 253–263.
74. Pummi K, Malminen M, Aho H, Karvonen S-L, Peltonen J, et al. (2001) Epidermal tight junctions: ZO-1 and occludin are expressed in mature, developing, and affected skin and in vitro differentiating keratinocytes. Journal of Investigative Dermatology 117: 1050–1058.
75. Ouban A, Hamdan H, Hakam A, Ahmed AA (2011) Claudin-1 Expression in Squamous Cell Carcinomas of Different Organs: Comparative Study of Cancerous Tissues and Normal Controls. Int J Surg Pathol Epub ahead of print.
76. Arabzadeh A, Troy TC, Turksen K (2007) Changes in the distribution pattern of Claudin tight junction proteins during the progression of mouse skin tumorigenesis. BMC Cancer 7: 196.
77. Yamamoto T, Kurasawa M, Hattori T, Maeda T, Nakano H, et al. (2008) Relationship between expression of tight junction-related molecules and perturbed epidermal barrier function in UVB-irradiated hairless mice. Arch Dermatol Res 300: 61–68.
78. Yuki T, Hachiya A, Kusaka A, Sriwiriyanont P, Visscher MO, et al. (2011) Characterization of tight junctions and their disruption by UVB in human epidermis and cultured keratinocytes. J Invest Dermatol 131: 744–752.

18

Loss of Grainy Head-Like 1 Is Associated with Disruption of the Epidermal Barrier and Squamous Cell Carcinoma of the Skin

Michal Mlacki[1], Charbel Darido[2], Stephen M. Jane[2,3], Tomasz Wilanowski[1]*

1 Laboratory of Signal Transduction, Nencki Institute of Experimental Biology, Warsaw, Poland, **2** Department of Medicine, Monash University Central Clinical School, Prahran, Victoria, Australia, **3** Alfred Hospital, Prahran, Victoria, Australia

Abstract

The Grainyhead-like 1 (GRHL1) transcription factor regulates the expression of desmosomal cadherin desmoglein 1 (*Dsg1*) in suprabasal layers of the epidermis. As a consequence, the epidermis of *Grhl1*-null mice displays fewer desmosomes that are abnormal in structure. These mice also exhibit mild chronic skin barrier defects as evidenced by altered keratinocyte terminal differentiation, increased expression of inflammatory markers and infiltration of the skin by immune cells. Exposure of $Grhl1^{-/-}$ mice to a standard chemical skin carcinogenesis protocol results in development of fewer papillomas than in wild type control animals, but with a rate of conversion to squamous cell carcinoma (SCC) that is strikingly higher than in normal littermates. The underlying molecular mechanism differs from mice with conditional ablation of a closely related Grhl family member, *Grhl3*, in the skin, which develop SCC due to the loss of expression of phosphatase and tensin homolog (PTEN) and activation of the phosphatidylinositol 3-kinase (PI3K)/AKT/mechanistic target of rapamycin (mTOR) signaling pathway.

Editor: Amanda Ewart Toland, Ohio State University Medical Center, United States of America

Funding: This work was supported by the European Molecular Biology Organization Installation Grant 2131 (http://www.embo.org/), the Marie Curie International Reintegration rant 256096 (FP7, EU)(http://ec.europa.eu/research/mariecurieactions/), the National Science Centre of Poland predoctoral grant 2011/03/N/NZ3/01957 (http://www.ncn.gov.pl/), supporting scholarship for PhD student in the Mazovia Region (Poland and European Social Fund, EU) (MM) (https://www.oeiizk.waw.pl/doktoranci/and http://ec.europa.eu/esf/), the National Health and Medical Research Council of Australia grant 628365 (http://www.nhmrc.gov.au/), the Association for International Cancer Research grant 11-0060 (http://www.aicr.org.uk/) and by the Victorian Cancer Agency Clare Oliver Fellowship (CD) (http://www.victoriancanceragency.org.au/). The funders had no role in study design, data collection and analysis, decision to publish, or preparation of the manuscript.

Competing Interests: The authors declare that they have no competing interests.

* E-mail: t.wilanowski@nencki.gov.pl

Introduction

Skin, a critical organ in terrestrial animals, constitutes the boundary between organism's interior and external environment, limiting water loss and protecting from mechanical, chemical and pathogenic insults. The functional barrier is formed by the epidermis – the most external layer of the skin. Keratinocytes, cells that make up the epidermis, undergo terminal differentiation – specific and tightly regulated form of cell death. During this process the remains of cells are cross-linked with proteins and lipids, forming hydrophobic and mechanically resistant layer. Proper barrier formation depends on cell-cell junctions, which include desmosomes, adherens junctions and tight junctions, and disruption of their protein content or architecture can cause abnormalities in skin function, eventually leading to diseases ranging from atopic skin reactions to more severe disorders such as palmoplantar keratoderma.

Desmosomes are composed of transmembrane cadherin family members – desmogleins (DSGs) and desmocollins (DSCs), as well as the proteins from plakin family (desmoplakin – DSP) and armadillo family (plakoglobin – JUP and plakophilins – PKPs). Cadherins form homo- and heterodimers with proteins on adjacent cells. Such complexes are connected via JUP, PKPs and DSP with cellular cytoskeleton – intermediate filaments, mainly from the keratin family. Because of their association with keratins, for many years desmosomes were assumed to be passive junctions, responsible only for mechanical endurance of the epidermis. Research of the last 10 years revealed their functions as "connectivity receptors". Today they are recognized as active players in cellular signaling pathways, many of which are linked to cancer development [1]. For instance, DSG1 suppresses the epidermal growth factor receptor (EGFR)/mitogen-activated protein kinase (MAPK) pathway during epidermal differentiation [2], DSC3 functions as a tumor suppressor by inhibiting the EGFR/extracellular signal-regulated kinase (ERK) signaling in human lung cancer [3], DSP acts as a tumor suppressor by inhibiting the wingless-type mouse mammary tumor virus integration site family (Wnt) signaling pathway in human lung cancer [4] and JUP indirectly inhibits Rous sarcoma oncogene (Src) kinase in prostate cancer [5]. Little is known about the involvement of desmosomal components in the development of skin cancers. The most likely candidates for suppressors or supporters of this type of malignancies are proteins responsible for the proper development of epidermis and formation of epidermal barrier.

The transcription factors from the Grainyhead-like (GRHL) family are highly expressed in the epidermis and are crucial for the accurate development and functional features of this organ, even in such evolutionarily distant organisms as insects and mammals. This family has three mammalian members, which are termed GRHL1-3 [6,7]. Previously we reported links between GRHL3 and skin cancer [8]. Mice with skin-specific ablation of *Grhl3* display increased propensity to chemically-induced skin tumorigenesis, and the expression of *GRHL3* is significantly reduced in human SCC samples, compared to the adjacent epidermis. The molecular mechanism underlying the role of GRHL3 in skin cancer is dependent on direct regulation of expression of tumor suppressor PTEN by GRHL3. In human skin tumors both *GRHL3* and *PTEN* are regulated by micro RNA miR-21 [8].

The role of GRHL1 in skin carcinogenesis has not been investigated before. Previously we reported that this transcription factor directly regulates the expression of *Dsg1* and in the epidermis of *Grhl1*$^{-/-}$ mice the desmosomes are fewer in numbers and have abnormal structure [9]. Consequently, epidermis of these animals is thicker and we observe perturbed expression of differentiation markers. On this basis we proposed a hypothesis that the *Grhl1*-null mice have altered susceptibility to the standard chemical skin carcinogenesis protocol. In this article we would like to present results concerning the role of GRHL1 transcription factor in maintenance of the epidermis, in the immunology of the skin, and in skin cancer development.

Materials and Methods

Ethics Statement

This study was carried out in strict accordance with the regulations of the Experiments on Animals Act (Act of 21 January 2005 on experiments on live animals, the Parliament of the Republic of Poland, Dz. U. Nr 33, poz. 289); as well as with the Directive 2010/63/EU of the European Parliament and of the Council of the European Union of 22 September 2010 on the protection of animals used for scientific purposes. All animal experiments were approved by the First Warsaw Local Ethics Committee for Animal Experimentation; permit number 1042/2009. All efforts were made to minimize suffering.

Skin Microscopic Sample Preparation

Mice of age about 6 months were sacrificed and shaved back skin sections were dissected, fixed in 4% paraformaldehyde (Acros Chemicals, Geel, Belgium) in phosphate-buffered saline (PBS) and embedded in paraffin (POCH, Gliwice, Poland). Samples were cut into 10 or 7 µm sections using microtome Hyrax M55 (Zeiss, Jena, Germany) and placed on Superfrost Ultra Plus microscope slides (Thermo Scientific, Waltham, MA, USA). Sections were then deparaffinized with xylene and decreasing concentrations of alcohols.

Immunohistochemistry and Immunofluorescence

Prepared 7 µm skin sections were incubated in citrate buffer at 60°C overnight (antigen retrieval). The endogenous peroxidase activity was blocked by incubation in 1% hydrogen peroxide in PBS for 15 minutes. The following rabbit polyclonal anti-mouse antibodies were used: anti-involucrin (PRB-140C), anti-filaggrin (PRB-417P), anti-loricrin (PRB-145P), anti-keratin 5 (PRB-160P), anti-keratin 6 (PRB-169P), anti-keratin 10 (PRB-159P) (all from Covance, Princeton, NJ, USA). The rabbit monoclonal anti-Ki67 antibody (ab16667) was purchased from Abcam (Cambridge, UK). For immunodetection the 3,3′-diaminobenzidine (DAB) Detection Kit (USA™ Ultra Streptavidin Detection System, Covance, SIG-32232) was used according to the manufacturer's instructions. For immunofluorescence, we followed the Immunofluorescence Standard Protocol published by the Cell Signaling Technology company. The results were documented using microscope (Eclipse 80i, Nikon, Tokyo, Japan) with digital camera.

Skin Infiltration by Mast Cells

Procedure as described in [10]. Skin samples from four *Grhl1*$^{-/-}$ and five *Grhl1*$^{+/+}$ mice were collected. Four different samples from every animal were paraffinized and cut to 10 µm sections. After deparaffinization they were incubated in acidic toluidine blue (Sigma-Aldrich, Munich, Germany) solution (0.1% toluidine blue, 7% ethanol, 1% sodium chloride, pH 2.3) for 5 minutes, thoroughly washed in water and dehydrated in increasing concentrations of alcohols, xylene and mounting medium (DePeX). Using microscope (Eclipse 80i, Nikon) purple mast cells between epidermis and dermal muscle layer were counted. Areas of interest were assessed using ImageJ software.

RNA and cDNA Preparation, Quantitative Real Time Polymerase Chain Reaction (Q-RT-PCR)

Mice of age about 6 months were sacrificed, their back skin dissected and immediately frozen in liquid nitrogen. The samples were ground in mortar in liquid nitrogen, the Ron's FastTRI Extraction Reagent (Bioron, Ludwigshafen, Germany) was added and the solution was homogenized using Polytron (PRO2000, PRO Scientific, Oxford, CT, USA). The RNA was isolated according to the manufacturer's instructions. The RNA was then reverse transcribed into cDNA using Moloney Murine Leukemia Virus (M-MuLV) reverse transcriptase (Bioron) according to the producer's protocol. The Q-RT-PCR reactions were carried out using SYBR Green PCR Mastermix on 7500 Real Time PCR System (Applied BioSystems, Grand Island, NY, USA). Used primers are listed in Table S3. Relative expression levels were standardized to hypoxanthine phosphoribosyltransferase (HPRT) expression, and statistical differences were determined by Student's t-test. In the assay of S100A8 expression, we used six *Grhl1*$^{-/-}$ and six *Grhl1*$^{+/+}$ animals; in the assay of S100A9 expression – five *Grhl1*$^{-/-}$ and five *Grhl1*$^{+/+}$ mice.

Thymic Stromal Lymphopoietin (TSLP) Level Assay

The blood level of TSLP was measured using enzyme-linked immunosorbent assay (ELISA) kit: Quantikine Mouse TSLP (R&D Systems, Minneapolis, MN, USA) according to the manufacturer's instructions, on groups of seven *Grhl1*$^{-/-}$ and five *Grhl1*$^{+/+}$ animals, at the age of about 4 months. Statistical differences were determined by Student's t-test.

Skin Carcinogenesis Protocol

To determine the role of GRHL1 transcription factor in skin carcinogenesis we utilized the well established protocol of chemically induced skin cancers [11]. Briefly, animals at 8–12 weeks of age (n = 15 per group) were shaved and topically treated with single application of tumor initiator 7,12-dimethylbenz[α]anthracene (DMBA) (25 µg dissolved in 150 µl of acetone) followed by twice weekly application of tumor promoter phorbol 12-tetradecanoate 13-acetate (TPA) (7.6 nanomoles dissolved in 200 µl of acetone). The treatment lasted for 30 weeks. Developing papillomas were counted when they reached at least 1 mm in diameter, their appearances were different from the adjacent tissue and remained visible for at least two weeks. Squamous cell carcinomas were counted as lesions that were at least 3.5 mm in diameter and acquired a round, crateriform shape. For ethical reasons mice which developed tumors larger than 1 cm in diameter were sacrificed. Measurements were performed using

ImageJ software. Representative groups of papillomas and carcinomas were histologically analyzed by a certified pathologist – Monika Durzynska, MD, from the Maria Sklodowska-Curie Memorial Cancer Center and Institute of Oncology in Warsaw.

Statistical Analysis

The statistical analysis was performed using Student's t-test incorporated into Microsoft Office Excel 2003 package.

Results

Keratinocytes in *Grhl1*$^{-/-}$ Epidermis Undergo Severely Deregulated Terminal Differentiation

To further characterize the functions of GRHL1 transcription factor, we carried out a detailed examination of the skin of *Grhl1*-null mice. In our previous work we investigated the expression of various keratins and involucrin only on the palmoplantar surfaces of the paws [9]. Now we focused our attention on the expression of relevant markers in the back skin. By histological analysis we showed that epidermis from the back skin of *Grhl1*$^{-/-}$ mice is thicker than in wild type littermates (Fig. 1A–B). Increased thickness of epidermis is recognized as one of the indicators of epidermal defects. To create functional barrier layer of the epidermis, which is formed between stratum granulosum and stratum corneum, it is crucial for epidermal keratinocytes to undergo proper terminal differentiation. To investigate this process in *Grhl1*$^{-/-}$ mice we performed immunohistochemical detection of specific markers (Fig. 1C–L). Epidermal cells of knockout animals undergo full program of terminal differentiation. Keratinocytes of basal layer (with additional cells in suprabasal layers, see later) express basal marker keratin 5, in suprabasal layers there is expression of early (keratin 10) and late differentiation markers (involucrin, filaggrin and loricrin). Cells with characteristic dense cytoplasmic granules, characteristic of stratum granulosum can be easily distinguished (Fig. 1B, F, red arrows). What is noteworthy, cells positive for keratin 5 (marker of basal keratinocytes) can also be detected in suprabasal layers of epidermis (Fig. 1D, black arrows). Furthermore, the expression of a proliferation marker Ki67 is increased in the *Grhl1*$^{-/-}$ epidermis (Fig. 1M–N). This suggests that the suprabasal keratinocytes in the skin of *Grhl1*-null mice exhibit severe deregulation of terminal differentiation program, which may lead to thickening of the epidermis and subacute impairment of epidermal barrier.

Grhl1$^{-/-}$ Mice Exhibit Mild Chronic Skin Barrier Defects

Mild impairments in epidermal barrier function are often accompanied by chronic activation of skin's immune system, hence specific markers of inflammation can serve as indicators of barrier function [12]. For that reason we investigated the activation of skin's immune system in *Grhl1*$^{-/-}$ mice. One of the markers of disrupted epidermal barrier and skin's allergic reaction is cytokine TSLP. Its high expression in keratinocytes and elevated level in blood is correlated with epidermal dysfunction and chronic inflammation [13]. Using ELISA we measured the level of this cytokine in the blood of *Grhl1*$^{-/-}$ mice and their wild type littermates. In the blood of knockout animals we detected significantly higher levels of TSLP than in the wild type controls (Fig. 2A; p = 0.0021). We employed the Q-RT-PCR method to measure the expression of other markers of subacute disruption of skin barrier – antimicrobial peptides S100A8 and S100A9 [14]. We detected significantly increased levels of expression of both these markers in knockout animals' epidermis. Relative expression of S100A8 in *Grhl1*$^{-/-}$ mice was 2.37, SD = 0.71; and in the wild

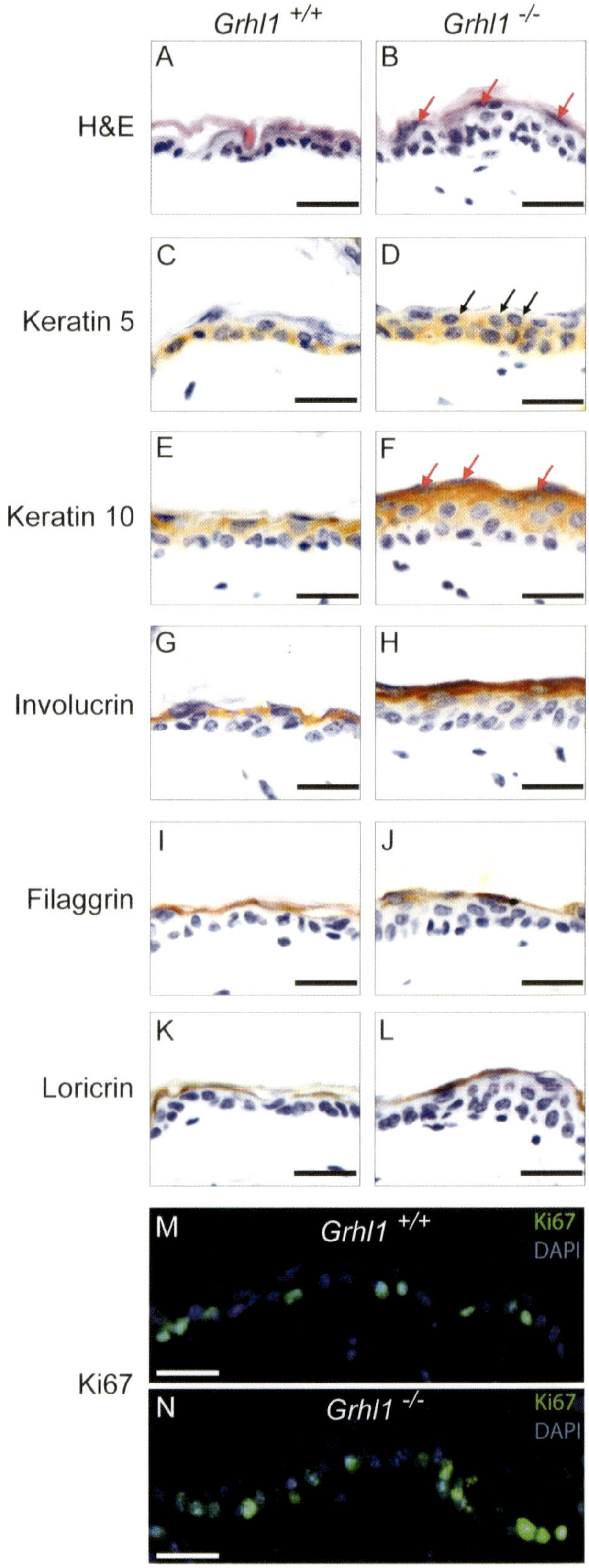

Figure 1. Histological analysis of the skin of *Grhl1*$^{-/-}$ mice (right panels) in comparison to wild type littermates *Grhl1*$^{+/+}$ (left panels). Scale bars represent 25 μm. (A–B) Hematoxylin and eosin (H&E) staining of epidermis of *Grhl1*$^{+/+}$ and *Grhl1*$^{-/-}$ mice; red arrows point to keratinocytes from granular layer of epidermis. (C–L)

Immunohistochemical analysis of markers of epidermal differentiation in the epidermis of *Grhl1*$^{+/+}$ and *Grhl1*$^{-/-}$ mice: marker of basal layer – keratin 5 (C, D, black arrows indicate suprabasal keratinocytes expressing keratin 5), marker of early terminal differentiation – keratin 10 (E, F, red arrows point to keratinocytes from the granular layer of epidermis), markers of late terminal differentiation – involucrin (G, H), filaggrin (I, J), loricrin (K, L). (M, N) Immunofluorescence staining of proliferation marker Ki67 in *Grhl1*$^{+/+}$ (M) and *Grhl1*$^{-/-}$ (N) mice.
doi:10.1371/journal.pone.0089247.g001

type controls 1.00, SD = 0.68 (p = 0.0066). In the case of S100A9, relative expression in *Grhl1*$^{-/-}$ mice was 5.52, SD = 3.15, and in the wild type controls 1.00, SD = 0.79 (p = 0.0091) (Fig. 2B).

Antimicrobial peptides and TSLP are known to act as chemoattractants and their elevated levels in the skin induce its infiltration with immune cells, as detailed in a recent review [15]. To detect immune cells in the dermis we stained skin sections with toluidine blue, which labels cells containing granules rich in histamine and heparin, mainly mast cells. After such staining they are visible as purple cells. Data was documented by photography (Fig. 2C). Results were quantified using ImageJ software as a number of cells per 1 mm^2 of 10 µm thick section of skin. *Grhl1*$^{-/-}$ mice have significantly more stained cells (79.8 cells/mm^2; SD = 18.5 cells/mm^2) than their wild type littermates (47.7 cells/mm^2; SD = 5.0 cells/mm^2) (p = 0.00001) (Fig. 2D). These results

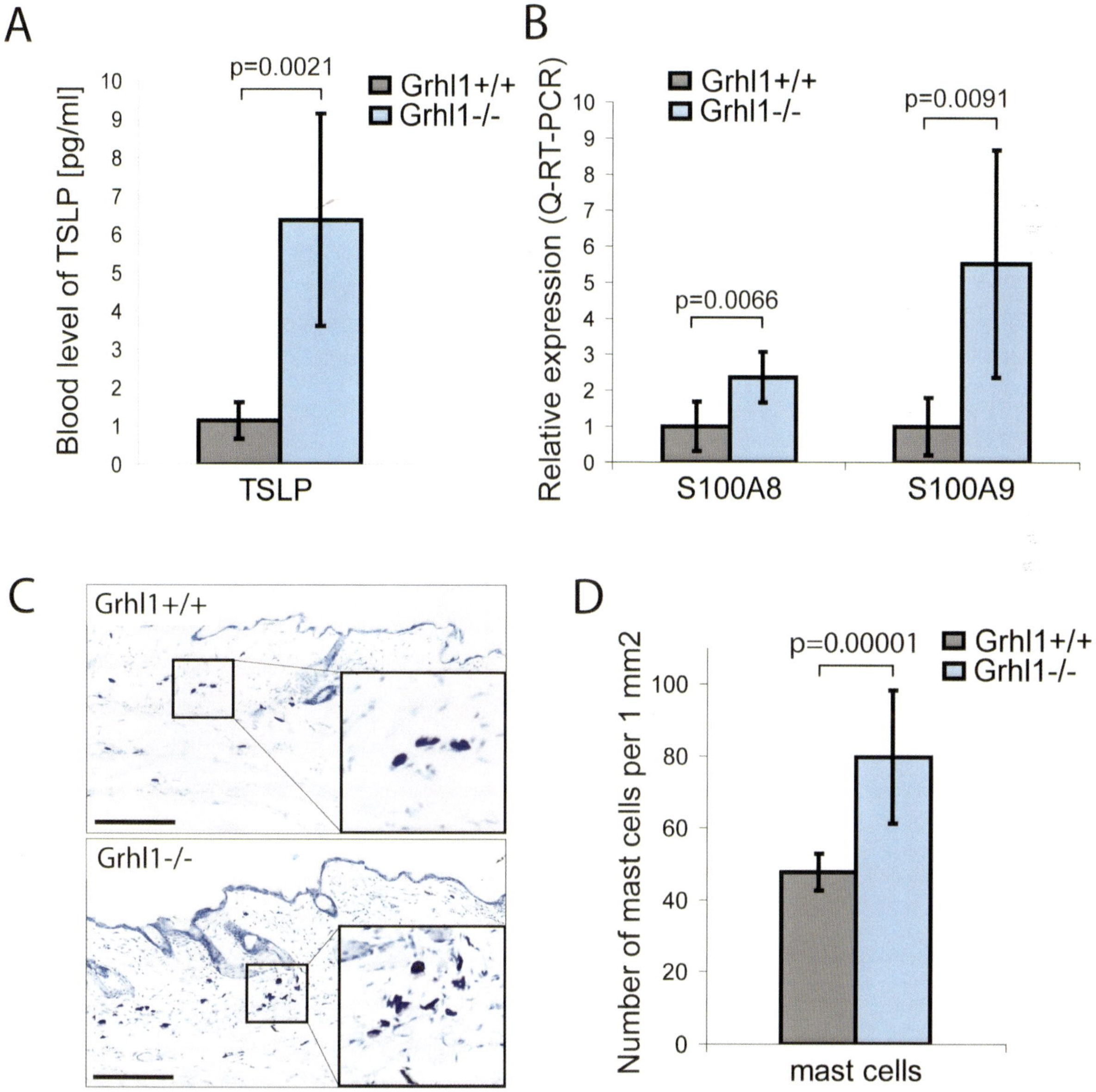

Figure 2. Skin inflammation in *Grhl1*$^{-/-}$ mice. (A) Blood levels of TSLP in *Grhl1*$^{+/+}$ (gray bar) and *Grhl1*$^{-/-}$ mice (blue bar), measured with ELISA kit. (B) Levels of expression of antimicrobial peptides S100A8 and S100A9 in the epidermis of *Grhl1*$^{+/+}$ (gray bar) and *Grhl1*$^{-/-}$ mice (blue bar), measured with Q-RT-PCR. (C) Representative skin sections of *Grhl1*$^{+/+}$ (top panel) and *Grhl1*$^{-/-}$ mice (bottom panel) stained with toluidine blue to visualize dermal mast cells (purple cells). Scale bars represent 200 µm. (D) Quantification of skin infiltration with mast cells for *Grhl1*$^{+/+}$ (gray bar) and *Grhl1*$^{-/-}$ mice (blue bar), estimated as numbers of stained cells per 1 mm^2 area of 10 µm thick skin section (using ImageJ software). (A, B, D) Significance (Student's t-test, p-value) is shown above bars.

indicate that the *Grhl1*$^{-/-}$ mice exhibit mild chronic skin inflammation.

Grhl1 −/− Mice Develop more Skin Tumors with Earlier Onset than Grhl1+/+ Littermates

It has recently been proposed that any mouse model with subacute skin barrier defects may display increased propensity to chemically-induced skin tumor development [16]. *Grhl1*$^{-/-}$ animals do not develop spontaneous tumors, even in old age, and the observable lifespan and activity of these mice in old age are the same as in control wild type littermates (Table S1). This suggests that loss of GRHL1 transcription factor alone is insufficient to induce cancerous transformation. However, the genetic background of *Grhl1* KO mice is C57BL/6 (Black 6), and this mouse strain is very resistant to skin tumorigenesis, which may explain why we did not observe spontaneous tumors in the *Grhl1*-null mice [17]. Therefore we applied the standard two-stage skin carcinogenesis protocol in *Grhl1*$^{-/-}$ and *Grhl1*$^{+/+}$ mice, using DMBA and TPA as tumor inducer and promoter, respectively (Fig. 3A) [11,18]. In this experiment we used 15 mice of each genotype, at the starting age of 2–3 months. The representative appearance of *Grhl1*$^{-/-}$ and *Grhl1*$^{+/+}$ mice after 30 weeks of TPA treatment is presented in Fig. 3B. The histological analysis was performed by certified pathologist – Monika Durzynska, MD, from the Maria Sklodowska-Curie Memorial Cancer Center and Institute of Oncology, Warsaw. This assay revealed no differences in types of lesions between control and *Grhl1*$^{-/-}$ mice, and all analyzed samples were papillomas or highly differentiated SCC. In the wild type mice, 26 overall lesions (28%) were examined by the certified pathologist, which included 10 SCC (100%). In the *Grhl1*-null mice, 32 overall lesions (65%) were examined by Ms Durzynska, which included 12 SCC (57%). The hematoxylin and eosin staining of a representative squamous cell tumor from a knockout animal is presented on Fig. 3C.

We did not observe significant differences between *Grhl1*$^{+/+}$ and *Grhl1*$^{-/-}$ mice in the onset of development of papillomas. In both groups the first papillomas appeared after 5 weeks of TPA treatment (Fig. 3E). In total the *Grhl1*$^{-/-}$ mice developed 49 papillomas, *Grhl1*$^{+/+}$ –94 papillomas ($p = 0.022$). The number of mice which developed papillomas was similar –14 and 13 mice, respectively, out of 15 mice in each group (Fig. 3D). These results suggest again that loss of GRHL1 transcription factor has no impact on timing of cancerous transformation of keratinocytes, but it reduces the occurrence of papillomas.

During the experiment some papillomas regressed. This affected 32 papillomas (34%) in *Grhl1*$^{+/+}$ mice and 4 papillomas (8%) in *Grhl1*$^{-/-}$ mice. Fig. 3D provides the sum total of all the papillomas that appeared on all the mice of a particular genotype during the experiment, and diagram 3E shows the average number of papillomas per mouse at given time points. Some papillomas progressed to SCC (Fig. 3D). In total *Grhl1*$^{-/-}$ mice developed 21 such tumors and wild type littermates –10; SCC arose in 10 *Grhl1*-null and 6 wild type mice. What is noteworthy, in *Grhl1*$^{-/-}$ mice almost 43% of papillomas progressed to SCC, whereas in the control animals – fewer than 11% ($p = 0.0031$). The onset of SCC was also accelerated – the first carcinomas in *Grhl1*-null mice were observed after 12 weeks of TPA treatment, and in *Grhl1*$^{+/+}$ mice – after 22 weeks ($p = 0.0007$) (Fig. 3F–G). Moreover, we also observed differences in size of carcinomas – in the case of *Grhl1*$^{+/+}$ mice only one animal developed SCC larger than 1 cm in diameter before the 30th week of experiment and had to be sacrificed for ethical reasons, whereas in *Grhl1*$^{-/-}$ mice – five animals had to be sacrificed for these reasons (Fig. 3D). This suggests that loss of *Grhl1* accelerates progression from benign papilloma to SCC, and positively influences the size of carcinomas.

Discussion

Our research interests concern the GRHL1 transcription factor and its role in the skin. Previously we demonstrated that this protein is confined to differentiating subrabasal keratinocytes in the epidermis and to the inner root sheath of hair follicle, but is absent from the dermal papilla [9]. The *Grhl1*$^{-/-}$ mice are viable and fertile, but they show initial delay in coat growth, and older mice have sparse fur and poor anchorage of hair shaft in the follicle which leads to extensive hair loss. They also display thickening of the epidermis on the palmoplantar surfaces of their paws, which is reminiscent of palmoplantar keratoderma, a disorder caused by mutations in the *DSG1* gene in human patients [19,20]. Accordingly, the epidermal desmosomes in *Grhl1*-null mice are shorter, less well organized and sensitive to ethylene glycol tetraacetic acid (EGTA), which is indicative of their reduced stability [9].

Here we present our results of a detailed analysis of epidermal function in the *Grhl1*$^{-/-}$ mice. Previously we reported that the GRHL1 transcription factor regulates the expression of a gene coding for desmosomal cadherin desmoglein 1 (*Dsg1*) [9]. This protein is a main constituent of cell-cell adhesion complexes between suprabasal keratinocytes – desmosomes, and is also a regulator of induction of terminal differentiation of keratinocytes [2]. What is noteworthy, we have shown before that the levels of expression of other markers of basal keratinocytes – DSG2 and DSG3– are increased in *Grhl1*-null mice [9]. These animals display the thickening of squamous layer. Thickening of the epidermis over areas exposed to mechanical forces is a typical response of healthy skin, but it may occur at low levels of mechanical stress if the mechanical endurance of the skin is compromised [21]. In the *Grhl1*$^{-/-}$ mice the level of DSG1 is insufficient for formation of properly composed suprabasal desmosomes, which results in numerous desmosomal defects and is likely to reduce the mechanical resistance of the skin. The observed epidermal response was exclusively dependent on changes in DSG1 expression, as the levels of components of other cell adhesion complexes are not altered in the *Grhl1*$^{-/-}$ mice [9]. GRHL1 is expressed in the same epidermal cells as DSG1, and in the *Grhl1*$^{-/-}$ animals the production of this cadherin is reduced, which leads to the thickening of innermost, keratin 5-positive cell layer. By study of other differentiation markers we demonstrated that the suprabasal keratinocytes in the skin of *Grhl1*-null mice exhibit severe deregulation of terminal differentiation program, which may lead to thickening of the epidermis and subacute impairment of epidermal barrier.

In our subsequent experiments we investigated whether the *Grhl1*$^{-/-}$ mice display symptoms of skin barrier defects. In the mutant animals we observed elevated blood levels of a marker of response to barrier defects TSLP, an interleukin-7-like cytokine. When secreted by epithelial cells, this factor stimulates tissue infiltration with immune cells and facilitates their activation [13]. Other markers of defective barrier are antimicrobial peptides S100A8 and S100A9. Genes coding for these Ca^{2+}-dependent alarm factors belong to epidermal differentiation complex (EDC) [22,23]. In the unaffected epidermis the expression of S100A8 and S100A9 is low, but it is strongly stimulated upon induction of chronic inflammation. These proteins act as chemoattractants and their elevated secretion by keratinocytes induces dermal infiltration by immune cells. In addition, S100 proteins are increasingly recognized as major regulators of tumor promoting inflammatory

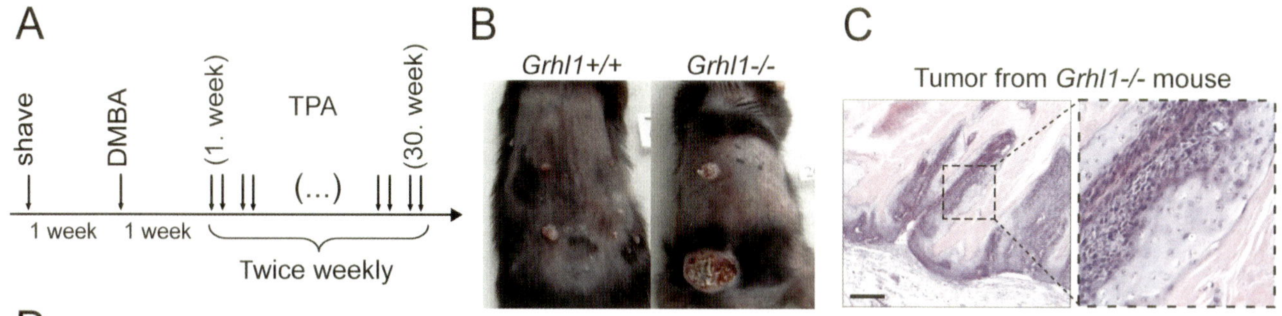

D

genotype	number of animals in the experiment	total number of papillomas	number of mice with papillomas	total number of SCC	number of mice with SCC	% of papillomas progressed to SCC	number of mice with SCC >1cm
Grhl1+/+	15	94	14	10	6	10.64%	1
Grhl1-/-	15	49	13	21	10	42.86%	5

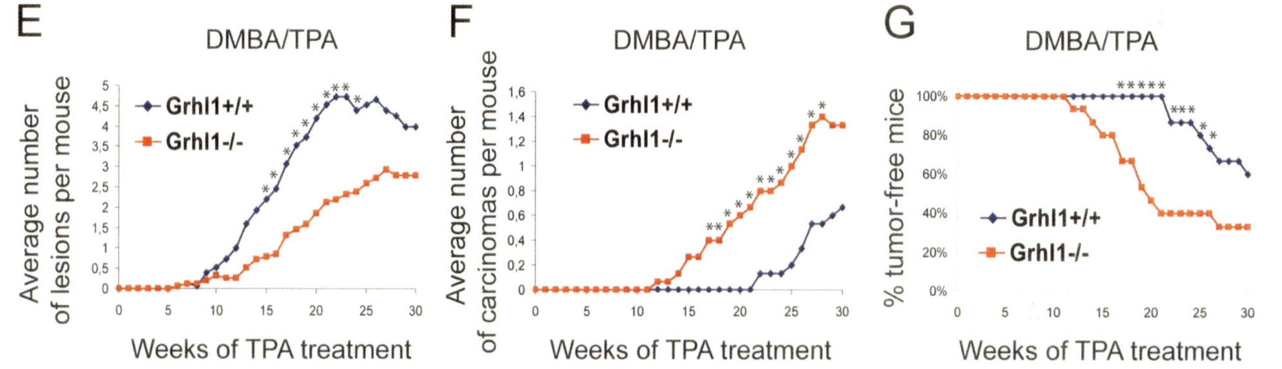

Figure 3. Skin carcinogenesis in *Grhl1*$^{-/-}$ and control mice. (A) Timeline of DMBA/TPA treatment in two-stage chemically-induced skin tumor development protocol. (B) Representative *Grhl1*$^{-/-}$ and *Grhl1*$^{+/+}$ mice after 30 weeks of TPA treatment. (C) Hematoxylin and eosin staining of a representative SCC tumor from a *Grhl1*$^{-/-}$ mouse at low (left panel) and high magnification (right panel); scale bar represents 200 µm. (D) Summary of the results. (E–F) Average number of: (E) papillomas; (F) squamous cell tumors; (G) Kaplan-Meier analysis presenting tumor free mice in relation to the time of experiment. *Grhl1*$^{-/-}$ – red lines; *Grhl1*$^{+/+}$ – blue lines. Asterisks indicate time points at which differences between the two groups of animals were statistically significant ($p<0.05$).

microenvironment [24]. Therefore we measured the levels of these markers in the epidermis of *Grhl1*$^{-/-}$ mice and we observed increased expression of S100A8 and S100A9. Moreover, the expressional microarray on whole skin (epidermis and dermis) of *Grhl1*$^{-/-}$ mice (Table S2 and [9]) revealed upregulation of genes from the small proline-rich family (SPRR) which also belong to EDC – *Sprr2d* (fold change more than 2), as well as *Sprr2g*, *Sprr2e*, *Sprr2a*, *Sprr1a* (fold change between 1 and 2). SPRR proteins form scaffold for other proteins in the cornified envelope of epidermis and are highly upregulated in the skin of barrier-deficient mouse models [22,25]. Furthermore, the upregulation of other genes associated with inflammation was also detected in this experiment, including the chemokines from chemokine C-X-C motif ligand (CXCL) family *Cxcl1*, *Cxcl9*, *Cxcl16*; beta-defensins *Defb4*, *Defb6*, *Defb14*; and others. Many of them have been associated with cancerous transformation (Table 1). Among the upregulated genes we also discovered genes coding for proteins specific for mast cells – multiple C2 domains, transmembrane 1 (*Mctp1*), *Mctp4* and protease, serine, 22 (*Prss22*) (Table S2). This prompted us to assess the number of immune cells infiltrating the skin. In the skin from *Grhl1*$^{-/-}$ mice we detected increased count of toluidine blue stained cells, that are recognized as mast cells. These are known to support the development of SCC [26]. The described gene signature and infiltration with immune cells agree with the notion that the *Grhl1*$^{-/-}$ mice exhibit mild skin barrier impairments.

Recent research showed that mice with subacute skin barrier defects may be more prone to chemically-induced skin tumor development [16]. The authors suggested that the underlying mechanism is general and is dependent on development of tumor-promoting chronic inflammatory microenvironment in the skin. Here we present data concerning the role of GRHL1 transcription factor in development of skin cancers. The *Grhl1*-null mice do not develop spontaneous tumors, even in old age, and their life span is the same as that of their *Grhl1*$^{+/+}$ littermates (Table S1). In the standard skin chemical carcinogenesis protocol the timing of papilloma development is the same in the *Grhl1*$^{-/-}$ mice and in their wild type littermates. This observation suggests that loss of *Grhl1* has no impact on timing of initiation of cancerous transformation of keratinocytes. However, the mutant mice developed significantly fewer papillomas, but the progression to

Table 1. List of some of the genes that are upregulated in the *Grhl1*$^{-/-}$ skin.

Gene name	Accession no.	Literature links to inflammation	Literature links to cancer
Cxcl1	NM_008176.1	[38]	[39,40]
Cxcl9	NM_008599.1	[38]	[41,42]
Cxcl16	NM_023158.3	[38,43]	[44,45]
Defb4	NM_019728.2	[46,47]	
Defb6	NM_054074.1	[48]	
Defb14/Defb3	NM_183026.1	[47]	[49]
Prss18/Klk6	NM_011177	[50,51]	[52,53]
Prss22	NM_133731.1	[54]	
Slpi	NM_011414.1	[55,56]	[57]
Stfa1	NM_001001332	[58]	[59,60]
Sprr2d	NM_011470.1	[61]	
Saa1	NM_009117.1	[62]	[63,64]
Saa3	NM_011315	[65]	[65]
Hpxn	NM_017371.1	[66]	
Hp	NM_017370.1	[66]	
Aldh3a1	NM_007436.1	[67]	
Serpina1b	NM_009244.2	[68]	[69]
Ier3	NM_133662.1	[70]	[70]

Full list of genes with fold changes higher than 2 is provided in Table S2.

squamous cell tumors was dramatically increased, with almost 43% of papillomas progressing to carcinomas, in comparison with wild type littermates, where the progression rate was under 11%. The tumors in knockout mice were also bigger in size and had earlier onset. In the light of these results we can state that loss of *Grhl1* supports the progression of papillomas to carcinomas in a mouse model.

The *Grhl1*$^{-/-}$ mice develop more carcinomas but fewer papillomas than their wild type littermate controls. This is a very unusual phenotype, but it is reminiscent of the *p53*-deficient mice [27]. p53 is a well known tumor suppressor [28]. Surprisingly, following the DMBA/TPA chemical skin carcinogenesis protocol, the *p53*$^{-/-}$ mice developed about five times fewer papillomas than their *p53*$^{+/+}$ and *p53*$^{+/-}$ littermates, and this result was statistically significant. In contrast, the frequency of conversion from papillomas to carcinomas was increased from 3% in wild type mice to 43% in *p53*-null mice. The onset of papillomas was the same in *p53*$^{-/-}$, *p53*$^{+/-}$ and *p53*$^{+/+}$ animals, but the onset of SCC in *p53*-null mice was much earlier than in their wild type and heterozygous littermates. The authors also reported regression of some papillomas in the *p53*$^{+/+}$ and *p53*$^{+/-}$ mice during the last five weeks of the experiment [27]. We obtained very similar results for the *Grhl1* knockout mice (Fig. 3D–G). The increased conversion rate from papillomas to SCC in the *p53*-null mice can be explained by the tumor suppressor properties of p53, while the decreased occurrence of papillomas in *p53*$^{-/-}$ mice is most likely caused by the activation of p53-independent apoptotic pathway [29]. It is thus possible that analogous mechanisms are responsible for the involvement of GRHL1 in skin carcinogenesis.

Yet another possible explanation for the decrease in the number of papillomas accompanied by an increased number of carcinomas is provided by recent research proposing different cells of origin of long-lived papillomas and papillomas progressing to carcinomas [30–33]. The former originate from the interfollicular epidermis, while the latter – from keratinocytes of the hair follicle. We have reported before that the epidermal defects in *Grhl1*$^{-/-}$ mice are relatively minor: the impermeability of skin barrier is not compromised; the Nikolsky sign for epidermal fragility is negative; and wound healing is unaffected. On the other hand, the impairments of hair follicles are much more severe: the hair anchoring is defective, and the structure of depilated hair follicles is completely different from the controls [9]. Thus the desmosomal defects in the *Grhl1*$^{-/-}$ mice are likely to have different effects on the keratinocytes in hair follicles and in interfollicular epidermis, which could explain why the mutant mice develop fewer papillomas but more carcinomas in skin carcinogenesis experiments.

There are several other mechanisms that may contribute towards the observed phenotype of *Grhl1*$^{-/-}$ mice, and these will need to be investigated in future studies. There may exist as yet unidentified additional target genes of GRHL1 regulation whose expression is dysregulated in the *Grhl1*-null mice, and this dysregulation may play a part in the decrease in papilloma incidence and increased conversion rate of papillomas to SCC. Another plausible mechanism involves changes to stem cells: the interfollicular stem cells may be impaired, while the hair follicle bulge stem cells may be expanded. The balance between proliferation and apoptosis may be disrupted in the *Grhl1*$^{-/-}$ epidermis as well. All these alternative mechanisms may be relevant to skin carcinogenesis in the *Grhl1*-null mice.

In our previous publication we described links between the GRHL3 transcription factor and skin cancer [8]. In that paper we reported that similarly to GRHL1, GRHL3 also has a protective role against skin carcinogenesis. Here we demonstrate that, even though GRHL1 and GRHL3 share a high degree of sequence homology, have almost identical target DNA binding sites and display very similar expression patterns in the epidermis [34], the molecular mechanisms linking them to cancer are very different.

GRHL3 inhibits epidermal tumorigenesis through direct regulation of tumor suppressor PTEN. Here we present evidence that GRHL1 does not regulate the expression of PTEN (Fig. S1), and that it protects against skin carcinogenesis by regulating the maintenance of skin barrier. This observation is consistent with our earlier report that, despite recognizing the same consensus DNA binding sequence, in living cells different GRHL factors regulate the expression of different target genes [35].

In summary, we report here that the *Grhl1*-null mice display increased susceptibility to chemically induced SCC. The underlying molecular mechanism is most likely related to the subacute skin barrier defects in these mice. Similar observations have been made using other mouse models; however, the molecular pathway has never been delineated that would link skin barrier impairments to increased tumor occurrence. At the present moment it is known that regardless of the cause of skin barrier disruption; whether it is brought about by alterations in the Notch signaling pathway [16], or in the Wnt signaling pathway [36], or by targeting a desmosomal component [37], or by ablation of the *Grhl1* gene (present study); in all these cases a not yet characterized skin barrier-dependent, tumor-promoting pathway is triggered which leads to increased cancer susceptibility. Characterizing this pathway presents a very important direction for future research.

Supporting Information

Figure S1 Relative expression of *Pten* gene in the epidermis of *Grhl1*-null mice and control animals, measured by Q-RT-PCR ($p = 0.96$).

Table S1 Age-related spontaneous cancer development in *Grhl1*-null mice and control animals.

Table S2 Upregulated genes (fold change min. 2.0) in *Grhl1*$^{-/-}$ mouse skin.

Table S3 List of primers used in Q-RT-PCR. The abbreviations are: R – reverse, F – forward.

Materials and Methods S1 Spontaneous cancers development. Microarray analysis of *Grhl1*$^{+/+}$ and *Grhl1*$^{-/-}$ mouse skin.

Acknowledgments

We thank Monika Durzynska for assistance with histopathological analyses; Carolyn de Graaf for help in analyzing the results of microarray experiments; Agnieszka Graczyk for supply of PCR primers; Lucjan Wyrwicz for helpful discussions; and the staff from the Nencki Institute Animal House for animal care.

Author Contributions

Conceived and designed the experiments: SMJ TW. Performed the experiments: MM CD. Analyzed the data: MM SMJ TW. Contributed reagents/materials/analysis tools: SMJ. Wrote the paper: MM TW.

References

1. Dusek RL, Attardi LD (2011) Desmosomes: new perpetrators in tumour suppression. Nature reviews Cancer 11: 317–323.
2. Getsios S, Simpson CL, Kojima S, Harmon R, Sheu LJ, et al. (2009) Desmoglein 1-dependent suppression of EGFR signaling promotes epidermal differentiation and morphogenesis. The Journal of cell biology 185: 1243–1258.
3. Cui T, Chen Y, Yang L, Knosel T, Huber O, et al. (2012) The p53 target gene desmocollin 3 acts as a novel tumor suppressor through inhibiting EGFR/ERK pathway in human lung cancer. Carcinogenesis 33: 2326–2333.
4. Yang L, Chen Y, Cui T, Knosel T, Zhang Q, et al. (2012) Desmoplakin acts as a tumor suppressor by inhibition of the Wnt/beta-catenin signaling pathway in human lung cancer. Carcinogenesis 33: 1863–1870.
5. Franzen CA, Todorovic V, Desai BV, Mirzoeva S, Yang XJ, et al. (2012) The desmosomal armadillo protein plakoglobin regulates prostate cancer cell adhesion and motility through vitronectin-dependent Src signaling. PLoS One 7: e42132.
6. Ting SB, Wilanowski T, Cerruti L, Zhao LL, Cunningham JM, et al. (2003) The identification and characterization of human Sister-of-Mammalian Grainyhead (SOM) expands the grainyhead-like family of developmental transcription factors. The Biochemical journal 370: 953–962.
7. Wilanowski T, Tuckfield A, Cerruti L, O'Connell S, Saint R, et al. (2002) A highly conserved novel family of mammalian developmental transcription factors related to Drosophila grainyhead. Mechanisms of development 114: 37–50.
8. Darido C, Georgy SR, Wilanowski T, Dworkin S, Auden A, et al. (2011) Targeting of the Tumor Suppressor GRHL3 by a miR-21-Dependent Proto-Oncogenic Network Results in PTEN Loss and Tumorigenesis. Cancer Cell 20: 635–648.
9. Wilanowski T, Caddy J, Ting SB, Hislop NR, Cerruti L, et al. (2008) Perturbed desmosomal cadherin expression in grainy head-like 1-null mice. The EMBO journal 27: 886–897.
10. Kitamura Y, Go S, Hatanaka K (1978) Decrease of mast cells in W/Wv mice and their increase by bone marrow transplantation. Blood 52: 447–452.
11. Nibbs RJ, Gilchrist DS, King V, Ferra A, Forrow S, et al. (2007) The atypical chemokine receptor D6 suppresses the development of chemically induced skin tumors. The Journal of clinical investigation 117: 1884–1892.
12. Segre JA (2006) Epidermal barrier formation and recovery in skin disorders. The Journal of clinical investigation 116: 1150–1158.
13. Demehri S, Liu Z, Lee J, Lin MH, Crosby SD, et al. (2008) Notch-deficient skin induces a lethal systemic B-lymphoproliferative disorder by secreting TSLP, a sentinel for epidermal integrity. PLoS biology 6: e123.
14. Aberg KM, Man MQ, Gallo RL, Ganz T, Crumrine D, et al. (2008) Co-regulation and interdependence of the mammalian epidermal permeability and antimicrobial barriers. The Journal of investigative dermatology 128: 917–925.
15. Bangert C, Brunner PM, Stingl G (2011) Immune functions of the skin. Clinics in dermatology 29: 360–376.
16. Demehri S, Turkoz A, Kopan R (2009) Epidermal Notch1 loss promotes skin tumorigenesis by impacting the stromal microenvironment. Cancer Cell 16: 55–66.
17. Sundberg JP, Sundberg BA, Beamer WG (1997) Comparison of chemical carcinogen skin tumor induction efficacy in inbred, mutant, and hybrid strains of mice: morphologic variations of induced tumors and absence of a papillomavirus cocarcinogen. Molecular carcinogenesis 20: 19–32.
18. Balmain A, Pragnell IB (1983) Mouse skin carcinomas induced in vivo by chemical carcinogens have a transforming Harvey-ras oncogene. Nature 303: 72–74.
19. Rickman L, Simrak D, Stevens HP, Hunt DM, King IA, et al. (1999) N-terminal deletion in a desmosomal cadherin causes the autosomal dominant skin disease striate palmoplantar keratoderma. Hum Mol Genet 8: 971–976.
20. Hunt DM, Rickman L, Whittock NV, Eady RA, Simrak D, et al. (2001) Spectrum of dominant mutations in the desmosomal cadherin desmoglein 1, causing the skin disease striate palmoplantar keratoderma. Eur J Hum Genet 9: 197–203.
21. Kottke MD, Delva E, Kowalczyk AP (2006) The desmosome: cell science lessons from human diseases. J Cell Sci 119: 797–806.
22. Patel S, Kartasova T, Segre JA (2003) Mouse Sprr locus: a tandem array of coordinately regulated genes. Mammalian genome : official journal of the International Mammalian Genome Society 14: 140–148.
23. Mischke D, Korge BP, Marenholz I, Volz A, Ziegler A (1996) Genes encoding structural proteins of epidermal cornification and S100 calcium-binding proteins form a gene complex ("epidermal differentiation complex") on human chromosome 1q21. The Journal of investigative dermatology 106: 989–992.
24. Lukanidin E, Sleeman JP (2012) Building the niche: the role of the S100 proteins in metastatic growth. Seminars in cancer biology 22: 216–225.
25. Koch PJ, de Viragh PA, Scharer E, Bundman D, Longley MA, et al. (2000) Lessons from loricrin-deficient mice: compensatory mechanisms maintaining skin barrier function in the absence of a major cornified envelope protein. The Journal of cell biology 151: 389–400.
26. Coussens LM, Raymond WW, Bergers G, Laig-Webster M, Behrendtsen O, et al. (1999) Inflammatory mast cells up-regulate angiogenesis during squamous epithelial carcinogenesis. Genes & development 13: 1382–1397.
27. Kemp CJ, Donehower LA, Bradley A, Balmain A (1993) Reduction of p53 gene dosage does not increase initiation or promotion but enhances malignant progression of chemically induced skin tumors. Cell 74: 813–822.
28. Hainaut P, Wiman KG (2009) 30 years and a long way into p53 research. Lancet Oncol 10: 913–919.

29. Greenhalgh DA, Wang XJ, Donehower LA, Roop DR (1996) Paradoxical tumor inhibitory effect of p53 loss in transgenic mice expressing epidermal-targeted v-rasHa, v-fos, or human transforming growth factor alpha. Cancer Res 56: 4413–4423.
30. Bailleul B, Surani MA, White S, Barton SC, Brown K, et al. (1990) Skin hyperkeratosis and papilloma formation in transgenic mice expressing a ras oncogene from a suprabasal keratin promoter. Cell 62: 697–708.
31. Brown K, Strathdee D, Bryson S, Lambie W, Balmain A (1998) The malignant capacity of skin tumours induced by expression of a mutant H-ras transgene depends on the cell type targeted. Current biology : CB 8: 516–524.
32. Frame S, Balmain A (2000) Integration of positive and negative growth signals during ras pathway activation in vivo. Current opinion in genetics & development 10: 106–113.
33. Blanpain C (2013) Tracing the cellular origin of cancer. Nat Cell Biol 15: 126–134.
34. Auden A, Caddy J, Wilanowski T, Ting SB, Cunningham JM, et al. (2006) Spatial and temporal expression of the Grainyhead-like transcription factor family during murine development. Gene Expr Patterns 6: 964–970.
35. Boglev Y, Wilanowski T, Caddy J, Parekh V, Auden A, et al. (2011) The unique and cooperative roles of the Grainy head-like transcription factors in epidermal development reflect unexpected target gene specificity. Developmental biology 349: 512–522.
36. Augustin I, Gross J, Baumann D, Korn C, Kerr G, et al. (2013) Loss of epidermal Evi/Wls results in a phenotype resembling psoriasiform dermatitis. J Exp Med 210: 1761–1777.
37. Beaudry VG, Jiang D, Dusek RL, Park EJ, Knezevich S, et al. (2010) Loss of the p53/p63 regulated desmosomal protein Perp promotes tumorigenesis. PLoS Genet 6: e1001168.
38. He D, Li H, Yusuf N, Elmets CA, Athar M, et al. (2012) IL-17 mediated inflammation promotes tumor growth and progression in the skin. PLoS One 7: e32126.
39. Kawanishi H, Matsui Y, Ito M, Watanabe J, Takahashi T, et al. (2008) Secreted CXCL1 is a potential mediator and marker of the tumor invasion of bladder cancer. Clinical cancer research : an official journal of the American Association for Cancer Research 14: 2579–2587.
40. Bolitho C, Hahn MA, Baxter RC, Marsh DJ (2010) The chemokine CXCL1 induces proliferation in epithelial ovarian cancer cells by transactivation of the epidermal growth factor receptor. Endocrine-related cancer 17: 929–940.
41. Walser TC, Ma X, Kundu N, Dorsey R, Goloubeva O, et al. (2007) Immune-mediated modulation of breast cancer growth and metastasis by the chemokine Mig (CXCL9) in a murine model. Journal of immunotherapy 30: 490–498.
42. Ohtani H, Jin Z, Takegawa S, Nakayama T, Yoshie O (2009) Abundant expression of CXCL9 (MIG) by stromal cells that include dendritic cells and accumulation of CXCR3+ T cells in lymphocyte-rich gastric carcinoma. The Journal of pathology 217: 21–31.
43. Oh ST, Schramme A, Tilgen W, Gutwein P, Reichrath J (2009) Overexpression of CXCL16 in lesional psoriatic skin. Dermato-endocrinology 1: 114–118.
44. Darash-Yahana M, Gillespie JW, Hewitt SM, Chen YY, Maeda S, et al. (2009) The chemokine CXCL16 and its receptor, CXCR6, as markers and promoters of inflammation-associated cancers. PLoS One 4: e6695.
45. Deng L, Chen N, Li Y, Zheng H, Lei Q (2010) CXCR6/CXCL16 functions as a regulator in metastasis and progression of cancer. Biochimica et biophysica acta 1806: 42–49.
46. Aldhous MC, Noble CL, Satsangi J (2009) Dysregulation of human beta-defensin-2 protein in inflammatory bowel disease. PLoS One 4: e6285.
47. Hollox EJ, Huffmeier U, Zeeuwen PL, Palla R, Lascorz J, et al. (2008) Psoriasis is associated with increased beta-defensin genomic copy number. Nature genetics 40: 23–25.
48. Hardman MJ, Waite A, Zeef L, Burow M, Nakayama T, et al. (2005) Macrophage migration inhibitory factor: a central regulator of wound healing. The American journal of pathology 167: 1561–1574.
49. Rohrl J, Huber B, Koehl GE, Geissler EK, Hehlgans T (2012) Mouse beta-defensin 14 (Defb14) promotes tumor growth by inducing angiogenesis in a CCR6-dependent manner. Journal of immunology 188: 4931–4939.
50. Christophi GP, Isackson PJ, Blaber S, Blaber M, Rodriguez M, et al. (2004) Distinct promoters regulate tissue-specific and differential expression of kallikrein 6 in CNS demyelinating disease. Journal of neurochemistry 91: 1439–1449.
51. Iwata A, Maruyama M, Akagi T, Hashikawa T, Kanazawa I, et al. (2003) Alpha-synuclein degradation by serine protease neurosin: implication for pathogenesis of synucleinopathies. Human molecular genetics 12: 2625–2635.
52. Breitenbach U, Tuckermann JP, Gebhardt C, Richter KH, Furstenberger G, et al. (2001) Keratinocyte-specific onset of serine protease BSSP expression in experimental carcinogenesis. The Journal of investigative dermatology 117: 634–640.
53. Borgono CA, Diamandis EP (2004) The emerging roles of human tissue kallikreins in cancer. Nature reviews Cancer 4: 876–890.
54. Yasuda S, Morokawa N, Wong GW, Rossi A, Madhusudhan MS, et al. (2005) Urokinase-type plasminogen activator is a preferred substrate of the human epithelium serine protease tryptase epsilon/PRSS22. Blood 105: 3893–3901.
55. Sallenave JM (2000) The role of secretory leukocyte proteinase inhibitor and elafin (elastase-specific inhibitor/skin-derived antileukoprotease) as alarm antiproteinases in inflammatory lung disease. Respiratory research 1: 87–92.
56. Meyer-Hoffert U (2009) Reddish, scaly, and itchy: how proteases and their inhibitors contribute to inflammatory skin diseases. Archivum immunologiae et therapiae experimentalis 57: 345–354.
57. Devoogdt N, Revets H, Ghassabeh GH, De Baetselier P (2004) Secretory leukocyte protease inhibitor in cancer development. Annals of the New York Academy of Sciences 1028: 380–389.
58. Jarvinen M, Rinne A, Hopsu-Havu VK (1987) Human cystatins in normal and diseased tissues–a review. Acta histochemica 82: 5–18.
59. Kos J, Krasovec M, Cimerman N, Nielsen HJ, Christensen IJ, et al. (2000) Cysteine proteinase inhibitors stefin A, stefin B, and cystatin C in sera from patients with colorectal cancer: relation to prognosis. Clinical cancer research : an official journal of the American Association for Cancer Research 6: 505–511.
60. Dang H, Trempus C, Malarkey DE, Wei SJ, Humble M, et al. (2006) Identification of genes and gene ontology processes critical to skin papilloma development in Tg.AC transgenic mice. Molecular carcinogenesis 45: 126–140.
61. Hoffjan S, Stemmler S (2007) On the role of the epidermal differentiation complex in ichthyosis vulgaris, atopic dermatitis and psoriasis. The British journal of dermatology 157: 441–449.
62. Booth DR, Booth SE, Gillmore JD, Hawkins PN, Pepys MB (1998) SAA1 alleles as risk factors in reactive systemic AA amyloidosis. Amyloid : the international journal of experimental and clinical investigation : the official journal of the International Society of Amyloidosis 5: 262–265.
63. Moshkovskii SA, Vlasova MA, Pyatnitskiy MA, Tikhonova OV, Safarova MR, et al. (2007) Acute phase serum amyloid A in ovarian cancer as an important component of proteome diagnostic profiling. Proteomics Clinical applications 1: 107–117.
64. Milan E, Lazzari C, Anand S, Floriani I, Torri V, et al. (2012) SAA1 is over-expressed in plasma of non small cell lung cancer patients with poor outcome after treatment with epidermal growth factor receptor tyrosine-kinase inhibitors. Journal of proteomics 76 Spec No.: 91–101.
65. Hiratsuka S, Watanabe A, Sakurai Y, Akashi-Takamura S, Ishibashi S, et al. (2008) The S100A8-serum amyloid A3-TLR4 paracrine cascade establishes a pre-metastatic phase. Nature cell biology 10: 1349–1355.
66. Hayes KR, Vollrath AL, Zastrow GM, McMillan BJ, Craven M, et al. (2005) EDGE: a centralized resource for the comparison, analysis, and distribution of toxicogenomic information. Molecular pharmacology 67: 1360–1368.
67. Pappas P, Sotiropoulou M, Karamanakos P, Kostoula A, Levidiotou S, et al. (2003) Acute-phase response to benzo[a]pyrene and induction of rat ALDH3A1. Chemico-biological interactions 143–144: 55–62.
68. Kushner I (1988) The acute phase response: an overview. Methods in enzymology 163: 373–383.
69. Karashima S, Kataoka H, Itoh H, Maruyama R, Koono M (1990) Prognostic significance of alpha-1-antitrypsin in early stage of colorectal carcinomas. International journal of cancer Journal international du cancer 45: 244–250.
70. Arlt A, Schafer H (2011) Role of the immediate early response 3 (IER3) gene in cellular stress response, inflammation and tumorigenesis. European journal of cell biology 90: 545–552.

Multiphoton Multispectral Fluorescence Lifetime Tomography for the Evaluation of Basal Cell Carcinomas

Rakesh Patalay[1,2]ᵠ, Clifford Talbot[1]ᵠ, Yuriy Alexandrov[1]ᵠ, Martin O. Lenz[1], Sunil Kumar[1], Sean Warren[1], Ian Munro[1], Mark A. A. Neil[1], Karsten König[4], Paul M. W. French[1], Anthony Chu[2], Gordon W. H. Stamp[5], Chris Dunsby[1,3]*

1 Photonics Group, Department of Physics, Imperial College London, South Kensington Campus, London, United Kingdom, **2** Department of Dermatology, Imperial College Healthcare NHS Trust, London, United Kingdom, **3** Department of Medicine, Imperial College Healthcare NHS Trust, London, United Kingdom, **4** JenLab GmbH, Jena, Germany, **5** CRUK London Research Institute, London, United Kingdom

Abstract

We present the first detailed study using multispectral multiphoton fluorescence lifetime imaging to differentiate basal cell carcinoma cells (BCCs) from normal keratinocytes. Images were acquired from 19 freshly excised BCCs and 27 samples of normal skin (*in & ex vivo*). Features from fluorescence lifetime images were used to discriminate BCCs with a sensitivity/specificity of 79%/93% respectively. A mosaic of BCC fluorescence lifetime images covering >1 mm^2 is also presented, demonstrating the potential for tumour margin delineation. Using 10,462 manually segmented cells from the image data, we quantify the cellular morphology and spectroscopic differences between BCCs and normal skin for the first time. Statistically significant increases were found in the fluorescence lifetimes of cells from BCCs in all spectral channels, ranging from 19.9% (425–515 nm spectral emission) to 39.8% (620–655 nm emission). A discriminant analysis based diagnostic algorithm allowed the fraction of cells classified as malignant to be calculated for each patient. This yielded a receiver operator characteristic area under the curve for the detection of BCC of 0.83. We have used both morphological and spectroscopic parameters to discriminate BCC from normal skin, and provide a comprehensive base for how this technique could be used for BCC assessment in clinical practice.

Editor: Irene Georgakoudi, Tufts University, United States of America

Funding: The authors gratefully acknowledge funding from the European Commission (SKINSPECTION, FP7-HEALTH-2007-A, 201577 and PHOTONICS-4-LIFE, FP7-ICT-2007-2, 224014), the Institute of Chemical Biology EPSRC funded Doctoral Training Centre (SW) and a Royal Society Wolfson Research Merit Award (PF). The funders had no role in study design, data collection and analysis, decision to publish, or preparation of the manuscript.

Competing Interests: KK is the CEO of JenLab GmbH. This does not alter the authors' adherence to all the PLoS ONE policies on sharing data and materials.

* E-mail: christopher.dunsby@imperial.ac.uk

ᵠ These authors contributed equally to this work.

Introduction

Basal cell carcinoma (BCC) is most common in caucasian populations and has a high prevalence in the western world [1,2] with a rising incidence in all age groups [3,4].

Initial assessment is currently made on clinical examination and uncertainty concerning the diagnosis can only be resolved by histology at present. The tumor must first be excised, fixed, processed, sectioned and stained before it can be reviewed. Biopsies can be both uncomfortable and cosmetically disfiguring to the patient and time-consuming and expensive to the clinician. The need for histological confirmation is also required in Mohs micrographic surgery to ensure clear margins and is often required in assessing clearance or recurrence following non-invasive topical therapy for malignancies. A non-invasive imaging modality capable of producing optically sectioned images *in situ* with high spatial resolution and correlation with histology is highly desirable. A number of label-free imaging modalities have been developed for dermatological applications [5] including high frequency ultrasound, optical coherence tomography, confocal laser scanning microscopy and multiphoton tomography (MPT).

MPT is an emerging optical imaging technique [6] that excites fluorescence from the sample through the simultaneous absorption of two or more photons of infrared light. This process requires a high intensity of excitation light and so is confined to the tightly focused excitation spot. Images are generated by raster-scanning the excitation spot across the specimen in two dimensions. MPT offers a spatial resolution similar to histopathology at high power magnification (<1 μm lateral, <2 μm axial) resolution [7] and is available for clinical use *in vivo*.

The skin contains naturally occurring fluorophores that can be imaged using MPT without the need for exogenous contrast agents. These include collagen, elastin, melanin, keratins, porphyrins, NAD(P)H and flavins. Fluorescence intensity imaging using MPT can be used to study skin morphology with subcellular resolution [8,9,10]. Further discrimination between fluorophores and thus tissues can be gained using the fluorescence emission spectrum [11,12] and fluorescence lifetime imaging (FLIM) [13,14,15,16], which measures the rate of decay of the fluorescence signal following a short pulse of excitation light.

The aim of this study is to evaluate multispectral FLIM MPT as a means to discriminate BCCs from normal skin. Fluorescence intensity and FLIM images were collected from normal skin (*in &*

ex vivo) and freshly excised BCCs using four emission spectral channels. The potential of this technique to provide improvements in diagnostic accuracy was then explored using visual architectural criteria together with cellular morphology and spectroscopic parameters. We identify the cellular morphology and spectroscopic parameters providing the greatest diagnostic discrimination and combine these to allow new semi- and fully-automated diagnostic algorithms to be tested for the first time.

Results

Table 1 summarizes the patients and data used in the analysis. 19 patients with normal skin were imaged *in vivo*, the remaining samples in the study were imaged *ex vivo*. Patients had skin phototypes I-IV with a mean of 2.5 and 2.2 for normal skin and BCCs respectively. All BCCs except 2 had nodular components and 8 were mixed subtypes including infiltrative, superficial and pigmented. Skin was imaged from the scalp, face, neck, chest, forearm and back for BCCs and face, forearm, back and lower leg for normal skin.

Figure 1a–n demonstrates typical fluorescence intensity and FLIM images (encoding mean fluorescence lifetimes using a false color scale) taken from normal skin. Images in Figures 1a–i have been taken from the same field of view of normal skin using the 4 spectral channels, (see Materials and Methods, Instrumentation). Figures 1a–d show the images recorded in the 4 spectral channels revealing contrast that is not visible in the calculated total fluorescence intensity image (Figure 1e). The second harmonic generation (SHG) signal from collagen, seen in the tips of the dermal papilla, dominates the blue spectral channel (Figure 1a) and can be visually separated from the weaker intracellular fluorophores (c.f. Figure 1b–d). It is however difficult to visually separate the multiple fluorophores contributing to the green, yellow and red channels (Figure 1b–d) using the fluorescence intensity images alone. The addition of the fluorescence lifetime information (Figures 1f–i) allows NAD(P)H autofluorescence (blue-green on false color scale), dominant in the green spectral channel to be easily distinguished from melanin (short lifetime [17] red on false color scale), which is dominant in the red spectral channel. The yellow spectral channel includes fluorescence from flavins, NAD(P)H and melanin. The multiple FLIM spectral channels also allow SHG from collagen (with an instantaneous decay) seen in the blue channel and elastin (with a long fluorescence lifetime [18]), seen in the green/yellow channels to be distinguished from the same spatial location within the dermal papilla.

Figures 1j–n show FLIM images acquired in the green spectral channel from different depths within the same sample. Dendritic processes containing melanin can be identified in Figure 1j,k between the keratinocytes in the s.granulosum and s.spinosum. Deeper in the skin, the nucleus to cytoplasm ratio increases and more cells contain intracellular melanin with a short fluorescence lifetime. The highest concentration of melanin can be seen in the cells of the basal cell layer surrounding the dermal papillae (Figure 1n). Corresponding images from all spectral channels can be found in Figure S1.

Figures 1o–x illustrate the visual architectural changes seen in BCCs using MPT. We observe features described previously [19,20] including 'detached cells with enlargement of intercellular spaces' (Figure 1o), 'cells with irregular contours' and 'random arrangement of cells' (both Figure 1p), 'aligned elongated cells' (Figure 1q, white arrow), 'double alignment of monomorphous cells' (Figure 1r, white arrows), 'palisading' (Figure 1w) and 'sheets of cells intermingled with fibres' (Figure 1v). The paired images in Figure 1w,x are taken from the green and blue channels respectively and show the proximity of BCC nests to the surrounding collagen fibres ('cell islands surrounded by fibres').

In addition to these features, we repeatedly saw a pattern of monomorphous cells, often heterogeneous in size, with large nuclear/cytoplasmic ratios, poorly defined cell margins and appearing to overlap. This new feature of 'merging cells' can be seen in Figure 1q,s,t,u and in the further image sets found in Figure S2.

All FLIM images were assessed by a dermatologist (RP) for the presence of at least one of the MPT diagnostic features for BCC described above and 'merging cells'. This yielded a sensitivity/specificity of 79%/93%.

A number of spectroscopic and cellular morphology parameters were calculated using manually defined regions of interest (ROI) corresponding to individual cells. The median ROI mean fluorescence lifetime is given for each spectral channel in Table 1, and the best discriminating parameters ranked by area under the curve (AUC) are listed in Table 2 together with the Cohen's d statistic. Histograms of several parameters are plotted in Figure 2a–f. A detailed description of all parameters, complete tables of all calculated values and their ranking by AUC are presented in Text S1, Table S1 and Table S2 respectively.

Figure 2a–c presents histograms of the three cellular morphology parameters, namely the flattening factor (ratio of minor to major axis length), orientation SD (the standard deviation of the ROI major axis angle of a cell and its neighbours), and the cell confluency (combined area of ROI and adjacent ROIs relative to intercellular space). The difference in the median value for the orientation SD and cell confluency between BCC and normal samples was found to be statistically significant at the 5% level using the Wilcoxon rank sum test ($p = 0.03$, 0.05 respectively), but was not significant for the flattening factor ($p = 0.33$). Both the

Table 1. Patient characteristics and median lifetimes for each spectral channel.

					Median τ_{mean} (ps) (Inter-quartile range)			
Diagnosis	**Patients (M/F)**	**Mean Age (Range)**	**Images**	**ROIs/Cells**	**Blue**	**Green**	**Yellow**	**Red**
BCC	19 (11/8)	64 (44–86)	110	4259	2419	2624	1908	1448
					(1759–2773)	(2412–2819)	(1582–2200)	(1240–2013)
Normal Skin	27 (15/12)	42 (17–80)	122	6203	1797	2189	1380	1036
					(1282–2175)	(1656–2709)	(888–1974)	(709–1428)
% difference from Normal					34.6	19.9	38.3	39.8

Abbreviations ROI-region of interest, τ_{mean} - mean fluorescence lifetime, ps - picoseconds.

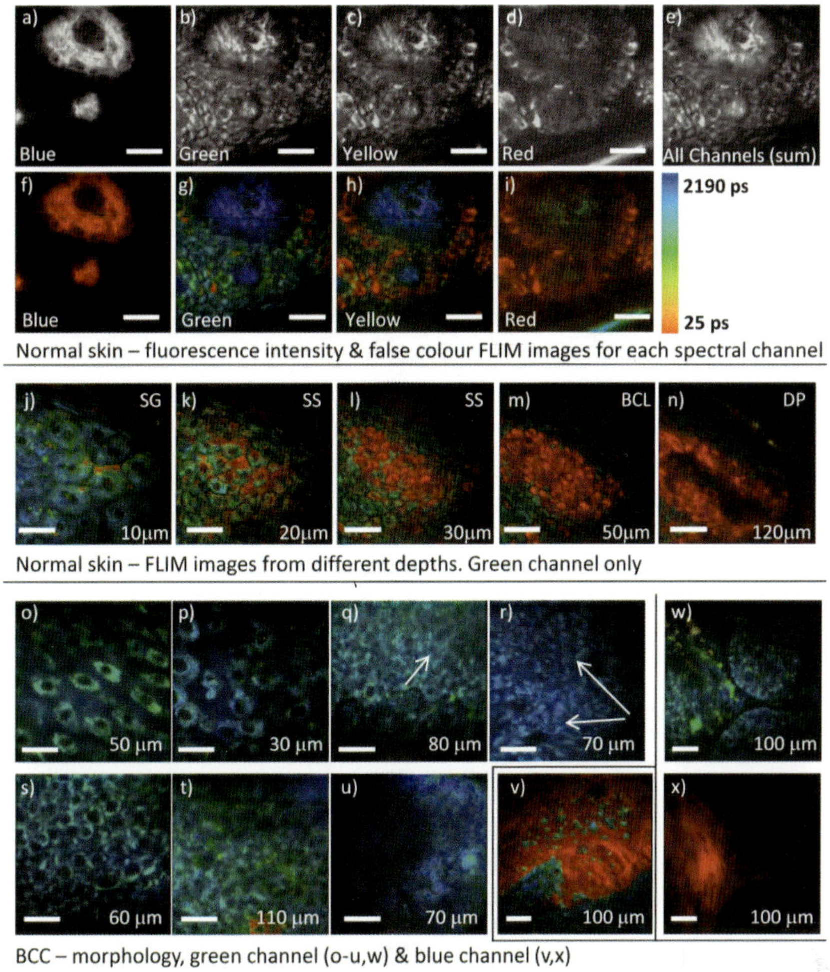

Figure 1. Multispectral fluorescence intensity and FLIM images acquired from normal skin and BCCs. (a–i) Fluorescence intensity and false color FLIM images from a single field of view acquired at a depth of 110 μm with all spectral channels taken near a dermal papilla from normal skin. (j–n) FLIM images taken from the green channel only of different depths within a sample of normal skin. (o–u) FLIM images taken from the green channel illustrating visual architectural features seen in BCC using MPT. (v) FLIM image taken from the blue channel of a BCC. (w,x) paired FLIM images taken from the green and blue channels respectively of a BCC nest. KEY SG-Stratum Granulosum, SS- Stratum Spinosum, BCL-Basal Cell Layer, DP-Dermal Papilla. Scale bar 25 μm.

AUC and Cohen's d statistics show that these distributions are not sufficiently separated for them to be used as the main components in multivariate discrimination. The difference in orientation SD reflects the increase in BCCs of aligned and elongated cells and of "palisade"-like structures. The cell confluency suggests that cells in BCCs are, on average, more sparsely arranged in an XY plane than those from normal skin. These differences are in accordance with visual assessments of tissue morphology discussed by Seidenari et al. [20] and above.

Histograms of spectroscopic and fluorescence lifetime parameters (Figure 2d–i) show a shift toward longer lifetimes for BCCs in τ_1 (short) and τ_2 (long fluorescence decay components) for all channels compared with normal skin. Strong peaks are seen in the BCC histograms at $\tau_1 = 450$ ps and $\tau_2 = 4000$ ps in the green channel, the peak in τ_2 shifts from 2400 ps to 3000 ps in the yellow channel and new peaks in τ_1 around 250 and 500 ps are present in the red channel in BCCs. The difference in median τ_{mean} between BCC and normal samples was found to be statistically significant to $p<0.01$ using the Wilcoxon rank sum test ($p = 0.0013$, 0.0049, 0.0061, 0.0006 in the blue, green, yellow and red channels respectively).

Analysis with respect to the fraction of the total fluorescence signal in each spectral channel (spectral contribution, Figure 2f) indicates a population of cells with a high contribution in the green channel in normal skin and a broader distribution in the yellow channel in normal compared to BCC. There is also an increase in spectral contribution in the red channel for BCCs, see also Table S1.

In order to develop a diagnostic algorithm using all of the spectroscopic and cellular morphology parameters, we employed principal component analysis based dimensionality reduction. Linear discriminant analysis was then applied to the first 4 principal components of the data, which allowed each ROI to be classified as either 'Normal' or 'BCC' using a leave one out approach, see Text S1. The fraction of cells/ROIs classified as 'BCC' was then determined for all patients. The separation of these variables' distributions (Figure S3a), as measured using the AUC, was 0.83. For example, if the threshold for classifying a patient as having BCC is set at having ≥30% of cells classified as BCC, then this yields a sensitivity/specificity of 89%/73%.

To further automate the discrimination we then replaced the step of manual segmentation with automatic ROI segmentation by

Table 2. The best discriminatory parameters ranked using the area under the curve (AUC).

Parameter	Index	Channel	Cohen's d	AUC
Spectroscopic	τ_1	Red	1.44	0.82
	τ_1	Blue	1.22	0.80
	τ_1	Yellow	1.00	0.77
	τ_2	Red	0.20	0.74
	τ_2	Green	0.87	0.73
	τ_2	Blue	0.38	0.73
	τ_1	Green	0.83	0.72
Cellular	Cell confluency (Gabriel)	-	0.02	0.60
morphology	Orientation SD (Gabriel)	-	0.12	0.53
	Flatting Factor (Gabriel)	-	0.17	0.52

Abbreviations AUC – area under the curve, τ_1 – short fluorescence lifetime decay component, τ_2 – long lifetime component.

the method of size-tuned non-linear top-hat detection [21]. This procedure identified 2343 BCC and 4034 normal ROIs. Here, the cellular morphology parameters were not included in the principal component analysis because the automatic ROI detection did not provide a clean outline of the cells (see figure 3(d)) and did not always correctly identify individual cells. However, the cellular morphology parameters only provide very weak discrimination between normal and BCC, see table 2, and so their exclusion is not expected to significantly affect the outcome. In fact, although the resulting fraction of cells/ROI's classified by this approach as 'BCC' (Figure S3b) is slightly different to that obtained with manual segmentation, the separation of these two distributions also yielded an AUC of 0.83. One might expect the discrimination based on automatically segmented ROIs to score lower than the one based on manual segmentation, due to the loss of information on the cellular morphology, the occasional grouping of more than one cell into the same ROI and erroneous inclusion of some extracellular fluorescence by the segmentation algorithm. In practice, however, we do not expect the exact shape of the ROI around a single cell to greatly affect the spatially integrated fluorescence decay from that ROI or the fluorescence lifetime parameters derived from it because the fluorescence decay profile is reasonably uniform across individual cells, see e.g. figure 1, and the erroneous inclusion of extracellular fluorescence makes only a small contribution to the total signal analysed. We note that, although the automatic segmentation is not perfect, it does allow bi-exponential fluorescence decay parameters to be measured at multiple regions across an image and is much less time-consuming than manual segmentation, which is important if this method is to be employed in a clinical setting. Further work and larger numbers of patients/samples will be required to compare the relative performance of these two methods more precisely. An analysis that

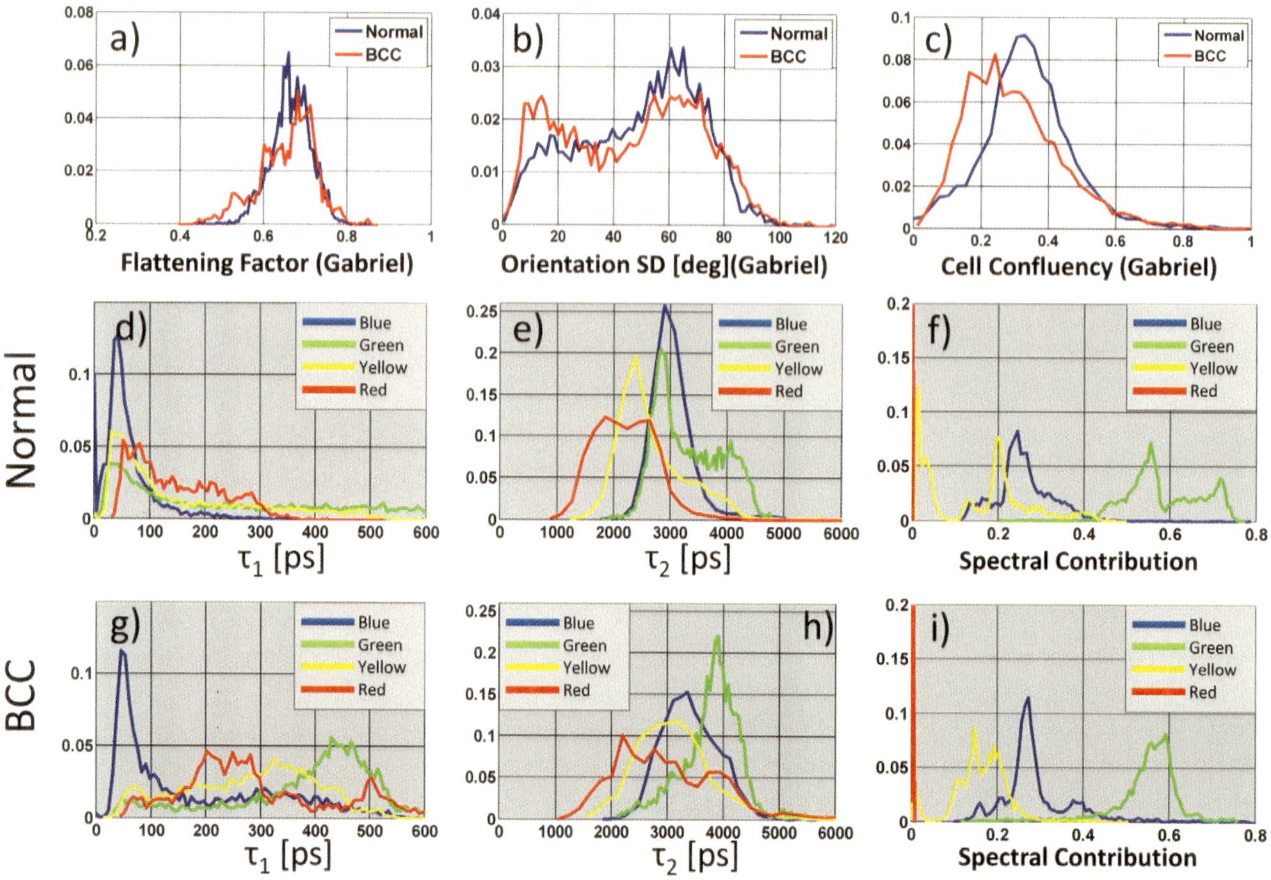

Figure 2. Histograms of morphology and fluorescence lifetime parameters for cells/ROIs in normal skin and BCCs. (a–c) Histograms of cellular morphology features demonstrating the difference between normal skin (coded Blue) and BCCs (Red) (d–i) Histograms of τ_1, τ_2, spectral contribution for all spectral channels for BCC and normal skin. Curves are color-coded according to channel "colors".

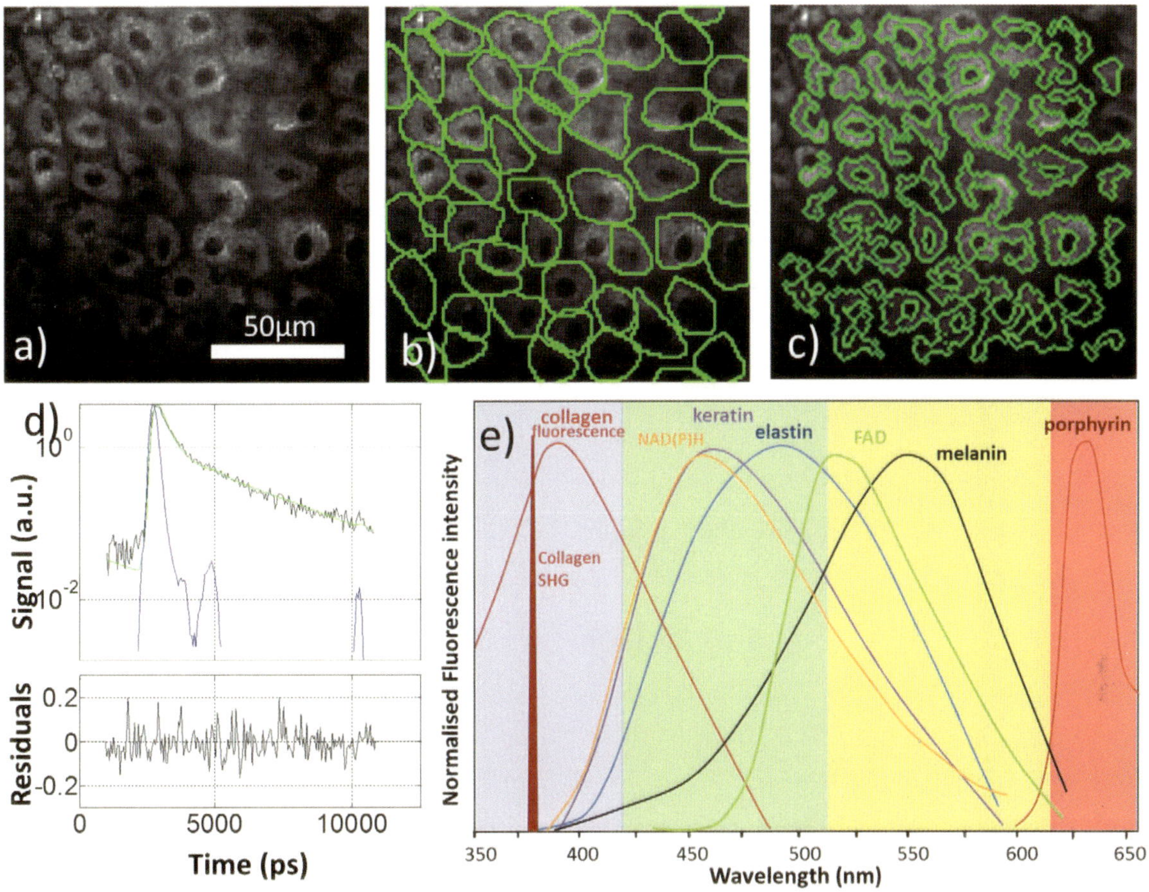

Figure 3. Exemplar segmented fluorescence intensity images, fitted fluorescence decay and fluorophore emission spectra. (a) Total fluorescence intensity image, same image with (b) manually and (c) automatically defined cellular regions of interest overlayed. (d) Top – exemplar fluorescence decay from one region of interest (black), biexponential fit to data (green) and instrument response function (blue). (d) Bottom – normalized residuals. (e) The emission spectra from endogenous fluorophores plotted in relation to the four spectral detection channels.

did not include any image segmentation (see Text S1) also resulted in a reasonable sensitivity/specificity of 72%/84% respectively.

To observe the variation of spectroscopic and morphological parameters of a lesion across a larger field of view than is possible with our MPT instrument (350 μm×350 μm^2), which is designed for use at high magnification, we employed a motorized stage to move *ex vivo* samples within the x,y plane and assembled mosaics of high resolution images. Figure 4 shows an example comprising 12×8 individual FLIM images from the green spectral channel acquired from a BCC, illustrating the potential of this technique to be used for high resolution label-free histology over a large field of view.

Discussion

We have shown that morphological features described by Seidenari et al. [20] together with the newly proposed feature of 'merging cells' provide a good specificity and sensitivity for identifying BCCs from FLIM images using a visual architectural analysis. The multispectral FLIM images aided the identification of many features, especially when assessing cells within fibres, see e.g. Figure 1v–x.

In our cell-based spectroscopic analysis, we observe longer mean fluorescence lifetimes in all spectral channels for BCC compared to normal in agreement with earlier non-spectrally resolved FLIM MPT studies of BCC [16,22,23]. It is important to note that since normal keratinocytes are present within BCC, many cells/ROIs in the BCC FLIM images will have actually been normal cells, yet statistically significant differences were observed between groups in spite of this. From a spectroscopic perspective, it could be argued that the observed fluorescence lifetime contrast is due to a higher concentration of melanin (with a short fluorescence lifetime) in normal samples. We do not believe this to be the case because our BCC dataset includes pigmented BCCs and we observe well matched spectral contributions between groups in the melanin dominated yellow and red spectral channels (see Table S1). It is interesting to note that the spectroscopic parameters providing the highest discrimination (AUC) between groups are the fluorescence lifetimes of the red and yellow channels. We speculate that this could be melanin changing its fluorescence lifetime or due to the presence of an additional fluorophore such as porphyrins in BCCs. Further research is required to elucidate the origin of this contrast and we believe that multispectral MPT FLIM provides a useful tool to address this.

Previous *in vivo* measurements in a hamster cheek pouch model of oral cancer by Skala et al. [24] show a decrease in the fluorescence lifetime of NAD(P)H and flavins associated with malignancy. Our measurements show the opposite trend, which may be due to differences between animal model and human, in

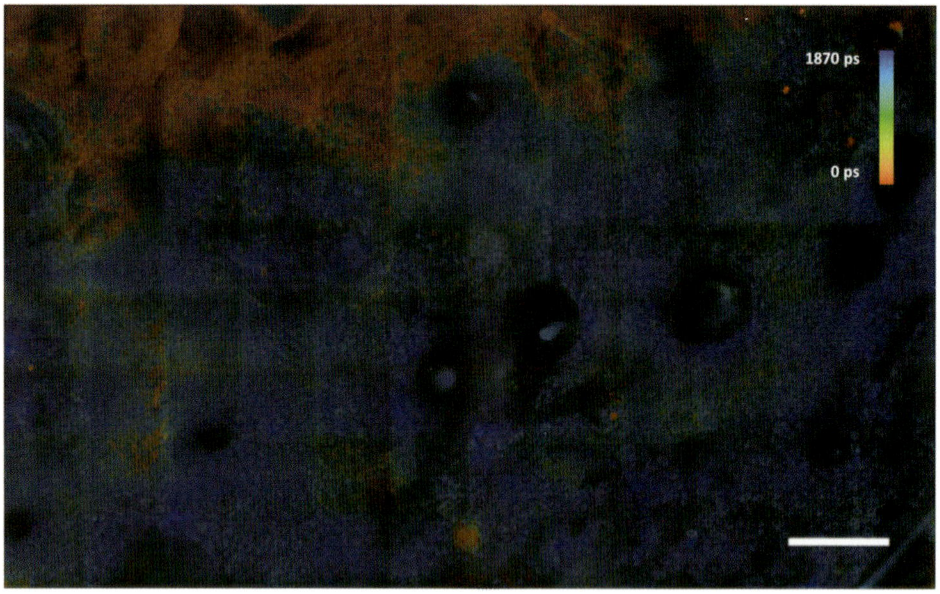

Figure 4. False color FLIM image from the green channel of a BCC consisting of 12×8 fields of view covering an area of 1.86×1.24 mm^2. Bar 0.2 mm.

disease pathophysiology or the absence of melanin in mucosal epithelium.

Potential confounding factors in fluorescence lifetime measurements include [13] imaging depth in the skin (τ_{mean} decreases with depth) and patient age (τ_{mean} increases with age). In our study, image depths were well matched between groups (62 v. 65 µm mean cell/ROI depth) and are not expected to influence the results significantly. In a previous study of two very distinct age populations (20–35 and >60 years) using a single spectrally broad FLIM channel [13], mean fluorescence lifetimes were observed to differ between age groups by 109 ps for upper skin layers and by 210 ps for lower layers. In our study the age disparity is much lower (mean age 42 v. 64, Table 1) and the observed changes in fluorescence lifetime between normal and BCC are much larger (394–584 ps, Table 1).

In order to verify that it is reasonable to combine data from normal skin acquired *in vivo* with that acquired *ex vivo*, we studied how the fluorescence lifetime changes with time following surgical excision. The only previous such study on human skin was performed by Sanchez et al. [15] and this paper provides a detailed discussion of the many factors that can affect the fluorescence lifetime. Sanchez et al. observed skin over a timescale of 7 days and showed that the fluorescence lifetime increased over this period. Therefore, in order to study these changes over the timescale of hours relevant for our study, we repeatedly imaged samples of freshly excised normal skin at the same field of view over a three hour period. The mean fluorescence lifetime averaged over four samples decreased from the initial value by 7.2%, 1.6%, 2.9% and 8.6% in the blue, green, yellow and red spectral channels respectively. These changes are in the opposite direction to the observations by Sanchez et al. (which were carried out over days rather than hours) and, importantly, are all much smaller than the differences seen between diagnostic groups (34.6, 19.9, 38.3 and 39.8% respectively, Table 1).

As a second step to verify that it is reasonable to combine normal skin imaged *ex vivo* and *in vivo*, we directly compared the median ROI/cell mean lifetime between these two groups and the *ex vivo* samples were found to have a longer fluorescence lifetime by 5.9%, 7.9%, 10% and 13% in the blue, green, yellow and red spectral channels respectively. However, these changes are again smaller than the differences seen between BCC and normal skin (see Table 1). When we consider the median mean fluorescence lifetime per sample, see Figure S5, the difference between *ex vivo* and *in vivo* measurements was found to be not statistically significant using the Wilcoxon rank sum test ($p = 0.98$, 0.70, 0.63 and 0.23 in the blue, green, yellow and red spectral channels respectively). As reported above, the difference in median mean lifetime between the BCC samples and the combined *in vivo* and *ex vivo* normals was found to be statistically significant using the same test ($p<0.01$ in all spectral channels).

Combining the subcellular resolution of multispectral MPT FLIM with a motorized stage to facilitate imaging over large fields of view provides a means to identify small nests of BCCs in normal skin, such as those seen with infiltrative BCCs, whose margins are notoriously difficult to define. Currently the manual acquisition and processing of montage data is slow with data acquisition, FLIM data analysis and montaging requiring approximately 100, 4 and 60 minutes respectively for 12×8 images. In the future, full automation of the image acquisition process would reduce the image acquisition time to ~45 minutes. Further reductions in image acquisition time may be possible by reducing the time required to acquire each sub-image, at the expense of signal-to-noise ratio in the final image. A wide range of sophisticated image stitching algorithms exist that could be used to greatly speed up the montaging compared to the current manual image stitching. While the current depth of penetration of MPT is too limited to assess the margins of many infiltrative BCCs *in vivo*, its high sensitivity, specificity and high spatial resolution can be exploited by stitching multiple images together to provide an extended multidimensional mosaic of such lesions. This could be useful for clinical *ex vivo* margin assessment, e.g. during Mohs procedures.

This work demonstrates the diagnostic potential of multispectral MPT FLIM for the evaluation of BCC and its margins. We have assessed existing MPT features and, together with a newly proposed feature ('merging cells'), demonstrated that visual assessment of the images provides a sensitivity/specificity of

79%/93%. In addition, we have used multispectral FLIM to perform the first detailed analysis of the discrimination afforded by a wide range of spectroscopic and cell-based morphologic parameters and ranked them by their discriminatory power (AUC). This information will be crucial to guide the development of more accurate, faster and lower cost imaging modalities.

We report the first semi- and fully-automated diagnostic algorithms based on manual and automatic segmentation of multispectral MPT FLIM images. Manual segmentation of cells followed by principal component analysis based dimensionality reduction and yielded an AUC of 0.83 for the discrimination of BCC from normal skin. In the future, the combination of automatically calculated spectroscopic information together with manually identified visual architectural features could lead to even higher diagnostic accuracies.

Materials and Methods

Ethics Statement

The study was approved by the Riverside NRES London ethics committee (Ref 09/H0706/28 & 83) and conformed to the Declaration of Helsinki protocols.

Instrumentation

Multiphoton imaging was performed using a modified DermaInspect® (JenLab GmbH, Jena, Germany), a CE marked two photon laser scanning tomograph [7]. Fluorescence was collected by four H7422P-40 photomultiplier tubes (Hamamatsu Photonics K.K., Japan) and recorded using time correlated single photon counting into 256 time bins (SPC-830, Becker & Hickl, GmbH, Germany). The four spectral channels were defined as 360–425 nm (blue), 425–515 nm (green), 515–620 nm (yellow) and 620–640/655 nm (red), see Figure 3e. Further description of the system is included in Text S1 and Figure S4.

Patients and Samples

Patients with suspected BCCs and volunteers attending clinics at the Department of Dermatology at Imperial College Healthcare NHS Trust were recruited. Patients gave written informed consent to participate. Patients with the following criteria were excluded: age 18 years or less, in state custody, carrying a blood borne infection, having a photosensitive skin disorder, or currently pregnant.

Freshly excised tissue samples were typically 5–10 mm in depth and always consisted of the whole epidermis and dermis, to the subcutaneous fat. Samples were rinsed with Hanks Balanced Salt Solution buffer without phenol red, calcium or magnesium (Gibco®, Invitrogen™, CA, USA), its surface moistened with the buffer solution and placed on damp gauze in an inverted glass bottomed petri dish (80–170 µm cover slip Matek®, MA,USA) immediately following excision.

Images of normal skin were taken from healthy patients *in vivo* and normal margins of *ex vivo* tumor samples. *Ex vivo* normal skin was only imaged from well-defined skin tumors that were excised with a wide surgical margin of normal skin. This normal skin was sufficiently distant from the tumor site to not be affected and appeared normal by clinical visual inspection of the surface. *Ex vivo* samples were kept at room temperature and imaged 66±38 mins (mean±s.d.) after excision.

The diagnoses of all excised samples were confirmed histologically.

Imaging

The excitation wavelength was fixed at 760 nm and the power was adjusted according to the depth of imaging (<50 mW). Images from several depths and sometimes more than one field of view were taken from within each lesion. Each FLIM image was either 128×128 or 256×256 pixels and was acquired over 25.5 s. The instrument response function was recorded daily from gold nanorods [25] in all spectral channels simultaneously.

The cellular layers of the epidermis were targeted for imaging. Images were taken at ~10 µm intervals until the dermis was reached or until the signal was too low to resolve a useful image. The mean depth imaged per sample was 65 µm for the BCCs and 62 µm for normal skin.

Data Analysis

FLIM images were generated by fitting a single exponential decay to the fluorescence from each spectral channel of each pixel in the image using software written in Matlab® (R2010b, The Mathworks Inc.,USA).

Regions of interest (ROI) were defined manually in each image corresponding to each cell using software written in Labview 7.1 (see Figure 3b,c) [26]. The spectral contribution was calculated for all ROIs. The spatially integrated fluorescence decay for each ROI in each channel (e.g. Figure 3d) was fitted to a double exponential model using non-linear least squares minimization. ROI fluorescence decay curves from a single spectral channel containing fewer than 1000 photons were excluded from the analysis as they contained too few photons to reliably fit to a double exponential model. ROIs containing <1000 photons in any spectral channel were excluded from the discriminant analysis for the same reason. Two patients (one normal, one BCC) did not have any ROIs with >1000 photons in all spectral channels and so were excluded from the discriminant analysis. See Text S1 for further details.

Automatic image segmentation was performed using size-tuned non-linear top-hat detection that has been described previously [21]. Briefly, this method applies a pixel-wise transformation to the image (formula A2.1 in [21]) that enhances the brightness of a pixel if its close vicinity is also bright and its distant vicinity is dim. The transformed image is then thresholded at a user defined value. The resulting binary images are then morphologically smoothed using the MATLAB 'imopen' function and spatially distinct regions identified. These regions are then size-sieved using standard MATLAB image processing functions to remove objects smaller than a user-defined threshold. The same procedure, including all thresholding parameters, was applied uniformly across all images.

Image montaging

A motorized microscope stage (Scan IM 120×80, Märzhäuser Wetzlar Gmbh, Germany) was used for the sequential acquisition of data from several fields of view from an *ex vivo* sample (without the use of the metallic coupling ring). A total of 12×8 fields were acquired. Each image in the montage was acquired over 25.5 s and using 256×256 pixels. The manual saving and initiation of stage translation required ~30 s therefore the total acquisition time for the montage of 12×8 images was ~100 minutes.

Fitting a single exponential decay model to every pixel in an image required approximately 2.5 s using an 8-core, 3.16 GHz PC with 32 GB RAM running MATLAB R2011a under Windows 7, 64 bit. Therefore the FLIM decay fitting process required a total of ~4 minutes for the entire montage in one spectral channel.

Due to backlash when reversing the direction of stage motion, fully automatic image stitching using the programmed stage translation distance did not provide satisfactory results. Therefore, semi-manual image registration was employed using a software package developed in-house in LabVIEW, which required approximately 1 hour to align the whole montage.

Statistics

Statistics were performed using SPSS 18 (SPSS Inc. IL, USA) and MATLAB®. See Text S1 for further details.

Supporting Information

Figure S1 Spectrally resolved FLIM images from a sample of normal skin taken at several depths. (Figure 1 j–n shows only the 425–525 nm (green) channel of this data).

Figure S2 ultispectral FLIM images taken at multiple depths from (a) a nodular/superficial BCC and (b) a nodular/pigmented BCC.

Figure S3 Histograms of the fraction of cells classified as BCC for the BCC and normal groups using both manual (a) and automatic (b) segmentation.

Figure S4 Schematic of instrument. Key-DCSP - dichroic short pass, DCLP – dichroic long pass.

Figure S5 Bar chart showing sample median ROI/cell mean fluorescence lifetime for BCCs, *in vivo* normal and *ex vivo* normal skin for the four spectral detection channels. Error bars indicate value of 25th and 75th percentile.

Table S1 Summary of all spectroscopic parameters calculated for each ROI/cell.

Table S2 The AUC for all calculated spectroscopic (a) and cellular morphology parameters (b).

Text S1 Supporting Materials and Methods.

Acknowledgments

The authors gratefully thank Fulvio Ratto, Paolo Matteini and Roberto Pini at the Istituto di Fisica Applicata, Consiglio Nazionale delle Ricerche, Italy for providing the sample of gold nanorods, Marcel Hofer, Rainer Bückle and Hans Georg Breunig from JenLab GmbH for their expert technical assistance and the Human Biomaterials Resource Centre of Imperial College Healthcare NHS Trust for their assistance in randomising and managing tissue for this study. This paper is dedicated to the memory of Dr. Hanno Wittig (SKINSPECTION project manager, tp21 GmbH).

Author Contributions

Conceived and designed the experiments: RP CT YA MN KK PF AC GS CD. Performed the experiments: RP CT CD. Analyzed the data: RP CT YA ML SK GS CD. Contributed reagents/materials/analysis tools: YA SW IM CD. Wrote the paper: RP CT YA SK MN KK PF AC GS CD.

References

1. Diepgen TL, Mahler V (2002) The epidemiology of skin cancer. Br J Dermatol 146 Suppl 61: 1–6.
2. Demers AA, Nugent Z, Mihalcioiu C, Wiseman MC, Kliewer EV (2005) Trends of nonmelanoma skin cancer from 1960 through 2000 in a Canadian population. Journal of the American Academy of Dermatology 53: 320–328.
3. Staples MP, Elwood M, Burton RC, Williams JL, Marks R, et al. (2006) Non-melanoma skin cancer in Australia: the 2002 national survey and trends since 1985. Med J Aust 184: 6–10.
4. Christenson LJ, Borrowman TA, Vachon CM, Tollefson MM, Otley CC, et al. (2005) Incidence of basal cell and squamous cell carcinomas in a population younger than 40 years. Jama-Journal of the American Medical Association 294: 681–690.
5. Mogensen M, Jemec GBE (2007) Diagnosis of Nonmelanoma Skin Cancer/Keratinocyte Carcinoma: A Review of Diagnostic Accuracy of Nonmelanoma Skin Cancer Diagnostic Tests and Technologies. Dermatologic Surgery 33: 1158–1174.
6. Denk W, Strickler JH, Webb WW (1990) Two-photon laser scanning fluorescence microscopy. Science 248: 73–76.
7. König K, Riemann I (2003) High-resolution multiphoton tomography of human skin with subcellular spatial resolution and picosecond time resolution. J Biomed Opt 8: 432–439.
8. Masters BR, So PT, Gratton E (1997) Multiphoton excitation fluorescence microscopy and spectroscopy of in vivo human skin. Biophys J 72: 2405–2412.
9. König K, Raphael AP, Lin L, Grice JE, Soyer HP, et al. (2011) Applications of multiphoton tomographs and femtosecond laser nanoprocessing microscopes in drug delivery research. Advanced Drug Delivery Reviews 63: 388–404.
10. Levitt JM, McLaughlin-Drubin ME, Munger K, Georgakoudi I (2011) Automated biochemical, morphological, and organizational assessment of precancerous changes from endogenous two-photon fluorescence images. PLoS ONE 6: e24765.
11. Palero JA, de Bruijn HS, van der Ploeg van den Heuvel A, Sterenborg HJ, Gerritsen HC (2007) Spectrally resolved multiphoton imaging of in vivo and excised mouse skin tissues. Biophys J 93: 992–1007.
12. Dimitrow E, Riemann I, Ehlers A, Koehler MJ, Norgauer J, et al. (2009) Spectral fluorescence lifetime detection and selective melanin imaging by multiphoton laser tomography for melanoma diagnosis. Exp Dermatol 18: 509–515.
13. Benati E, Bellini V, Borsari S, Dunsby C, Ferrari C, et al. (2011) Quantitative evaluation of healthy epidermis by means of multiphoton microscopy and fluorescence lifetime imaging microscopy. Skin Research and Technology 17: 295–303.
14. Cicchi R, Sestini S, De Giorgi V, Massi D, Lotti T, et al. (2008) Nonlinear laser imaging of skin lesions. J Biophotonics 1: 62–73.
15. Sanchez WY, Prow TW, Sanchez WH, Grice JE, Roberts MS (2010) Analysis of the metabolic deterioration of ex vivo skin from ischemic necrosis through the imaging of intracellular NAD(P)H by multiphoton tomography and fluorescence lifetime imaging microscopy. Journal of Biomedical Optics 15: 046008–046011.
16. Seidenari S, Arginelli F, French P, König K, Magnoni C, et al. (2012) Multiphoton laser tomography and fluorescence lifetime imaging of basal cell carcinoma: Morphologic Features for Non-Invasive Diagnostics. Experimental Dermatology (accepted for publication).
17. Teuchner K, Freyer W, Leupold D, Volkmer A, Birch DJ, et al. (1999) Femtosecond two-photon excited fluorescence of melanin. Photochem Photobiol 70: 146–151.
18. König K, Schneckenburger H (1994) Laser-induced autofluorescence for medical diagnosis. Journal of fluorescence 4: 17–40.
19. Paoli J, Smedh M, Wennberg AM, Ericson MB (2008) Multiphoton laser scanning microscopy on non-melanoma skin cancer: morphologic features for future non-invasive diagnostics. J Invest Dermatol 128: 1248–1255.
20. Seidenari S, Arginelli F, Bassoli S, Cautela J, Cesinaro A, et al. (2012) Diagnosis of BCC by multiphoton laser tomography. Skin Research and Technology: doi: 10.1111/j.1600-0846.2012.00643.x. [Epub ahead of print].
21. Santos AF, Zaltsman AB, Martin RC, Kuzmin A, Alexandrov Y, et al. (2008) Angiogenesis: An Improved In Vitro Biological System and Automated Image-Based Workflow to Aid Identification and Characterization of Angiogenesis and Angiogenic Modulators. Assay and Drug Development Technologies 6: 693–710.
22. Cicchi R, Massi D, Sestini S, Carli P, De Giorgi V, et al. (2007) Multidimensional non-linear laser imaging of Basal Cell Carcinoma. Opt Express 15: 10135–10148.
23. De Giorgi V, Massi D, Sestini S, Cicchi R, Pavone FS, et al. (2009) Combined non-linear laser imaging (two-photon excitation fluorescence microscopy, fluorescence lifetime imaging microscopy, multispectral multiphoton microscopy) in cutaneous tumours: first experiences. J Eur Acad Dermatol Venereol 23: 314–316.
24. Skala MC, Riching KM, Gendron-Fitzpatrick A, Eickhoff J, Eliceiri KW, et al. (2007) In vivo multiphoton microscopy of NADH and FAD redox states, fluorescence lifetimes, and cellular morphology in precancerous epithelia. Proceedings of the National Academy of Sciences of the United States of America 104: 19494–19499.
25. Talbot CB, Patalay R, Munro I, Warren S, Ratto F, et al. (2011) Application of ultrafast gold luminescence to measuring the instrument response function for

multispectral multiphoton fluorescence lifetime imaging. Optics Express 19: 13848–13861.
26. Patalay R, Talbot C, Alexandrov Y, Munro I, Neil MAA, et al. (2011) Quantification of cellular autofluorescence of human skin using multiphoton tomography and fluorescence lifetime imaging in two spectral detection channels. Biomed Opt Express 2: 3295–3308.

Depletion of Cutaneous Macrophages and Dendritic Cells Promotes Growth of Basal Cell Carcinoma in Mice

Simone König[1], Frauke Nitzki[1], Anja Uhmann[1], Kai Dittmann[2], Jennifer Theiss-Suennemann[2], Markus Herrmann[3], Holger M. Reichardt[2], Reto Schwendener[4], Tobias Pukrop[5], Walter Schulz-Schaeffer[6], Heidi Hahn[1]*

1 Institute of Human Genetics, University Medical Center, Goettingen, Germany, **2** Institute of Cellular and Molecular Immunology, University Medical Center, Goettingen, Germany, **3** Department of Radiation Oncology, University Medical Center, Goettingen, Germany, **4** Institute of Molecular Cancer Research, University of Zurich, Zurich, Switzerland, **5** Department of Hematology and Oncology, University Medical Center, Goettingen, Germany, **6** Department of Neuropathology, University Medical Center, Goettingen, Germany

Abstract

Basal cell carcinoma (BCC) belongs to the group of non-melanoma skin tumors and is the most common tumor in the western world. BCC arises due to mutations in the tumor suppressor gene *Patched1* (*Ptch*). Analysis of the conditional *Ptch* knockout mouse model for BCC reveals that macrophages and dendritic cells (DC) of the skin play an important role in BCC growth restraining processes. This is based on the observation that a clodronate-liposome mediated depletion of these cells in the tumor-bearing skin results in significant BCC enlargement. The depletion of these cells does not modulate Ki67 or *K10* expression, but is accompanied by a decrease in collagen-producing cells in the tumor stroma. Together, the data suggest that cutaneous macrophages and DC in the tumor microenvironment exert an antitumor effect on BCC.

Editor: Amanda Ewart Toland, Ohio State University Medical Center, United States of America

Funding: This work was supported by the Deutsche Forschungsgemeinschaft (http://www.dfg.de/; FOR942 HA 2197/5-2 to Heidi Hahn). The funders had no role in study design, data collection and analysis, decision to publish, or preparation of the manuscript.

Competing Interests: The authors have declared that no competing interests exist.

* E-mail: hhahn@gwdg.de

Introduction

BCC is the most commonly diagnosed tumor among people in the western world and arises due to mutations in the tumor suppressor gene *Ptch*. Although BCC rarely metastasizes it can cause significant morbidity due to local aggressiveness and recurrences [1]. Interestingly, approximately 20% of BCCs show signs of spontaneous regression [2]. BCC regression is associated with significantly increased numbers of T cells and the expression of the IL-2 receptor, which is an early activation marker for T cells [3]. Furthermore, a role of T-helper 1 type cytokines such as INFγ, IL-2 and TNFβ has been suggested [4]. In addition, the immune modulator imiquimod that is used for topical treatment of BCC results in a massive peri- and intratumoral increase in macrophages [5].

In the skin, several types of antigen-presenting immune cells exist. In the mouse these are mainly macrophages and DC. DC that populate the basal and suprabasal layers of the epidermis are often called Langerhans cells (LC), while DC in the dermis are often called dermal DC (dDC) [6,7]. Common to these cells is the potential to internalize particulate macromolecules and to display migratory properties [8]. In addition, these cells can express MHCII and/or F4/80 [6].

There is growing evidence that interactions between tumor cells and the surrounding stroma plays an important role in tumor progression. Several reports have demonstrated that DC including LC are essential in the generation of an antitumor immunity in the skin (e.g. [9,10]). Given the rich network of these cells in the skin they are often thought to be the first immune cells to encounter tumor antigens from cutaneous cancers (for review see [11]). This also has been demonstrated for macrophages in extra-cutaneous cancers where macrophages can exert a beneficial role due to cytotoxicity to tumor cells but not to normal cells [12]. However, high macrophage numbers also have been linked to reduced survival of patients with solid cancers, indicating that the presence of macrophages could also be advantageous for tumor growth and metastasis [13]. Therefore, macrophages probably can have contrasting roles in cancer depending on their phenotype (for review see [14]).

Using the conditional $Ptch^{flox/flox}ERT2^{+/-}$ knockout mouse model for BCC [15], we now provide evidence that macrophages and DC are involved in growth restraining processes in this tumor entity.

Materials and Methods

Mice and induction of BCC

Animals were sacrificed at the indicated end points of the experiments or if necessary due to the health conditions (e.g. weight loss >15%, apathy) by CO2 anesthesia followed by cervical dislocation. The mice used in the study were handled in accordance with the German animal protection law and the experiments were approved by the Niedersächsisches Landesamt für Verbraucherschutz und Lebensmittelsicherheit (permit numbers: 33.14.42502-04-026/09 and 33.14.42502-04-111/09). All experiments using animals were performed in compliance with all legal and ethical requirements. $Ptch^{flox/flox}$ mice have *loxP* sites in *Ptch* introns 7 and 9 [16]. *Rosa26CreERT2(ERT2)* mice express a tamoxifen-inducible cre recombinase under the control of the endogenous and ubiquitously expressed *Rosa26*-promoter [17]. $Ptch^{flox/flox}ERT2^{+/-}$ mice were on a mixed C57BL/6 x Balb/c background. Genotyping of the $Ptch^{flox}$ and the Cre-mediated $Ptch^{del}$ alleles and of *ERT2* was performed as described [18]. All primers used for genotyping are listed in Table S1.

BCCs were induced in 8 week-old conditional $Ptch^{flox/flox}ERT2^{+/-}$ mice by intramuscular (i.m.) injection of 100 µg tamoxifen as described [18,19].

Depletion of macrophages in mice using clodrolip

Liposome-encapsulated clodronate termed clodrolip was essentially prepared as described previously [20]. For depletion of macrophages in mice, clodrolip was injected intraperitoneally (i.p.) in $Ptch^{floxflox}ERT2^{+/-}$ mice (n = 7) 15 days after tamoxifen-mediated BCC induction. The initial clodronate dose was 2 mg/20g body weight. Subsequently clodrolip was injected every fourth day at a dose of 1 mg/20 g and the treatment was continued for 75 days. The same amount of empty liposomes served as a control (n = 4). Clodrolip and empty liposomes were freshly diluted each time in PBS to obtain the desired drug dose in 120 µl for each animal. Animals were sacrificed 24 h after the last clodrolip or liposome dose. Spleen and skin samples were excised. Parts of the samples were either used for FACS analyses or RNA isolation, or were formalin-fixed and embedded in paraffin for immunohistological analyses.

Cell culture experiments

The murine BCC cell line ASZ001 was established from UV-induced BCC of *Ptch* mutant mice and was cultured as described [21].

Cell viability/metabolic activity of ASZ001 was determined by addition of WST-1 reagent (Roche Diagnostics, Mannheim, Germany) according to the manufacturer's recommendations after incubation with 0.1 mg/ml clodrolip or the same amount of empty liposomes for 24–72 h.

FACS analyses of tissue macrophages

FACS analysis of immune cells was performed on single cell suspensions of skin that were obtained as recently described [22]. Cells (1×10^6) were stained with monoclonal antibodies against Mac1 (anti CD11b-FITC, BD Biosciences #557396) and F4/80 (anti F4/80-Cy5, eBiosciences 15-4801). At least 2×10^5 viable cells were acquired on the basis of forward and side scattering and quantified by using a BD LSRII cytometer. Data acquisition and analysis were performed using the software BD FacsDiva (BD Biosciences Pharmingen) and FlowJo (Treestar, Ashland, OR).

Gene expression analysis

Total RNA from skin was isolated using the RNeasy Fibrous Tissue Mini Kit (Qiagen, Hilden, Germany) and cDNA was synthesized using Superscript II and random hexamers (Invitrogen, Karlsruhe, Germany). Gene expression was analyzed by SYBR-green-based qRT-PCR assays on the ABI Prism HT 7900 Detection System instrument and software (Applied Biosystems, Darmstadt, Germany). The data was analyzed using the standard curve method for relative quantification. All primer pairs were intron-flanking and are shown in the Table S1. Amplification of *18S rRNA* served to normalize the amount of sample cDNA. Each sample was reverse transcribed twice and analyzed in triplicates. The mean value of each sample was used for analysis.

Immunohistochemistry

Formalin-fixed tail skin was embedded in paraffin and sectioned at 5 µm for histological analyses. The identity of BCC was confirmed by examination of hematoxylin and eosin (H&E) stained sections. The paraffin sections were stained using a monoclonal anti-MHCII antibody (rat anti-mouse I-A/I-E #107602 from BioLegend; for antigen retrieval boric acid was used) that detects DC and to a lesser extend macrophages. In addition, an anti-F4/80 antibody (rat anti mouse #MCA497GA from Serotec; no antigen retrieval necessary) was employed that labels macrophages and to a lesser extend DC [6]. A biotinylated polyclonal antibody from Dako (# E0468, rabbit anti rat) served as secondary antibody. Following incubation with Streptavidin/HRP (#P0397, from Dako) and several washing steps, 3-Amino-9-Ethylcarbazol was used as a substrate. For Ki67 stainings the anti-Ki76 antibody #556003 from BD Pharmingen was used (antigen retrieval with citrate buffer pH 6). For detection of the primary antibody the Envision Polyclonal rabbit/mouse HRP kit (Dako, #K5007) was used. For TUNEL staining the DeadEnd Colorimetric TUNEL System (Promega, Germany) was applied according to the manufacturer's instructions. Staining was visualized with 3-Amino-9-Ethylcarbazol. After counterstaining with haematoxylin the sections were covered using glycergel (Dako GmbH, Hamburg).

$MHCII^+$ cells were counted separately both in the epidermis (representing LC) and the dermis (representing mostly dDC) of 7 clodrolip treated and 4 liposome treated mice. $F4/80^+$ cells were counted in the BCC stroma of 4 clodrolip treated and 3 liposome treated mice. For this purpose 2 independent paraffin-embedded skin samples (sample length and width app. 2.0 cm and 0.1 cm, respectively) from each mouse were sectioned and positive cells were counted on at least 3 microscopic fields of vision per sample. The analyzed stromal or epidermal areas (at least 3.6 mm^2/field of vision or 1 mm^2/field of vision, respectively) were measured using the software cellSens Dimension (*Olympus* Soft Imaging Solutions GmbH; Germany). Given are the numbers of F4/80 positive cells per mm^2 stroma and MHCII positive cells per mm^2 stroma or epidermis.

All $Ki67^+$ cells of at least 1000 BCC cells on 2 independent paraffin sections of 7 clodrolip treated and 4 liposome treated mice were counted and the percentage of $Ki67^+$ BCC cells was calculated.

$TUNEL^+$ BCC cells were very rare. Thus all $TUNEL^+$ cells of 2 independent paraffin sections each of 7 clodrolip treated and 4 liposome treated mice were counted.

Goldner staining was performed to visualize components of the connective tissue in the tumor stroma as described by Goldner [23]. This staining labels collagen in green, cell nuclei in brownish-red, and keratin in red color. Since most cells embedded in collagen are fibroblasts, calculation of the number of cell nuclei embedded in the collagen allows for quantification of fibroblasts localized in the tumor-adjacent stroma. In order to compare the amount of fibroblasts in liposome- and clodrolip-treated BCC-bearing skin (n = 4 and n = 7, respectively), 16 and 23 fields of vision (0.4 mm^2 each) were analyzed, respectively. The stromal area (in green) was measured using the software cellSens Dimension (*Olympus* Soft Imaging Solutions GmbH; Germany). Subsequently, all cellular nuclei in this region were counted and $MHCII^+$ and $F4/80^+$ cells (counted on adjacent slides) were subtracted. Given is the number of cells per mm^2 stroma.

Measurement of tumor size

BCC size was measured on H&E stained sections using the area calculation tool of the software cellSens Dimension (*Olympus* Soft

Imaging Solutions GmbH; Germany). For this purpose 6 independent skin samples (each sample at app. 2.0 cm length and 0.1 cm width) of 7 clodrolip treated and 4 liposome treated mice were sectioned at 5 µm. The tumor area was calculated by summing up the individual tumor area measured from each sample and consecutive normalization to the total skin area analyzed.

Statistical analyses

If not otherwise indicated, statistical differences were analyzed using Mann-Whitney testing. Data was considered significant when $P<0.05$.

Results

Stromal areas in BCC-bearing skin of $Ptch^{flox/flox}ERT2^{+/-}$ mice are infiltrated with MHCII$^+$ cells

We recently showed that the stroma of BCC of $Ptch^{flox/flox}ERT2^{+/-}$ mice is infiltrated with F4/80$^+$ tumor-associated macrophages [19]. Using paraffin sections, we first confirmed this observation and stained paraffin embedded tissue sections with a MHCII antibody that marks dDCs and also LC in the murine skin and to lesser extent cutaneous macrophages [6]. As shown in Figure 1, the BCC stroma shows many MHCII$^+$ cells, indicating that the tumor-bearing skin is abundantly infiltrated with the above-mentioned cell populations.

Systemic clodrolip treatment of $Ptch^{flox/flox}ERT2^{+/-}$ mice results in depletion of macrophages, dDC and LC and in an enhancement of BCC growth

In order to determine whether the network of cutaneous DC and macrophages are involved in growth-regulating processes in BCC we depleted these cells in BCC-bearing $Ptch^{flox/flox}ERT2^{+/-}$ mice by treating the animals with clodrolip. Empty liposomes were used as vehicle-control. The treatment scheme was as previously published by Zeisberger and colleagues [20] and was started 15 days after tamoxifen-mediated induction of BCC. The treatment was continued for 75 days.

Successful macrophage depletion was first demonstrated by reduced F4/80 immunoreactivity of the spleens of clodrolip treated mice (Figure S1). Next we performed FACS analysis of single cell suspensions of the skin using Mac1 and F4/80 antibodies. Whereas Mac1 is expressed on granulocytes, T-, B- and NK-cells, DC and monocytes [24], macrophages are double positive for Mac1 and F4/80 [25]. For the analyses 3 clodrolip- and 3 vehicle-treated animals were sacrifized. As shown in Table 1, the numbers of Mac1$^+$, F4/80$^+$ and Mac1$^+$F4/80$^+$ double positive cells were generally lower in the skin of the clodrolip-treated cohort when compared to the controls (Table 1). As also shown in Table 1, the depletion was highly efficient in two of the clodrolip-treated mice (mouse 2 and mouse 3 in Table 1). These results were similar to those reported by Zeisberger and colleagues who showed that clodrolip treatment caused depletion of F4/80$^+$ and Mac1$^+$ cells [20].

A reduction of F4/80$^+$ cells in the clodrolip-treated cohort was also revealed by immunohistochemistry (Fig. 2A). In addition, MHCII$^+$ cells in the BCC stroma were almost entirely depleted in the clodrolip-treated group when compared to the vehicle-treated group (Fig. 2B). The clodrolip-treatment also resulted in a significant decrease in epidermal MHCII$^+$ LC (Fig. 2B). Together these results show that clodrolip-treatment resulted in an efficient depletion of macrophages, dDC (i.e. DC in the dermis) and LC (i.e DC in the basal and suprabasal layers of the epidermis). With respect to macrophages and dDC the results are in accordance with the current literature, which describes depletion of these cells by clodronate. However, they are in contrast to published data showing that LC are resistant towards the drug [26–28].

Next, we studied the effects of clodrolip on BCC growth. For this purpose the BCC area was analyzed on H&E stained paraffin

Table 1. Systemic application of clodrolip decreases the numbers of macrophages in the skin.

		BCC-bearing skin		
	mouse	Mac1$^+$	F4/80$^+$	Mac1$^+$F4/80$^+$
	liposomes	M1	5.98	4.30
4.40				
	M2	4.97	4.82	3.57
	M3	3.02	3.77	2.52
	mean (SEM)	4.66 (0.87)	4.30 (0.30)	3.50 (0.54)
	clodrolip	M1	4.69	2.41
2.38				
	M2	1.00	0.82	0.64
	M3	1.74	0.96	0.85
	mean (SEM)	2.48 (1.13)	1.40 (0.51)	1.29 (0.55)

The percentage of Mac1$^+$, F4/80$^+$ and Mac1$^+$F4/80$^+$ double-positive cells in tumor-bearing skin of $Ptch^{flox/flox}ERT2^{+/-}$ mice was determined by FACS. M1 to M3: mouse 1 to mouse 3.

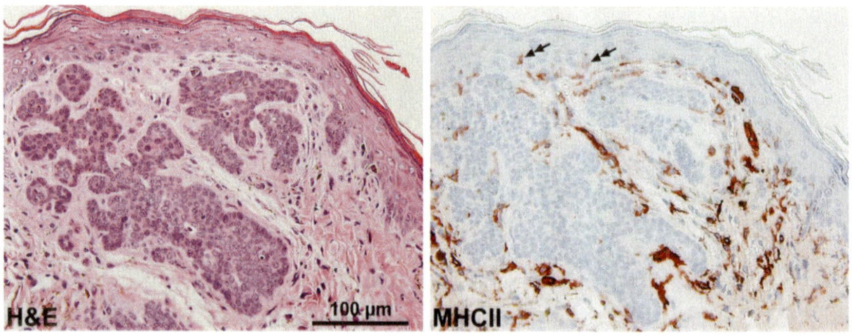

Figure 1. MHCII expression in BCC-bearing skin of $Ptch^{flox/flox}ERT2^{+/-}$ mice. H&E staining and immunohistochemical analysis of MHCII expression on paraffin sections derived from BCC-bearing skin of $Ptch^{flox/flox}ERT2^{+/-}$ mice. The secondary antibody alone did not result in any staining, hence the MHCII signals were specific (data not shown). double arrows: intraepidermal MHCII$^+$ LC.

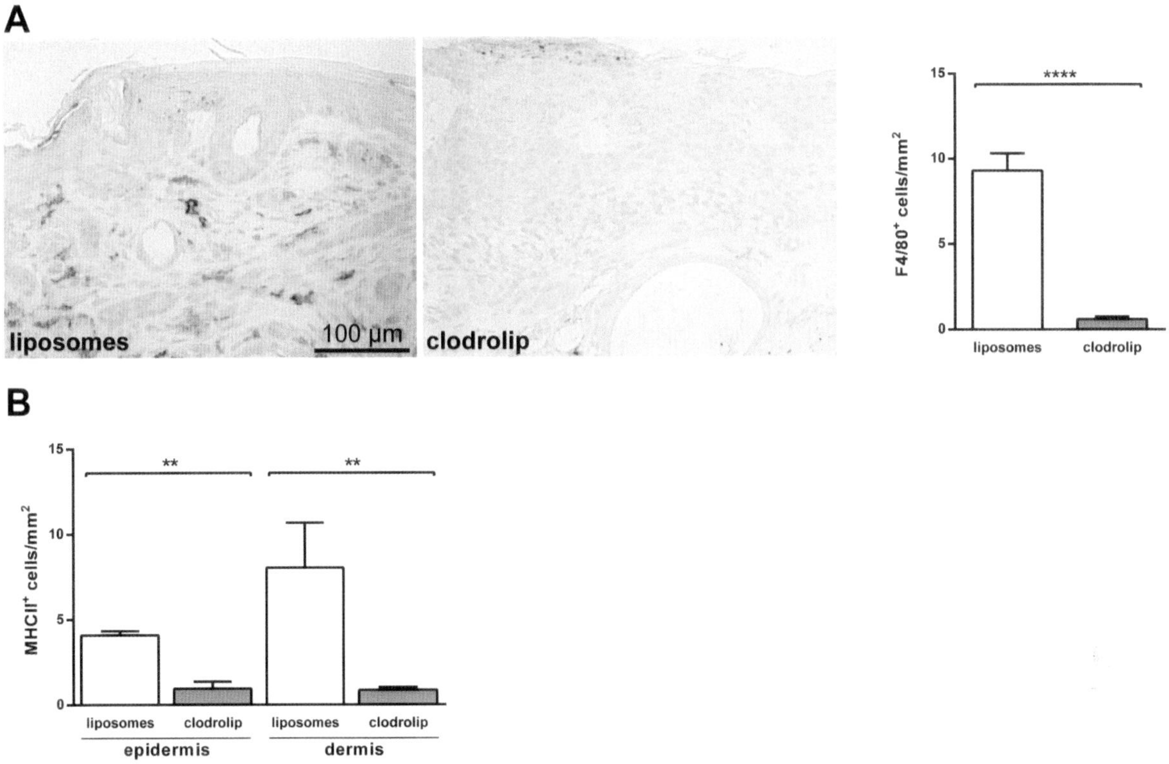

Figure 2. Clodrolip treatment results in depletion of cutaneous phagocytic cells in BCC-bearing skin of *Ptch*$^{flox/flox}$*ERT2*$^{+/-}$ mice. (A) Immunohistochemical analysis of F4/80 expression on paraffin-sections of BCC-bearing skin derived from liposome- or clodrolip-treated *Ptch*$^{flox/flox}$*ERT2*$^{+/-}$ mice. Left panel shows micrographs; right panel shows the absolute number of F4/80$^+$ cells per square millimeter of BCC-bearing tissue. **** $P<0.0001$ (mean +SEM). (B) Absolute numbers of MHCII$^+$ cells per square millimeter of BCC-bearing tissue as counted on stained paraffin-sections from liposome- or clodrolip-treated *Ptch*$^{flox/flox}$*ERT2*$^{+/-}$ mice. MHCII$^+$ cells were counted separately both in the epidermis (representing LC) and the stroma (representing DC). ** $P<0.01$.

sections derived from 7 clodrolip- and 4 vehicle-treated mice. The tumor area was calculated by summing up the individual tumor area measured from each sample (see material and methods) and normalization to the total area of the skin analyzed. The data revealed that the BCC of the clodrolip-treated group were significantly enlarged when compared to the vehicle-treated group (Fig. 3A; Fig. 3B left panel). This was also obvious when comparing the BCC size of the vehicle-treated group with that of the 2 animals (mouse 2 and mouse 3 in Table 1) in which the clodrolip-treatment resulted in efficient depletion of macrophages in the skin (Fig. 3B right panel).

In order to examine whether clodrolip or empty liposomes directly influenced tumor cell growth, we also investigated the toxic effects of clodrolip on BCC cells *in vitro*. For this purpose, the BCC cell line ASZ001 was incubated with 0.1 mg/ml clodrolip for 24 h to 72 h. The same amounts of empty liposomes or of PBS alone were used as controls. As shown in Figure 3C clodrolip significantly reduced the viability of ASZ001 when compared to the controls (Fig. 3C). These data indicate that clodrolip has direct tumoricidal activity. Therefore the *tumor-promoting* activity of clodrolip *in vivo* might be an indirect effect of the drug on the tumor cells.

Together these data show that macrophages and DC including LC in BCC-bearing skin were efficiently depleted after treatment with clodrolip. This depletion was accompanied by a significant enhancement of tumor growth.

Clodrolip treatment of BCC-bearing skin of *Ptch*$^{flox/flox}$*ERT2*$^{+/-}$ mice decreases the number of collagen-producing stromal cells

In order to analyze whether the clodrolip-mediated enhancement of BCC growth was associated with a decrease in proliferation or with increased apoptosis, we performed immunohistochemical analysis of the proliferation marker Ki67 and TUNEL staining, respectively. However, neither the numbers of Ki67$^+$ nor of TUNEL$^+$ cells were different between the cohorts (Figure 4A and 4B, respectively). In addition, a first expression analysis of the differentiation marker *K10* that is solely expressed by epidermal cells did not reveal any significant difference (data not shown). However, we found that the clodrolip treatment resulted in a decrease in collagen-producing stromal cells. This became obvious by a Goldner staining (see Figure S2). As shown in Fig 4C (left panel) the number of collagen-producing cells that are mainly fibroblasts was significantly lower in the clodrolip-treated cohort when compared to the liposome-treated cohort. This was in line with qRT-PCR data showing that the expression of the fibroblast markers *vimentin* and *prolyl-4-hydroxylase beta* (*P4hb*) was decreased in the clodrolip-treated samples (Fig. 4C, middle and right panel). Together, these data suggest that the clodrolip-treatment, besides lowering the F4/80$^+$ and MHCII$^+$ cells in the tumor microenvironment, also decreases the numbers of collagen-producing cells, which are in all likelihood stromal fibroblasts.

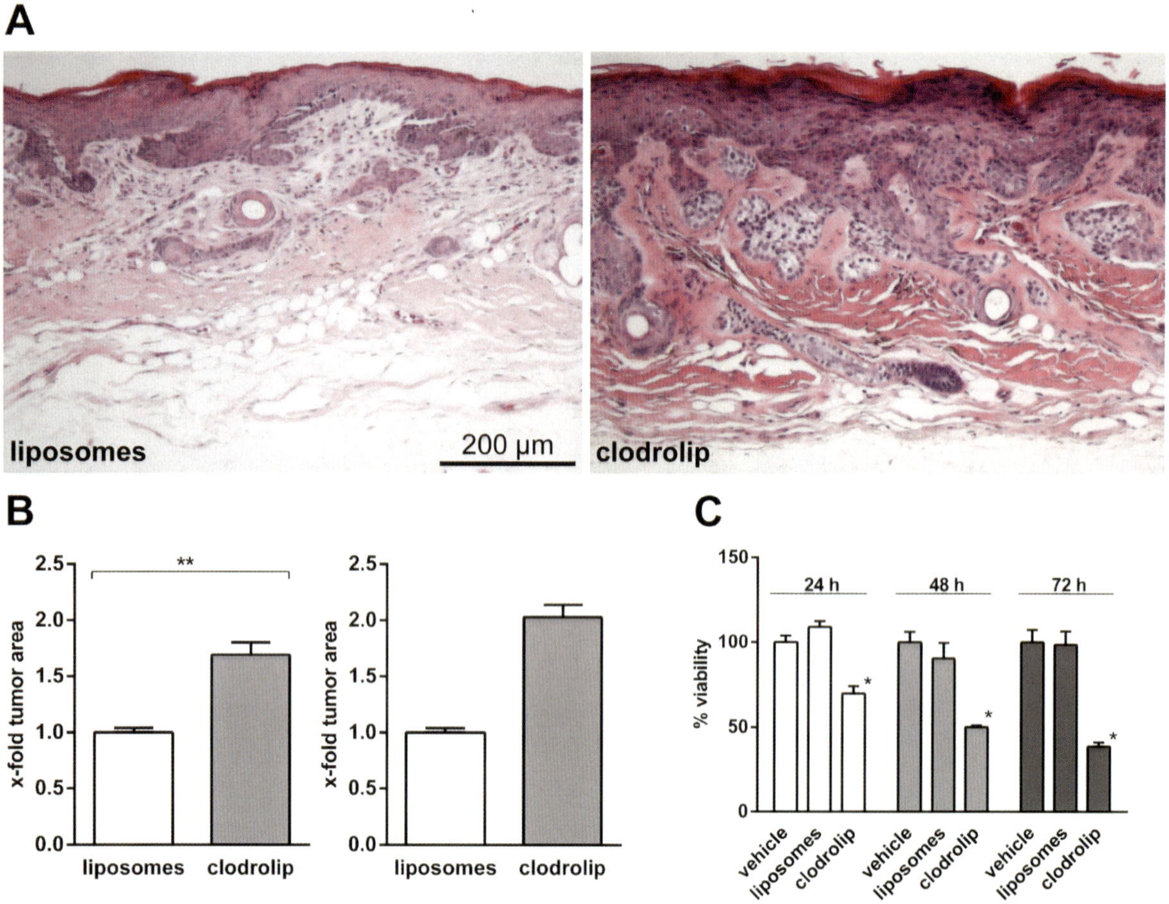

Figure 3. Clodrolip enhances BCC growth in *Ptch*$^{flox/flox}$*ERT2*$^{+/-}$ mice. (A) H&E stainings of paraffin-sections derived from BCC-bearing skin of liposome- or clodrolip-treated *Ptch*$^{flox/flox}$*ERT2*$^{+/-}$ mice. (B) Relative tumor areas of H&E-stained BCC-bearing skin samples of liposome- or clodrolip-treated *Ptch*$^{flox/flox}$*ERT2*$^{+/-}$ mice. The mean value of the liposome-treated controls was normalized to 1. Left panel shows the mean value (+SEM) of all liposome- and clodrolip-treated animals $^{**}P<0.01$; right panel shows the mean value (+SEM) of all liposome-treated animals in comparison with 2 clodrolip-treated mice (mouse 2 and mouse 3 in Table 1), in which the phagocytic cells have been very efficiently depleted (due to the small sample size, statistical analysis was omitted). (C) Viability/metabolic activity of the BCC cell line ASZ001 after treatment with PBS, liposomes or clodrolip. Mean value of the PBS-treated controls was set to 100%. $^{**}P<0.01$.

Discussion

Our data suggest that cutaneous macrophages and DC are necessary for tumor growth restraining processes in the *Ptch*$^{flox/flox}$*ERT2*$^{+/-}$ mouse model for BCC. This assumption is based on the observations that the BCC stroma is infiltrated with these cells and that a clodronate-liposome mediated depletion enhances BCC growth. In addition, the clodrolip treatment was accompanied by a decrease in collagen-producing cells. Because the fibroblast markers *vimentin* and *P4hb* were downregulated as well, it is likely that the respective cells were fibroblasts. The reduction of fibroblasts was probably not a direct toxic effect of clodronate because i) liposome-encapsuled clodronate is not internalized by non-phagocytic cells [29] and ii) clodronate in cell culture only marginally affects fibroblast growth [30]. Instead, the decrease of the collagen-expressing cells might be directly associated with the loss of macrophages that have been shown to enhance fibroblast proliferation [31], probably by the secretion of TNFα, PDGF or IL-1β [31,32]. However, these assumptions are pure speculations and need more investigation in the future.

Together, our experiments demonstrate a very important role of macrophages and DC in growth restraining processes in BCC. In our experiments application of liposome-encapsulated clodronate resulted in effective depletion of these cells as demonstrated by loss of MHCII^{+} cells that is expressed by professional immune antigen-presenting cells. In addition depletion of macrophages was also demonstrated by loss of Mac1^{+}F4/80^{+} cells. This is in accordance to other reports that demonstrated elimination of DC and macrophages upon treatment with clodronate [26,33]. We observed a significant reduction of epidermal LC. This is in contrast to other reports showing that LC are resistant to clodronate [28]. However, since the skin in our setting was highly loaded with BCC it is possible that the LC were activated and thus phagocytosed this toxic drug at higher avidity.

The clodronate-liposome mediated loss of DC and the accompanying enhancement of BCC growth in our model match the established role of these cells in non-melanoma cutaneous cancer. Thus, specific subsets of DC inclusive LC are beneficial for tumor eradication in the skin. This is due to their ability to either recognize, process and present foreign (tumor) antigens to T cells or to stimulate T cell proliferation and enhance T cell activity, respectively. In addition, DC including both LC and dDC can produce IFN-α in response to foreign (tumor) antigens. Accordingly, it has been shown that elevated amounts of dDC subsets are indeed associated with increased clearance of BCC lesions

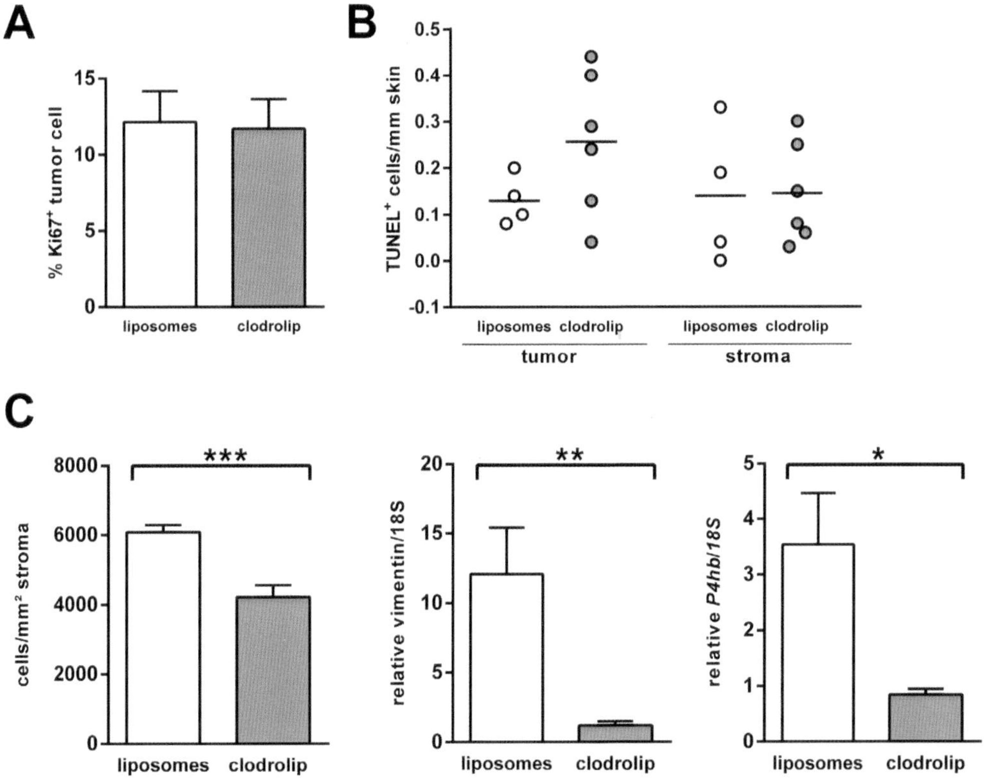

Figure 4. Clodrolip decreases the number of collagen-producing cells and the mRNA expression of the fibroblast markers *vimentin* and *P4hb* in BCC-bearing skin of *Ptch*$^{flox/flox}$*ERT2*$^{+/-}$ mice. (A) Percentage of Ki67^{+} BCC cells in liposome- or clodrolip-treated *Ptch*$^{flox/flox}$*ERT2*$^{+/-}$ mice. (B) TUNEL^{+} BCC cells per mm BCC-bearing skin in liposome- or clodrolip-treated *Ptch*$^{flox/flox}$*ERT2*$^{+/-}$ mice. (C) Collagen-producing cells (mainly fibroblast) as estimated by Goldner staining (left panel; see main manuscript for detailed informations) and qRT-PCR analysis of *vimentin* (middle panel) and of *P4hb* (right panel) in BCC-bearing skin of *Ptch*$^{flox/flox}$*ERT2*$^{+/-}$ mice treated with liposomes or clodrolip. Data shows the mean value (+SEM). * $P<0.05$, ** $P<0.01$, *** $P<0.001$.

following treatment with imiquimod (for review see [11]). In addition to dDC and LC, macrophages can play beneficial roles in cancer [34]. Thus, in contrast to tumor-promoting M2 macrophages, these so-called M1 macrophages act by defending the host from infections and also from tumors. Therefore, depletion of the latter cells can result in tumor-promoting effects, which also may have contributed to the enhancement of BCC growth in our model as well.

In the clinics, bisphosphonates such as clodronate are frequently used to delay the spread of bone metastases. This is due to the fact that bisphosphonates strongly bind to mineralized bone surfaces and are ingested by osteoclasts, wherein they inhibit osteolysis, thereby preventing the release of growth factors from the bone matrix [35]. In addition, bisphosphonates also revealed direct killing of different cancer cells, including myeloma, breast cancer, prostate cancer, and lung cancer *in vitro* (reviewed in [36]). Indeed, also in our experiments the drug efficiently decreased the viability of the BCC cell line ASZ001. Furthermore, bisphosphonates encapsulated in nanocarriers such as liposomes can inhibit angiogenesis and can deplete tumor-promoting macrophages, whereas the free drug mainly inhibits osteolysis. In line with all these effects many studies on a variety of tumors thus report that administration of bisphosphonates generates an antitumor activity [36]. However, despite these data there are also several reports showing *protumoral* effects of clodronate administered as free drug. For example, a study of 299 women with breast cancer demonstrated a significantly increased rate of non-skeletal metastases and a significantly lower overall survival rate after clodronate therapy [37]. Furthermore, cases of esophagus carcinoma have been described after oral bisphosphonate use [38]. These studies show that, as in our study, clodronate can also result in enhancement of cancerous malignancies.

In summary, in our BCC model the tumor-promoting effects of liposome-encapsulated clodronate may result from various processes. These include a decrease in antigen-presenting cells of the skin (i.e. of DC including LC and macrophages), a decrease in collagen-producing cells and most likely other so far unknown molecular processes such as modulation of T cell numbers, modulation of dermal angiogenesis, and the induction of a wide palette of cytokines such as IFNγ, IL-17, IL-1, IL-6, TNFα and IL-23 that are all modulated in the skin upon treatment with clodronate [39]. An elucidation of the exact mechanisms underlying the tumor-promoting effects of clodrolip presented here will be further complicated by the fact that empty liposomes themselves can induce antitumor effects (see Figure S3) that are likewise associated with macrophage responses such as e.g. the induction of *iNOS*, *Arg1* and *Trem2* [22]. Nevertheless, our data strongly suggest that macrophages and DC of the skin play an important role in skin cancer pathogenesis in that they exert antitumor effects on BCC, the most common tumor in humans.

Supporting Information

Figure S1 Depletion of F4/80-expressing cells in spleens derived from clodrolip-treated $Ptch^{flox/flox}ERT2^{+/-}$ mice. Immunohistochemical analysis using an anti-F4/80 antibody of paraffin-embedded spleens of $Ptch^{flox/flox}ERT2^{+/-}$ mice treated with empty liposomes or clodrolip.

Figure S2 Evaluation of amounts of fibroblasts by the Goldner method. The Goldner method labels collagen in green and the nuclei and keratin in red color. Calculation of the number of cell nuclei embedded in the collagen (in the lower panel, the coloring of the tumor-bearing epidermis was attenuated using the software FreeHand MX (Macromedia Inc.) to better visualize the collagen-producing stromal cells) allows for quantification of fibroblasts localized in the tumor-adjacent stroma. As demonstrated by the figures, the amount of nuclei embedded in the collagen is lower in the clodrolip-treated BCC when compared to the liposome-treated BCC.

Figure S3 Empty liposmes themselves can induce antitumor effects in BCC-bearing $Ptch^{flox/flox}ERT2^{+/-}$ mice. HE-stained skin sections of liposome-treated mice (left panel) and PBS-treated mice (right panel). The analysis of the tumor-bearing skin revealed that tumors of PBS-treated mice are larger when compared to liposome-treated mice.

Table S1 Oligonucleotides used for genotyping and reverse-transcription polymerase chain reaction.

Acknowledgments

We are grateful to Susan Peter for excellent animal care and Anke Frommhold for technical assistance.

Author Contributions

Conceived and designed the experiments: SK FN AU KD JT MH HH TP RS. Performed the experiments: SK FN AU KD JT MH. Analyzed the data: SK FN AU KD JT MH HH WSS. Contributed reagents/materials/analysis tools: HH HR RS. Wrote the paper: HH.

References

1. Epstein EH (2008) Basal cell carcinomas: attack of the hedgehog. Nat Rev Cancer 8: 743–54.
2. Curson C, Weedon D (1979) Spontaneous regression in basal cell carcinomas. J Cutan Pathol 6: 432–7.
3. Hunt MJ, Halliday GM, Weedon D, Cooke BE, Barnetson RS (1994) Regression in basal cell carcinoma: an immunohistochemical analysis. Br J Dermatol 130: 1–8.
4. Wong DA, Bishop GA, Lowes MA, Cooke B, Barnetson RS, et al. (2000) Cytokine profiles in spontaneously regressing basal cell carcinomas. Br J Dermatol 143: 91–8.
5. Urosevic M, Maier T, Benninghoff B, Slade H, Burg G, et al. (2003) Mechanisms underlying imiquimod-induced regression of basal cell carcinoma in vivo. Arch Dermatol 139: 1325–32.
6. Ginhoux F, Ng LG, Merad M (2012) Understanding the murine cutaneous dendritic cell network to improve intradermal vaccination strategies. Current topics in microbiology and immunology 351: 1–24.
7. Nestle FO, Filgueira L, Nickoloff BJ, Burg G (1998) Human dermal dendritic cells process and present soluble protein antigens. J Invest Dermatol 110: 762–6.
8. Valladeau J, Saeland S (2005) Cutaneous dendritic cells. Seminars in immunology 17: 273–83.
9. Fuertes MB, Kacha AK, Kline J, Woo SR, Kranz DM, et al. (2011) Host type I IFN signals are required for antitumor CD8+ T cell responses through CD8{alpha}+ dendritic cells. J Exp Med 208: 2005–16.
10. Romano E, Rossi M, Ratzinger G, de Cos MA, Chung DJ, et al. (2011) Peptide-loaded Langerhans cells, despite increased IL15 secretion and T-cell activation in vitro, elicit antitumor T-cell responses comparable to peptide-loaded monocyte-derived dendritic cells in vivo. Clin Cancer Res 17: 1984–97.
11. Yanofsky VR, Mitsui H, Felsen D, Carucci JA (2013) Understanding dendritic cells and their role in cutaneous carcinoma and cancer immunotherapy. Clinical & developmental immunology 2013: 624123.
12. Biswas SK, Mantovani A (2010) Macrophage plasticity and interaction with lymphocyte subsets: cancer as a paradigm. Nat Immunol 11: 889–96.
13. Lewis CE, Pollard JW (2006) Distinct role of macrophages in different tumor microenvironments. Cancer Res 66: 605–12.
14. Mosser DM, Edwards JP (2008) Exploring the full spectrum of macrophage activation. Nat Rev Immunol 8: 958–69.
15. Nitzki F, Becker M, Frommhold A, Schulz-Schaeffer W, Hahn H (2012) Patched knockout mouse models of Basal cell carcinoma. Journal of skin cancer 2012: 907543.
16. Uhmann A, Dittmann K, Nitzki F, Dressel R, Koleva M, et al. (2007) The Hedgehog receptor Patched controls lymphoid lineage commitment. Blood 110: 1814–23.
17. Hameyer D, Loonstra A, Eshkind L, Schmitt S, Antunes C, et al. (2007) Toxicity of ligand-dependent Cre recombinases and generation of a conditional Cre deleter mouse allowing mosaic recombination in peripheral tissues. Physiol Genomics 31: 32–41.
18. Zibat A, Uhmann A, Nitzki F, Wijgerde M, Frommhold A, et al. (2009) Time-point and dosage of gene inactivation determine the tumor spectrum in conditional Ptch knockouts. Carcinogenesis 30: 918–26.
19. Nitzki F, Zibat A, Konig S, Wijgerde M, Rosenberger A, et al. (2010) Tumor stroma-derived Wnt5a induces differentiation of basal cell carcinoma of Ptch-mutant mice via CaMKII. Cancer Res 70: 2739–48.
20. Zeisberger SM, Odermatt B, Marty C, Zehnder-Fjallman AH, Ballmer-Hofer K, et al. (2006) Clodronate-liposome-mediated depletion of tumour-associated macrophages: a new and highly effective antiangiogenic therapy approach. Br J Cancer 95: 272–81.
21. So PL, Langston AW, Daniallinia N, Hebert JL, Fujimoto MA, et al. (2006) Long-term establishment, characterization and manipulation of cell lines from mouse basal cell carcinoma tumors. Exp Dermatol 15: 742–50.
22. Konig S, Regen T, Dittmann K, Engelke M, Wienands J, et al. (2013) Empty liposomes induce antitumoral effects associated with macrophage responses distinct from those of the TLR1/2 agonist PamCSK (BLP). Cancer Immunol Immunother.
23. Goldner J (1938) A modification of the masson trichrome technique for routine laboratory purposes. Am J Pathol 14: 237–43.
24. Rasmussen JW, Cello J, Gil H, Forestal CA, Furie MB, et al. (2006) Mac-1+ cells are the predominant subset in the early hepatic lesions of mice infected with Francisella tularensis. Infection and immunity 74: 6590–8.
25. Ferron M, Vacher J (2005) Targeted expression of Cre recombinase in macrophages and osteoclasts in transgenic mice. Genesis 41: 138–45.
26. Kataru RP, Jung K, Jang C, Yang H, Schwendener RA, et al. (2009) Critical role of CD11b+ macrophages and VEGF in inflammatory lymphangiogenesis, antigen clearance, and inflammation resolution. Blood 113: 5650–9.
27. Kurimoto I, van Rooijen N, Dijkstra CD, Streilein JW (1994) Role of phagocytic macrophages in induction of contact hypersensitivity and tolerance by hapten applied to normal and ultraviolet B-irradiated skin. Immunology 83: 281–7.
28. Wang H, Peters T, Kess D, Sindrilaru A, Oreshkova T, et al. (2006) Activated macrophages are essential in a murine model for T cell-mediated chronic psoriasiform skin inflammation. J Clin Invest 116: 2105–14.
29. Claassen I, Van Rooijen N, Claassen E (1990) A new method for removal of mononuclear phagocytes from heterogeneous cell populations in vitro, using the liposome-mediated macrophage 'suicide' technique. Journal of immunological methods 134: 153–61.
30. Walter C, Klein MO, Pabst A, Al-Nawas B, Duschner H, et al. (2010) Influence of bisphosphonates on endothelial cells, fibroblasts, and osteogenic cells. Clinical oral investigations 14: 35–41.
31. Fleming JM, Miller TC, Kidacki M, Ginsburg E, Stuelten CH, et al. (2012) Paracrine interactions between primary human macrophages and human fibroblasts enhance murine mammary gland humanization in vivo. Breast cancer research: BCR 14: R97.
32. Chow FY, Nikolic-Paterson DJ, Atkins RC, Tesch GH (2004) Macrophages in streptozotocin-induced diabetic nephropathy: potential role in renal fibrosis. Nephrol Dial Transplant 19: 2987–96.
33. Handoko HY, Rodero MP, Boyle GM, Ferguson B, Engwerda C, et al. (2013) UVB-Induced Melanocyte Proliferation in Neonatal Mice Driven by CCR2-Independent Recruitment of Ly6c(low)MHCII(hi) Macrophages. J Invest Dermatol 133: 1803–12.
34. Solinas G, Germano G, Mantovani A, Allavena P (2009) Tumor-associated macrophages (TAM) as major players of the cancer-related inflammation. Journal of leukocyte biology 86: 1065–73.
35. Gnant M, Dubsky P, Hadji P (2012) Bisphosphonates: prevention of bone metastases in breast cancer. Recent results in cancer research. Fortschritte der Krebsforschung. Progres dans les recherches sur le cancer 192: 65–91.
36. Morgan G, Lipton A (2010) Antitumor effects and anticancer applications of bisphosphonates. Seminars in oncology 37 Suppl 2: S30–40.

37. Saarto T, Blomqvist C, Virkkunen P, Elomaa I (2001) Adjuvant clodronate treatment does not reduce the frequency of skeletal metastases in node-positive breast cancer patients: 5-year results of a randomized controlled trial. J Clin Oncol 19: 10–7.
38. Wysowski DK (2009) Reports of esophageal cancer with oral bisphosphonate use. N Engl J Med 360: 89–90.
39. Ward NL, Loyd CM, Wolfram JA, Diaconu D, Michaels CM, et al. (2011) Depletion of antigen-presenting cells by clodronate liposomes reverses the psoriatic skin phenotype in KC-Tie2 mice. Br J Dermatol 164: 750–8.

21

Altered Prostanoid Signaling Contributes to Increased Skin Tumorigenesis in Tpl2 Knockout Mice

Kathleen L. DeCicco-Skinner[1]⁹, Sabrina J. Nolan[1]⁹, Monika M. Deshpande[2], Erika L. Trovato[1,2], Taylor A. Dempsey[1], Jonathan S. Wiest[2]*

1 Department of Biology, American University, Washington, DC, United States of America, **2** Laboratory of Cancer Biology and Genetics, National Cancer Institute, National Institutes of Health, Bethesda, Maryland, United States of America

Abstract

Squamous cell carcinoma is the second most common form of skin cancer with the incidence expected to double over the next 20 years. Inflammation is believed to be a critical component in skin cancer progression. Therefore, understanding genes involved in the regulation of inflammatory pathways is vital to the design of targeted therapies. Numerous studies show cyclooxygenases (COXs) play an essential role in inflammation-associated cancers. *Tpl2 (MAP3K8)* is a protein kinase in the MAP Kinase signal transduction cascade. Previous research using a two-stage skin carcinogenesis model revealed that $Tpl2^{-/-}$ mice have significantly higher tumor incidence and inflammatory response than wild-type (WT) controls. The current study investigates whether cyclooxygenase-2 (COX-2) and COX-2- regulated prostaglandins and prostaglandin receptors drive the highly tumorigenic state of $\text{Tpl2}^{-/-}$ mice by investigating the relationship between Tpl2 and COX-2. Keratinocytes from newborn WT or $Tpl2^{-/-}$ mice were treated with 12-*O*-tetradecanoylphorbol-13-acetate (TPA) for various times over 24 hours. Western analysis revealed significant differences in COX-2 and COX-2 dependent prostanoids and prostanoid receptors. Additionally, *in vivo* experiments confirmed that COX-2 and COX-2 downstream factors were elevated in TPA-treated $\text{Tpl2}^{-/-}$ skin, as well as in papillomas from $Tpl2^{-/-}$ mice. Use of the selective COX-2 inhibitor Celecoxib showed the increased tumorigenesis in the $\text{Tpl2}^{-/-}$ mice to primarily be mediated through COX-2. These experiments illustrate COX-2 induction in the absence of Tpl2 may be responsible for the increased tumorigenesis found in $Tpl2^{-/-}$ mice. Defining the relationship between Tpl2 and COX-2 may lead to new ways to downregulate COX-2 through the modulation of Tpl2.

Editor: Soheil S. Dadras, University of Connecticut Health Center, United States of America

Funding: This research was supported in part by the Intramural Research Program of the National Cancer Institute, National Institutes of Health and by grant number UA5CA152907 from the National Cancer Institute. The funders had no role in study design, data collection and analysis, decision to publish, or preparation of the manuscript

Competing Interests: The authors have declared that no competing interests exist.

* E-mail: jwiest@mail.nih.gov

⁹ These authors contributed equally to this work.

Introduction

Deregulation in mitogen activated protein kinase (MAPK) signaling is a common alteration in the development or progression of skin cancer [1]. *Tumor Progression Locus 2 (Tpl2)*, also known as *MAP3K8*, is a MAP3K serine/threonine kinase in the MAPK signal transduction cascade [2]. *Tpl2* resides upstream of the MAPK ERK where it functions to phosphorylate MEK, the ERK kinase [3]. In addition to participating in ERK signaling, Tpl2 cross-talks with numerous other pathways including JNK, p38, NFAT, and nuclear factor kappa B (NF-κB) [4–8]. In non-stimulated cells, Tpl2 is held in complex with ABIN2 and the NF-κB precursor protein p105 [9]. This interaction stabilizes the Tpl2 protein but also prevents Tpl2 and NF-κB from activating their downstream signaling cascades by inhibiting the kinase activity of Tpl2 and the proteolysis of NF-κB p105 [10]. Upon activation of Tpl2 by various pro-inflammatory stimuli, IκB kinase (IKK) phosphorylates p105, releasing Tpl2 and p105 from the complex. This newly liberated Tpl2 now phosphorylates substrates in the ERK and JNK pathways. Additionally, p105 is subsequently degraded into p50 by the proteosome. p50 can now dimerize with other NF-κB family members and translocate to the nucleus where the active NF-κB complex can regulate over 400 genes. The overall result is an upregulation of diverse genes involved in growth, differentiation, and inflammation.

The *Tpl2/MAP3k8* gene was first isolated from thyroid tumors as a gene capable of inducing morphological transformation of NIH3T3 and SHOK cells [11]. Early reports in rodents showed *Tpl2* truncation of the C-terminus, resulting from provirus insertion, to be associated with T-cell lymphoma [12]. Subsequently several reports have found elevated *MAP3K8* activity in a number of human cancers including breast, endometrial, thymomas, lymphomas, lung, Hodgkin's disease, and nasopharyngeal carcinoma [4,12–15]. Additionally, recent reports correlate heightened *MAP3K8* expression levels with acquired resistance to drug therapy in melanoma [16]. However, the exact role of *Tpl2* in carcinogenesis has remained an enigma. Overexpression of *Tpl2/MAP3k8 in vivo* is weakly oncogenic and *Tpl2* mutations in humans are rarely found [12,17]. However, recent evidence suggests that under certain conditions *Tpl2* may serve a tumor suppressor role. $\text{Tpl2}^{-/-}$ mice, when crossed with the T cell receptor transgene, develop a high incidence of T cell lymphomas, whereas wild type mice remain cancer free [18]. Moreover, our laboratory recently reported that nearly 80% of Tpl2$^{-/-}$ mice developed chemically induced skin tumors compared to 16% of wild type mice, providing the first evidence in a *de novo* cancer model that *Tpl2* may serve as a tumor suppressor [19]. Therefore, the role of Tpl2 in tumorigenesis is complex, as either over-expression or reduced expression of this gene can promote a tumorigenic state depending on the cancer type [17].

Numerous reports suggest inflammation in the microenvironment contributes to the development or progression of skin cancer [20]. Among other inflammatory enzymes, cyclooxygenases (COXs) play an essential role in inflammation-associated cancers [21,22]. COXs catalyze the conversion of arachidonic acid (AA) to the intermediate product prostaglandin H_2 (PGH_2) [21,22]. PGH_2 can then be converted to the biologically active prostanoids PGE_2, PGD_2, $PGF_{2\alpha}$, PGI_2 and TXA_2 through prostanoid synthases. Human cells contain two primary COX isoforms, namely COX-1 and COX-2 [21]. Both isoforms catalyze the same reaction, but differ in their expression patterns. *COX-1* is expressed constitutively in most tissues, and is involved in a number of normal physiological processes, including maintenance of the gastric

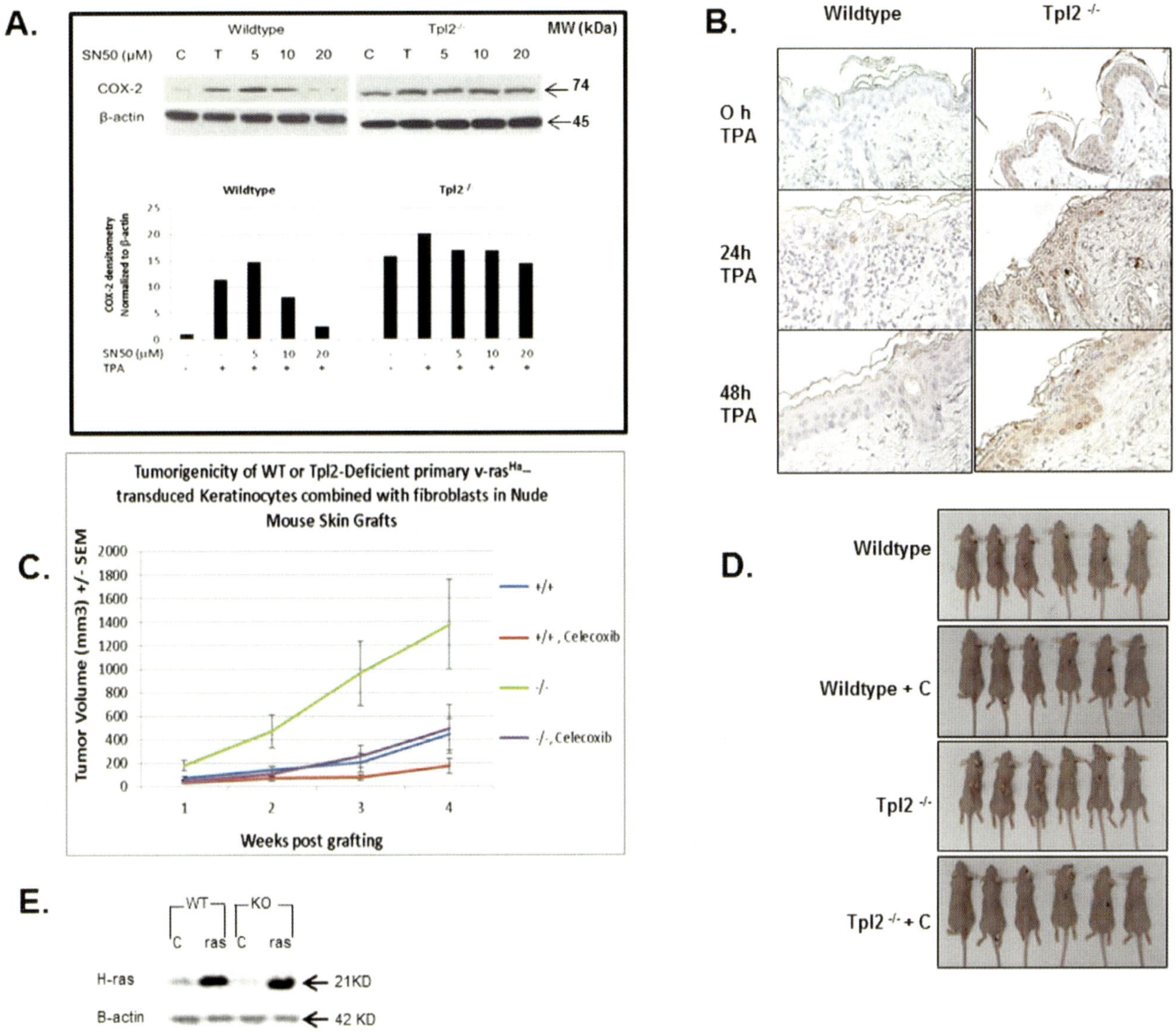

Figure 1. COX-2 signaling is augmented in keratinocytes and skin from Tpl2$^{-/-}$ mice. (A) Primary keratinocytes were treated with DMSO control (Lane C), TPA (Lane T) (10 ng/ml), or TPA +5 μM, 10 μM, or 20 μM of the NF-κB inhibitor, SN50, and COX-2 expression measured 18 h later by western blot analysis. Densitometry of COX-2 after normalizion to β -actin is shown. (B) Immunohistochemical analysis of COX-2 in wildtype (WT) and Tpl2$^{-/-}$ mouse skin. Normal WT and Tpl2$^{-/-}$ skin as well as TPA-treated skin (24 or 48 hours) from WT and Tpl2$^{-/-}$ mice was stained for COX-2 (1:200 dilution). Magnification = 10X. (C) Tumorigenicity of keratinocytes expressing oncogenic v-ras^{Ha} in nude mouse grafts. Data are expressed as means +/− SEM of approximate tumor volume in mm^3. Statistical differences were found between mice grafted with v-ras^{Ha} transformed WT (+/+) or those grafted with v-ras^{Ha} transformed KO (−/−) keratinocytes as well as between mice grafted with Tpl2$^{-/-}$ keratinocytes and those grafted with Tpl2$^{-/-}$ keratinocytes and fed 500 ppm Celecoxib in their diets ($p<0.01$). No statistical difference was found when comparing mice grafted with Tpl2$^{-/-}$ keratinocytes and fed Celecoxib and mice grafted with WT cells. (D) Clinical appearance of mice grafted with v-ras^{Ha} transformed WT or v-ras^{Ha} transformed Tpl2$^{-/-}$ keratinocytes fed AIN-93G diet +/−500 ppm Celecoxib. (E) Western blotting of basal H-ras levels of WT or KO keratinocytes and H-ras levels post ras^{Ha} retrovirus transduction.

mucosa, platelet aggregation, and regulation of renal blood flow [22]. In contrast, *COX-2* expression is undetectable in most normal tissues but highly inducible. It is expressed rapidly and transiently in response to inflammatory or mitogenic stimuli. Elevation in *COX-2* mRNA and protein levels has been documented in cancers of the prostate, colon, breast, lung, cervix, pancreas, skin, intestine, and stomach [23–26]. Additionally, constitutive overexpression of COX-2 has been observed in chemically-induced papillomas and carcinomas [27].

In keratinocytes COX-2 exerts much of its effects through its product PGE_2 [28]. PGE_2 is the major prostaglandin produced in skin where it has numerous functions including wound healing, keratinocyte proliferation and localized edema [29–30]. It acts on skin cells in an autocrine or paracrine manner due to its rapid metabolic breakdown. Additionally, PGE_2 has been reported to autoregulate its own synthesis by transcriptionally activating *COX-2* in a cAMP-dependent manner [30]. Although PGE_2 facilitates skin homeostasis, it can also act as a tumor promoter, causing many of the hallmarks characteristic of cancer cells. Several reports have shown that overexpression of PGE_2 increases tumor cell growth and progression [29–31]. Increased binding of cAMP response element binding protein (CREB), activator protein-1 (AP-1) and NF-κB to the promoter regions of cyclin D1 and vascular endothelial growth factor *(VEGF)* may be partially responsible for this heightened tumorigenesis [29–31].

PGE_2 manifests its biological activity by binding to four different transmembrane receptors; EP1, EP2, EP3 and EP4 [23]. These G-protein coupled receptors appear to have different binding affinities for PGE_2, different downstream signaling pathways, and are differentially expressed in tissues and cells [23]. EP1 receptors are coupled to G_q and when activated increase intracellular calcium levels. Conversely, EP3 receptors are most often linked to G_i proteins and therefore can inhibit cAMP production. EP2 and EP4 receptors, by binding G_s proteins, are both coupled to adenylate cyclase (AC) [29,32]. Activation of AC results in the conversion of ATP to cyclic AMP (cAMP) which in turn binds to protein kinase A (PKA), NF-κB, or CREB. Deregulation of cAMP pathways and aberrant activation of cAMP-controlled genes is linked to carcinoma growth, angiogenesis and resistance to apoptosis [33].

The purpose of this study was to determine whether COX-2 and COX-2- regulated prostaglandins and prostaglandin receptors drive the highly tumorigenic state of $Tpl2^{-/-}$ mice by investigating the relationship between Tpl2 and COX-2. In this article we show that $Tpl2^{-/-}$ mice have increased expression of cyclooxygenase-2 (COX-2) and COX-2- downstream factors including PGE_2, EP2, EP4, and cAMP. Additionally, through the use of the selective COX-2 inhibitor Celecoxib, we found the increased tumorigenesis in the $Tpl2^{-/-}$ mice to be mediated through COX-2. These experiments illustrate that COX-2 induction in the absence of Tpl2 may be responsible for the increased tumorigenesis found in $Tpl2^{-/-}$ mice.

Materials and Methods

Wildtype and Transgenic Mice

Male and female $Tpl2^{-/-}$ mice were engineered as previously described [12]. C57BL/6 wildtype control mice were generated from the same colony as the $Tpl2^{-/-}$ mice. All mice were bred and maintained at the NIH Animal Facility (Bethesda, MD). $Tpl2^{-/-}$ status was regularly confirmed by PCR. All animal work was performed following NIH guidelines under an approved animal protocol.

Immunoblotting

Primary keratinocytes and fibroblasts were isolated from $Tpl2^{-/-}$ and C57Bl6 mice pups at 1–2 days of age as previously described and plated in 6 well dishes [34]. At the time of treatment, cells received 10 ng/ml 12-*O*-tetradecanoylphorbol-13-acetate (TPA) or Dimethyl Sulfoxide (DMSO) as the vehicle control. For the EP receptors, lysates were collected after 1, 3, 6, 12 and 24 hours of TPA treatment. For the COX-2 immunoblot,

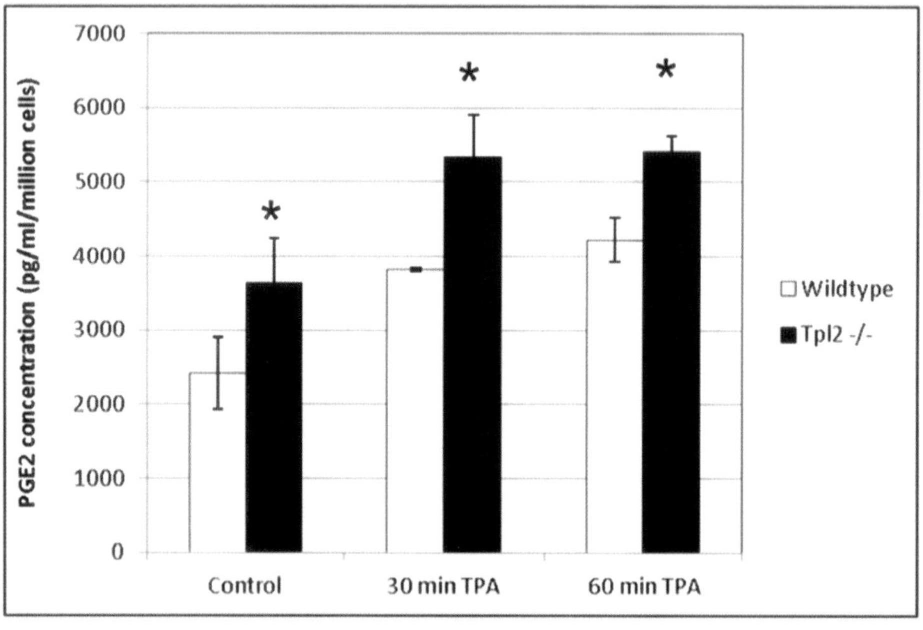

Figure 2. PGE_2 production is higher in keratinocytes from $Tpl2^{-/-}$ mice. Wildtype or $Tpl2^{-/-}$ keratinocytes received vehicle (DMSO) or TPA (10 ng/ml). Supernatants were collected after 30 or 60 minutes of TPA treatment. PGE_2 concentration was determined using a PGE_2 immunoassay kit. Significant differences were found between genotypes at all time points ($p<0.003$).

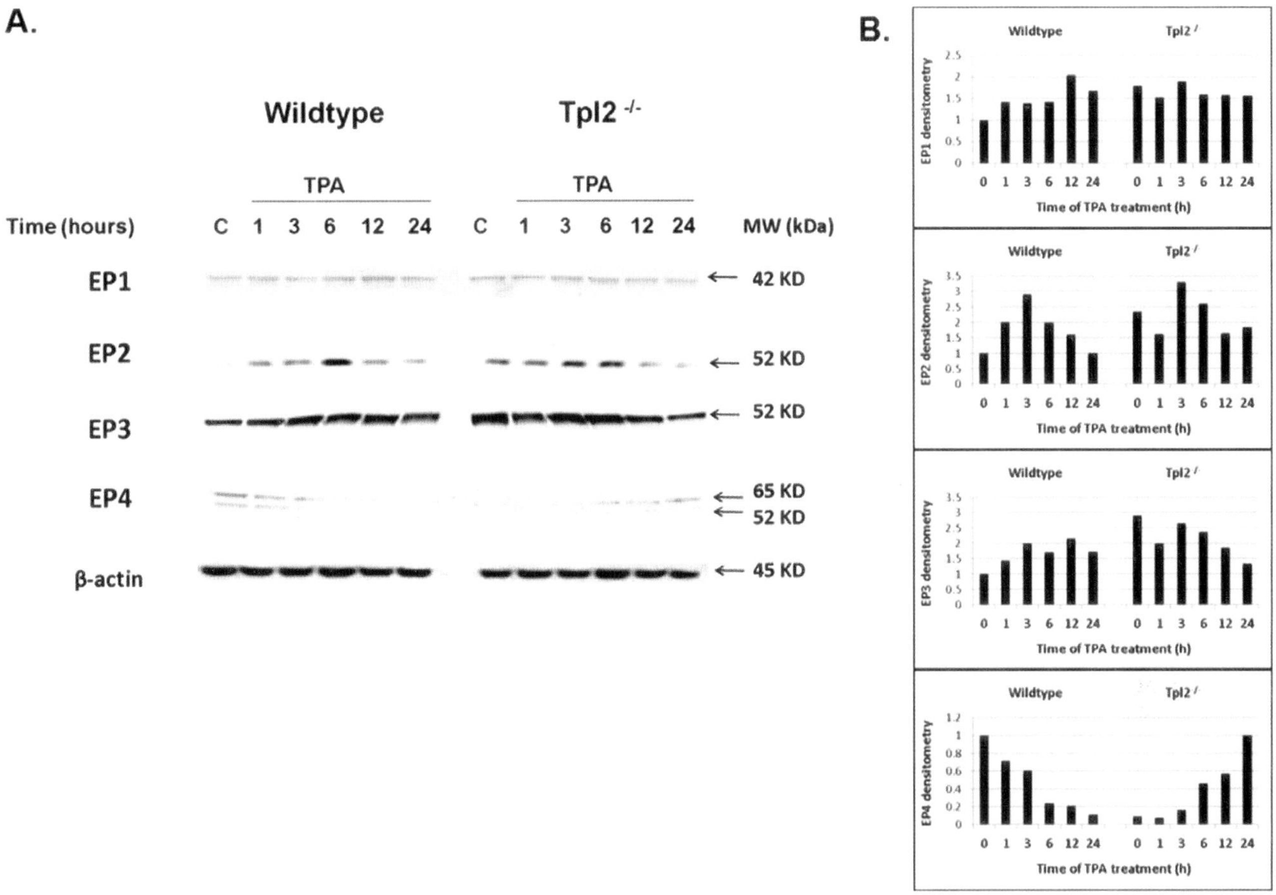

Figure 3. Western blotting of prostanoid receptor expression in wildtype and Tpl2$^{-/-}$ mouse keratinocytes. Wildtype or Tpl2$^{-/-}$ keratinocytes received DMSO only (labeled C) or TPA (10 ng/ml) for 1, 3, 6, 12, or 24 hours. Western blotting analysis was used to determine the levels of EP1, EP2, EP3, EP4, and β -actin. Bands were quantified through densitometry (Image J) and normalized to β -actin.

keratinocytes were primed with 5, 10, or 20 μM of the NF-κB inhibitor SN50 (Calbiochem, San Diego, CA) for 30 minutes prior to TPA treatment and again at time of TPA treatment. Total protein lysates were collected 18 hours post TPA treatment. For the H-ras blot, lysates were collected from WT or Tpl2$^{-/-}$ keratinocytes prior to and five days after infection with the v-ras^{Ha} retrovirus. Lysates were prepared using M-PER reagent (Thermo Fisher Scientific, Rockford, IL) containing complete protease inhibitor (Roche, Indianapolis, IN) and Halt phophastase inhibitor (Thermo Fisher Scientific, Rockford, IL) in accordance with the manufacturer's protocol. Proteins were separated using NuPAGE 4–12% Bis-Tris gradient gels (Invitrogen, Carlsbad, CA), then electrophoretically transferred onto PVDF membrane followed by immunoblotting. Membranes were incubated overnight at 4°C with EP1, EP2, EP3, β-actin (1:1000) or EP4 (1:400) primary rabbit antibodies (Cayman Chemical Company, Ann Arbor, MI), or H-ras antibody (1:1000; EMD Millipore, Billerica, MA). Anti-rabbit HRP secondary antibody was applied at a dilution of 1:2000 (Cell Signaling, Danvers, MA). West Dura Cemillumines-cent substrate (Thermo, Rockland, Il) was used for signal detection. Membranes were visualized using a ChemiDoc-It imaging system (UVP, Upland, CA). Densitometry was performed on all western blots using the Image J program and signal normalized to β -actin.

Immunohistochemistry

Papillomas and mouse skin treated with TPA for 4, 8, 12, or 24 hours were fixed in 10% normal buffered formalin (NBF) overnight and processed into paraffin blocks from which 4 μm sections were cut and stained with hematoxylin and eosin (H&E). The slides were rehydrated followed by antigen retrieval and endogenous peroxidase activity was quenched using methanol and hydrogen peroxide. Following washing and protein block (DAKO, Carpinteria, CA) the slides were incubated overnight at 4°C with COX2, EP2 or EP4 primary antibodies at dilutions ranging from 1:200 to 1:500 (Cayman Chemical Company, Ann Arbor, MI). Negative controls were acquired by substituting primary antibody with buffer. Following washing, the slides were incubated for 40 minutes at room temperature with Donkey anti-Goat biotinylated secondary antibody (Thermo Scientific, Rockford, IL). ABC reagent (Vector Labs Inc, Burlingame, CA) was then applied for amplification of primary antibody binding and 3,3-diaminobenzi-dine (DAB) was applied for visualization. Sections were melanin-bleached, and counterstained with Gill's hematoxylin. The sections were dehydrated through graded alcohols, immersed in xylene, and mounted with coverslips. For the immunohistochem-istry studies for EP2 or EP4, mice were treated with TPA for 0, 4, 8 12, 24, or 48 hours (n = 4/group). A minimum of four sections were stained for each time point and staining was repeated a minimum of three times. Representative areas were photo-

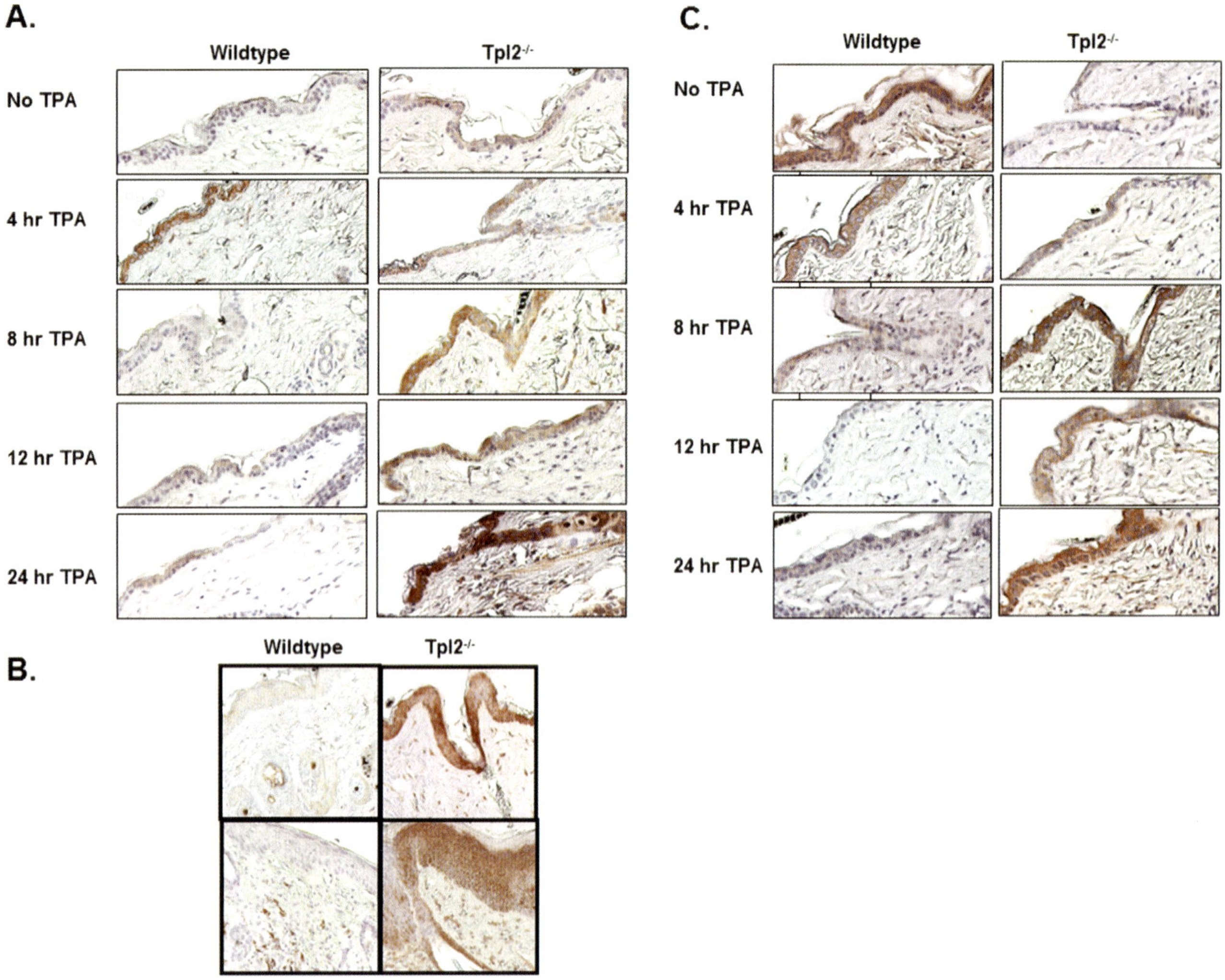

Figure 4. EP2 and EP4 receptor expression is heightened in epidermis and papillomas from Tpl2$^{-/-}$ mice. Shaved wildtype and Tpl2$^{-/-}$ mice were treated with TPA (10 μg) for 0, 4, 8, 12, or 24 hours and analyzed for expression of EP2 (Figure 4A) or EP4 (Figure 4C). Additionally, papillomas from wildtype and Tpl2$^{-/-}$ mice were analyzed for expression of EP2 (Figure 4B). Magnification = 10X.

graphed using an Eclipse E800 digital camera (Nikon, Melville, NY) at 10× magnifications.

PGE_2 Assay

Wildtype or Tpl2$^{-/-}$ keratinocytes received vehicle (DMSO) or TPA (10 ng/ml). Supernatants were collected after 30 or 60 minutes of TPA treatment. PGE_2 concentration was determined using a PGE_2 immunoassay kit from R&D Systems (Minneapolis, MN) per manufacturer's instructions. Briefly, supernatants from control or treated keratinocytes were plated in a 96-well plate. Other wells received buffer only or standards supplied by the manufacturer. PGE_2 antibody solution was added to wells followed by PGE_2 conjugate and the plate was incubated for 2 hours. After four washes, substrate was added to wells and the plate was incubated for 30 minutes. Stop solution was added to each well and absorbance was read at 570 nm using a MultiSkan FC microplate reader (Thermo Scientific, Rockford, IL). The concentration of PGE_2 was calculated from a standard curve and normalized to total cell number. The results presented are averages from triplicate samples ± standard deviation of two independent experiments.

cAMP Assay

Five million wildtype or Tpl2$^{-/-}$ keratinocytes received vehicle (DMSO) or TPA (10 ng/ml). Protein lysates were isolated after 60 minutes of TPA treatment. A cAMP assay was performed per manufacturer's instructions using a kit from R&D Systems (Minneapolis, MN). Briefly, lysates from control or treated keratinocytes were plated in a 96-well plate. Other wells received buffer only or standards provided by the manufacturer. cAMP conjugate was added to wells followed by cAMP antibody solution and the plate was incubated for 2 hours. After three washes, pNPP substrate was added to wells and the plate was incubated for one hour. Stop solution was added to each well and absorbance was read at 570 nm using a MultiSkan FC microplate reader (Thermo Scientific, Rockford, IL). The concentration of cAMP was calculated from a standard curve. The results presented are averages from triplicate samples ± standard deviation of two independent experiments.

Grafting Cells on Athymic Nude Mice

Tpl2$^{-/-}$ or wildtype (WT) primary keratinocytes isolated from newborn mice were infected with the v-ras^{Ha} retrovirus, then

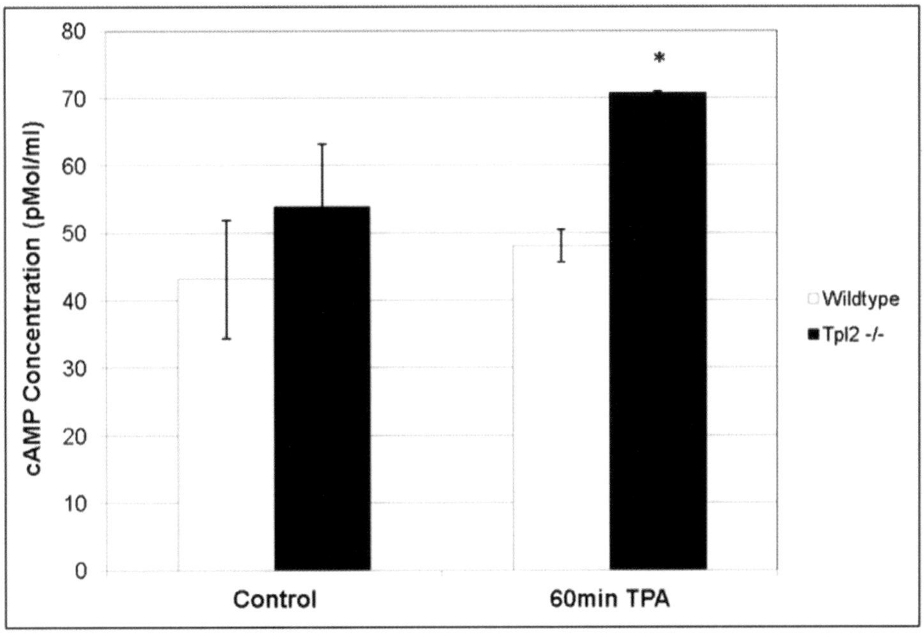

Figure 5. cAMP production is higher in keratinocytes from Tpl2$^{-/-}$ mice. Wildtype or Tpl2$^{-/-}$ keratinocytes received DMSO only (control) or TPA (10 ng/ml). Lysates were collected after 60 minutes of TPA treatment. cAMP concentration was determined using a cAMP immunoassay kit. Significant differences were found between genotypes following TPA treatment ($p<0.002$).

trypsinized and used for grafting on day 8 as described previously [34]. Briefly, 24 eight week old athymic nude mice were equally divided into four groups ($n=6$) and a graft site was prepared on their backs. Mice received six million keratinocytes (either WT or Tpl2$^{-/-}$) mixed with six million fibroblasts (either WT or Tpl2$^{-/-}$). The four groups of mice received the following combinations: a) wildtype keratinocytes plus wildtype fibroblasts, AIN-93G diet, b) wildtype keratinocytes plus wildtype fibroblasts, AIN-93G diet +500 ppm Celecoxib, c) Tpl2$^{-/-}$ keratinocytes plus Tpl2$^{-/-}$ fibroblasts, AIN-93G diet, or d) Tpl2$^{-/-}$ keratinocytes plus Tpl2$^{-/-}$ fibroblasts, AIN-93G diet +500 ppm Celecoxib. Tumor measurements began 10 days after grafting and continued once a week for 28 days. Tumor volume was calculated using the height multiplied by the length along the spinal column and the width at right angles to the length. Data are expressed as means ± SEM of approximate tumor volume in mm^3.

Statistical Analysis

PGE_2, grafting data and cAMP levels were analyzed through two-way ANOVA analysis with PASW Statistics software (IBM, Armonk, NY). P-values <0.05 were considered significant and LSD Post-hoc tests were performed to identify the significant interaction.

Results

TPA-treated Mouse Skin and TPA-treated Keratinocytes from Tpl2$^{-/-}$ Mice have Elevated COX-2 Signaling

We recently reported Tpl2$^{-/-}$ mice have increased inflammatory responses and this is primarily mediated through exaggerated NF-κB signaling [19]. COX-2 is an NF-κB regulated gene whose elevated expression is documented in a variety of neoplastic tissues. Using western analysis we assessed the basal expression of COX-2 in keratinocytes from wildtype and Tpl2$^{-/-}$ mice. Basal expression of COX-2 is nearly 15 fold higher in Tpl2$^{-/-}$ keratinocytes compared to wildtype cells, whose expression is barely detectable (Figure 1A). As expected, TPA treatment induced COX-2 protein in both genotypes. However, in wildtype mice this induction could be reversed in a dose-dependent manner when SN50, an NF-κB inhibitor, was added to the keratinocytes. In knockout mice, the heightened COX-2 expression remained high upon the addition of SN50, only beginning to slightly decrease with the highest dose of SN50. Additionally, using immunohistochemistry we assessed the level of COX-2 in TPA-treated mouse skin and found significant increases in Tpl2$^{-/-}$ skin treated with TPA for 24 or 48 hours compared with skin from control animals (Figure 1B).

Celecoxib Inhibits Tumors Developed on Nude Mice with v-ras^{Ha} Transduced Tpl2$^{-/-}$ Cells

To show an upregulation in COX-2 correlates with the heightened tumorigenesis found in Tpl2$^{-/-}$ mice, we grafted nude mice with v-ras^{Ha} -transduced keratinocytes from Tpl2$^{-/-}$ or wildtype mice mixed with fibroblasts from the same genotype, and fed a subset of these animals the COX-2 selective inhibitor Celecoxib. We found nude mice grafted with v-ras^{Ha} transduced keratinocytes and fibroblasts from Tpl2$^{-/-}$ mice developed four times larger tumors than mice grafted with v-ras^{Ha} transduced keratinocytes and fibroblasts from wildtype animals (Figure 1C, 1D). Administration of Celecoxib to nude mice grafted with v-ras^{Ha} transduced keratinocytes and fibroblasts from Tpl2$^{-/-}$ mice decreased the size of the tumors to a level that was indistinguishable from untreated control mice. These differences were statistically significant ($p<0.01$). However, there were not statistical differences in tumor sizes between mice fed Celecoxib and grafted with Tpl2$^{-/-}$ keratinocytes and mice grafted with wildtype keratinocytes (Figure 1C, 1D). The level of v-ras^{Ha} expression in each genotype following transduction was confirmed by Western blot (Figure 1E).

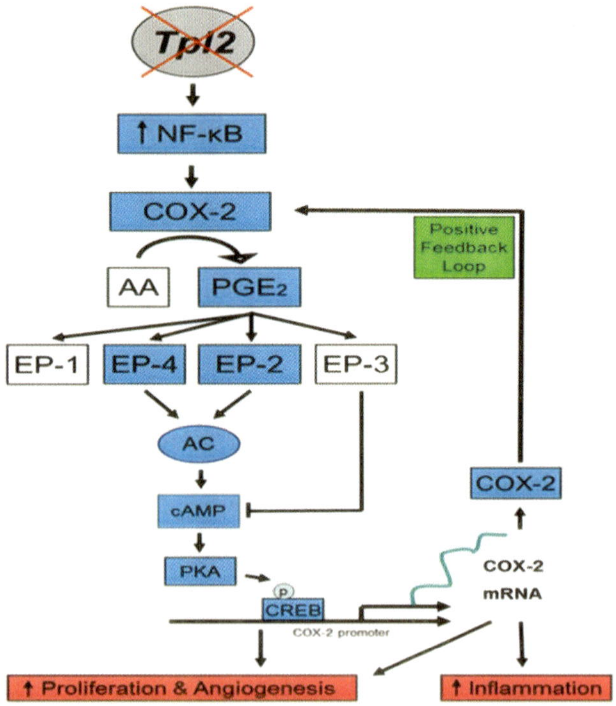

Figure 6. Proposed model describing how loss of Tpl2 results in increased inflammation and tumorigenesis. Tpl2 is normally held in complex with p105 NF-κB, preventing proteolysis and activation of the NF-κB and MAPK signaling pathways. Without Tpl2, NF-κB activity increases (see reference 19), resulting in increased production of NF-κB target genes such as COX-2. COX-2 activation results in the conversion of arachidonic acid to PGE_2, which then can bind to one of four G-protein linked receptors (EP1–EP4). EP2 and EP4 receptor activation causes the formation of cAMP from ATP. cAMP can then bind to cAMP response genes such as CREB and PKA. The end result is an increase in inflammatory and cell survival proteins, ultimately contributing to both tumorigenesis and inflammation.

$Tpl2^{-/-}$ Keratinocytes have Enhanced PGE_2 Signaling

COX-2 catalyzes the first committed step in prostanoid synthesis, resulting in the production of several prostaglandins including PGE_2, the primary prostanoid found in skin. To assess whether $Tpl2^{-/-}$ keratinocytes had elevated PGE_2 levels, an immunoassay was performed. We found basal production of PGE_2 was 35% higher in $Tpl2^{-/-}$ keratinocytes than in wildtype cells (Figure 2). TPA treatment for 30 or 60 minutes exaggerated PGE_2 release in both genotypes, but the PGE_2 released from $Tpl2^{-/-}$ keratinocytes remained significantly ($p<0.003$) greater than in wildtype cells.

$Tpl2^{-/-}$ Keratinocytes have Increased Expression of the PGE_2 Receptors EP2 and EP4

PGE_2 is a major product of COX-2 activation and binds to one of four G-protein coupled receptors. Activation of two of these receptors, EP2 and EP4, is linked to increased skin tumor development and cancer cell migration [29,35]. Western analysis with TPA-treated keratinocytes assessed if EP2 and EP4 receptors are differentially regulated in our wildtype and $Tpl2^{-/-}$ model (Figure 3). We found $Tpl2^{-/-}$ keratinocytes had 2.5 times higher basal expression of EP2 when compared to keratinocytes from wildtype mice. Interestingly, we also found TPA-treatment increased expression of EP4 in $Tpl2^{-/-}$ keratinocytes, whereas TPA-treatment decreased expression of EP4 in wildtype cells. It is interesting to note that EP3 has been reported to oppose EP2 and EP4 as induction of EP3 receptor decreases cAMP [29,32]. Our data suggests EP3 may work in an opposing fashion to EP4 in our model. As the levels of EP4 increase in our $Tpl2^{-/-}$ cells the levels of EP3 decline. We found no differences in the expression of EP1, agreeing with previous literature that suggests EP1 does not have a major role in skin tumor formation [35].

TPA-treated Skin Sections from $Tpl2^{-/-}$ Mice Exhibit Increased EP2 and EP4 Expression

We performed immunohistochemistry to correlate our *in vitro* results with the expression levels of EP2 and EP4 in TPA-treated mouse skin and papillomas. Within 8 hours of TPA treatment, there was markedly higher staining of EP2 in $Tpl2^{-/-}$ skin and this heightened staining was maintained over the course of 24 hours (Figure 4A). However, the wildtype mice showed relatively weak basal staining with an induction at the 4 hour time point. By 8 hours this induction has subsided. Additionally, we found higher levels of EP2 in papillomas from $Tpl2^{-/-}$ mice supporting its role in tumorigenesis (Figure 4B). EP4 expression in TPA-treated wildtype and $Tpl2^{-/-}$ mouse skin was also similar to what was observed *in vitro* in mouse keratinocytes. In wildtype mice, expression of this receptor is highest in untreated skin and declines with TPA treatment, being nearly undetectable after 8 hours of TPA treatment (Figure 4C). Expression of EP4 is low at basal levels in $Tpl2^{-/-}$ mice but increases with TPA treatment over the course of 24 hours.

TPA-treated Keratinocytes from $Tpl2^{-/-}$ Mice Show Elevated cAMP Levels

As demonstrated both *in vitro* and *in vivo*, $Tpl2^{-/-}$ mice display heightened EP2 and EP4 receptor levels upon stimulation with TPA. As previously reported, EP2 and EP4 activation increases cAMP levels [29,32]. As a second messenger, cAMP can induce numerous genes involved in cancer growth and progression [33]. We performed an immunoassay to determine if keratinocytes from our $Tpl2^{-/-}$ mice had elevated cAMP levels compared to keratinocytes from wildtype mice. Although basal cAMP levels were approximately 20% higher in untreated $Tpl2^{-/-}$ keratinocytes, the differences were not significant. However, the level of cAMP produced by TPA-treated $Tpl2^{-/-}$ keratinocytes was 46% higher than the level of cAMP produced by TPA-treated WT keratinocytes (70.8 pmol/ml vs. 48.4 pmol/ml) (Figure 5).

Discussion

The incidence of squamous cell carcinoma, the second most common form of skin cancer, is rising each year and expected to double in the next 20 years [36]. Reports over the last several years suggest inflammation in the tumor microenvironment contributes to the development or progression of skin cancer [37–38]. The persistent recruitment of inflammatory cells found in the tumor microenvironment can enhance proliferation, survival and migration of keratinocytes. Additionally, chemokines, selectins, and their receptors found on tumor cells can facilitate late stages of cancer progression, including invasion, migration and metastasis [37–38].

We recently identified a tumor suppressor function of *Tpl2* in skin cancer, with the absence of Tpl2 contributing to both DMBA/TPA-induced tumorigenesis and inflammation [19]. In this model, $Tpl2^{-/-}$ mice showed augmented nuclear factor-kappa B (NF-κB) signaling, neutrophil recruitment, expression of pro-inflammatory cytokines, and edema [19]. The current study was conducted to determine if the enhanced inflammatory response found in $Tpl2^{-/-}$ mice contributes to their heightened tumorigenesis. We found TPA-treated keratinocytes, TPA-treated skin, and papillomas from Tpl2$^{-/-}$ mice have increased expression of COX-2 and its downstream signaling pathways. COX-2, an inducible enzyme involved in prostaglandin biosynthesis, is overexpressed in numerous epithelial cancers [39]. COX-2 overexpression can inhibit apoptosis, while stimulating angiogenesis and invasion, in several cancer types [40]. Additionally, the peroxidase function of COX-2 can aid in the conversion of pro-carcinogens to carcinogens and initiate tumorigenesis [40]. In the case of skin cancer several laboratories have used genetic means to document a cause-effect relationship between COX-2 expression and tumorigenesis [27,39,41–43]. In this regard, chemically-induced papillomas and carcinomas constitutively overexpress COX-2. Interestingly COX-2 transgenic mice develop skin tumors without the need for a promoting agent such as TPA [39]. In contrast, deleting the *COX-2* gene or treating mice with COX-2 inhibitors suppresses the development or progression of chemically or UV-induced skin tumors in mice [42–43]. Consequently, the use of non-steroidal anti-inflammatory drugs (NSAIDs), which primarily work through the inhibition of cyclooxygenases, has been associated with a reduced risk in numerous cancers [44].

We grafted nude mice with v-ras^{Ha} -transduced keratinocytes from Tpl2$^{-/-}$ or wildtype mice mixed with fibroblasts from the same genotype and fed subsets of these animals the COX-2 selective inhibitor Celecoxib to show an upregulation in COX-2 is correlated with increased tumorigenesis seen in Tpl2$^{-/-}$ mice. We found nude mice grafted with keratinocytes and fibroblasts from Tpl2$^{-/-}$ mice developed significantly larger tumors than mice grafted with keratinocytes and fibroblasts from wildtype animals. Administration of Celecoxib to nude mice grafted with keratinocytes and fibroblasts from Tpl2$^{-/-}$ mice decreased the size of the tumors to a level indistinguishable from untreated wild type control mice. Thus, these data implicate COX-2 as a causative agent in the high skin tumorigenesis found in these animals.

Activation of COX-2 results in the conversion of arachidonic acid to PGE_2. In our report we found production of PGE_2 was significantly higher (both basally and upon TPA-treatment) in Tpl2$^{-/-}$ keratinocytes than in wildtype keratinocytes. *In vitro* and *in vivo* studies correlate PGE_2 levels with enhanced keratinocyte proliferation [31,45–46]. Reports also show tumor promoting agents such as TPA directly increase the release of PGE_2 in keratinocytes, and released PGE_2 is associated with increased DNA synthesis [45–47]. Additionally, treatment with the NSAID indomethacin inhibits TPA-stimulated keratinocyte proliferation but this effect is reversed by addition of exogenous PGE_2 [45]. Despite having important effects on the normal growth of epidermal tissue, increased PGE_2 has been associated with tumorigenesis. This is presumably due to the ability of PGE_2 to activate multiple signaling pathways including EGFR, cAMP, PI3/AKT, and MAPK [31]. Activation of these signaling pathways results in elevated promoter binding to genes such as cyclin D1 and VEGF. This can cause increases in cancer cell growth and angiogenesis [31].

As mentioned earlier, PGE_2 binds to one of four transmembrane receptors, EP1, EP2, EP3, or EP4. In our report, using both *in vitro* and *in vivo* techniques, we found significantly higher expression of EP2 and EP4 receptors in Tpl2$^{-/-}$ mice compared with wildtype mice. In the case of EP2, TPA-treated keratinocytes, TPA-treated skin, and papillomas from Tpl2$^{-/-}$ mice all had elevated EP2 protein levels compared with wildtype mice. As previously reported, EP2 mRNA is elevated in human squamous cell carcinomas compared to normal skin, as well as in UV-treated skin [29,48,49]. Additionally, whereas EP2 -transgenic mice have enhanced skin tumor development, survival, proliferation, angiogenesis, and inflammation, ablation of EP2 leads to a decrease in TPA-induced inflammation and skin tumorigenesis [29,35]. Moreover, EP2 knockout mice have significant decreases in skin tumorigenesis, keratinocyte proliferation, epidermal thickness, and inflammatory parameters [50–52].

In our study, we also found differences in the expression pattern of the EP4 receptor between genotypes. In TPA-treated skin and TPA-treated keratinocytes, wildtype mice have moderate basal expression levels of the EP4 receptor with expression declining after TPA treatment. This is in contrast to the Tpl2$^{-/-}$ mice where expression of this receptor is low at basal levels but increases with TPA treatment, peaking at 24 hours. Others have found increased expression of EP4 in papillomas and squamous cell carcinomas compared with normal and UV-irradiated skin [49]. EP2 and EP4 both function through the same cAMP-mediated pathway. In the current study we found TPA-treated Tpl2$^{-/-}$ cells produce 46% higher cAMP levels than TPA-treated wildtype keratinocytes. EP3 works in an opposing manner to EP2 and EP4 as it can inhibit production of cAMP. Interestingly in our study, EP3 expression increases with TPA treatment in wildtype mice and decreases with TPA treatment in knockout animals. Thus, the induction of EP2 and EP4 in TPA-treated keratinocytes in Tpl2$^{-/-}$ mice, as well as the reduction in EP3 in TPA-treated keratinocytes in knockout animals both may contribute to the enhanced cAMP levels. Overall, increases in cAMP and cAMP-mediated pathways together with aberrant activation of cAMP-controlled genes are linked to carcinoma growth, angiogenesis and resistance to apoptosis [33].

In summary, using both *in vitro* and *in vivo* experiments we demonstrated that *Tpl2* knockout mice have elevated cyclooxygenase-2 (COX-2) and COX-2 downstream factors including PGE_2, EP2, EP4, and cAMP. These results suggest one possible mechanism to explain how deletion in Tpl2 can lead to enhanced skin tumorigenesis (Figure 6). The notion that inhibition of COX-2 and its downstream factors is chemopreventative has led to the design of COX-2 selective inhibitors. However, there are safety concerns regarding COX-2 inhibitors, as long-term use may predispose to cardiovascular events [53]. As we begin to unveil the factors in the COX-prostaglandin pathway contributing to tumorigenesis it is critical to understand how these factors are regulated. Identifying how Tpl2 and COX-2 interact may lead to new ways to downregulate COX-2, an enzyme often overexpressed in skin cancer, through the modulation of Tpl2.

Author Contributions

Conceived and designed the experiments: KD JW SN. Performed the experiments: KD SN ET MD TD. Analyzed the data: KD SN JW. Contributed reagents/materials/analysis tools: JW KD. Wrote the paper: KD JW.

References

1. Khavari TA, Rinn J (2007) Ras/Erk MAPK signaling in epidermal homeostasis and neoplasia. Cell Cycle 6: 2928–2931.

2. Aoki M, Akiyama T, Miyoshi J, Toyoshima K (1991) Identification and characterization of protein products of the cot oncogene with serine kinase activity. Oncogene 6: 1515–1519.

3. Patriotis C, Makris A, Chernoff J, Tsichlis PN (1994) Tpl-2 acts in concert with Ras and Raf-1 to activate mitogen-activated protein kinase. Proc Natl Acad Sci U S A 91: 9755-9759.
4. Salmeron A, Ahmad TB, Carlile GW, Pappin D, Narsimhan RP, et al. (1996) Activation of MEK-1 and SEK-1 by Tpl-2 proto-oncoprotein, a novel MAP kinase kinase kinase. EMBO J 15: 817-826.
5. Patriotis C, Makris A, Bear SE, Tsichlis PN (1993) Tumor progression locus 2 (Tpl-2) encodes a protein kinase involved in the progression of rodent T-cell lymphomas and in T-cell activation. Proc Natl Acad Sci U S A 90: 2251-2255.
6. Chiariello M, Marinissen MJ, Gutkind JS (2000) Multiple mitogen-activated protein kinase signaling pathways connect the Cot oncoprotein to the c-jun promoter and to cellular transformation. Mol Cell Biol 20: 1747-1758.
7. Tsatsanis C, Patriotis C, Tsichlis PN (1998)Tpl-2 induces IL-2 expression in T-cell lines by triggering multiple signaling pathways that activate NFAT and NF-kappa B. Oncogene 17: 2609-2618.
8. Belich MP, Salmerón A, Johnston LH, Ley SC (1999) TPL-2 kinase regulates the proteolysis of the NF-kappaB-inhibitory protein NF-kappaB1 p105. Nature 397: 363-368.
9. Lang V, Symons A, Watton S J, Janzen J, Soneji Y, et al. (2004) ABIN-2 forms a ternary complex with TPL-2 and NF-κB1 p105 and is essential for TPL-2 protein stability. Mol Cell Biol 24: 5235-5248.
10. Beinke S, Deka J, Lang V, Belich MP, Walker PA, et al. (2003) NF-kappaB1 p105 negatively regulates TPL-2 MEK kinase activity. Mol Cell Biol 23: 4739-4752.
11. Miyoshi J, Higashi T, Mukai H, Ohuchi T, Kakunaga T (1991) Structure and transforming potential of the human cot oncogene encoding a putative protein kinase. Mol Cell Biol 11: 4088-4096.
12. Ceci JD, Patriotis CP, Tsatsanis C, Makris AM, Kovatch R, et al. (1997) Tpl-2 is an oncogenic kinase that is activated by carboxy-terminal truncation. Genes Dev 11: 688-700.
13. Tsatsanis C, Spandidos DA (2000) The role of oncogenic kinases in human cancer. Int J Mol Med 5: 583-590.
14. Sourvinos G, Tsatsanis C, Spandidos DA (1999) Overexpression of the Tpl-2/Cot oncogene in human breast cancer. Oncogene 18: 4968-4973.
15. Clark AM, Reynolds SH, Anderson M, Wiest JS (2004) Mutational activation of the MAP3K8 protooncogene in lung cancer. Genes Chromosomes Cancer 41: 99-108.
16. Johannessen CM, Boehm JS, Kim SY, Thomas SR, Wardwell L, et al. (2010) COT drives resistance to RAF inhibition through MAP kinase pathway reactivation. Nature 468: 968-972.
17. Vougioukalaki M, Kanellis DC, Gkouskou K, Eliopoulos AG (2011) Tpl2 kinase signal transduction in inflammation and cancer. Cancer Lett 304: 80-89.
18. Tsatsanis C, Vaporidi K, Zacharioudaki V, Androulidaki A, Sykulev Y, et al. (2008) Tpl2 and ERK transduce antiproliferative T cell receptor signals and inhibit transformation of chronically stimulated T cells. Proc Natl Acad Sci U S A 105: 2987-2992.
19. DeCicco-Skinner KL, Trovato EL, Simmons JK, Lepage PK, Wiest JS (2011) Loss of tumor progression locus 2 (Tpl2) enhances tumorigenesis and inflammation in two-stage skin carcinogenesis. Oncogene 30: 389-397.
20. de Visser KE, Eichten A, Coussens LM (2006) Paradoxical roles of the immune system during cancer development. Nat Rev Cancer 6(1): 24-37.
21. Funk CD (2001) Prostaglandins and leukotrienes: advances in eicosanoid biology. Science 294: 1871-1875.
22. Dempke W, Rie C, Grothey A, Schmoll HJ (2001) Cyclooxygenase-2: a novel target for cancer chemotherapy? J Cancer Res Clin Oncol 127: 411-417.
23. Cao Y, Prescott SM (2002) Many actions of cyclooxygenase-2 in cellular dynamics and in cancer. J Cell Physiol 190: 279-286.
24. Trifan OC, Hla T (2003) Cyclooxygenase-2 modulates cellular growth and promotes tumorigenesis. J Cell Mol Med 7: 207-222.
25. An KP, Athar M, Tang X, Katiyar SK, Russo J, et al. (2002) Cyclooxygenase-2 expression in murine and human nonmelanoma skin cancers: implications for therapeutic approaches. Photochem Photobiol 76: 73-80.
26. Chun KS, Surh YJ (2004) Signal transduction pathways regulating cyclooxygenase-2 expression: potential molecular targets for chemoprevention. Biochem Pharmacol 68: 1089-1100.
27. Müller-Decker K, Kopp-Schneider A, Marks F, Seibert K, Furstenberger G (1998) Localization of prostaglandin H synthase isozymes in murine epidermal tumors: Suppression of skin tumor promotion by inhibition of prostaglandin H synthase-2. Mol Carcinogenesis 23: 36-44.
28. Greenhough A, Smartt HJ, Moore AE, Roberts HR, Williams AC (2009) The COX-2/PGE2 pathway: key roles in the hallmarks of cancer and adaptation to the tumour microenvironment Carcinogenesis 30: 377-386.
29. Sung YM, He G, Fischer SM (2005) Lack of expression of the EP2 but not EP3 receptor for prostaglandin E2 results in suppression of skin tumor development. Cancer Res 65: 9304-9311.
30. Maldve RE, Kim Y, Muga SJ, Fischer SM (2000) Prostaglandin E(2) regulation of cyclooxygenase expression in keratinocytes is mediated via cyclic nucleotide-linked prostaglandin receptors. J Lipid Res 41: 873-881.
31. Ansari KM, Rundhaug JE, Fischer SM (2008) Multiple signaling pathways are responsible for prostaglandin E2-induced murine keratinocyte proliferation. Mol Cancer Res. 6: 1003-1016.
32. Klein T, Shephard P, Kleinert H and Kömhoff M (2007) Regulation of cyclooxygenase-2 expression by cyclic AMP. Biochimica et Biophysica Acta 1773: 1605-1618.
33. Abramovitch R, Tavor E, Jacob-Hirsch J, Zeira E, Amariglio N, et al. (2004) A Pivotal Role of Cyclic AMP-Responsive Element Binding Protein in Tumor Progression. Cancer Res 64: 1338-1346.
34. Lichti U, Anders J, Yuspa SH (2008) Isolation and short-term culture of primary keratinocytes, hair follicle populations and dermal cells from newborn mice and keratinocytes from adult mice for in vitro analysis and for grafting to immunodeficient mice. Nat Protoc 3: 799-810.
35. Sung YM, He G, Hwang DH, Fischer SM (2006) Overexpression of the prostaglandin E2 receptor EP2 results in enhanced skin tumor development. Oncogene 25: 5507-5516.
36. Xie J (2008) Molecular biology of basal and squamous cell carcinomas. Adv Exp Med Biol 624: 241-251.
37. Mueller MM (2006) Inflammation in epithelial skin tumours: old stories and new ideas. Eur J Cancer 42: 735-744.
38. Coussens LM, Werb Z (2002) Inflammation and cancer. Nature 420: 860-867.
39. Müller-Decker K, Fürstenberger G (2007) The cyclooxygenase-2-mediated prostaglandin signaling is causally related to epithelial carcinogenesis. Mol Carcinog 46: 705-710.
40. Ghosh N, Chaki R, Mandal V, Mandal SC (2010) COX-2 as a target for cancer chemotherapy. Pharmacol Rep 62: 233-244.
41. Müller-Decker K, Neufang G, Berger I, Neumann M, Marks F, et al. (2002) Transgenic cyclooxygenase-2 overexpression sensitizes mouse skin for carcinogenesis. Proc Natl Acad Sci USA 99: 12483-12488.
42. Fischer SM (2002) Is cyclooxygenase-2 important in skin carcinogenesis? J Environ Pathol Toxicol Oncol 21: 183-191.
43. Tiano HF, Loftin CD, Akunda J, Lee CA, Spalding J, et al. (2002) Deficiency of either cyclooxygenase (COX)-1 or COX-2 alters epidermal differentiation and reduces mouse skin tumorigenesis. Cancer Res 62: 3395-3401.
44. Hussain M, Javeed A, Ashraf M, Al-Zaubai N, Stewart A, et al. (2012) Non-steroidal anti-inflammatory drugs, tumour immunity and immunotherapy. Pharmacol Res 66: 7-18.
45. Furstenberger G, Marks F (1978) Indomethacin inhibition of cell proliferation induced by the phorbol ester TPA is reversed by prostaglandin E2 in mouse epidermis in vivo. Biochem Biophys Res Commun 84: 1103-1111.
46. Pentland AP, Needleman P (1986) Modulation of keratinocyte proliferation in vitro by endogenous prostaglandin synthesis. J Clin Invest 77: 246-251.
47. Aizu E, Yamamoto S, Nakadate T, Kato R (1990) Differential effects of various skin tumor-promoting agents on prostaglandin E2 release from primary cultures of mouse epidermal cells. Eur J Pharmacol 182: 19-28.
48. Rundhaug JE, Fischer SM (2010) Molecular Mechanisms of Mouse Skin Tumor Promotion. Cancers (Basel) 2: 436-482.
49. Lee JL, Kim A, Kopelovich L, Bickers DR, Athar M (2005) Differential expression of E prostanoid receptors in murine and human non-melanoma skin cancer. J Invest Dermatol 125: 818-825.
50. Brouxhon S, Konger RL, VanBuskirk J, Sheu T-j, Ryan J, et al. (2007) Deletion of prostagandin E2 EP2 receptor protects against ultraviolet-induced carcinogenesis, but increases tumor aggressiveness. J Invest Dermatol 127: 439-446.
51. Ansari KM, Sung YM, He G, Fischer SM (2007) Prostaglandin receptor EP2 is responsible for cyclooxygenase-2 induction by prostaglandin E2 in mouse skin. Carcinogenesis 28: 2063-2068.
52. Chun KS, Lao HC, Trempus CS, Okada M, Langenbach R (2009) The prostaglandin receptor EP2 activates multiple signaling pathways and β- arrestin 1 complex formation during mouse skin papilloma development. Carcinogenesis 30: 1620-1627.
53. Dajani EZ, Islam K (2008) Cardiovascular and gastrointestinal toxicity of selective cyclo-oxygenase-2 inhibitors in man. J Physiol Pharmacol 59: 117-133.

Permissions

All chapters in this book were first published in PLOS ONE, by The Public Library of Science; hereby published with permission under the Creative Commons Attribution License or equivalent. Every chapter published in this book has been scrutinized by our experts. Their significance has been extensively debated. The topics covered herein carry significant findings which will fuel the growth of the discipline. They may even be implemented as practical applications or may be referred to as a beginning point for another development.

The contributors of this book come from diverse backgrounds, making this book a truly international effort. This book will bring forth new frontiers with its revolutionizing research information and detailed analysis of the nascent developments around the world.

We would like to thank all the contributing authors for lending their expertise to make the book truly unique. They have played a crucial role in the development of this book. Without their invaluable contributions this book wouldn't have been possible. They have made vital efforts to compile up to date information on the varied aspects of this subject to make this book a valuable addition to the collection of many professionals and students.

This book was conceptualized with the vision of imparting up-to-date information and advanced data in this field. To ensure the same, a matchless editorial board was set up. Every individual on the board went through rigorous rounds of assessment to prove their worth. After which they invested a large part of their time researching and compiling the most relevant data for our readers.

The editorial board has been involved in producing this book since its inception. They have spent rigorous hours researching and exploring the diverse topics which have resulted in the successful publishing of this book. They have passed on their knowledge of decades through this book. To expedite this challenging task, the publisher supported the team at every step. A small team of assistant editors was also appointed to further simplify the editing procedure and attain best results for the readers.

Apart from the editorial board, the designing team has also invested a significant amount of their time in understanding the subject and creating the most relevant covers. They scrutinized every image to scout for the most suitable representation of the subject and create an appropriate cover for the book.

The publishing team has been an ardent support to the editorial, designing and production team. Their endless efforts to recruit the best for this project, has resulted in the accomplishment of this book. They are a veteran in the field of academics and their pool of knowledge is as vast as their experience in printing. Their expertise and guidance has proved useful at every step. Their uncompromising quality standards have made this book an exceptional effort. Their encouragement from time to time has been an inspiration for everyone.

The publisher and the editorial board hope that this book will prove to be a valuable piece of knowledge for researchers, students, practitioners and scholars across the globe.

List of Contributors

Lieke M. C. Gijezen, Marigje Vernooij, Herm Martens Charlene E. U. Oduber and Charles J. M. Henquet
Department of Dermatology, GROW School for Oncology and Developmental Biology, Maastricht University Medical Centre+, Maastricht, The Netherlands

Maurice A. M. van Steensel
Department of Dermatology, GROW School for Oncology and Developmental Biology, Maastricht University Medical Centre+, Maastricht, The Netherlands
Department of Clinical Genetics, GROW School for Oncology and Developmental Biology, Maastricht University Medical Centre+, Maastricht, The Netherlands
Institute of Medical Biology, Singapore, Singapore

Theo M. Starink
Department of Dermatology, VU University Medical Centre, Amsterdam, The Netherlands

Martin H. Prins and Patty J. Nelemans
Department of Epidemiology, CAPHRI Research School for Public Health Primary Care, Maastricht University Medical Centre+, Maastricht, The Netherlands

Fred H. Menko
Department of Clinical Genetics, VU University Medical Centre, Amsterdam, The Netherlands

Kazuhiro Okumura, Megumi Saito Eriko Isogai and Yuichi Wakabayash
Department of Carcinogenesis Research, Division of Experimental Animal Research, Chiba Cancer Center Research Institute, Chiba, Chiba, Japan

Ikuo Miura and Shigeharu Wakana
Technology and Development Team for Mouse Phenotype Analysis, Japan Mouse Clinic, Riken Bioresource Center, Tsukuba, Ibaraki, Japan

Ryo Kominami
Department of Molecular Genetics, Graduate School of Medical and Dental Sciences, Niigata University, Niigata, Niigata, Japan

Jasmine George, Madhulika Singh, Amit Kumar Srivastava, Kulpreet Bhui, Preeti Roy, Pranav Kumar Chaturvedi and Yogeshwer Shukla
Proteomics Laboratory, Indian Institute of Toxicology Research, Council of Scientific and Industrial Research (CSIR), Uttar Pradesh, India

Donggou He and Hui Li
Department of Dermatology, University of Alabama at Birmingham, Birmingham, Alabama, United States of America

Mohammad Athar
Department of Dermatology, University of Alabama at Birmingham, Birmingham, Alabama, United States of America, Skin Disease Research Center, University of Alabama at Birmingham, Birmingham, Alabama, United States of America

Nabiha Yusuf, Craig A. Elmets, Santosh K. Katiyar and Hui Xu
Department of Dermatology, University of Alabama at Birmingham, Birmingham, Alabama, United States of America
Skin Disease Research Center, University of Alabama at Birmingham, Birmingham, Alabama, United States of America
Birmingham VA Medical Center, Birmingham, Alabama, United States of America

Zhenghua Gong, Yaowei Shi, Ze Zhu, Xuan Li, Yang Ye, Jianbing Zhang, Aiping Li and Jianwei Zhou
Department of Molecular Cell Biology and Toxicology, the Key Laboratory of Modern Toxicology, Ministry of Education and Department of Occupational Medicine and Environmental Health, School of Public Health; Nanjing Medical University, Nanjing, People's Republic of China
Jiangsu Key Lab of Cancer Biomarkers, Prevention and Treatment, Cancer Center; Nanjing Medical University, Nanjing, People's Republic of China

Gang Li
Department of Dermatology and Skin Science, Jack Bell Research Centre, Vancouver Coastal Health Research Institute, University of British Columbia, Vancouver, British Columbia, Canada

Zhihai Ma and Andrew Fire
Department of Genetics, Stanford University School of Medicine, Stanford, California, United States of America

Helen Swede
Department of Community Medicine and Health Care, University of Connecticut Health Center, Farmington, Connecticut, United States of America

David Cassarino
Department of Pathology, Southern California Permanente Medical Group, Los Angeles, California, United States of America

Elizabeth Fleming
Department of Genetics/Developmental Biology, University of Connecticut Health Center, Farmington, Connecticut, United States of America

Soheil S. Dadras
Department of Genetics/Developmental Biology, University of Connecticut Health Center, Farmington, Connecticut, United States of America
Department of Dermatology, University of Connecticut Health Center, Farmington, Connecticut, United States of America

Olinda C. Luiz and José Eluf-Neto
Laboratório de Epidemiologia e Imunobiologia - LIM38, Departamento de Medicina Preventiva da Faculdade de Medicina da Universidade de São Paulo, Sao Paulo, Brazil

Reinaldo José Gianini
Laboratório de Processamento de Dados Biomédicos-LIM39, Departamento de Medicina Preventiva da Faculdade de Medicina da Universidade de São Paulo, Sao Paulo, Brazil
Pontifícia Universidade Católica de São Paulo, Sorocaba, Brazil

Fernanda T. Gonçalves and Gilka J. F. Gattas
Laboratório de Imuno-hematologia e Hematologia Forense - LIM40, Departamento de Medicina Legal, Ética Médica, Medicina Social e do Trabalho, Faculdade de Medicina da Universidade de São Paulo, Sao Paulo, Brazil

Guilherme Francisco and Roger Chammas
Laboratório de Oncologia Experimental - LIM24, Departamento de Radiologia, Faculdade de Medicina da Universidade de São Paulo, Sao Paulo, Brazil

Cyro Festa-Neto and José Antonio Sanches
Departamento de Dermatologia, Faculdadede Medicina da Universidade de São Paulo, Sao Paulo, Brazil

Liljana Mervic
Department of Dermatology, Center of Dermatooncology, University of Tüebingen, Germany, Department of Dermatovenereology, University Medical Centre Ljubljana, Slovenia

Hyunmi Kim and Angela M. Christiano
Department of Genetics and Development, Columbia University, College of Physicians and Surgeons, New York, New York, United States of America
Department of Dermatology, Columbia University, College of Physicians and Surgeons, New York, New York, United States of America

Alexandre Casta
Institute of Human Nutrition, Columbia University, College of Physicians and Surgeons, New York, New York, United States of America

Xiuwei Tang, Courtney T. Luke, Arianna L. Kim, David R. Bickers and Mohammad Athar
Department of Dermatology, Columbia University, College of Physicians and Surgeons, New York, New York, United States of America

Salma Dabiri and E. Scott Seeley
Department of Pathology, Stanford University Medical Center, Stanford, California, United States of America

Jinah Kim
Department of Pathology, Stanford University Medical Center, Stanford, California, United States of America
Department of Dermatology, Stanford University Medical Center, Stanford, California, United States of America

Synnøve Magnussen, Elin Hadler-Olsen, Nadezhda Latysheva, and Robert Hanes, Jan-Olof Winberg and Gunbjørg Svineng
Department of Medical Biology, Faculty of Health Sciences, UiT - The Arctic University of Norway, Tromsø, Norway

Sonja E. Steigen and Lars Uhlin-Hansen
Department of Medical Biology, Faculty of Health Sciences, UiT - The Arctic University of Norway, Tromsø, Norway
Diagnostic Clinic - Department of Clinical Pathology, University Hospital of North Norway, Tromsø, Norway

Emma Pirila
Department of Diagnostics and Oral Medicine, Institute of Dentistry, University of Oulu, and Medical Research Center, Oulu University Hospital, Oulu, Finland

Tuula Salo
Department of Diagnostics and Oral Medicine, Institute of Dentistry, University of Oulu, and Medical Research Center, Oulu University Hospital, Oulu, Finland
Institute of Dentistry, University of Helsinki, Helsinki, Finland

Shang Brian Jiang, Julie A. Gladsjo, Monika Gerber and Tissa Hata
Division of Dermatology, University of California San Diego, La Jolla, California, United States of America

Beda Muehleisen
Division of Dermatology, University of California San Diego, La Jolla, California, United States of America
Department of Dermatology, Zurich University Hospital, Zurich, Switzerland

Richard L. Gallo
Division of Dermatology, University of California San Diego, La Jolla, California, United States of America
Department of Medicine, University of California San Diego, La Jolla, California, United States of America
Veterans Administration San Diego Healthcare System, San Diego, California, United States of America

Otmar Elsaeßer, Ulrike Leiter, Thomas K. Eigentler, Friedegund Meier, Benjamin Weide, Gisela Metzler and Helmut Breuninger
Center for Dermatooncology, Department of Dermatology, and Central Malignant Melanoma Registry of the German Dermatological Society, Eberhard-Karls-University of Tuebingen, Tuebingen, Germany

Claus Garbe
Center for Dermatooncology, Department of Dermatology, and Central Malignant Melanoma Registry of the German Dermatological Society, Eberhard-Karls-University of Tuebingen, Tuebingen, Germany
Skin Cancer Research Group, School of Public Health and Tropical Medicine, James Cook University, Townsville, Queensland, Australia

Petra G. Buettner
Skin Cancer Research Group, School of Public Health and Tropical Medicine, James Cook University, Townsville, Queensland, Australia

Linan Ha, Roshini M. Ponnamperuma, M. Stacey Ricci and Wendy C. Weinberg
Division of Monoclonal Antibodies, Center for Drug Evaluation and Research/Food and Drug Administration (CDER/FDA), Bethesda, Maryland, United States of America

Steven Jay
SAIC-Frederick, Inc., Frederick, Maryland, United States of America

Jan Hönnemann Adrián Sanz-Moreno and Hans-Peter Elsässer
Department of Cytobiology, Philipps-University Marburg, Germany

Elmar Wolf and Martin Eilers
Theodor-Boveri-Institute, Biocentre, University of Würzburg, Germany

Josefa P. Alameda, Rodolfo Moreno-Maldonado, Manuel Navarro, Angustias Page, José L. Jorcano, Ángel Ramírez and M. Llanos Casanova
Division of Epithelial Biomedicine, CIEMAT, Madrid, Spain

M. Jesús Fernández-Aceñero
Department of Pathology, Fundación Jiménez Díaz, Madrid, Spain

Ana Bravo
Department of Veterinary Clinical Sciences, Veterinary Faculty, University of Santiago de Compostela, Lugo, Spain

Michaela Zorn-Kruppa, Ulrich Ohnemus, Nina Kirschner, Sabine Vidal-y-Sy, Christian Börnchen, Ingrid Moll and Johanna M. Brandner
Department of Dermatology and Venerology, University Hospital Hamburg-Eppendorf, Hamburg, Germany

Susanne Rachow
Department of Dermatology and Venerology, University Hospital Hamburg-Eppendorf, Hamburg, Germany
Tabea Clinics GmbH, Hamburg, Germany

Peter von den Driesch
Dermatological Center, Klinikum Stuttgart, Stuttgart, Germany,

Jürgen Eberle
Department of Dermatology, Venerology and Allergology, Skin Cancer Center, Charité, Berlin, Germany

Michael Mildner
Department of Dermatology, Medical University of Vienna, Vienna, Austria

Eik Vettorazzi
Department of Medical Biometry and Epidemiology, University Hospital Hamburg-Eppendorf, Hamburg, Germany

Rita Rosenthal
Institute of Clinical Physiology, Charité-Universitätsmedizin Berlin, Berlin, Germany

Michal Mlacki and Tomasz Wilanowski
Laboratory of Signal Transduction, Nencki Institute of Experimental Biology, Warsaw, Poland

Charbel Darido
Department of Medicine, Monash University Central Clinical School, Prahran, Victoria, Australia

Stephen M. Jane
Department of Medicine, Monash University Central Clinical School, Prahran, Victoria, Australia
Alfred Hospital, Prahran, Victoria, Australia

Clifford Talbot, Yuriy Alexandrov, Martin O. Lenz, Sunil Kumar, Sean Warren, Ian Munro, Mark A. A. Neil and Paul M. W. French
Photonics Group, Department of Physics, Imperial College London, South Kensington Campus, London, United Kingdom

Rakesh Patalay
Photonics Group, Department of Physics, Imperial College London, South Kensington Campus, London, United Kingdom
Department of Dermatology, Imperial College Healthcare NHS Trust, London, United Kingdom

Karsten König
JenLab GmbH, Jena, Germany

Anthony Chu
Department of Dermatology, Imperial College Healthcare NHS Trust, London, United Kingdom

Gordon W. H. Stamp
CRUK London Research Institute, London, United Kingdom

Chris Dunsby
Photonics Group, Department of Physics, Imperial College London, South Kensington Campus, London, United Kingdom
Department of Medicine, Imperial College Healthcare NHS Trust, London, United Kingdom

Simone König, Frauke Nitzki, Anja Uhmann and Heidi Hahn
Institute of Human Genetics, University Medical Center, Goettingen, Germany

Kai Dittmann Jennifer Theiss-Suennemann and Holger M. Reichardt
Institute of Cellular and Molecular Immunology, University Medical Center, Goettingen, Germany

Markus Herrmann
Department of Radiation Oncology, University Medical Center, Goettingen, Germany

Reto Schwendener
Institute of Molecular Cancer Research, University of Zurich, Zurich, Switzerland

Tobias Pukrop
Department of Hematology and Oncology, University Medical Center, Goettingen, Germany

Walter Schulz-Schaeffer
Department of Neuropathology, University Medical Center, Goettingen, Germany

Kathleen L. DeCicco-Skinner, Sabrina J. Nolan and Taylor A. Dempsey
Department of Biology, American University, Washington, DC, United States of America

Erika L. Trovato
Department of Biology, American University, Washington, DC, United States of America
Laboratory of Cancer Biology and Genetics, National Cancer Institute, National Institutes of Health, Bethesda, Maryland, United States of America

Monika M. Deshpande and Jonathan S. Wiest
Laboratory of Cancer Biology and Genetics, National Cancer Institute, National Institutes of Health, Bethesda, Maryland, United States of America

Index

A
Ablative Laser, 2
Adjuvant Therapy, 124
Allele-specific Alteration, 9
Angiofibromas, 1-2, 6-8
Autosomal Dominant Disorder, 1

B
Basal Cell Carcinoma (BCC), 55-56, 112-117, 119, 121-122, 189-196, 198-204
Bcl-6, 145
Birt-hogg-dube Syndrome (BHD), 1-3, 5-8
Brdu-lrcs, 9-10, 12, 15-16
Breslow's Depth of Invasion, 49, 56

C
Cancer Chemoprevention, 18-19
Cancer Susceptibility, 9, 187
Cdkn1a, 145-147, 149, 151, 153
Cell Senescence, 132-133, 135-139, 143-144
Chemopreventive Agents, 18
Cldn-4, 167-173, 175-176, 178
Congenic Mapping, 9, 13, 17
Cosmetic Improvement, 1-5
Cox, 17, 28, 30, 32-33, 35-38, 68-69, 74, 78, 83-86, 94, 124, 127, 129, 139, 144, 165, 206-208, 211-214
Cutaneous Melanoma, 49-51, 53, 55-57, 59-62, 64-68, 70-72, 74, 76-77, 89-94, 124, 127, 129-131

D
Dicer, 49-53, 55-60
Dnp63a, 132-143
Dsg1, 180-181, 184

E
E-cadherin, 156, 162, 166-169, 173-175, 177-178
Electrocoagulation, 2

F
Facial Surgery, 2
Fibrofolliculomas, 1-2, 4-8
Flcn, 2, 4-7
Flim, 189-191, 193-196

G
Gfi-1, 145, 155
Grhl1, 180-187

I
Immunohistochemistry, 17-18, 49-50, 52, 59, 82, 86, 106, 108, 110, 132-133, 146, 149, 151, 154, 157, 163, 181, 199-200, 209, 211-212
Immunosuppressive Treatment, 2
In Vitro, 6, 8, 18, 39, 45, 49, 56, 58, 79, 81, 84, 96-98, 101-102, 105, 110-111, 132-133, 139, 141, 143, 155, 176, 178-179, 196, 201, 203-204, 212-214
Inflammation, 2, 19, 30-38, 55, 79, 83, 85, 88, 110-111, 123, 161-162, 166, 182-186, 188, 204, 206-207, 212-214

K
Kaplan-meier, 20, 42, 68-69, 124-125, 127, 129, 153, 185
Keratinocytes, 39, 41, 44-48, 50, 52, 55, 57, 59, 79-81, 84-86, 88, 112, 121, 123, 132-147, 149, 151, 153, 156, 158-165, 167-168, 170, 174-180, 182-186, 189-190, 193, 206-214

L
Lentivirus Infection, 133-134, 140-141
Lmcg, 2, 7
Lung Cysts, 1
Lymph Node Ultrasound, 127
Lymphadenectomy, 124, 130-131

M
M. Spretus, 9, 12
Malignant Tumors, 19, 52, 122, 132, 162, 175
Mapks, 18-19, 22, 26-29, 39, 44, 47
Median Tumor Thickness, 124, 127
Micrometastases, 124, 127, 129-131
Miz1, 145-147, 149, 151, 154-155
Mtor, 1-2, 5-8, 121, 137, 144, 180
Multivariate Cox Proportional Hazard, 124, 127, 129

N
Non-melanoma Skin Cancer, 115-117, 119, 121-122, 156, 196

P
P53, 18-19, 25-26, 28-29, 132-134, 137, 139, 143-144, 146, 149, 151, 153-155, 166, 186-188
Papillomagenesis, 9-10, 12, 22
Pcna, 19-20, 24-25, 27, 37, 41-44, 46-47, 83-86
Pigmented Lesion Removal, 61, 63-66
Placebo, 1-7
Pneumothorax, 1, 7
Ptch, 198-199, 204

Q

Quiescent Stem Cells, 9-10, 15

R

Randomisation, 2-3

Rapamycin, 1-8, 121-122, 180

S

Sa-b-gal, 132, 137, 140-141

Scarring, 2

Screening, 2-3, 124

Skin Carcinogenesis, 9-10, 12, 18, 26, 31, 34-36, 38-39, 46-48, 78, 83-84, 121, 144, 147, 149, 155-156, 162-166, 180-181, 185-187, 206, 214

Skin Papillomas, 9-10, 39, 41-45, 47, 145, 147, 153, 165

Skin Pigmentation, 61-62, 66

Skin Tumour, 17, 109

Slnb, 124-125, 127, 129-130

Split-face Trial, 1-2

Squamous Cancer, 133, 137

Stmm1, 9-16

Sun Exposure, 61-62, 66

T

Tuberous Sclerosis Complex, 1, 7-8

Tumor Incidence, 18, 21, 31, 139, 143, 149, 206

Tumor Mitotic Index, 49, 55

Tumor Regression, 22, 112, 127

Tumorigenesis, 8, 22, 24, 28-29, 35, 38-39, 78-81, 84-85, 87, 123, 132-133, 139, 143, 145-147, 149, 151, 155, 161-163, 165-168, 176, 178-179, 184, 206-208, 211-214

U

Ulceration, 50, 55, 57, 68, 70, 73-76, 124-125, 127, 129-130

UV Index, 66-67

UV Radiation, 29, 61, 63, 67